Families, Infants, & Young Children at Risk

PATHWAYS TO BEST PRACTICE

by

Gail L. Ensher, Ed.D.
Syracuse University
New York

David A. Clark, M.D.
Children's Hospital at Albany Medical Center
New York

and

Nancy S. Songer, M.S.
Syracuse University
New York

with invited contributors

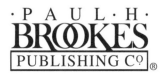

·P·A·U·L·H·
BROOKES
PUBLISHING Co.®

Baltimore · London · Sydney

KH

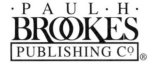

Paul H. Brookes Publishing Co.
Post Office Box 10624
Baltimore, Maryland 21285-0624
USA

www.brookespublishing.com

Typeset by Integrated Publishing Solutions, Grand Rapids, Michigan.
Manufactured in the United States of America by
Versa Press, Inc., East Peoria, Illinois.

The information provided in this book is in no way meant to substitute for a qualified health care professional's advice or expert opinion. Readers should consult a qualified health care professional if they are interested in more information. This book is sold without warranties of any kind, express or implied, and the publisher and authors disclaim any liability, loss, or damage caused by the contents of this book.

The individuals described in this book are composites or real people whose situations are masked and are based on the authors' experiences. Poems and parent quotes are used with permission; as applicable, names and identifying details have been changed to protect confidentiality.

As applicable, the photographs that appear throughout the book and on the cover are used by permission of the individuals pictured or their parents or guardians.

Permission to reprint extracts from the following in Chapters 1 and 22 is gratefully acknowledged: Shonkoff, J.P., & Phillips, D.A. (2000). *From neurons to neighborhoods: The science of early childhood development.* Washington, DC: National Academies Press. Reprinted with permission from the National Academies Press, Copyright © 2000, National Academy of Sciences.

Library of Congress Cataloging-in-Publication Data

Ensher, Gail L.
    Families, infants, and young children at risk : pathways to best practice /
by Gail L. Ensher, David A. Clark and Nancy S. Songer ; with invited contributors.
        p.   cm.
    Includes bibliographical references and index.
    ISBN-13: 978-1-55766-806-6 (pbk.)
    ISBN-10: 1-55766-806-X (pbk.)
    1. Children with disabilities—Development.   2. Developmentally disabled children—
Education.   3. Infants with disabilities.   4. Newborn infants—Diseases.
I. Clark, David A. (David Albert)   II. Songer, Nancy S.   III. Title.
[DNLM: 1. Infant, Newborn, Diseases—therapy. 2. Child. 3. Developmental Disabilities—
rehabilitation. 4. Disabled Children—education. 5. Early Intervention (Education)
6. Education, Special. 7. Family Health. 8. Infant. 9. Sensation Disorders—therapy.
WS 421 E59f 2009]
RJ137.E57 2009
618.92—dc22   2008028232

British Library Cataloguing in Publication data are available from the British Library.

2012   2011   2010   2009   2008
10   9   8   7   6   5   4   3   2   1

4/15/13

Families,
Infants, &
Young Children
at Risk

Contents

I Beginnings

1 Families, Infants, and Young Children:
New Challenges to Best Practice
Gail L. Ensher

New Faces and New Languages
Caregivers in a Working World
The Influences of Media
Continuing Agendas and New Challenges for Families
Ethical Issues in Perinatal-Neonatal Medicine
Realities of Federal Department of Education Mandates

2 Pregnancy, Labor, and Delivery
David A. Clark

Overview of Pregnancy
Problem Pregnancies
The Fetus
Labor and Delivery

3 Evaluation and Care of the Neonate
David A. Clark

Delivery Room Management
Birth Injuries
The Physiology and Behavior of Transition
Assessment of Gestational Age
Neurological Evaluation
Growth and Gestational Age
Routine Newborn Care
Newborn Screening
Discharge Planning

4 The Family as Foreground
Jill R. Weldum, Nancy S. Songer, and Gail L. Ensher

Careful Assumptions
The Significance of a Personal Lens
Experiences of Families Who Have Children with Special Needs
Collaborative Care as a Best Practice
The Family as Context
Contemporary Families
Family Roles
Life Cycle Changes
Family Systems
Stressors and Resiliency
Child Development

     Mandates of Statewide and Federal Legislation
     Early Intervention in the State of New York
     Transitions to New Settings and New Programs
     Programs of Promise

     What Have We Learned About Pathways to Best Practices?

           Organizations Providing Obstetric, Pediatric, and Health Care Information
           Information on Intervention and Early Childhood Special Education

About the Authors

Gail L. Ensher, Ed.D., Professor of Education, Teaching and Leadership Program, School of Education, Syracuse University, 155 Huntington Hall, Syracuse, New York 13244

In addition to her work as Professor of Education, Gail L. Ensher is Coordinator of two master's degree programs in the School of Education at Syracuse University: Early Childhood Special Education and the Inclusive Program on Severe Disabilities. She received her doctorate in special education from Boston University in 1971. Prior to receiving her doctoral degree, she taught for 3 years in Hanover, New Hampshire, and Quincy, Massachusetts. She later assumed a position on the faculty at the Pennsylvania State University in State College prior to taking a position on the faculty at Syracuse University.

For many years, Dr. Ensher has been actively involved in teaching, writing and research, and community service related to families and young children who are at risk and have developmental disabilities. At Syracuse University, she teaches courses at the undergraduate and graduate levels about methods and curriculum in early childhood special education, families of young children with special needs, the assessment of infants and young children, and the theoretical foundations of early childhood special education. She has extensive experience in clinical work with infants, young children, and their families and continues to train graduate students in this area of expertise. She has authored play-based assessments for infants and toddlers, most recently *Partners in Play: Assessing Infants and Toddlers in Natural Contexts* (Thomson/Delmar Learning, 2007). In addition, Dr. Ensher co-authored with Dr. David Clark the first and second editions of *Newborns at Risk: Medical Care and Psychoeducational Intervention* (Aspen Publishers, 1986, 1994).

Dr. Ensher is a single mother of two daughters adopted from Calcutta, India—Kimberly and Lindsey—now respectively 25 and 21 years of age.

David A. Clark, M.D., Professor and Martha Lepow Chairman of Pediatrics, Professor of Obstetrics and Gynecology, Albany Medical College, Director, Children's Hospital at Albany Medical Center, 43 New Scotland Avenue, Albany, New York 12208

David A. Clark is a pediatrician and neonatologist who trained at North Carolina Memorial Hospital, University of North Carolina at Chapel Hill, and completed a Neonatology Fellowship at Rainbow Babies and Children's Hospital, Case Western Reserve University in Cleveland, Ohio, and State University of New York, Upstate Medical Center in Syracuse. Dr. Clark's certifications include Diplomate, American Board of Pediatrics; the American Board of Pediatrics, Sub-Board of Neonatal-Perinatal Medicine; and the Neonatal Resuscitation Program, Regional Instructor.

Dr. Clark is a member of 25 professional societies, including the American Academy of Pediatrics—Fellow, Section on Perinatal Pediatrics, Section of Gastroenterology and Nutrition, Section on Transport Medicine, and Critical Care Section; the Society of Pediatric Research; American College of Nutrition; American Pediatric Society; and the New York Academy of Sciences.

Dr. Clark's curriculum vitae includes a total of 103 peer-reviewed publications; four books; more than 200 abstracts; and numerous invited chapters, reviews, and presentations.

Dr. Clark is the father of three daughters and a grandfather of five, including William David (WD), who tragically died at the age of 4 years during Hurricane Katrina.

xii About the Authors

Nancy S. Songer, M.S., Director, Early Childhood Direction Center, Center on Human Policy, School of Education, Syracuse University, Hoople Building, 805 South Crouse Avenue, Syracuse, New York 13244; Educational Specialist, Center for Children's Cancer and Blood Disorders, Upstate Medical University, 750 East Adams Street, Syracuse, New York 13210

Nancy S. Songer is a graduate of Syracuse University, where she received an undergraduate degree in music education and in 1998 earned a graduate degree in early childhood special education. She taught in the Solvay School District in Solvay, New York, for 5 years and was a home visitor for many years as part of the FIRST LOOK project, a project dedicated to serving young children with behavioral and social emotional challenges and their families.

Ms. Songer is the parent of five children, two of whom received special education services during both their preschool and school-age years. She serves on several disabilities-related community boards and was appointed as the chairperson of the New York State Interagency Coordinating Council by Governor Mario Cuomo, where she served from 1990–1992. As an adjunct faculty member, she has taught graduate courses related to guiding children with challenging behaviors.

Ms. Songer is a frequent keynote speaker and conference presenter. Her areas of expertise are children with challenging behaviors, working collaboratively with families, understanding the importance of observation during assessment, and using sensory strategies in early childhood settings.

Contributors

Heidi Baldwin, M.S.
High School Special Education Teacher
Madison Central School
7303 State Route 20
Madison, New York 13402

Ellen B. Barnes, Ph.D.
Director
Jowonio School
3049 East Genesee Street
Syracuse, New York 13224

Dona Bauman, Ph.D.
Assistant Professor
Education Department
University of Scranton
800 Jefferson Avenue
Scranton, Pennsylvania 18510

Toni S.P. Bell, B.A.
Graduate Student
School of Education
Syracuse University
Huntington Hall
Syracuse, New York 13244

Deborah A. Bryden, M.S., CAS
Referral Coordinator
North Syracuse Early Education Program
205 South Main Street
North Syracuse, New York 13212

Michelle L. Eastman, M.S., RNC, NNP-BC
Neonatal Nurse Practitioner
Children's Hospital at Albany Medical Center
43 New Scotland Avenue
Albany, New York 12208

Marilyn A. Fisher, M.D., M.S.
Associate Professor of Pediatrics
Albany Medical College
Children's Hospital at Albany Medical Center
43 New Scotland Avenue
Albany, New York 12208

Susan Arana Furdon, M.S., RNC, NNP-BC
Neonatal Clinical Nurse Specialist/
    Nurse Practitioner
Children's Hospital at Albany Medical Center
43 New Scotland Avenue
Albany, New York 12208

Gretchen Kinnell, B.S.
Education Director
Child Care Solutions
6724 Thompson Road
Syracuse, New York 13211

Ava E. Kleinmann, Ph.D.
Assistant Professor of Psychology
Western New England College
1215 Wilbraham Road
Springfield, Massachusetts 01119

Linda J. Levy, M.S., RNC, NNP
Neonatal Nurse Practitioner
Children's Hospital at Albany Medical Center
43 New Scotland Avenue
Albany, New York 12208

Upender K. Munshi, M.D. (Paed.), M.B.B.S.
Associate Professor
Albany Medical College
Children's Hospital at Albany Medical Center
43 New Scotland Avenue
Albany, New York 12208

Margo A. Nish, M.S., CAS
Coordinator for Early Childhood Education
Syracuse City School District
220 West Kennedy Street
Syracuse, New York 13205

Janet O'Flynn, M.S., OTR/L
Adjunct Faculty
School of Education
Syracuse University
Huntington Hall
Syracuse, New York 13244

Christy Cook Pica, B.S.
Graduate Student
School of Education
Syracuse University
230 Huntington Hall
Syracuse, New York 13244

Carol Reinson, Ph.D., OTR/L
Assistant Professor in Occupational Therapy
University of Scranton
800 Linden Street
Scranton, Pennsylvania 18510

Angel Rios, M.D.
Professor of Pediatrics
Albany Medical College
Children's Hospital at Albany Medical Center
43 New Scotland Avenue
Albany, New York 12208

Lori Saile, M.S.
Special Education Teacher
Jowonio School
3049 East Genesee Street
Syracuse, New York 13224

Jill R. Weldum, M.A., LMFT
Licensed Marriage and Family Therapist
Weldum Family Therapy Services
7030 East Genesee Street
Fayetteville, New York 13066

Preface

Future pathways to best practice in the fields of early childhood special education and pediatrics will compel society to examine new visions for young children and their families. We anticipate dramatic changes in our own professional work and partnerships with colleagues, as well as more imaginative approaches to early education. Although we have learned much about technology and the "science of neurons" in early development, many of the ills of person-to-person relationships, neighborhoods, communities, and social and mental health issues remain to be addressed in effective and substantive ways. Furthermore, the world of education is becoming ever more complex, thus expanding the parameters of what we need to know and how early intervention can be best woven into the fabric of daily lives for families. Infants and young children at risk and those with special needs represent a remarkable opportunity for the pathways to best practice in medicine, education, and related clinical fields to converge in ways that can maximize knowledge, resources, service delivery systems, and human potential.

AUDIENCE OF THE BOOK

Families, Infants, and Young Children at Risk: Pathways to Best Practice was written for families, professionals from multiple disciplines, and graduate students in teacher- and clinical-preparation programs. The book speaks to medical, cultural, psycho-social, developmental, and educational issues that confront families of infants and young children with special needs and of those who are at risk for developmental delay. These concerns are addressed within the multiple contexts of hospital, home, educational settings, and the community at large. Professionals, including nurses, physicians, teachers, psychologists, and other clinical personnel, will find essential information on family-centered practices, federal legislation, assessment, exemplary early childhood programs, collaboration and teamwork, and much

more. Finally, students in training from the fields of teaching, physical and occupational therapy, communication sciences and disorders, medicine, social work, psychology, and other human services will want to use this book as a vital text and professional reference as they learn about disabilities, environments, the diversity of families, and the significant roles of various professionals who deliver services within the context of home, hospital, and educational programs.

GOALS AND FOCUS OF THE BOOK

When writing this book, the authors had several goals in mind:

- To offer a readable text containing up-to-date information that is relevant and accessible to different disciplines working with young children and their families

- To offer a readable text that is family centered, with information that is relevant and accessible to families

- To illustrate pathways to best practice through vignettes and child–family studies

- To highlight issues and strategies that facilitate partnerships among disciplines and enhance best practices in serving young children and their families

- To discuss new avenues of research and education for young children and their families that demonstrate the interconnectedness of neuroscience, the creation of environments, collaboration, and relationship-based practices

ORGANIZATION OF THE BOOK

Families, Infants, and Young Children at Risk: Pathways to Best Practice is organized into four sections and includes several noteworthy features for the reader. First, each chapter opens with specific goals and objectives, which are intended to help the reader focus on relevant topics, and closes with a Conclusion section, which is designed for reinforcement of salient points. Throughout the book, the referencing and manuscript format of the American Psychological Association is used because this is a widely accepted style of writing among professionals and training institutions. Related web sites are included in the Appendix at the close of the book for further reader information and investigation. Finally, chapters are arranged around four primary themes. These themes should aid the reader in moving through, understanding, and remembering the breadth of medical, clinical, and educational information contained in the text.

Section I, "Beginnings," includes Chapters 1 through 4. The section is introduced with a discussion of new challenges to best practices in early childhood special education and pediatrics and then is followed by chapters focusing on pregnancy and the fetus, labor and delivery, evaluation and care of the neonate, and family systems and environments. Section I covers fundamental medical, developmental, and family-centered information, which serves as a reference point for discussions and considerations throughout the remainder of the book.

Section II, "Early Problems and Developmental Courses," includes Chapters 5 through 14. This section focuses on neonatal neurology, new trends in authentic assessment of young children and the importance of developmental surveillance, new paradigms in the education of children with autism spectrum and sensory processing disorders, the respiratory system, nutrition, physical development and impairments, and infection and immunity. Section II concludes with a discussion of the interface of physiology and medical environments and the management of pain in neonatal intensive care units.

Section III, "Families as the Social Foundation for Growing and Learning," deals with several prominent issues in today's U.S. society that affect the lives of infants, young children, and their families. Chapters 15 through 19 center on cultural diversity and the different perspectives of families relative to child rearing and having a child with a disability, the realities of substance abuse, the web of family abuse and neglect, parents with developmental disabilities, and teen parents.

Section IV, "The Intersection of Best Practice in Medical Treatment and Early Education" is the final section of the book and includes Chapters 20 though 22, as well as an Appendix of helpful resources. The primary theme of Section IV is environments—in hospitals and neonatal intensive care units, in homes, and in educational settings. Pathways to best practice are discussed within the contexts of meeting families in the midst of a neonatal crisis and thereafter; working with families during the referral, assessment, and early intervention and preschool education processes; and addressing educational transitions and programming as young children and their families move from preschool services into kindergarten and the early primary grades.

As authors, we bring to this text a breadth of backgrounds and experience. We believe that the best practice for serving young children who are at risk and have developmental delays lies within the context of home and community and requires a broader perspective for thinking and application. It is this philosophy, woven throughout, that distinguishes *Families, Infants, and Young Children at Risk: Pathways to Best Practice* from other books.

Acknowledgments

Families, Infants, and Young Children at Risk: Pathways to Best Practice would not have been written without the encouragement, support, and understanding of many people. First and foremost, we thank our respective families, who have taught us the true meaning of parenting, child development, patience, love, compassion, and best practice, who have given of themselves so unselfishly on behalf of our endeavors over the years.

Second, several colleagues have made a special difference in our professional lives. Those still active in our professional work include Douglas Biklen, Joseph Shedd, Corinne Smith, and Jeff Thompson. Many are not with us any longer, but they have left an enduring handprint on our work and the contributions that we have been able to make in our individual fields of scholarship and practice. The latter include Burton Blatt, Eric Gardner, Ernest Kraybill, and Margaret Williams, who were faithful mentors, friends, and examples of the very best in our respective fields.

A number of colleagues contributed to the writing of this book and are listed in the opening pages. They persevered through numerous rewrites and requests over the past 5 years. To them, we owe a tremendous debt of gratitude.

Several individuals participated in the preparation of the manuscript for this book—offering their time and effort in terms of typing and technological expertise. In this regard, we thank Kristen Evans, Janis Keehan, Renae Wilkins, and Rachael Zubal-Ruggieri.

Finally, over the years, countless families, students, and friends listened to and shaped our ideas, offered feedback, and contributed photos. As these people have come and gone from our lives, it is doubtful that they will ever know how important their time, eyes, ears, and advice have been in the development and completion of this work—nonetheless, we wish to recognize the invaluable gifts that they have given to each of us.

My name is William David Pardo, but you can call me WD.
I was born in Metarie, Louisiana, just outside of New Orleans.
I'm a special child, as all children should be.
In fact, I'm extra special because my parents, Jenny and Bill, love me,
even though I was not born perfect; they call me God's Gift.
I just happen to be missing a small piece of a chromosome that
must be important, because there are so many things I have a hard time doing.

I had extra fluid in my brain and had to have a shunt to drain it.

But I can smile.

I could never suck and swallow good enough and had surgery
for a permanent feeding tube into my stomach.

But I can smile.

Despite surgery on my hip, I never did develop enough strength to walk.

But I can still smile.

I've had the chance to meet many people who have helped me, nurses and doctors
in intensive care nurseries, teachers, physical therapists, speech therapists, and many others.
I smiled at all of them (when I didn't hurt), and they smiled back at me.

Maybe that's how I got one of my nicknames, Sweet William.

I had to leave sooner than I expected, but I know I was loved
and will be remembered by many, especially Mama and Dada.

Thank you.

This book my Grandpa helped write is dedicated to
the thousands of children who are "extra special" like me,
and to the many professionals who devote their lives to help us.

SMILE!

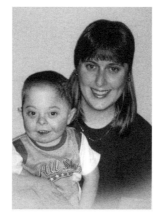

William David Pardo (WD)
April 18, 2001–September 1, 2005

Beginnings

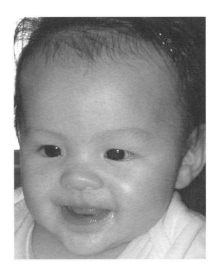

CHAPTER 1

Families, Infants, and Young Children

NEW CHALLENGES TO BEST PRACTICE

Gail L. Ensher

At the conclusion of this chapter, the reader will

- *Understand the context of contemporary child, family, cultural, community, and professional issues that most challenge early education services for young children and their families in the United States*

- *Understand the educational requirements of current federal legislation for children at risk for and with developmental disabilities, birth to age 8, and their families*

- *Be able to envision the potential of early education on behalf of young children and their families within the context of 21st-century research and best practice*

As parents, educators, and health care professionals join together to search for pathways to best practice on behalf of young children with and without disabilities, they will face major cultural, economic, and environmental changes. These conditions will have a profound effect on the ways in which we raise, educate, and provide services for children in the 21st century. This chapter addresses just a few of the significant challenges that continue to dominate the social and educational systems in the United States and influence the growth and emotional well-being of our youngest partners in the developmental process.

New Faces and New Languages

Families of young children in America represent a weaving of many colors and threads. Diversity spans every dimension of daily life, and it shapes how families raise their children, how they think about the education of their children, how they perceive themselves as participants within educational systems, and how they engage in partnerships with their professional peers.

It is a well-recognized fact that families with two parents and those with nonworking mothers are becoming a minority in contemporary society. Family structure and membership have changed dramatically, and single mothers assuming full responsibility for the financial and parenting support of their children constitute an ever-increasing norm (Hanson & Lynch, 2004).

Middle-class Anglo-European families have been largely outnumbered by families of varied cultures, ethnicities, religions, and languages in both urban and suburban communities across America (Hanson & Lynch, 2004; Harkness & Super, 2002; Lynch & Hanson, 2004). Although barriers are not insurmountable, these differences inevitably affect communication, family comfort levels regarding sharing information, receptivity to and acceptance of help, and abilities

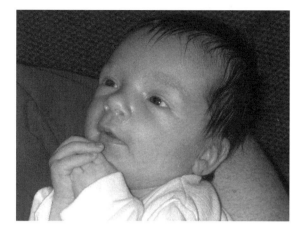

of families to negotiate pathways through "professional" legacies and agendas. For particularly young parents (younger than the age of 20 years), another layer of education in caregiving may be added to the challenges of engagement and participation when infants are born at risk for developmental difficulties or with identified impairments. Current legislation (Individuals with Disabilities Education Improvement Act [IDEA] of 2004 [PL 108-446]) requires that young children be offered early intervention services within a family-centered context. How those services are delivered to families across Latino (Harwood, Leyendecker, Carlson, Asencio, & Miller, 2002), African American (McAdoo, 2002), Asian, Anglo-European, or other cultures, however, will need to translate into uniquely tailored partnerships and relationships in hospital, home, and school settings.

Hanson and Lynch (2004) described the magnitude of these cultural issues in the United States:

Data from the 2000 Census present a picture of increasing diversity within the United States. Words such as "majority" are no longer meaningful when the population statistics are examined. In California, for example, no cultural or ethnic group constitutes a majority, with 46.7% of the population white, 32.4% Latino, 10.8% Asian and Pacific Islander, and 6.4% African American ("Diverse, Yet Distinct," 2001). Although the changes may be less dramatic in other parts of the country, the whole nation is growing and being enriched by increased diversity. (p. 21)

The first author's extensive experience working in a school district indicates that it is not unusual to find that many urban preschools, for example, consist of classes in which more than 50% of the children come from Spanish-speaking families or kindergartens in which more than 95% of the students are African American. These statistics prevail despite a frequently marked absence of diversity among teachers and professionals, largely Caucasian, who are responsible for providing services.

Complicating concerns around issues of diversity in culture and language are the persistent questions of the differences in how young children are prepared for formal educational experiences before they enter school. U.S. early childhood programs for children birth through second grade vary greatly in terms of resources, opportunities afforded to families, and quality of administrators and teaching staff (Pianta & Cox, 1999). Unfortunately, and not surprisingly, such inequities in the earliest years may have compounding effects that may endure throughout a child's lifelong school experience and beyond. Entwisle and Alexander explained that

Evidence is mounting that social stratification in the larger society is affected strongly by the nature of children's elementary schooling, especially by events and experiences in the first grade or just before. All else being equal, repeating a grade or getting poor marks in elementary school increases the likelihood that students will drop out (see Alexander et al., 1994; Entwisle et al., 1997). The other side of the coin is that attending preschool or kindergarten can improve reading and math achievement in elementary school (Barnett, 1996; Entwisle, Alexander, Pallas, & Cadigan, 1987; Lazar & Darlington, 1982) and long-term follow-ups of attending preschool show that positive preschool effects apparently persist or at least predict better outcomes in adulthood (Barnett, 1996; Consortium of Longitudinal Studies, 1983). (1999, p. 29)

Clearly, early education from birth through the earliest years and then into the primary grades holds great potential for framing the most critical foundation for young children and their families. Understanding the changing diversities of individual child and collective family scenarios is proving to be an emerging challenge for professionals across all disciplines. Detailing how these issues might be addressed within the context of best practices is one of the major objectives of this book.

Caregivers in a Working World

The fact that the majority of parents and other caregivers in the 21st century are working full time outside of their homes to "make ends meet" has had a profound effect on the lives of young children in the United States (Shonkoff & Phillips, 2000). Furthermore, economic pressures in the future will drive the number of families in the workplace higher and higher. Shonkoff and Phillips (2000) noted that the relationship between maternal employment and children's development is not a simple one to understand.

> We have learned that maternal employment is too complex a phenomenon for simple comparisons between young children with and without working mothers to reveal consistent differences. Rather, it is the circumstances of work, such as the income it generates, the proportion of the day the infant is spending in the presence of a security-giving, trusted caregiver, and related effects on family functioning that lie at the heart of how maternal employment affects young children. In particular, there is now evidence that nonstandard working hours—which now make up a major share of jobs for poor working women—pose risks for children; and that going to work for long hours during the child's first year poses a risk to child development perhaps especially when trade-offs are involved from time in sensitive and stable parental care at home to time in poorer quality alternative care, as they often are. (2000, p. 296)

It is important to note that although Shonkoff and Phillips commented in particular on the potentially negative effects for children of lower income families, other research has revealed a similarly adverse impact on cognitive functioning of children by 36 months within a large sample of European American families in which mothers

worked 30 or more hours per week outside the home during the first 9 months of life (Brooks-Gunn, Han, & Waldfogel, 2002). The related conclusions of these two studies raise the challenging issue that increasing numbers of very young children are now spending significant periods of time in their earliest years of life with caregivers outside of the family (Tout, Zaslow, Papillo, & Vandivere, 2001). The quality of this care often is cited as being variable and probably questionable, at best. Concerns about early child care continue to include the quality of teacher–child and caregiver–child interactions, staff–child ratios, the nature of programming and curricula, and the quality of family participation.

For families with children who have special needs and who also receive child care in home- or center-based settings, additional considerations need to be taken into account. For example, are the child care staff sufficiently knowledgeable to carry out differentiated program objectives within an inclusive group of young children? Are the staff able to adapt activities to accommodate diverse styles of learning that fully include the child with special needs? Is there consistency among the staff in terms of positive approaches to guiding challenging child behavior? Do the staff have the time and willingness to communicate positively with families about child behavior and progress in the setting?

In addition to concerns about appropriate child care for infants and young children, working families are confronted with numerous other daily pressures and responsibilities. Contemporary families in the fast pace of life often find themselves stretched for time, energy, and finances. Resilient families must have opportunities to renew their resources and connect with other families for a sense of community. In the absence of such relationships, parents (and, likewise, their children) may become isolated, even in the midst of working 30–40 hours per week. Such situations may leave families even more vulnerable to other problems. Developing and sustaining supports in the face of common, daily adversity and living is a critical part of the well-being of families and favorable developmental outcomes for young children.

The Influences of Media

Another major source of influence in the everyday lives of young children today is the media culture. Beginning at birth, children are immersed in environments that are filled with television, computers, and video games. The amount of time that is devoted to watching television, using computers, and playing video games; the content of the media; and the patterns of media involvement established in relation to later learning and achievement in school all have come under scrutiny by educators, researchers, and parents. Debates about the impact of the media on young children continue to rage with little consensus on academic and social outcomes.

For the youngest children, 10–36 months, questions have focused on the emotional reactions of infants and toddlers as onlookers and the inferences that they may or may not draw from exposure to various television scenarios (Mumme & Fernald, 2003). For example, researchers have found that infants as young as 12 months "were able to use social information presented on television" (Mumme & Fernald, 2003, p. 235) in shows such as *Sesame Street*. Although such information can be used in beneficial ways for educational purposes, especially as infants advance in age into their toddler years, this media-acquired social information can also influence behavior, future learning, and achievement patterns of very young children. In addition, if parents themselves are significant consumers of television viewing to the neglect of play, social interactions, and time devoted to creating literacy-rich environments, negative consequences may ensue for their children (e.g., an inability to relate well to caregivers and siblings in age-appropriate ways). Accordingly, both the amount of time spent viewing television and the child-specific, educational content of programs have been the target of numerous research studies with toddlers and preschoolers between the ages of 2 and 5 years. For example, Wright et al. (2001) looked at two cohorts of children from low- to moderate-income families. Not surprisingly, these researchers found the following:

Viewing child-audience informative programs between ages 2 and 3 predicted high subsequent performance on all four measures of academic skills. For both cohorts, frequent viewers of general-audience programs performed more poorly on subsequent tests than did infrequent viewers of such programs. Children's skills also predicted later viewing, supporting a bidirectional model. Children with good skills at age 5 selected more child-audience informative programs and fewer cartoons in their early elementary years. Children with lower skills at age 3 shifted to viewing more general-audience programs by ages 4 and 5. The results affirm the conclusion that the relations of television viewed to early academic skills depend primarily on the content of the programs viewed. (p. 1347)

Writing about parenting in a multimedia society, Dorr, Rabin, and Irlen (2002) echoed similar findings, as well as the need for parents to be actively engaged with their young children in print- and language-rich activities at home (Snow, Burns, & Griffin, 1998). This conclusion does not negate the importance of child-specific television programming, such as *Sesame Street*, which has been associated with better achievement later in school, but it reinforces the need for attention to quality interaction that is developmentally appropriate for young children.

The genuine challenge for parents living with their children in a technological, media culture often is one of balance and effective monitoring of exposure. With large numbers of families with both caregivers working, time together is often in short supply. Sorting out the pieces of a complex interaction of environmental and later academic and social-emotional outcomes is a difficult research agenda (Clarke & Kurtz-Costes, 1997). Families often find themselves out of control in the process of trying to monitor what their children see and hear through the media. This is a critical issue across all ages, with television and computer audiences of younger children increasing (Anderson & Evans, 2001) at home, in child care, and even in preschool programs. Television in American families—either as background or foreground exposure—is on approximately 6 hours per day (Anderson & Evans, 2001).

At the forefront of concerns about the media is the amount of violence that young children now witness routinely on the screen (Levin, 1998). Modeling is a powerful "teacher," and young children may learn from the media that the primary way to solve conflict and problems is through aggression and hurting others without visible consequences (Levin, 1998). Frequently, such acts are portrayed by role models in child cartoons and other general audience programming that is readily available to children from preschool on. In addition, violence in the real world is reflected in almost every morning and nightly news broadcast about war, terrorism, and natural disasters. For weeks after the catastrophe of September 11, 2001, children were bombarded with the realities of devastation and horror that left their families and teachers speechless as they tried to explain the situation and answer their questions (Thomas, 2001, 2002). Scenes of devastation from natural disasters that affected the lives of children torn from their families during the 2004 Indian Ocean tsunami and the 2005 U.S. Hurricanes, Katrina and Rita, were inescapable on the television screen.

Advancements in the technological world, for better or worse, have brought the realities of all aspects of our society into our homes. Helping young children make sense of these realities is a developmental and mental health imperative shared by parents, teachers, and health care professionals. It is a challenge of the 21st century that cannot be ignored.

Continuing Agendas and New Challenges for Families

Poverty (Magnuson & Duncan, 2002), substance abuse (Mayes & Truman, 2002), teen pregnancy (Moore & Brooks-Gunn, 2002; Rais-Bahrami & Short, 2007), and child abuse and neglect (Azar, 2002) are not new to families. They are serious concerns that have been studied for years, and, unfortunately, continue to be active challenges for families across the United States. Over time, each of these factors has demonstrated a negative impact on the development of infants and young children; yet, as many educators and researchers have pointed out, they are closely related and often interact as causal connections in the cultures of American families. Having acknowledged this evidence, we need to be mindful that although individuals included in many studies were drawn from lower income populations and underrepresented groups, the issues of substance abuse, teen pregnancy, and child abuse and neglect affect families of all income and education levels. Moreover, a common thread shared by numerous families in difficulty is a prominent feeling of isolation with little sense of empowerment to change the trajectory of their lives.

The underlying contributors to less advantageous outcomes for young children may be evidenced in multiple and confluent ways. For example, although numbers since the late 1990s have declined, the United States still remains at the top of the list of industrialized nations in adolescent pregnancies (see Chapter 19 for more information). To further complicate this issue, young mothers in their teens often do not receive adequate prenatal care and are subsequently prone to deliver premature and small-for-dates newborns (Ensher & Clark, 1994; Rais-Bahrami & Short, 2007). In turn, such infants often are more difficult to care for and parent, which may cause families to be more vulnerable to child abuse and neglect. Lack of parenting skills to address challenging toddler and preschool behavior may be an issue. Furthermore, in the contemporary culture of American schools, alcohol and other illegal substances are readily available to teens, thus adding further elements of risk to teen pregnancies and family situations. Such difficult scenarios are not unusual in the process of raising young children today in a society where social-emotional supports and family networks may be in short supply.

In light of these stressors, an ongoing need for families facing hardships and adversity is the development of nurturing relationships, sensitive parenting, and the fostering of resilience in their young children. Shonkoff and Phillips (2000) spoke to the complexity of parent intervention and efforts to change patterns of behavior in families.

The question is not whether interventions focused on parents can be effective, but rather what does it take to change parenting behavior in ways that will be sufficient to produce improved child outcomes. . . . The complex evidence on parenting interventions suggests that this is not an easy task for which success can be readily assumed. The challenges become even more daunting in light of the multiple problems that face many at-risk families today. The committee agrees with others (see Cowan et al., 1998; Teti, 1999) who have suggested that these families are likely to require more intensive services than the typical parenting intervention program provides, interventions that go beyond the enhancement of parenting skills to address the serious life issues (e.g., poverty, hopelessness, depression, substance abuse, troubled relationships) they face and involve adults other than just the mother and utilize program staff who are specifically qualified to work with multiproblem families. The growing diversity of families with young children also raises profoundly important questions about how best to match programs to the needs, values, and goals of various ethnic and cultural groups. A final challenge to parenting interventions is posed by the demographics and circumstances of working parents, for whom finding the time to participate in these programs is exceedingly difficult. (pp. 263–264)

Clearly, the increasing complexity of our families, larger communities, and the difficult circumstances that confront parents daily has greatly altered the parameters of raising healthy children with positive developmental outcomes. Moreover, we still have much to learn about the ways in which the dimensions of poverty and its associated connections interact with biology and genetics, or how environmental factors outside the home act to protect children in their earliest years from short- and long-term negative consequences.

In addition to ongoing, systemic challenges, families now face new issues that involve developing and negotiating growing numbers of relationships outside the home environment. These new interactions have emerged as a result of several medical, legislative, economic, and demographic factors. Due to the large number of families in which the only caregiver or both are now working, infants and young children, on average, are spending more hours per day in child care. These environments require new relationships among children and nonfamily member caregivers, as well as among parents and child care providers. Such child care communities exert tremendous influences on the development and well-being of young children and have been the subject of intense research study in recent years (Ahnert & Lamb, 2003; Johnson, Jaeger, Randolph, Cauce, Ward, & National Institute of Child Health and Human Development Early Child Care Research Network, 2003; Loeb, Fuller, Kagan, & Carrol, 2004; National Institute of Child Health and Human Development Early Child Care Research Network, 2003; Votruba-Drzal, Coley, & Chase-Lansdale, 2004).

Quality child care for children with special needs in addition to existing early intervention and preschool services is often lacking in communities and has expanded the need for collaboration among professionals across agencies and among parents (Markos-Capps & Godfrey, 1999). Communication among the involved adults has become an essential component of service delivery to young children who demonstrate increasingly complex behavioral, technological, and physical and/or therapeutic needs beyond typical caregiving requirements. Greater numbers of children are being identified with pervasive developmental disorders and autism in the toddler and preschool years in programs and schools across the country. Meaningful, accessible inclusion of young children and families in natural community environments of the 21st century will depend upon the development of innovative models (Stayton & Bruder, 1999) to facilitate closer collaboration among families and professionals of diverse disciplines. Such models will require major changes in how regular and special education early childhood personnel are taught to work in partnership with parents and with one another.

Despite data on the potentially positive effects of quality child care on short- and long-term developmental and/or academic outcomes of young children from families with the fewest resources (Shonkoff & Phillips, 2000), there still remains little research including young children with special needs. Undoubtedly this absence of data reflects diminished numbers of young children and families being included in natural community environments, which is a growing challenge for parents who need to return to work within the early years of their young families. Shonkoff and Phillips summarized some of the challenges for early childhood programs in addressing the needs of families with a genuine sense of community, acceptance, and understanding.

> Traditional program formats and strategies (both for children who are labeled at risk and for those with diagnosed disabilities) need to be reconciled with the values and cultural practices of an increasingly diverse population. For many families, including both immigrant and native-born families with widely varying cultural and linguistic backgrounds, involvement in an early intervention program can be a complex challenge. The potential complications may include different perceptions of: (1) parenting roles and functions, (2) expectations of young children and beliefs about appropriate developmental goals, (3) views about needing and accepting "help" from nonfamily members, (4) fears about being judged unfavorably, and (5) barriers imposed by language. Although major strides have been made in adapting traditional service formats to the needs and beliefs of an increasingly diverse array of families, such as those achieved by Head Start, the design of interventions that are perceived as relevant, engaging, and needed by the full spectrum of targeted families remains a central challenge to the field. (p. 401)

Finally, a new population of families has emerged as a result of terrorist acts against the United States and subsequent U.S. military action. Specifically, with the devastating loss of life on September 11, 2001, and many American troops situated in Iraq and Afghanistan, numerous families now find themselves without fathers and/or mothers on a temporary or permanent basis. The years ahead will reveal the full implications of this new group of young children who are growing up in single-parent families with the advent of these unfortunate events.

Ethical Issues in Perinatal-Neonatal Medicine

Ethical issues in perinatal-neonatal medicine are not new. However, rapid developments in the technology of saving newborns at much earlier gestational ages and smaller birth weights, mothers working longer before starting their families, increases in the use of fertility drugs, increases in multiple gestation pregnancies, and intrauterine therapy, among other issues, have had a substantial impact on the landscape of ethical issues now confronting families and medical personnel. Several authors (Boyle, 2001; Ensher & Clark, 1994; Silber, 2007) have noted that decision making is never "black and white" and it becomes even more difficult in light of the possibility of severe special needs, questionable abilities of families to care for children who are ill or who have severe disabilities, and limited family resources. Both mortality and morbidity rates have dropped dramatically since the late 1990s, weighing in favor of much better developmental outcomes for children. However, families who have had newborns admitted to neonatal intensive care units, preterm or full term, almost universally agree that such experiences are fraught with anxiety and concern, regardless of the duration of time in the hospital.

Decisions regarding the treatment of infants born early are always complex. According to Ensher and Clark,

> When a family turns to health care professionals—obstetricians, pediatricians, neonatologists, or nurses—the family members have certain expectations regarding nonscientific aspects of care. First and most obvious is the belief that the health care professional is acting on behalf of the best interests of the child. In recent years, this responsibility has been broadened in the intensive care nursery to the anticipation that the health care professional is acting in the best interests of both the child and the family. Sometimes inappropriately, this expectation presupposes that these professionals, as individuals and as team members, are capable of making unbiased, objective decisions without regard to the social or economic status of the family. The deliberations and care rendered are supposed to be confidential and are assumed to be based on societal concepts of moral and ethical standards. This situation raises many difficult questions with respect to the use of technology. In particular, it is easy to initiate, and charge for, the use of technological systems (e.g., for life support), but it is sometimes extremely difficult to withhold or withdraw such systems, even from neonates with obviously irreversible fatal illness, when individuals in the society often expect "everything be done." (1994, pp. 190–191)

In addition to the obvious confusion for families, critical decisions inevitably are affected by legal, social, religious, and economic factors. Families always should be given as much information as possible under the circumstances. Often, however, in the high tension of the moment, they may not understand or *hear* what is being said to them. Having been thrust into an unknown and frightening situation, they may not be able to comprehend the long-term consequences of immediate options. Furthermore, ultimate outcomes for children invariably are imprecise and unpredictable. Medical professionals, at best, can offer guidance, based on statistical data; however, there are no absolutes or guarantees.

Decision making in intensive care nurseries is never easy for families or for the medical care personnel, but the process in all situations needs to be collaborative and with a commitment to best outcome on behalf of the mother and the child. There are times when conflicts arise between survival of the infant and the well-being of the mother (Ensher & Clark, 1994). In such instances, short-term and long-term consequences need to be carefully weighed for both mother and child by the family and professional team. Hopefully, resolutions can be achieved with mutual respect for all parties concerned with the use of plain language, a mutually agreeable course of action and treatment, and decisions that are open to change (should circumstances deem that to be necessary). Technology has raised the level of difficulty in making life-saving decisions today; however, within the constraints of the law and wise practice, the precious sense of human cost should not be lost in the midst of turmoil and open access to medical treatment.

Realities of Federal Department of Education Mandates

Since the mid-1980s, a notable amount of federal legislation focused directly on authorization of services for infants and young children with special needs. In 1986, the Education of the Handicapped Act Amendments (PL 99-457) that amended the Education for All Handicapped Children Act of 1975 (PL 94-142) mandated free and appropriate public education for 3- to 5-year-old children with disabilities (Part B, Section 619). Part H of PL 99-457 added incentives for states to develop programs to serve infants and toddlers (birth through 2 years of age). In 1990, the Education for All Handicapped Children Act was reauthorized and became the Individuals with Disabilities Education Act (IDEA) of 1990 (PL 101-476). In 1991, the Individuals with Disabilities Education Act Amendments (PL 102-119) reauthorized, amended, and extended Part H of PL 99-457 on behalf of infants and toddlers and amended Part B, Section 619, on behalf of 3- to 5-year-olds. In 1997, IDEA was further amended (becoming PL 105-17), which changed Part H on behalf of infants and toddlers to Part C, ensured access for children with special needs to the general education curriculum, mandated the involvement of families in the education of their children, and emphasized the need for accountability (McLean, 2004). Subsequently, IDEA 2004 (PL 108-446) redefined the age range of developmental delay to apply to young children 3–9 years of age, including any subset of that age range (e.g., 3- to 5-year-olds). Finally, on a broader scale, on December 13, 2001, the House approved President George W. Bush's reform legislation, the No Child Left Behind Act of 2001 (PL 107-110). This legislation, which interfaces with services provided under IDEA, was designed to initiate the following changes (U.S. House of Representatives, Committee on Education and Labor, 2005):

- Increase accountability within public schools by requiring annual testing in kindergarten through Grade 12 to ensure that all children are learning.

- Give parents "report cards" on school performance.

- Offer additional resources for "underachieving" schools and provide new options to families of children attending chronically underachieving and dangerous schools.

- Streamline the number of federal K–12 education programs.

- Extend funding for literacy programs with demonstrated effectiveness, based on research findings.

- Revise bilingual programs to assist children with learning English as a second language.

- Strengthen state mandates for highly qualified teachers.

- Increase resources for special education services and quality special education teachers.

- Expand the flexibility of local public schools in the use of federal education funding.

Clearly, each of these pieces of legislation has been passed with high hopes and expectations for improving services for infants, young children, and beyond. The increased focus on partnerships with families has been a landmark addition as professionals attempt to define priorities within homes and educational program settings. To the degree that this alliance genuinely and openly takes place for young children, the power of early intervention and early childhood is strengthened. Likewise, the availability of services at much earlier ages is a significant step forward in reaching both families and children in terms of prevention and proactive educational intervention. In the process, professionals of all disciplines need to be accountable for their work with families and their impact on child learning.

Having acknowledged these advantages, there remain many challenges with implementing services for infants, toddlers, and 3- to 9-year-olds under IDEA (Danaher, 2005; Shackelford, 2005), as well as for older children under the terms of the No Child Left Behind legislation. Definitions and guidelines for establishing eligibility under Part C and Part H of IDEA have been a continuing source of difficulty, despite amendments and clarifications of recent years. There is a great deal of variability across states in terms of lead funding agencies for Part C on behalf of infants and toddlers, and often these agencies change when and/or if children move into preschool programs. For example, many states have designated state health departments as being responsible for programs focusing on children birth to age 3, and state education departments as being responsible for programs focusing on 3-

to 9-year-olds. Funding mechanisms and delivery of services for these two agencies are very different, and frequently transitions from early intervention to preschool education programs are not smooth. Some states have elected a model of itinerant services for infants and toddlers, with providers across disciplines drawn from disparate programs, thus making the coordination of services for families somewhat fragmented. In some situations, there have been tendencies for heavier service provision by one agency versus the other, thus causing discrepancies and possible conflicts for families. In addition, as a result of excessive cost of funding programming for their youngest constituents, local programs not surprisingly in recent years have elected to opt out of serving infants and toddlers. Last, but not insignificantly, a number of states and professionals still rely considerably on norm-referenced assessments for establishing eligibility for service, an approach which has a demonstrated record of unreliability within the preschool years, especially with young children with special needs.

Historically, norm-referenced assessments have been used with populations of children who have been carefully selected out of research and/or standardization processes. Fortunately, these historical practices (now criticized by the National Association for the Education of Young Children) are now giving way to a greater reliance on natural environments as primary settings for evaluation of young children; the use of criterion- and/or curriculum-based assessment; the inclusion of informed clinical judgment; and teaming across disciplines, including partnerships with parents (Ensher et al., 2007; McLean, 2004; Sandall, McLean, & Smith, 2000). If the precedence of the past is any predictor for the future, further changes are close at hand, hopefully in favor of greater coherence of service for families and young children.

On the surface it is difficult to challenge the goals of the No Child Left Behind legislation. Schools and teachers need to be accountable for their impact on child learning; bilingual education is an ever-expanding need for increasingly diverse populations of children in American schools, as is the heightened focus on literacy;

and schools have always needed closer ties between their practice and research. However, not unlike the preschool legislation, the realities of implementation leave room for concern and improvement. Especially with respect to children with special needs, educators and families find themselves very worried about the heavy emphasis placed on passing tests. Only children with the most severe disabilities are exempt under this new legislation, and, in fact, rather than enhancing the quality of education for all, the actual result may be the selective exclusion of children with mild and moderate special needs (e.g., those with attention-deficit/hyperactivity disorder) who have extreme difficulty with testing as the primary yardstick.

Related to this issue is the concern that schools with large populations of underachieving students may be making excellent progress in addressing problems of poor performance in terms of literacy, math, and other academic areas; however, these changes may not be reflected in smaller increments of change in schools that are forced to take on added burdens in the face of insufficient funding. Again, one standard is not appropriate for everyone, and, unfortunately, under the new legislation those schools most in need of additional funding ultimately may be penalized, and the gap between disadvantaged and advantaged will widen.

Another point to consider is the dominant emphasis on academic achievement, perhaps to the neglect of other important dimensions of education, such as the social-emotional development and behavior of students. Schools in the United States are struggling with the academic and social values of their students. High-quality education needs to focus on both. New Early Reading First programs are laudable in terms of their goals to develop language-rich home and school environments, but the reality is that many preschool children are developmentally far from being ready to take advantage of such exposure, needing to focus instead on attending abilities, behaving in socially appropriate ways with their peers, learning how to participate in groups, and numerous other learning to learn capacities.

In the end, many educators, politicians, administrators, and parents predict that the imple-

mentation of No Child Left Behind will fall far short of accomplishing its laudable objectives because of its punitive nature. In the future, revisiting the legislation to strengthen schools and open up access to quality education for all children might be better accomplished with the following:

- Offering incentives for partnerships of parents, educators, and administrators at the local level to make policy decisions regarding accountability of schools

- Developing multiple, innovative strategies for assessing student progress and school achievement, including goals of adaptive, socially appropriate behavior that are responsive to diverse cultures

- Minimizing reliance on standardized testing that is least appropriate for children of all ages who are challenged by learning

- Building incentives for learning by children at all levels of ability through strengthening collaboration between home and school

- Increasing in-service opportunities for teachers in high-risk schools and offering appropriate incentives for improved quality of teaching, which should be determined by respective local teaching administrative staffs of schools

- Using proficiency standards with developmental and achievement benchmarks rather than standardized tests as measures of improvement and anticipated goals (However, these benchmarks would be separate from specific requirements for students in terms of graduation and would examine, in particular, the needs of students from underrepresented groups and children with disabilities.)

- Increasing requirements that teachers be certified in both regular and special education that could help educators meet the growing needs of serving more diverse populations of students.

- Increasing the flexibility of the No Child Left Behind legislation by relaxing the rigid annual schedules of testing and meeting standard benchmarks (Such changes hopefully would lessen the strong tendencies of teachers to teach to tests and focus more appropriately on the quality of education that students are receiving and on identifying additional supports.)

• Investing federal funds in all aspects of educational programs, such as extracurricular activities that can serve to keep children and families engaged, including those for students who demonstrate special talents and abilities

In summary, the legislation since the mid-1980s has been passed to improve the quality of education and specialized services for all children. The challenge of the 21st century will be how best to achieve these goals within the realistic context of implementation.

Conclusion

This chapter has focused on just a few of the challenges that confront families, young children, and professionals in the 21st century. These include increasing diversity within our schools, the effect of the media, family and ethical issues, and the implementation of recently passed legislation to improve education for all children. In many respects, the social ills of the past continue to live on, and the struggles for many American families in raising young children are greater than ever. At the same time, the potentials for change have never been better.

The chapters that follow explore and provide some principles for best practice that will make a difference for families, their children, and professionals who are dedicated to children's medical, physical, social-emotional, and educational well-being. At the least, the authors of this book believe that new visions will need to include ways to address the following:

• Adult to adult collaborations on behalf of young children that are shared by families, communities, and professionals

• Ways for addressing the exposure of infants and young children to violence in our communities

• Transdisciplinary education that addresses delivery of services for families of increasingly diverse cultures

• Transdisciplinary education that addresses the delivery of health, social, and education services to young children with increasingly complex special needs from infancy onward

• New strategies for evaluating child development and progress in programs and schools that examine educational, social-emotional, and behavioral change

• Examination of fragmentation of services and transition within educational programs and schools

• Reconsideration of ways in which legislation on behalf of infants and young children is implemented in terms of cost, program and school incentives, equal care for all families, and appropriate training support for professionals

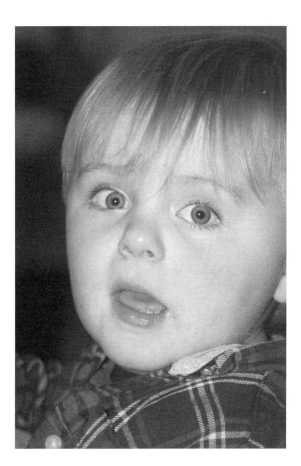

Research has demonstrated remarkable progress in both the medical and educational fields on behalf of families and their young children. New possibilities are continuing to emerge as, for example, medical professionals explore closer links between neurobiology and outcome in newborns, researchers seek new treatments for human immunodeficiency virus/acquired immunodeficiency syndrome (HIV/AIDS), and empirical research in education attempts to define more explicitly the questions about intervention with families that are at risk and children who have developmental delays. The fundamental challenge of many of the issues discussed in this chapter is the constant search for ways to turn "knowledge into action" (Shonkoff & Phillips, 2000, p. 381) and, in the process, to nurture the diverse pathways to best practice.

REFERENCES

Ahnert, L., & Lamb, M.E. (2003). Shared care: Establishing a balance between home and child care settings. *Child Development, 74*(4), 1044–1049.

Anderson, D.R., & Evans, M.K. (2001, October/November). Peril and potential of media for infants and toddlers. *Zero to Three,* 10–16.

Azar, S.T. (2002). Parenting and child maltreatment. In M.H. Bornstein (Ed.), *Handbook of parenting: Vol. 4* (2nd ed., pp. 361–388). Mahwah, NJ: Lawrence Erlbaum Associates.

Batshaw, M.L., Pellegrino, L., & Roizen, N.J. (Eds.). (2007). *Children with disabilities* (6th ed.). Baltimore: Paul H. Brookes Publishing Co.

Boyle, R.J. (2001). Ethics in the neonatal intensive care unit and beyond. *Infants and Young Children, 13*(3), 36–46.

Brooks-Gunn, J., Han, W.J., & Waldfogel, J. (2002). Maternal employment and child cognitive outcomes in the first three years of life: The NICHD study of early child care. *Child Development, 74*(4), 1052–1073.

Clarke, A.T., & Kurtz-Costes, B. (1997). Television viewing, educational quality of the home environment, and school readiness. *The Journal of Educational Research, 90*(5), 279–285.

Danaher, J. (2005). Eligibility policies and practices for young children under Part B of IDEA. *NECTAC Notes, 15,* 1–18.

Dorr, A., Rabin, B.E., & Irlen, S. (2002). Parenting in a multimedia society. In M. H. Bornstein (Ed.), *Handbook of parenting: Vol. 5* (2nd ed., pp. 349–373). Mahwah, NJ: Lawrence Erlbaum Associates.

Education for All Handicapped Children Act of 1975, PL 94-142, 20 U.S.C. §§ 1400 *et seq.*

Education of the Handicapped Act Amendments of 1986, PL 99-457, 20 U.S.C. §§ 1400 *et seq.*

Ensher, G.L., Bobish, T.P., Gardner, E.F., Reinson, C.L., Bryden, D.A., & Foertsch, D.J. (2007). *Partners in play: Assessing infants and toddlers in natural contexts.* Clifton Park, NY: Thomson Delmar Learning.

Ensher, G.L., & Clark, D.A. (1994). *Newborns at risk: Medical care and psychoeducational intervention* (2nd ed.). Gaithersburg, MD: Aspen Publishers.

Entwisle, D.R., & Alexander, K.L. (1999). Early schooling and social stratification. In R.C. Pianta & M.J. Cox (Eds.), *The transition to kindergarten* (pp. 13–38). Baltimore: Paul H. Brookes Publishing Co.

Hanson, M.J., & Lynch, E.W. (2004). *Understanding families: Approaches to diversity, disability, and risk.* Baltimore: Paul H. Brookes Publishing Co.

Harkness, S., & Super, C.M. (2002). Culture and parenting. In M.H. Bornstein (Ed.), *Handbook of parenting: Vol. 2* (2nd ed., pp. 253–280). Mahwah, NJ: Lawrence Erlbaum Associates.

Harwood, R., Leyendecker, B., Carlson, V., Asencio, M., & Miller, A. (2002). Parenting among Latino families in the U.S. In M.H. Bornstein (Ed.), *Handbook of parenting: Vol. 4* (2nd ed., pp. 21–46). Mahwah, NJ: Lawrence Erlbaum Associates.

Individuals with Disabilities Education Act Amendments of 1991, PL 102-119, 20 U.S.C. §§ 1400 *et seq.*

Individuals with Disabilities Education Act Amendments of 1997, PL 105-17, 20 U.S.C. §§ 1400 *et seq.*

Individuals with Disabilities Education Act (IDEA) of 1990, PL 101-476, 20 U.S.C. §§ 1400 *et seq.*

Individuals with Disabilities Education Improvement Act (IDEA) of 2004, PL 108-446, 20 U.S.C. §§ 1400 *et seq.*

Johnson, D.J., Jaeger, E., Randolph, S.M., Cauce, A.M., Ward, J., & National Institute of Child Health and Human Development Early Child Care Research Network. (2003). *Child Development, 74*(5), 1227–1244.

Levin, D.E. (1998). *Remote control childhood? Combating the hazards of media culture.* Washington, DC: National Association for the Education of Young Children.

Loeb, S., Fuller, B., Kagan, S.L., & Carrol, B. (2004). Child care in poor communities: Early learning effects of type, quality, and stability. *Child Development, 75*(1), 47–65.

Lynch, E.W., & Hanson, M.J. (Eds.). (2004). *Developing cross-cultural competence: A guide for working with children and their families* (3rd ed.). Baltimore: Paul H. Brookes Publishing Co.

Magnuson, K.A., & Duncan, G.J. (2002). Parents in poverty. In M.H. Bornstein (Ed.), *Handbook of parenting: Vol. 4* (2nd ed., pp. 95–121). Mahwah, NJ: Lawrence Erlbaum Associates.

Markos-Capps, G., & Godfrey, A.B. (1999). Availability of day care services for preschool children with special health care needs. *Infants and Young Children*, *11*(3), 62–78.

Mayes, L.C., & Truman, S.D. (2002). Substance abuse and parenting. In M.H. Bornstein (Ed.), *Handbook of parenting: Vol. 4* (2nd ed., pp. 329–359). Mahwah, NJ: Lawrence Erlbaum Associates.

McAdoo, H.P. (2002). African American parenting. In M.H. Bornstein (Ed.), *Handbook of parenting: Vol. 4* (2nd ed., pp. 47–58). Mahwah, NJ: Lawrence Erlbaum Associates.

McLean, M. (2004). Assessment and its importance in early intervention/early childhood special education. In M. McLean, M. Wolery, & D.B. Bailey, Jr., *Assessing infants and preschoolers with special needs* (3rd ed., pp. 1–21). Upper Saddle, NJ: Pearson/Merrill Prentice Hall.

Moore, M.R., & Brooks-Gunn, J. (2002). Adolescent parenthood. In M.H. Bornstein (Ed.), *Handbook of parenting: Vol. 3* (2nd ed., pp. 173–214). Mahwah, NJ: Lawrence Erlbaum Associates.

Mumme, D.L., & Fernald, A. (2003). The infant as onlooker: Learning from emotional reactions observed in a television scenario. *Child Development*, *74*(1), 221–237.

National Institute of Child Health and Human Development Early Child Care Research Network. (2003). Does amount of time spent in child care predict socioemotional adjustment during the transition to kindergarten? *Child Development*, *74*(4), 976–1005.

No Child Left Behind Act of 2001, PL 107-110, 115 Stat. 1425, 20 U.S.C. §§ 6301 *et seq.*

Pianta, R.C., & Cox, M.J. (Eds.). (1999). *The transition to kindergarten*. Baltimore: Paul H. Brookes Publishing Co.

Rais-Bahrami, K., & Short, B.L. (2007). Premature and small-for-dates infants. In M.L. Batshaw, L. Pellegrino, & N.J. Roizen (Eds.), *Children with disabilities* (6th ed., pp. 107–122). Baltimore: Paul H. Brookes Publishing Co.

Sandall, S., McLean, M., & Smith, B.J. (Eds.). (2000). *DEC recommended practices in early intervention/early childhood special education*. Longmont, CO: Sopris West Educational Services.

Shackelford, J. (2005). State and jurisdictional eligibility definitions for infants and toddlers with disabilities under IDEA. *NECTAC Notes*, *18*, 1–15.

Shonkoff, J.P., & Phillips, D.A. (2000). *From neurons to neighborhoods: The science of early childhood development*. Washington, DC: National Academies Press.

Silber, T.J. (2007). Ethical dilemmas. In M.L. Batshaw, L. Pellegrino, & N.J. Roizen (Eds.), *Children with disabilities* (6th ed., pp. 591–600). Baltimore: Paul H. Brookes Publishing Co.

Snow, C.E., Burns, M.S., & Griffin, P. (Eds.). (1998). *Preventing reading difficulties in young children*. Washington, DC: National Academies Press.

Stayton, V., & Bruder, M.B. (1999). Early intervention personnel preparation for the new Millennium. *Infants and Young Children*, *12*(1), 59–69.

Thomas, J.M. (2001, 2002, December/January). A long walk together: Children's world learning center—Pentagon. *Zero to Three*, 5–8.

Tout, K., Zaslow, M., Papillo, S.R., & Vandivere, S. (2001). *Early care and education: Work support for families and developmental opportunity for young children*. Washington, DC: The Urban Institute.

U.S. House of Representatives, Committee on Education and Labor. (2005). Bill summary: The No Child Left Behind Act (H.R. 1): Closing the achievement gap in America's public schools. Retrieved October 28, 2005, from http://edworkforce.house.gov/issues/108th/education/nelb/billsummary.htm

Votruba-Drzal, E., Coley, R.L., & Chase-Lansdale, P.L. (2004). Child care and low-income children's development: Direct and moderated effects. *Child Development*, *75*(1), 296–312.

Wright, J.C., Huston, A.C., Murphy, K.C., St. Peters, M., Pinon, M., Scantlin, R., & Kotler, J. (2001). The relations of early television viewing to school readiness and vocabulary of children from low-income families: The early window project. *Child Development*, *72*(5), 1347–1366.

CHAPTER 2

Pregnancy, Labor, and Delivery

David A. Clark

At the conclusion of this chapter, the reader will

- *Understand the functions and conditions associated with typical pregnancies*

- *Understand the potential maternal and environmental problems that could lead to abnormal pregnancies and complications in newborns*

- *Understand the potential problems associated with the fetus that may lead to later fetal health and/or developmental problems*

- *Have a basic understanding of ways of assessing fetal health and therapy*

It is often taken for granted when a healthy full-term baby is born as a result of a "normal" pregnancy. The reality, however, is that there are many genetic and environmental factors that may alter the course of a pregnancy and fetus, resulting in serious injury to the mother or in a newborn who is premature or has physical malformations. The health and nutritional status of the mother is crucial in promoting a healthy full-term pregnancy.

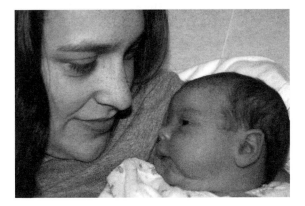

Overview of Pregnancy

The emphasis of prenatal care is to identify conditions that would place the mother or fetus at risk for problems. (See Table 2.1 for a list of antepartum high-risk pregnancy screenings.) Prepregnancy care identifies pregnancies that are at increased risk of fetal abnormalities. These conditions include mothers with a family history of an inherited disorder, a previous birth of an abnormal child, a mother greater than 35 years old (which prompts screening for trisomy 21), consanguinity of the parents, and parents who are known carriers of a chromosomal recessive disorder (e.g., thalassemia) (Lissauer & Fanaroff, 2006). In addition, there may also be specific risks with certain ethnic groups (e.g., African Americans and sickle cell disease; Ashkenazi Jews and Tay-Sachs disease—a neurodegenerative disorder). (See Table 2.2 for a list of possible antepartum genetic screenings.)

In addition to these intrinsic risks of the pregnancy, specialists in obstetrics and high-risk

Table 2.1. Medical conditions that suggest a high-risk pregnancy and warrant antepartum screening

Autoimmune disorder (e.g., lupus)
Blood transfusions
Depression or other psychiatric illness
Diabetes
Gynecological surgery
Heart disease
History of abnormal Pap smear
Hypertension
Infertility
Kidney disease (e.g., urinary tract infection)
Liver disease (e.g., hepatitis)
Neurological disease (e.g., seizures)
Pulmonary disease (e.g., asthma)
Thyroid dysfunction (e.g., hyperthyroidism)

Source: The American College of Obstetricians and Gynecologists. (2007a).

obstetrics (i.e., specialists in maternal fetal medicine) routinely counsel mothers to avoid smoking, to avoid alcohol and drug abuse, and to consume only essential prescribed medications (The American College of Obstetricians and Gynecologists, 2005b). Mothers also should avoid exposure to cats, which carry toxoplasmosis (i.e., a parasite). Nonpasteurized dairy products and soft ripe cheeses should be eliminated during pregnancy to help minimize the risk of Listeria infection. Finally, all mothers are advised to take folic acid supplements to reduce the risk of neural tube defects and to be routinely screened for preexisting conditions, especially diabetes mellitus, which is discussed later in this chapter.

Table 2.2. Reasons to conduct antepartum screening for potential genetic disease

Congenital heart defect
Cystic fibrosis
Hemophilia
Intellectual disabilities
Maternal age greater than 35
Muscular dystrophy
Neural tube defects (e.g., meningomyelocele)
Recurring pregnancy loss
Tay-Sachs disease
Thalassemia (Italian, Greek, Asian descent)
Sickle cell disease or trait

Source: The American College of Obstetricians and Gynecologists. (2007a).

Conception and Fertility

Failure to conceive may be due to factors related to the mother or the potential father. Despite apparently normal menses, some women do not ovulate. In addition, the sperm of the potential father may be too few in number or have poor motility.

Once fertilized, the egg begins to develop with several cell divisions prior to implantation. As many as one third of the developing embryos that implant are potentially lost before placental tissue develops, and another 10% are lost because of failure of the placenta to develop properly. Some of these early pregnancy losses are associated with chromosome abnormalities.

Fetal Growth and Maturity

Excess fertility is the primary cause for the increase of low birth weight (LBW) infants in the United States. Many couples who have difficulty conceiving use an array of methods that improve fertility, which leads to a much higher incidence of multiple births. Virtually all quadruplets, the majority of triplets, and nearly half of all twin gestations are now a result of induced fertility (National Institutes of Health, 2007). In general, the maximum size for a single newborn at term is 12 pounds. This weight, divided by the number of fetuses, results in ever smaller babies who deliver even more prematurely. In other words, the vast majority of twins deliver several weeks prior to term, triplets deliver earlier, and quadruplets deliver even earlier. Although these babies may be genetically healthy, the intrauterine environment does not provide for the same sufficient quality nutrition for multiple gestations as it does for a single birth.

Placenta

In mammals, the placenta has three essential functions (Kaufman & Scheffen, 1998). The first is to provide and transfer essential nutrients from the mother to the fetus. The second is to remove waste products produced by the fetus. The third function is the protection of the fetus from maternal rejection. This is accomplished by placental hormones that help to sustain the pregnancy, and at term interact with the mother to initiate labor (Gilbert & Machlin, 2005).

All the basic nutrients for fetal growth must be transferred from the mother to the baby (Sibley & Boyd, 1998). These include glucose, amino acids, fats, minerals, and vitamins. In general, each of these nutrients is in higher concentration in the maternal blood circulation than in the baby. Because the placenta is a living tissue, its own metabolism and growth extracts some of the nutrients prior to passage to the fetus. Initially there are only 10 layers of cells of connective tissue between maternal and fetal blood circulation. As the pregnancy proceeds, the placenta increases in weight and diameter. This greater weight and diameter form an ever larger surface area for the transfer of nutrients to the fetus, who demands an increased supply of nutrients and is producing waste products in greater quantity. The waste products eliminated by the placenta include carbon dioxide and the breakdown of products of protein, such as urea. Carbon dioxide is excreted by the mother's lungs and the urea (a water soluble compound) is eliminated by the mother's kidneys.

There are many factors that determine the rates at which nutrients reach the fetus and waste products are eliminated. The first is the adequacy of the mother's blood supply to the uterus and placenta. Maternal diseases that affect blood flow are hypertension and diabetes. Placenta malformations or poor placement of the placenta in the uterus may lead to inefficient flow and mixing of maternal blood, yielding a poor gradient for nutrients.

During pregnancy, the placenta produces a plethora of hormones, including human chorionic gonadotropin (hCG), placenta lactogen, progesterone, and estrogen. These hormones aid in establishing the initial conditions for pregnancy by preventing the cyclic shedding of the endometrium, as well as increasing the blood flow to the uterus. Other placental hormones (insulin-like growth factor) secreted by the fetus assist in growth of not only the placenta but also the fetus.

Because one half of fetal genes are derived from the father and, therefore, many proteins in the baby's cells and cell surfaces could be recognized as foreign tissue by the mother, the placenta acts as an intermediary in protecting the fetus from rejection by the mother and in preventing spontaneous pregnancy loss. The placenta creates a barrier that is both physical and immunologic. This barrier minimizes the mixing of fetal and maternal blood and helps to block the mother's immune response, allowing her to better tolerate the fetal proteins (Benirschke & Kaufman, 1991).

Amniotic Fluid

The amnion is the innermost layer of the placental membranes and is the primary source of amniotic fluid in the early gestation period. A small portion of amniotic fluid arises from transudates (i.e., fluid movement) through immature fetal skin and across the umbilical cord in the first and second trimesters. However, in the third trimester the prominent source of amniotic fluid is fetal urine and, in late gestation, fetal pulmonary secretions. The amniotic fluid has multiple roles—the most important is the protection of the fetus against trauma (Ostergard, 1970). Amniotic fluid allows a gravity-free environment in which delicate structures, such as hands, feet, and face, can grow without compression from the very muscular uterus. There is a slow circulation of amniotic fluid.

In the third trimester, the fetus swallows amniotic fluid, and the amniotic protein induces intestinal tract enzymes that digest proteins that are similar to the whey proteins of breast milk. The fluid portion of the amniotic fluid is absorbed into the intestine and enters the bloodstream, which allows waste products to be exchanged with the mother once again.

An excess of amniotic fluid suggests the possibility of obstruction of the proximal small intestine, a blockage of the duodenum, or atresia of the esophagus (the most common gastrointestinal obstruction to result in excess amniotic fluid). However, severe fetal neurological disease may result in poor swallowing and excess amniotic fluid. Oligohydramnios, which is insufficient amniotic fluid, occurs in the third trimester if there are no kidneys or if there is a blockage of the fetal urinary tract. Severely depleted amniotic fluid leads to compression of the fetus and maldevelopment of the lungs.

Amniotic fluid can be sampled to assess fetal genetic disease, to detect inherited metabolic abnormalities, and to assess fetal well-being and fetal lung maturity. See Chapters 9 and 11 for more information.

Problem Pregnancies

As previously mentioned, lack of prenatal care prevents detection of potential problems that could result in an abnormal pregnancy (Harmon, 1993). A prenatal screening involves physical assessment of the mother, blood sampling for a variety of diseases, and, commonly, ultrasound assessment. (See Table 2.3 for a list of common antepartum tests.)

Although screening tests vary geographically, they commonly include assessment for a number of infections that are of great risk to the fetus. These include hepatitis B and C, syphilis, rubella, and HIV infection. A maternal serum alpha-fetoprotein that is elevated may be due to a neural tube defect (meningomyelocele) in the fetus. The mother's blood type antibodies for red blood cells are determined, and the maternal hemoglobin may be analyzed (The American

College of Obstetricians and Gynecologists, 2007b).

There has been an increased use of the prenatal ultrasound, especially in the first trimester, to date pregnancies more precisely and to identify multiple gestation pregnancies. In addition, 50%–70% of major congenital malformations should be identified by ultrasound, including congenital heart disease and malformations of the back, face, and extremities. Fetal growth is monitored by serial measurements of the abdominal circumference, head circumference, and femur length. Amniotic fluid volume is calculated and, if too great or too little, may be associated with internal anomalies of the fetus.

Hypertensive Disorders

With the increase of type II diabetes and obesity in the United States, there is a concomitant increase in hypertension. The blood volume of the mother increases during the pregnancy, and this increase can exacerbate the hypertension. In addition, there is pregnancy-associated hypertension, which is commonly known as *preeclampsia*. The clinical syndrome of preeclampsia includes excess excretion of protein in the urine, edema, neurological signs, and an exaggerated response of the deep tendon reflexes (hyperreflexia).

Primary hypertension, especially with superimposed pregnancy-induced hypertension, may result in catastrophic neurological disease in the mother. The most common approach is to infuse intravenous magnesium sulfate, which usually decreases the hypertension and improves the neurological symptoms. If this condition cannot be managed medically, often the fetus is delivered prematurely.

Maternal Metabolic Disease

Although there may be numerous metabolic conditions in the mother, the most important one is diabetes mellitus (The American College of Obstetricians and Gynecologists, 2001). Intrauterine death and congenital malformations are increased with maternal insulin-dependent diabetes (type I). Both mortality and morbidity are improved with strict control of the diabetes. With

Table 2.3. Items included in comprehensive antepartum screenings

Blood type
Complete blood count (e.g., hematocrit)
Infectious screening
Bacterial
Group B streptococcus
Urine culture
Gonorrhea
Viral
Hepatitis B and C
HIV
Rubella
Varicella (i.e., chicken pox)
Other
Syphilis
Chlamydia
Pap smear

Source: The American College of Obstetricians and Gynecologists. (2007a).

less adequate control, the maternal hypergly-cemia results in fetal hyperglycemia and a fetal insulin response. The fetal insulin is a primary growth factor, which potentially results in mal-formations as well as excess growth of the fetus. All malformations are four times more common in babies born to diabetic mothers. Cardiac mal-formations also are more common. Macrosomia (i.e., an overgrown baby), which commonly oc-curs as a result of maternal diabetes, results in preterm birth and an increased risk for birth trauma. With severe diabetes affecting placental function, intrauterine growth restriction is also seen. Other metabolic endocrine conditions in-clude those of the thyroid. If the mother has hy-perthyroidism and is well controlled, the fetus and newborn usually are unaffected. However, a less-controlled mother may deliver a baby with transient hyperthyroidism, including tachycar-dia, heart failure, and goiter. The infant of a treated mother also may suffer from hypothy-roidism and require supplementation until his or her own thyroid can recover. Maternal hypothy-roidism is most commonly caused by a defi-ciency of iodine. It is very important to monitor for this condition, because congenital hypothy-roidism leads to short stature and severe learning difficulties.

Multiple Gestations

As previously mentioned, most multiple gesta-tions are commonly caused by assisted fertility (Martin, MacDorman, & Mathews, 1997). For ex-ample, the majority of twins are delivered at 35 weeks' gestation or less, triplets at an average of 32 weeks' gestation, and quadruplets at an aver-age of 29 weeks' gestation or less. Although a vast majority of these fetuses are genetically nor-mal, they have increased morbidity and mortal-ity as a result of lower gestational ages. There also may be asymmetrical growth in multiple gestations, resulting in one fetus of twins grow-ing less or having growth restriction (see Figure 2.1). This condition is commonly due to inade-quate nutrition from the placenta or poor placen-tal placement for the smaller twin. With identical twins that may share a common circulation, there

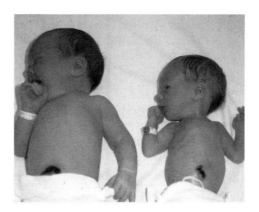

Figure 2.1. Asymmetrical growth can occur in multiple gestations. The newborn twin on the right displays discordant growth restriction. (From Clark, D.A., private collection; reprinted by permission.)

is an increased risk of twin–twin transfusion syndrome. This occurs when blood flows from one fetus to the other across placental arteriove-nous anastomoses (shunts). The donor fetus de-velops anemia and hypoalbuminemia (low serum albumin) from blood loss and has growth restric-tion and inadequate urine production, leading to insufficient amniotic fluid (oligohydramnios). The receiving twin experiences increased blood volume and polycythemia (increase in red cell mass), which may result in heart failure, excess urine production, and polyhydramnios (or ex-cess amniotic fluid). This combination may result in preterm labor or intrauterine death of one or both fetuses.

Since 2000, laser surgery intrauterine treat-ment has become available to coagulate the pla-cental blood vessels, which precludes transfusion from one fetus to the other. On rare occasions, there may be intrauterine death of a twin, which results in premature labor. If twins are identical, an activated clotting factor transfers to the live fetus and may initiate widespread clotting and destruction of tissue, including neurological im-pairment or death (Benirschke, 1998).

Postterm Pregnancy

The due date that the mother is given, also known as the estimated date of confinement (EDC) or es-timated date of delivery (EDD), is 40 weeks of completed gestation, based initially on the last menstrual period. With the widespread use of early pregnancy ultrasound, the dating of pregnancy has become much more precise. A term pregnancy is considered between 37 and 42 weeks of gestation. Pregnancies lasting greater than the 42 weeks' gestation are considered to be postterm. They comprise 3%–5% of all pregnancies (The American College of Obstetricians and Gynecologists, 2004).

The permanent complications of postdate pregnancies have to do with fetal growth and maternal complications. Compared to 10% of term infants, 25% of postterm infants weigh more than 4 kilograms. These large babies have a greater incidence of birth trauma (due to their size) and shoulder dystocia (i.e., the baby's shoulder is trapped in the mother's pelvis). Mothers with postterm pregnancies also have more cesarean section deliveries.

Oligohydramnios, decreased amniotic fluid, is more common in postterm gestation (assessed by ultrasound), and may result in compression deformities, especially of the ankles. In addition, meconium, the intestinal contents of the fetus, may be shed into the amniotic fluid, which becomes thicker because of the lack of volume. This is a much more common occurrence in the case of fetal distress. This condition increases the risk of severe meconium aspiration syndrome, in which the newborn aspirates meconium into the lungs, which results in severe respiratory distress.

Postmaturity syndrome occurs beyond term gestation when the placenta is no longer functioning, providing fewer nutrients and eliminating waste products less effectively. The fetus typically has flat fetal growth, loss of subcutaneous tissue (dried wrinkled skin), and a shriveling umbilical cord. Postterm babies typically have hypothermia and hypoglycemia due to decreased fat and less carbohydrate stored in the liver.

The postterm pregnancy continues to be a dilemma in management. If the pregnancy is appropriately confirmed as postdate, induction of labor with Pitocin may be initiated if the cervix is mature. The status of the fetus must be carefully monitored, and if distress is detected, delivery by cesarean section is common.

The Fetus

Fetal growth is dependent on maternal nutrition throughout the pregnancy. Mothers with a prepregnancy weight of less than 100 pounds have more than twice as many low birth weight newborns than mothers with a prepregnancy weight of 120 pounds or greater. Women who lose weight or fail to gain weight during pregnancy have a three-fold increase in low birth weight infants compared to those who gain 20 pounds or more during gestation. Approximately one third of the typical 20 pounds weight gain during pregnancy is attributed to the fetus. The placenta, amniotic fluid, and uterus account for one third of the additional weight gain. The remaining weight gain comes from an increase in maternal blood volume, breast enlargement, and fats and other maternal stores held in reserve for breast feeding (10%–15%).

Abnormal Fetal Growth

Macrosomia or excess fetal growth is associated with postdate pregnancies in infants born to diabetic mothers (The American College of Obstetricians and Gynecologists, 2001). Their large size makes them more prone to birth injury with a vaginal delivery. Many of these babies are born by cesarean section because they are too large to deliver vaginally. As neonates, they are more prone to hypoglycemia. Many of these large babies deliver somewhat prematurely and may be poor feeders.

Fetal growth restriction or intrauterine growth retardation is the failure of the fetus to achieve his or her genetic growth potential. Intrauterine growth restriction has been classified as *symmetrical* and *asymmetrical*, although there may be overlap (Gross & Sokol, 1989). Symmetrical growth failure affects weight, length, and head circumference. This is commonly caused by fetal factors such as chromosomal disorders, syndromes, or congenital infection. Even if genetically normal, infants are likely to be small throughout childhood and have a greater chance of developmental delay.

Asymmetrical failure means that head growth and, therefore, brain growth are relatively preserved. Weight and length may be disproportionately small. This condition usually is caused by utero-placental insufficiency with reduced nutrient and oxygen transfer to the fetus. The fetal adaptation to hypoxia is to reserve blood supply to organs, such as the brain, heart, and adrenal glands, at the expense of the kidney, gastrointestinal tract, liver, limbs, and subcutaneous tissues. Intrauterine growth retardation may be due to maternal or fetal factors. Fetal factors resulting in growth restriction include chromosomal disorders, such as trisomy 18, structural malformations, and congenital infections (e.g., cytomegalovirus, rubella, toxoplasmosis) that may alter the growth of a genetically healthy fetus.

Maternal nutrition factors (e.g., mothers with eating disorders, mothers experiencing famine in developing countries) may result in poor fetal growth. Maternal hypoxia (low oxygen tension) results in fetal restriction. Maternal conditions may include cyanotic heart disease, chronic respiratory disease, as well as pregnancies that proceed at high altitudes, such as the Andes Mountains. External influences that may affect fetal growth include the use of cigarettes (which may decrease average fetal weight at term by as much as 8 oz), alcohol, and illicit drugs.

Assessment of Fetal Health

Indirect assessment of the fetus has become more common with improved technology (The American College of Obstetricians and Gynecologists, 1999). Growth of the fetus is evaluated clinically at each prenatal visit by assessing the growth of the uterus. If there is poor growth of the fetus, an obstetric ultrasound is used to assess the position and growth of the placenta, as well as the amniotic fluid volume and fetal growth and development. If abnormalities are detected, advanced imaging is used to define the extent of the abnormality. Fetal echocardiography provides a detailed analysis of any abnormality of the fetal heart. The majority of infants with significant heart disease are diagnosed prior to birth and commonly delivered in regional perinatal centers. More sophisticated imaging by magnetic resonance imaging (MRI) may be used to identify the extent of an anomaly of the brain, spinal column, lung, and abdominal malformations (Cuniff, 2004).

Fetal maturity may be estimated from weight, head size, and fetal femur length. The most important index of maturity of a well-grown fetus is that of fetal lung maturity. This is determined by analysis of amniotic fluid for the presence of various fats, such as lecithin, phosphatidyl glycerol, and phosphatidyl inositol, in the amniotic fluid. As these rise in the amniotic fluid, they predict surfactant (i.e., a chemical in the lung that decreases surface tension and allows for easier breathing) sufficiency of the maturing fetal lung.

A biophysical profile of the fetus is measured in pregnancies at risk (Alfirevic & Neilson, 1996). It includes fetal gross body movements, fetal breathing, fetal tone, reactive heart rate, and measurement of amniotic fluid volume. Heart rate, breathing, and tone are similar to components of the Apgar score.

Chorionic villus sampling (CVS) of early gestation or amniocentesis in the second trimester for fetal white blood cells in the amniotic fluid yields cells that can be analyzed for chromosomal abnormalities or specific defects in the DNA. Amniocentesis also can be used to analyze for fetal infection, using the polymerase chain reaction (PCR) for toxoplasmosis, cytomegalovirus, and other viruses. Fetal skin biopsy may be used for other severe congenital disorders (The American College of Obstetricians and Gynecologists, 2007c).

Fetal Therapy

The earliest form of fetal therapy is available to the baby with severe fetal anemia resulting from maternal antibodies against fetal red blood cells. The severe anemia can be blunted by a transfusion, when red blood cells are injected into the fetal umbilical vein. The use of RhoGAM with Rh– mothers has greatly decreased the incidence of fetuses at risk for this disorder.

Fetal surgery is commonly in the news. As a cutting edge technology, the results of these procedures are commonly poor because the malformations that justify fetal surgery are so severe that there is a very high risk of premature onset of labor. Therefore, such procedures are restricted to randomized clinical trials at only a few centers.

Surgery (opening the uterus, or hysterotomy) at 22–24 weeks' gestation to repair a diaphragmatic hernia or spina bifida has been performed. There is very little evidence that the clinical outcome is significantly improved. Instead, many infants are born prematurely.

Catheters have been inserted into the bladder and are connected to the amniotic cavity in cases where the fetus has had obstruction of the outlet of the bladder. This seems to do little in terms of improving renal function.

With fetal hydrocephalus, the shunting from the enlarged cerebral ventricles into the amniotic fluid in utero has been largely abandoned because of a high rate of severe disability and premature birth.

Environmental Risks to the Fetus

Fetal health is totally dependent on the health and well-being of the mother. Mothers with hypertension, severe renal disease, heart disease, diabetes, sickle cell disease, drug addiction and alcoholism, and other conditions are at great risk for pregnancy loss or giving birth to babies with disabilities. Severe anemia in the mother may result in poor fetal oxygenation and spontaneous abortion.

The fetal metabolic rate is considerably higher than that of the mother, and thus the byproducts of metabolism heat, metabolic acid, and protein breakdown must be transferred to the mother. The typical fetal temperature is approximately 1° C higher than the mother's temperature. If she has a fever, especially during early gestation, the mother is less capable of dissipating the heat, and the fetal temperature is even higher. If this situation occurs early in the first trimester, there is an increased incidence of cleft lip and cleft palate.

Environmental chemicals create a particular hazard for the fetus. Tobacco smoking results in fetal growth retardation, as well as increased incidence of placental abruption. Maternal alcohol use, illicit drugs (especially cocaine), and even prescription drugs for serious maternal illnesses all pose a threat to the fetus. Excellent prenatal care includes adjusting medications appropri-

ately and substituting less hazardous medications (and perhaps more inexpensive medications) to protect the developing fetus.

Labor and Delivery

Fetal-maternal medicine (perinatology) has rapidly developed since the late mid-1980s. The focus of this field is to identify high-risk situations (with both the mother and the baby) and to intervene, if possible, to produce best outcomes. (See Table 2.4 for a list of issues requiring antepartum counseling.)

An example of this is early detection and management of pregnancy-induced hypertension in the mother, which could otherwise result in adverse newborn neurological outcome. The management of preterm labor to prolong fetal growth and development is also a priority (Goldenberg & Rouse, 1998). This section explains the events surrounding labor and delivery and subsequent problems that may arise.

Labor

Uterine contractions can be detected throughout the normal pregnancy. They are irregular, uncoordinated, of variable intensity, and usually not felt by the mother. As the uterus stretches with the fetal and placental growth, this activity continues throughout the pregnancy until approaching term gestation, which is defined as a range of 37–42 weeks' gestation post menstrual age. Near term, the cervix begins to dilate and shorten in

Table 2.4.   Issues requiring antepartum counseling

Activity
Breast feeding
Domestic violence
Environmental and/or work hazards
   Exposure to cats (toxoplasmosis)
   Exposure to toxins
   Handling raw meat
Fetal activity
Medications
   Herbal
   Prescriptions
Nutrition (diet) (e.g., appropriate weight gain)
Postpartum depression
Use and possible abuse of tobacco, alcohol, or illicit drugs

Source: The American College of Obstetricians and Gynecologists. (2007a).

preparation for coordinated labor. The precise timing of the labor is difficult to determine, which prompts the terms *false labor* and a *prolonged latent phase of labor.*

Labor remains a complex process that includes a delicate biochemical interaction between hormones produced in the mother's brain, the placenta, and fetal hormones as well as the mechanical stretch of the uterus. Conventionally, labor has been divided into three stages. The first stage is from onset of labor to full dilation of the cervix. The first stage is also divided into two phases, which are 1) the latent phase from the onset of irregular contractions to the beginning of the active phase; and 2) the active phase, which is the time when the rate of cervical dilation begins to change rapidly until full dilation. The active phase usually begins at 3–4 centimeters dilation of the cervix.

The second stage of labor is from full dilation of the cervix to the delivery of the infant. The third stage is from the delivery of the infant to the delivery of the placenta. Some clinicians describe an additional stage of labor (the fourth stage) as the hour following delivery of the placenta in which rapid changes are occurring in the mother.

Data from several thousand patients documenting cervical dilation and stations of the presenting fetal head throughout labor are used to establish normal limits for a mother's pregnancy for the first time, as well as the mother who has delivered successfully previously (multiparous). As would be surmised, the latent and active phases of the first hours of labor are longer in mothers with a first pregnancy compared to mothers who have been pregnant two or more times. The latent phase of the first stage in the first pregnancy averages 6.4 hours, with an active phase averaging 4.6 hours, for an approximate total first stage of 11 hours. This is compared to multiparous women who have an average latent phase of 4.8 hours and an active phase of 2.4 hours, for an average total of 7.2 hours. As is to be expected, the descent of the fetus is much more rapid in the multiparous mother than in the mother delivering for the first time.

The mechanical energy of the contracting uterus during labor is a significant stress to the fetus. Prior to rupture of the membranes, the amniotic fluid provides a cushion and helps to distribute the intrauterine pressure evenly across the fetus, including into the lungs. In the second stage of labor, intrauterine pressure increases approximately 5–8 times that of the resting phase, and, if the mother *bears down*, pressure may rise to 12–15 times that of the quiet, first phase.

There can be variation from mother to mother regarding the frequency, intensity, and duration of uterine contractions. Once the membranes rupture and amniotic fluid escapes, the fetus typically orientates head down in preparation for delivery. In 90% of pregnancies, the head, which is the largest body part of the fetus, is the presenting part for delivery.

A breech presentation occurs when the buttocks or feet are engaged first. In either case, the greatest pressure is exerted on the presenting parts located in the narrowest portion of the uterus and its outlet. In preterm babies, the compression of the skull with the immature vessels in the brain is, in part, responsible for intracranial hemorrhage (see Chapter 5 for a discussion on neonatal neurology). Pressure on the head during this time also results in a fetal neurological response with decreased heart rate. There is no evidence that this response (decreased heart rate) is deleterious if the duration is short and there is a prompt return to a normal heart rate once the contraction has subsided. In addition, there are changes in blood flow to the uterus with contractions as placental blood flow is decreased. This is important because nutrients and fetal waste products must be exchanged through the placenta. The oxygen content of the fetal blood lowers during labor and carbon dioxide (a waste product) is somewhat higher. The transient metabolic challenges are readily handled by term infants but are less well tolerated by premature babies. A prolonged labor and intense contractions may lead to severe distress for the infant. The field of obstetrics and the subspecialty of fetal-maternal medicine look to avoid undue stress on the fetus by identifying those at greater risk and delivering them as safely as possible. This has led to the increase of cesarean section deliveries in complicated pregnancies, especially of the very small preterm infant.

Pain Management of Labor

Historically, very little was offered for pain management for mothers in labor. Narcotics and other forms of sedation were used, and many of these have effects on the fetus as the medication can be transferred across placenta and is less well metabolized by the fetus. Narcotic suppression of newborn muscle tone and respiratory effort was common with the use of narcotics during the mid-1990s.

If labor proceeds fairly well and the mother is reasonably comfortable, pain management may not be necessary. In these mothers with a vaginal delivery, local anesthesia may be used during descent through the birth canal and the delivery itself.

However, modern anesthetic techniques are being used routinely, even in facilities with relatively few deliveries. Spinal anesthesia, which provided a Novocain-like medication to block the nerve sensation from the contracting uterus, was commonly used for cesarean section delivery. One of the primary complications of spinal anesthesia was protracted numbness of the lower abdomen and extremities, which took hours for recovery. In addition, a small leak of spinal fluid commonly resulted in headaches.

Since the 1990s, epidural anesthesia has been used very effectively. The epidural space is an area outside of the outer membrane of the spinal cord where the nerves that supply the abdomen and uterus intersect and where their transmissions can be effectively blocked with medication. Much less medication is required for an epidural than spinal anesthesia, and the adverse effect on the mother is much shorter, with little medication passing on to the fetus. Therefore, epidural anesthesia can be used throughout the late first and through the second stage of labor safely for both mother and baby.

Complications of Delivery

There can be abnormalities of any phase of labor and delivery. The arrest of labor when the cervix fails to dilate and the head fails to descend for more than 2 hours is a very serious matter. Many of these conditions are associated with a head that is too large to move through the pelvis appropriately. This is called cephalopelvic dispro-

portion. This is, in part, a consequence of humans becoming larger, especially in mothers with diabetes whose fetuses grow disproportionately large. This commonly leads to delivery by cesarean section.

Cesarean section is also performed for abnormal presentation, including a transverse lie, in which the shoulder is a presenting part and the baby is in a U-shaped position with the head and feet toward the top of the uterus, and with a compound presentation where a hand and foot present simultaneously. A frank breech presentation occurs in approximately 3–4% of all deliveries. These may be delivered safely by an experienced obstetrician. More commonly, however, these are preterm babies, and a combination of prematurity and breech presentation nearly always results in a cesarean section delivery. Some infants with breech presentations also have various congenital disorders, including neuromuscular disease and hydrocephalus. (Specific complications of delivery that result in compromising the newborn are discussed in Chapter 3.)

The mother may be at risk for blood loss once the placenta detaches. It is shed relatively rapidly after delivery, and occasionally Pitocin (oxitocin) is given to decrease blood flow to the uterus in an effort to limit postpartum bleeding. Rarely, fragments of placenta may be retained and require surgical removal via the vagina 1–2 days after delivery.

Typically mothers will shiver after delivery. This is a normal physiologic adaptation to produce heat. This results because prior to delivery the fetus and placenta have a high metabolic rate and are transferring that heat to the mother. Following delivery, the loss of heat source from the uterus results in a compensatory mechanism for the mother to maintain her body temperature by producing heat from muscular activity. This effect is not a result of anesthesia.

Conclusion

In summary, conception, embryonic development, fetal growth, labor, and delivery are all an intricate series of biologic processes with multiple opportunities to go wrong. The birth of a full-term, healthy baby is truly a miracle.

REFERENCES

Alfirevic, Z., & Neilson, J.P. (1996). Biophysical profile for fetal assessment in high-risk pregnancies. *Cochrane Database of Systematic Reviews*, Issue 1. (Article No. CD000038. DOI:10.1002/14651858)

The American College of Obstetricians and Gynecologists. (1999). Antepartum fetal surveillance. *ACOG Practice Bulletin, 9*, 1–10.

The American College of Obstetricians and Gynecologists. (2001). Gestational diabetes. *ACOG Practice Bulletin, 30. Obstetrics and Gynecology, 98*, 525–538.

The American College of Obstetricians and Gynecologists. (2004). Management of postterm pregnancy. *ACOG Practice Bulletin, 55. Obstetrics and Gynecology, 104*, 639–646.

The American College of Obstetricians and Gynecologists. (2005). Smoking and women's health. In *Special Issues in Women's Health*, 151–167.

The American College of Obstetricians and Gynecologists. (2005). Substance use: Obstetric and gynecologic implications. In *Special Issues in Women's Health*, 105–150.

The American College of Obstetricians and Gynecologists. (2007a). *ACOG antepartum record*. Washington, DC: Author.

The American College of Obstetricians and Gynecologists. (2007b). Hemoglobinopathies in pregnancy. *ACOG Practice Bulletin, 78. Obstetrics and Gynecology, 109*, 229–237.

The American College of Obstetricians and Gynecologists. (2007c). Screening for fetal chromosomal abnormalities. *ACOG Practice Bulletin, 77. Obstetrics and Gynecology, 109*, 217–227.

Benirschke, K. (1998). Multiple pregnancy. In R.A. Polin & W.W. Fox (Eds.), *Fetal and neonatal physiology: Vol. 1* (pp. 115–124). Philadelphia: W.B. Saunders.

Benirschke, K., & Kaufman, P. (1991). *The pathology of the human placenta* (2nd ed.). New York: Springer.

Cuniff, C. (2004). Prenatal screening and diagnosis for pediatricians. *Pediatrics, 114*, 889-894.

Gilbert, W.M., & Machlin, G.A. (2005). Placental function and diseases: The placenta, fetal membranes, and umbilical cord. In H.W. Tauesch, R. Ballard, & C. Gleason (Eds.), *Avery's diseases of the newborn* (8th ed., pp. 23-31). Philadelphia: Elsevier.

Gross, T.J., & Sokol, R.J. (1989). *Intrauterine growth retardation: A practical approach.* Chicago: Year Book Material.

Goldenberg, R., & Rouse, D. (1998). Prevention of preterm birth. *New England Journal of Medicine, 339*, 313–320.

Harmon, J. (1993). High-risk pregnancy. In C. Kenner, A. Brueggeyemer, & L.P. Gunderson (Eds.), *Comprehensive neonatal nursing* (pp. 157–170). Philadelphia: W.B. Saunders.

Kaufman, P., & Scheffen, I. (1998). Placental development. In R.A. Polin & W.W. Fox (Eds.), *Fetal and neonatal physiology: Vol. 1* (pp. 59–70). Philadelphia: W.B. Saunders.

Lissauer, T., & Fanaroff, A. (Ed.). (2006). *Neonatology at a glance.* Oxford, United Kingdom: Blackwell Publishing.

Martin, J.A., MacDorman, M.F., & Mathews, T.J. (1997). Triplet births: Trends and outcomes, 1971-94. *Vital Health Stat, 21*(55), 1–20.

National Institutes of Health. (2007, May). Presentation at Pediatric Academic Societies, Toronto.

Ostergard, D.R. (1970). The physiology and clinical importance of amniotic fluid: A review. *Obstetrical and Gynecological Survey, 25*, 297-319.

Sibley, C.P., & Boyd, R.D. (1998). Mechanisms of transfer across the human placenta. In R.A. Polin & W.W. Fox (Eds.), *Fetal and neonatal physiology: Vol. 1* (pp. 77–88). Philadelphia: W.B. Saunders.

CHAPTER 3

Evaluation and Care of the Neonate

David A. Clark

At the conclusion of this chapter, the reader will

- *Understand the basics of delivery room management of the newborn*

- *Understand basic assessment of the newborn that is carried out immediately following delivery*

- *Understand the newborn's transition to life after delivery*

- *Understand routine care and screening of the newborn prior to discharge*

The transition of a baby from the womb to the outside world is a complex process. Crucial elements of newborn care are anticipation of problems prior to birth, serial evaluation over the first few days, and careful attention to the details of newborn screening.

Delivery Room Management

The vast majority of newborns are born healthy and require little intervention at birth. The neonate is wet with amniotic fluid and will lose heat rapidly; therefore, the child needs to be dried quickly and placed on a heat source. The child should be stimulated to cry by the gentle flicking of the feet or stimulation of the chest. Once the baby has been assessed and is breathing appropriately, the umbilical cord is clamped and vitamin K is given. The child can then be wrapped and given to the family (American Academy of Pediatrics Committee on Fetus and Newborn and The American College of Obstetricians and Gynecologists Committee on Obstetric Practice, 2007).

Some infants will have difficulty at birth and require resuscitation. A scoring system known as the Apgar score was developed in 1953 by Dr. Virginia Apgar, an anesthesiologist who proposed rating the five characteristics of the infant that correlate with intrauterine stress and perinatal difficulties (Apgar, 1953). These parameters include in descending order of importance: heart rate, respiratory effort, muscle tone, reflex irritability, and color. Table 3.1 shows how these scores are rated.

Each of the characteristics is scored on a scale of 0–2. A 0 is given if there is no response, such as no heart rate, no respiratory effort, or a total blue color (cyanosis). A 2 is given for the best response, such as a heart rate that is greater than 100 beats per minute, a regular sustained respiratory effort, and a totally pink color. An Apgar score of 1 in each category indicates a response between 0 and 2. These scores are assigned at 1 and 5 minutes and then in 5-minute intervals until a total score of 6 or greater is attained. The 1-minute Apgar score is some indication of the severity of in-utero distress and how well the child will respond to resuscitation. The

Table 3.1. Explanation of Apgar scores

	0	1	2
Heart rate	Absent	< 100 bpm	> 100 bpm
Respiratory effort	Absent	Slow, irregular	Good
Muscle tone	Limp	Some flexion of extremities	Active motion
Reflex irritability (nose suction)	No response	Grimace	Cough or sneeze
Color	Blue, pale	Acrocyanosis	Completely pink

Source: Apgar (1953).
Key: bpm = beats per minute.

5-minute Apgar score correlates more predictability to morbidity and mortality. Although many individuals have tried to modify and improve the scoring, there is little consensus, and most of these more precise evaluations continue to be used as research tools rather than aids to clinical practice (The American College of Obstetricians and Gynecologists & American Academy of Pediatrics, 2006).

There are serious difficulties with the use of Apgar scores to predict outcome. Many infants are born with distress and may not be evaluated accurately in the hectic activity of the resuscitation effort. Despite the simplicity of the Apgar score, it is helpful in offering the general description of the state of the newborn that can be shared among facilities.

Neonatal resuscitation is a rapid sequence of events that needs to be performed if a baby's respiratory effort or circulation is impaired. The aim is to clear the airway and to optimize breathing

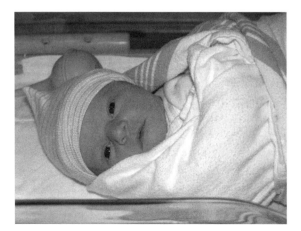

and circulation as quickly as possible. The vast majority of infants who require resuscitation can be anticipated. Many of these neonates are born prematurely, are multiple gestation babies, have a low fetal heart rate by antepartum assessment, or have congenital anomalies (Lissauer & Fanaroff, 2006). The resuscitation process has been standardized by the well-established, Neonatal Resuscitation Program (NRP), which is a joint effort of the American Academy of Pediatrics and the American Heart Association. This program is an educational effort and not a certification. It includes didactic lessons, workbooks, periodic tests, and hands-on skill demonstrations as part of the training (American Academy of Pediatrics and American Heart Association, 2006).

Resources can be marshaled when antepartum risk factors have been identified. A team of skilled, health care professionals must be available to resuscitate the child properly. As with healthy children, all infants are assessed at birth, kept warm, and dried. The airway is cleared, and the child is stimulated to breathe. If the baby's heart rate and respiratory effort are poor, the next step is to establish effective ventilation with mask ventilation or intubation and positive pressure. If the child is being appropriately ventilated and the heart rate remains low, the next step is chest compression followed by the use of medications, especially epinephrine if the child is still not responding appropriately. The vast majority of resuscitation efforts are successful, and only 3%–5% of babies who have an Apgar score of 3 or less at 5 minutes have long-term, neurological disabilities (National Institute of Child Health and Human Development, 1996). Many of these are preterm infants.

There are times when resuscitation is inappropriate. International guidelines for withholding care are established. These include not initiating resuscitation if the child is a very preterm fetus of less than 23 weeks' gestation or has a birth weight of less than 400 grams. It may be withheld if the child has a major lethal anomaly, such as anencephaly or previously diagnosed trisomy 13. Resuscitation should also be stopped if there has been no heartbeat or respiratory effort after 5 minutes of effective resuscitation. The more difficult ethical decision arises if the baby is born at 23–25 weeks' gestation. This raises the issues of high mortality, expensive and prolonged neonatal intensive care hospitalization, and the high risk of short-term morbidity and long-term disabilities (Davis, 1993).

Birth Injuries

Labor and vaginal delivery are stressful and traumatic to nearly every newborn (Kendig, 1992). All newborns have edema of the scalp. Some may acquire a cephalohematoma (see Figure 3.1), which is caused by bleeding under the outer surface of the bones of the lateral skull and results from being scraped across the pelvic ischial spines. Cephalohematomas commonly enlarge within several days of the birth as additional fluid is drawn into the area due to breakdown of the red blood cells. They resolve slowly by calcifying along the outer edge until a firm mass is formed. As the infant's head grows during the first year of life, the skull remolds the lump on the side of the head and it becomes less obvious.

Most other injuries are to the head and neck. They include paralysis of the 7th cranial nerve, which is the facial nerve. This nerve may be damaged by pressure, especially application of forceps near the point where the nerve emerges from the skull at the edge of the jaw as it articulates with the skull. Such trauma frequently leads to paralysis of the involved muscles. Clinically, when the infant cries, the infant's mouth is drawn to the normal side. Droopy eyelids and loss of wrinkles are often seen on the affected

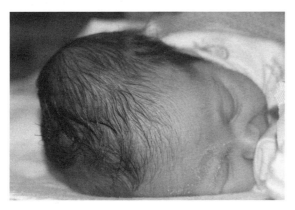

Figure 3.1. Infant with cephalohematoma. (From Clark, D.A., private collection; reprinted by permission.)

side when the nerve is damaged. The child also may have difficulty closing the eyelid on the affected side. The majority of these facial palsies begin to diminish spontaneously within several days. Total recovery takes from weeks to months.

Any prominence of the head may be traumatized during delivery. Eyes and eyelids may become damaged and bruised, there may be hemorrhage in the sclera of the eye, and corneal abrasions may occur. In addition, ears are prone to abrasions, hematomas, and occasionally lacerations. The majority of these insults resolve within the first several weeks with little residual effect.

The more serious injuries are those that occur in the neck. For example, the lateral neck swelling seen in newborns may result from bleeding into the belly of the sternocleidomastoid muscle that connects the sternum and clavicle (cleido-) to the mastoid area of the skull. Contraction of this muscle allows for turning of the head. As a hematoma in this muscle begins to resolve, it may cause scarring and foreshortening and contraction of the muscle, which leads to torticollis (stiffening of the neck). If this condition is not recognized early and appropriate physical therapy initiated, it may become a very severe problem that is difficult to correct, even with surgery.

The various nerves of the neck are especially susceptible to injury. The brachial plexus includes the nerves extending from the neck to the arm. Erb's palsy, paralysis of the shoulder and upper arm, results from injury to the 5th and 6th cervical nerve roots. Klumpke palsy, paralysis of the lower arm, results from injury to the 8th cervical and the 1st thoracic roots. (See Figure 3.2 for an example of Erb's palsy.)

The injuries to various nerves usually follow a prolonged and somewhat difficult labor. Commonly, the infant is large and has had severe fetal distress. The increased pressure applied to the head and shoulders to assist with delivery may result in trauma. The principle treatment for these conditions is the maintenance of an appropriate range of motion for the affected joints. Treatment consists of partial immobilization followed by an active physical therapy program by 7–10 days of age. If the nerve roots are intact, function may return within a brief period of time

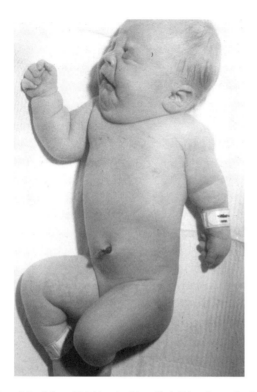

Figure 3.2. Infant with Erb's palsy. (From Clark, D.A., private collection; reprinted by permission.)

as local edema and hemorrhage resolve. Although the rate of recovery varies with the degree and location of the injury, most infants return to normal function within 3–6 months. However, an infant with severe injury may show continued improvement over several years. In particular, paralysis of the lower arm has a poor prognosis with the possibility that a claw deformity of the hand will develop.

Several other nerves of the neck may be affected as well. The most important of these is the phrenic nerve, which innervates the diaphragm. Injury to this nerve may result in a paralyzed diaphragm and asynchronous respiratory effort. In addition, there may be trauma to the recurrent laryngeal nerve leading to unilateral vocal paralysis, which is associated with hoarse crying and respiratory distress.

Other potential birth injuries include fractured clavicle or extremity; rupture of the liver or spleen; hemorrhage into the adrenal gland; and, in a breech presentation, trauma to the genitalia. The prognosis of each of these injuries varies considerably; however, most of these conditions are treatable and have a very good return of func-

tion in a relatively short time period. Whenever any form of birth trauma has been identified, it is important to examine the infant carefully for other injuries.

Babies born prematurely, those with anomalies or major malformations, and those diagnosed with significant perinatal injury usually require a higher level of specialty care than is often available in a community hospital. Regional perinatal centers and children's hospitals offer the range of consultants and personnel to evaluate these children and develop a comprehensive plan of intervention (Stark, 2004).

The Physiology and Behavior of Transition

The transition from fetal to extrauterine existence is one of the most physiologically traumatic experiences of life (Lissauer & Fanaroff, 2006). The baby is disconnected from his or her life support system and must make a very rapid transfer to air breathing, which requires major changes in the circulatory system. The lungs, which have been filled with fluid, must expel or absorb the fluid to allow adequate exchange of oxygen as a nutrient and carbon dioxide as a waste product. The central nervous system must deal with stimuli that have not been present or have been muted within the uterus, including touch, smell, taste, and vision. The kidneys begin to concentrate and dilute the body's waste products in order to excrete them. Furthermore, the upper gastrointestinal tract must digest food properly to provide optimal nutrition to continue the rapid growth of the baby.

One of the most profound changes is the rapid transition of the circulation. Prior to birth, less than 5% of blood pumped by the heart enters the lungs. Blood returning from the placenta has sufficient oxygen for fetal needs. As it enters the right side of the heart, this blood may cross directly to the left side and travel to the body, or it may be pumped by the right muscular chamber (ventricle) out toward the lungs. Most of this blood bypasses the lungs through a vessel called the patent ductus arteriosus, which connects the pulmonary and the systemic circulations. At

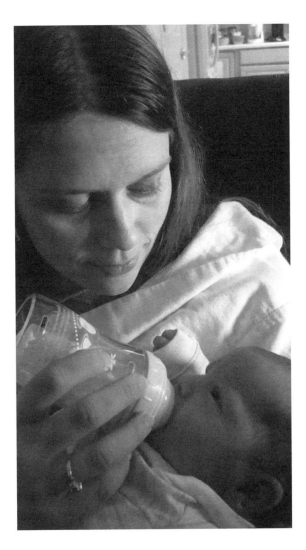

tive to the experience of being born. A characteristic series of changes in vital signs and clinical appearances takes place. These include the first period of reactivity, a relatively unresponsive interval, and the second period of reactivity. The first reactive phase begins shortly after birth and may last as long as 6 hours. The newborn is alert, exploratory, and responds quickly to various stimuli. The second phase is a sleep state and commonly lasts 3–6 hours. The third phase (i.e., a second reactive phase) follows, by which time the healthy infant has established complete control of respiration and circulation.

There is marked variability in the behavior of newborns during transition. Failure to respond in accordance with described patterns is not suggestive of infant brain damage or even temporary compromise. Labor and delivery pose an especially stressful time for the infant. In most cases, however, anticipation of potential problems and their correction leads to a smooth transition of the fetus from intrauterine existence to the environmental challenges of the outer world.

birth, the lungs expand rapidly and blood flow must match lung expansion for the baby to survive. Resistance in the lung blood vessels drops rapidly in the first 24–48 hours, and thus there may be some back flow of small amounts of blood from the systemic circulation into the pulmonary circulation that now has the lower pressure. This increase in blood oxygen level typically leads to a contraction of muscles in the walls of the patent ductus arteriosus and obliteration of this vessel usually within 1 week. In many preterm infants, this vessel may not close and may result in excess activity of the heart with heart failure.

During the transition to extrauterine life, there are three phases of newborn behavior. Upon delivery, the infant is vigorous and reac-

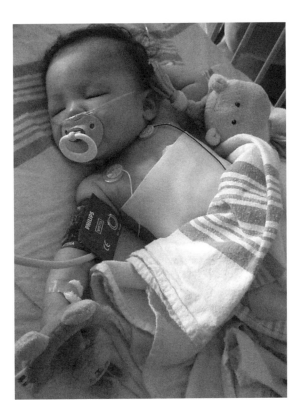

Assessment of Gestational Age

The assessment of gestational age begins with appropriate dating of the pregnancy. Due to increasingly precise early fetal ultrasound assessments in the first trimester, obstetrical dating has become ever more accurate. Growth can be followed closely, and the size of the head, length of long bones, and other parameters can be used to assess continuous fetal growth.

Several methods have been developed to assess gestational age of the newborn that are based on physical and neurological characteristics (Dubowitz, Dubowitz, & Goldberg, 1970). Many external physical characteristics progress in an orderly fashion during the third trimester period (Dubowitz & Dubowitz, 1977). These include the following:

- There is a progressive disappearance of vernix, a cheeselike material that initially appears at 24 weeks' gestation, that covers the body of the fetus and begins to diminish at 36 weeks. In a full-term infant, it generally is found only in the creases of the body.

- The skin of the extremely premature infant is thin and translucent with blood vessels prominent. With increasing gestation, the vessels become less apparent as a result of deposition of fat and thickening of the skin.

- The lanugo, which is a fine hair that covers the entire body as early as 22 weeks of gestation, vanishes from the face only 3–4 weeks prior to birth and commonly may be seen on the shoulders of many newborns.

- The areola, the nipple and surrounding tissue, are not visible or barely visible in a very premature infant. At 34 weeks' gestation, the areola begins to rise, and in response to maternal hormones, fat is deposited in the breast. By term, a 5–6 millimeter nodule can be felt.

- The ear of the term infant has a well-defined incurving of the outer edge. It is firm with well-developed cartilage and stands erect from the head. The ear of the 28-week infant is flat and shapeless and does not spring back when it is folded because little cartilage is present.

- Genitalia development is most easily traced in males with descent of the testes, which begin as intraabdominal organs that first appear at the beginning of the inguinal canal at 28 weeks' gestation. They descend into the scrotum and are pendulous. In response to this development, the scrotum manifests increased folds and becomes more pigmented. In the female, deposition of fat plays a role. In a 32-week baby, the clitoris is prominent and the labia majora are small and widely separated. As the fetus approaches term with the fatty deposition in the labia, the labia minora and clitoris are completely covered.

- The sole of the foot is smooth at 28 weeks' gestation. As the pregnancy proceeds, there is a progressive increase of sole creases with the anterior two thirds of the foot covered with creases by 36 weeks' gestation.

In general, these physical characteristics should be documented within the first 24 hours. With predictable loss of extracellular fluid, the characteristics of the skin and appearance of sole creases may be altered after that time. Once the infant is cleaned, vernix is no longer useful as an adjunct to assess gestational age.

Neurological Evaluation

Although determination of gestational age by physical criteria should be performed immediately after birth, the neurological evaluation should not be performed until later when the infant's condition is stable. With the events of transition, this assessment cannot usually be done until the end of the first day. Numerous perinatal factors may affect the neurological assessment, including perinatal asphyxia, maternal anesthesia, maternal medication, and various illnesses and syndromes that affect the newborn (Dubowitz & Dubowitz, 1977).

Neurological development of the fetus during the last trimester is characterized by an increase of muscle mass and tone, as well as changes in reflexes and joint mobility in the extremities. Several neurologists have provided details of neurological examinations of gestational age.

Infants born at 28 weeks' gestational age or less have very poor muscle tone, known as hypotonia, with a resting posture that fully extends the arms and legs. Flexor tone begins at 30 weeks' gestation and increases first in the lower extremities. At 35–36 weeks' gestational age, the infant has good muscle tone in the lower extremities but only partial flexion in the arms. By full term, the resting posture should include full flexion of all the joints and both upper and lower extremities. The extremely preterm infant, however, does not resist various passive maneuvers, such as movement of the heel to the ear (the scarf sign).

By 36 weeks, the neck extensors and flexors begin to function, and by 38 weeks many infants can hold their heads for a few seconds when pulled to a sitting position. The tone of the trunk can be measured by ventral suspension. Premature infants at 28 weeks' gestation or less have very poor trunk tone and will appear to be draped over an outstretched hand. At 32–34 weeks, the back has straightened. By full-term, the head rises above the straightened back.

A number of primitive reflexes, such as the Moro reflex, crossed extension reflex, and rooting and sucking reflexes, have been used to determine gestational age. However, most of these reflexes are absent prior to 32 weeks' gestation and are well established by term. In the interval between 32 and 36 weeks, they are not sufficiently discriminating to assess gestational age accurately. Most of these reflexes disappear in the first year of life.

In general, gestational age assessment of newborns is accomplished most commonly with a combination of detailed prenatal information and confirmatory physical and neurological findings.

Growth and Gestational Age

Once the gestational age of the newborn has been established, the growth characteristics are exam-

ined to determine whether intrauterine growth has been appropriate. Babies that are in less than the 10th percentile in the major growth parameters of weight, length, and head circumference are considered small-for-gestational-age (SGA) infants. Those babies whose weight, length, and head circumference are greater than the 90th percentile are considered large-for-gestational-age (LGA) infants. These indicators are based on normative curves, which predict the weight, length, and head circumference for the growth of fetuses at each gestational age beyond 24 weeks' gestation. SGA babies, despite their degree of gestational age, are more likely to have syndromes and chromosomal abnormalities. LGA babies are more likely to be born to parents that are large and/or to mothers who have diabetes.

Routine Newborn Care

Following resuscitation and stabilization, a number of things are done with each infant receiving specific prophylactic health care. This includes proper identification, care of the umbilical cord, eye care, administration of vitamin K, and newborn screening.

Umbilical Cord Care

At delivery, the cord is clamped to prevent blood loss. It then dries and at approximately 7–10 days is spontaneously shed. The dried cord is shed by enzymatic action of white blood cells that have been attracted to the site in response to normal bacterial colonization. Antibacterial substances are no longer applied to the cord because they delay colonization and prolong the time until the cord is shed (Zupan & Garner, 1999).

Eye Prophylaxis

Ophthalmia neonatorum (conjunctivitis) of the newborn can be caused by a variety of infectious agents. In the early 1900s, gonorrhea was a common cause of newborn conjunctivitis, which commonly resulted in severe vision loss. Newborn eye care, known as Credé's method, involves instilling a prophylactic agent into the eyes of all newborns. The recommended solutions are erythromycin or tetracycline, both of which may be somewhat effective against chlamydia, which causes a less serious eye infection (Bell, Grayston, Krohn, & Kronmal, 1993). For the few infants who do develop conjunctivitis, a specific infectious agent should be sought and treatment administered to prevent vision loss.

Vitamin K

Hemorrhagic disease of the newborn was first described in 1894 as generalized bleeding that occurred in the first week of life in otherwise healthy infants. It is well known to be caused by severe depression of the coagulation factors II, VII, IX, and X, which is due to a deficiency of vitamin K (Zipursky, 1999). Vitamin K is typically produced by bacteria within the intestine; however, the newborn has a sterile intestine and will not be sufficiently colonized with vitamin K–producing organisms until approximately 1 week of age (Hey, 1999). The administering of vitamin K intramuscularly or orally at birth allows improved coagulation during this very specific interval (American Academy of Pediatrics Committee on Fetus and Newborn, 2006).

Newborn Screening

Screening of the newborn has become much more complicated and extensive since the mid-1990s (Maternal and Child Health Bureau, 2006). Rapid advances in technology have allowed for many more diseases to be detected and treated prior to any clinical symptoms (Wiley, Carpenter, & Wilcken, 1999). The overall goal of newborn screenings is to detect as early as possible children that may be affected and to intervene and produce a healthier child. There are many diseases that can be detected by screening, some of which are very difficult to treat and others that have no treatment. Some of those difficult to treat (e.g., Krabbe disease) may be treated with bone marrow transplant and still have very limited survival at a great cost. Debate will continue on the appropriateness and efficacy of these more complex screening programs.

In general, newborn screening falls into a number of categories, including metabolic, endo-

crine, hematology, infection, cystic fibrosis, and hearing (Cunniff, 2004).

Metabolic Screening

Tandem mass spectrometry is a technology that includes the pairing of a mass spectrometer with a second mass spectrometer to analyze in detail various chemicals produced within the body (Zytkovicz et al., 2001). The vast majority of inborn errors of protein and fat metabolism may be detected with this technology. The majority of these are treatable by diet or medication. One of the most common of these is phenylketonuria, which is the inability to handle the amino acid phenylalanine. Untreated, this disease causes growth retardation and poor neurological development. By simply minimizing the amino acid phenylalanine, these children can develop without difficulty.

Endocrine Disease Screening

The prominent endocrine diseases being screened for in newborns include hypothyroidism and congenital adrenal hypoplasia. Hypothyroidism has an incidence of approximately 1 in 4,000 newborns. If they are not treated with the thyroid hormone (thyroxine), they are at great risk for abnormal neurological development that is irreversible. Congenital adrenal hypoplasia is a disease in which there is a defect of an enzyme in the adrenal gland, which results in failure to produce key hormones. Affected newborns lose excessive amounts of salt in the urine and may die of hyponatremia (low blood sodium). Newborn females may have ambiguous genitalia.

Hematology and Infection Screening

Hematology screening is confined primarily to detect abnormal hemoglobin. The prototype is sickle cell disease. Although it does not directly affect newborns because their hemoglobin is primarily a fetal hemoglobin, infants with sickle cell disease are at great risk for infection in the first 6 months of life and require special surveillance and immunizations.

Infectious screenings are limited. As of 2008, only New York and New Jersey screen all newborns for HIV, although other states are considering this surveillance. Other potential perinatal infections being screened for include toxoplasmosis and cytomegalovirus.

Cystic Fibrosis and Specific Gene Defect Screening

Screening for cystic fibrosis is done by analyzing the blood for immunoreactive trypsin (IRT), an enzyme that would not be in the blood in high concentration if the disease were absent. Children with a high level of IRT are examined for specific gene defects. Although the disease cannot be cured, its effects may be ameliorated by early aggressive management of nutrition that promotes fat absorption in these infants.

Hearing Screening

A newborn hearing screening is the only infant test that is performed at individual hospitals (Erenberg, Lemons, Sia, Trunkel, & Ziring, 1999). Therefore, it has wide variability because it is based on multiple testers. The purpose is to identify hearing difficulties in infants as early as possible so that intervention can occur to modify speech and language development.

Discharge Planning ____

Preparation for discharge includes ensuring that the baby is able to consume adequate calories for growth, is able to maintain body temperature, and is free of medical conditions.

Breast Feeding

Breast milk from the mother of the baby remains the best possible nutrition for the newborn (Fomon, 1993). It is superior to any formula preparation in the quality of nutrients, especially proteins, as well as various nutrients that help the newborn to control the bacterial colonization of the intestines (Weimer, 2001). (See Chapter 10 for more information.)

Circumcision

Routine newborn male circumcision is still commonly practiced only in the United States. Europe, Asia, Africa, South America, and Australia do not circumcise newborn males unless it is for religious custom. The procedure is unnecessary, painful, and often results in injury (Patel et al., 2001). In general, pediatricians and many obstetricians are counseling parents of its risks (ACOG, 2001; AAP Committee on Fetus and Newborn, 2004).

Conclusion

This chapter has described the basics regarding assessment of newborns and the transition to life after delivery. Evaluation and care of the newborn form a detailed and multistep process. Each component is critical to the success of the infant's ability to thrive and develop.

REFERENCES

American Academy of Pediatrics and The American College of Obstetricians and Gynecologists. (2007). Care of the neonate. In *Guidelines for perinatal care* (6th ed.). (pp. 205–249). Elk Grove Village, IL: American Academy of Pediatrics; Atlanta: The American College of Obstetricians and Gynecologists.

American Academy of Pediatrics and the American Heart Association. (2006). *Textbook of neonatal resuscitation* (5th ed.). Elk Grove Village, IL: American Academy of Pediatrics; Dallas: American Heart Association.

American Academy of Pediatrics Committee on Fetus and Newborn. (2004). Hospital stay for healthy term newborns. *Pediatrics, 113*, 1434–1436.

American Academy of Pediatrics Committee on Fetus and Newborn. (2006). Controversies concerning vitamin K and the newborn. *Pediatrics, 112*, 191–192.

The American College of Obstetricians and Gynecologists. (2001). Circumcision. *ACOG Committee Opinion No. 260. Obstetrics and Gynecology, 98*, 707–708.

The American College of Obstetricians and Gynecologists & American Academy of Pediatrics. (2006). *ACOG Committee Opinion No. 333. Obstetrics and Gynecology, 107*, 1209–1212.

Apgar, V. (1953). A proposal for a new method of evaluation of the newborn infant. *Anesthesia Analgesia, 32*, 260–264.

Bell, T.A., Grayston, J.T., Krohn, M.A., & Kronmal, R.A. (Eye Prophylaxis Study Group). (1993). Randomized trial of silver nitrate, erythromycin, and no eye prophylaxis for the prevention of conjunctivitis among newborns not at risk for gonococcal ophthalmitis. *Pediatrics, 92*, 755–760.

Cunniff, C. (American Academy of Pediatrics Committee on Genetics). (2004). Prenatal screening and diagnosis for pediatricians. *Pediatrics, 114*, 889–894.

Davis, D.J. (1993). How aggressive should delivery room cardiopulmonary resuscitation be for extremely low-birth-weight neonates? *Pediatrics, 92*, 447.

Dubowitz, L.M.S., & Dubowitz, V. (1977). *Gestational age of the newborn.* Boston: Addison Wesley.

Dubowitz, L.M.S., Dubowitz, V., & Goldberg, C. (1970). Clinical assessment of gestational age in the newborn infant. *Journal of Pediatrics, 77*, 1–10.

Erenberg, A., Lemons, J., Sia, C., Trunkel, D., & Ziring, P. (1999). Newborn and infant hearing loss: Detection and intervention. American Academy of Pediatrics Task Force on Newborn and Infant Hearing. *Pediatrics, 103*(2), 527–530.

Fomon, S.J. (1993). Human milk and breastfeeding. In S.J. Foman (Ed.), *Nutrition of normal infants* (pp. 409–423). St. Louis: Mosby.

Hey, E. (1999). Prevention of vitamin K deficiency in newborns. *British Journal of Haematology, 106*, 255–256.

Hittner, H., Hirsch, N., & Rudolph, A. (1977). Assessment of gestational age by examination or the anterior vascular capsule of the lens. *Journal of Pediatrics, 91*, 455–458.

Kendig, J.W. (1992). Care of the normal newborn. *Pediatrics in Review, 13*(7), 262–268.

Lissauer, T., & Fanaroff, A. (2006). Neonatal resuscitation. In T. Lissauer & A. Fanaroff (Eds.), *Neonatology at a glance* (pp. 34–37). Oxford, United Kingdom: Blackwell Publishing.

Maternal and Child Health Bureau. (2006). *Newborn screening: Toward a uniform screening panel and system. Report for public comment.* Rockville, MD: Author. Retrieved December 11, 2007, from http://mchb.hrsa.gov/screening.

National Institute of Child Health and Human Development. (1996). *Report of the workshop on acute perinatal asphyxia in term infants* (NIH publication 96-3823). Washington, DC: Author.

Patel, H.I., Moriarty, K.P., Brisson, P.A., & Feins, N.R. (2001). Genitourinary injuries in the newborn. *Journal of Pediatric Surgery, 36*, 235–239.

Stark, A.R. (American Academy of Pediatrics Committee on Fetus and Newborn). (2004). Levels of neonatal care. (published erratum) (appears in *Pediatrics*, 2005, *115*, 1118). *Pediatrics, 114*, 1341–1347.

Weimer, J. (2001). The economic benefits of breastfeeding: A review and analysis. U.S. Department of Agriculture. Economic Research Service. *ERS Food Assistance and Nutrition Research Report, 13*, 1–20.

Wiley, V., Carpenter, K., & Wilcken, B. (1999). Newborn screening with tandem mass spectrometry: 12 months' experience in NSW Australia. *Acta Paediatrica Supplements, 88*, 48–51.

Zipursky, A. (1999). Prevention of vitamin K deficiency bleeding in newborns. *British Journal of Haematology, 104*, 430–437.

Zupan, J., & Garner, P. (1999). Topical umbilical cord care at birth. *The Cochrane Library, Issue 2.* Oxford, United Kingdom: Update Software.

Zytkovicz, T.H., Fitzgerald, E.F., Marsden, D., Larson, C.A., Shih, V.E., Johnson, D.M., et al. (2001). Tandem mass spectrometric analysis for amino, organic, and fatty acid disorders in newborn dried blood spots: A two-year summary from the New England Newborn Screening Program. *Clinical Chemistry, 47*, 1945–1955.

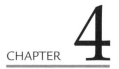

CHAPTER 4

The Family as Foreground

Jill R. Weldum, Nancy S. Songer, and Gail L. Ensher

At the conclusion of this chapter, the reader will

- *Be sensitive to the ways in which biases and personal lenses affect working with families*

- *Understand the importance of professional, collaborative relationships when working with families who have children with special needs*

- *Understand cornerstone principles of best practices when working with families who have children with special needs*

- *Understand commonalities and the uniquenesses of families who have children with special needs, including individual stressors and resiliency in daily living*

- *Understand how life cycles of children and families change over time and have an impact on working with families who have children with special needs*

This chapter considers several aspects of working with children with special needs, including family life and child development; how the professional relationship with families and children affects, and is affected by, the family system; and some best ways to engage with families to promote systemwide support of children. To achieve best practices with children and their families, two basic principles are helpful. First, every family is unique and potentially open to change. Second, the beliefs, assumptions, and training of professionals determine how effective they are with children with special needs and their families.

The terms *special needs, delays*, and *disabilities* are used interchangeably in this chapter to describe children with physical, developmental, and emotional needs that distinguish them from children with no health, cognitive, emotional, or trauma-related issues. These include children with life-threatening illness; chronic disease; physical disabilities, such as speech, sight, or hearing difficulties; developmental disabilities, such as au-

tism; and mental health and/or emotional challenges.

This chapter is directed toward professionals, such as speech therapists, physicians, counselors, and teachers who work with children, as well as concerned families. The best practices of these professionals begin with the notion that using a collaborative, team approach is most effective because it emphasizes that family members and professionals are contributors who bring unique, equally important perspectives and knowledge to the care of children with disabilities. From this principle, it follows that goals are mutually defined and need to reflect family priorities. Professionals need to demonstrate flexibility and sensitivity in order to successfully collaborate with families. This family-centered care approach takes into consideration the dynamics that affect and organize each of the children concerned and invites those in the system to participate as equal members in achieving the best possible outcome for children with disabilities.

39

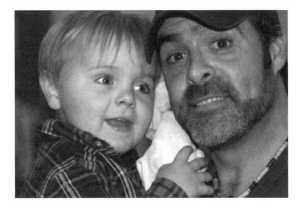

Historically, the parents of children with disabilities were seen as the source of problems. Often blamed, parents were seen as barriers to the children being served. This perspective has gradually shifted as parents have created organizations that challenge the original paradigm. The power of these organizations has affected available services, schooling, and legal issues.

Because of these pioneers, today's parents can potentially be learners, teachers, advocates, and decision makers. Now, their roles are dictated by their desires, the systems they are involved in, and the individuals they encounter as their children receive and participate in services. By understanding the unique family landscape and each child's individual development, professionals in the field of disabilities can work most effectively with families. Furthermore, they need to be personally aware of how their own personal lens affects what they see and respond to when working with others. Awareness of our personal lens allows us to recognize when our own issues are contributing to problematic situa-

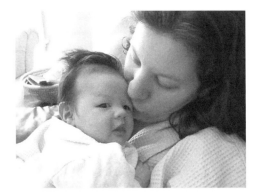

tions, connect with others who are not as reactive to the situation, and be more successful with identifying strengths and supporting families in their self-care.

Careful Assumptions

Much of what we do as humans is to categorize. This helps us create order as we move through the world and helps us make sense of situations. However, by categorizing, assumptions are made that limit and negate relationships. Categorizing relationships causes us to overlook and ignore unique aspects and strengths about the people with whom we work. Two issues pertinent to this discussion of working with families of children with special needs are the notion of the nuclear family and the ways in which professionals use theories.

Many of us continue to hold onto the premise of the nuclear family. From this assumption of the one man, one woman, and children composite of a family, we inevitably create a comparison of other family compilations. There is no such standard; that is, every family, including those consisting of one man, one woman, and children, have relationships, dysfunctions, dynamics, and experiences that render them unique. It is important to resist the urge to compare families and, instead, to consider each family separately, as well as their strengths and their challenges. This frees us to see families as individuals, rather than looking at their achievements and failures in comparison to a given standard.

Care providers are susceptible to perceiving families automatically through the medical model (i.e., through a medical or health care lens). At its worst, the medical model encourages focusing on a person's illness, disability, or dysfunction. This is in part necessary to investigate the so-called problem, but typically any strengths or exceptions to the problem go unnoticed. There are strengths and resiliencies in every person and system, and it is important to investigate those resiliencies with as much energy as the dysfunctions and disorders. The popular culture of the United States has internalized this medical model as part of each individual's personal lens. Humans inevitably view others from their own personal perspective. Even with the most extensive training, it is unavoidable that our experiences, perceptions, values, and beliefs color our relationships with others. For best practices to prevail, it is necessary to understand our personal lenses and their limitations.

Anyone who works with children also works with families. What we as professionals learn from the theories of child development and family systems provides structure for understanding the dynamics that occur within family systems. We look at families through these structures. Theories can provide insight into systems and children that help us connect with them. However, theories about family systems and child development are just that—theories. Theories can help us understand internal and system dynamics, and they can limit us if we adhere to them too steadfastly. Common theories are presented in this chapter, but assumptions about families should not be made based on these theories alone. Family and internal dynamics are in a continual flux and are constructed differently depending on socioeconomic factors, ethnicity, gender, personality, life experiences, life cycle stages, and current circumstances. Although it may be tempting to assume that families with similar socioeconomic status, ethnicity, and disability experience are the same, they are not. Recognized and accepted theories can be valuable in providing a general framework for understanding families, but they are seldom facts about any single family.

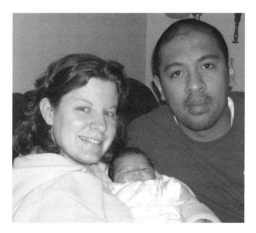

The Significance of a Personal Lens

When we meet a new family, we typically encounter several layers or aspects of that family system simultaneously. We process rapidly who we think the family is; that is, it is the rare professional who gives much more organized thought about a family beyond initial impressions. Most of us tend to focus on the child and see the family in the background as either helpful or a hindrance. Our professional identity and our assumptions dictate where we focus our attention and define our perceptions and practice. Speech therapists tune into how the communication process works between child and family members, and physicians attend to the physiological aspects. Our lens is also formed by our personal characteristics, including gender, ethnicity, socioeconomic status, and the impact these characteristics have had on our lives, as well as by the situations and relationships we have encountered throughout our lives. Last but not least, our lens is informed by the values we hold—values that may have originated from our culture, family, or ourselves.

Across professions over time, awareness has increased regarding the impossibility of being completely neutral. Our personal lens has tremendous potential to help us understand everyone we encounter. It can tell us our initial feelings about the parent who denies the cognitive delay of his or her child. For example, those initial feelings may be frustration because the parent's denial inhibits our ability to help, leaving us to feel powerless. At the other extreme, we may have deep empathy as we recall our own feelings of denial when we watched a loved one of our own experience an illness or face a challenge, and we begin to reexperience the helplessness we felt in that situation. From either of these directions, we can work with parents struggling with a child's limitations as long as we recognize what is happening within ourselves.

Humans tend to feel safe when they experience a balance of closeness and distance that seems familiar and comfortable. These boundaries strongly define professional relationships with families, especially when they take us to the homes of families. Our sense and a family's sense of safety are also affected by the numbers and kinds of roles we play (Nelson, Summers, & Turnbull, 2004). When service providers play more than a professional role in a family's life, the relationships can become more complicated. To varying degrees, professional associations as well as legal necessity define the kinds of roles professionals can play with families. These guidelines are intended to protect the consumer (i.e., family and child), and they also act to protect the relationship between the professional and the consumer. Three themes have been identified through research as potential problem areas: 1) accessibility of the provider to families; 2) the provider's responsiveness to families (i.e., going beyond one's job description); and 3) dual relationships (Nelson et al., 2004).

Maintaining appropriate and healthy relationships with families and the children served is of paramount importance. Our personal sense of appropriate boundaries varies depending on the relationships we are in and our own preferences regarding closeness and distance with others. Some of us are more comfortable with complicated, multiple roles, and some of us are more comfortable with clearly defined, fairly structured boundaries. A number of issues are of paramount importance when considering boundaries and best practices with families:

1. Know and follow the ethical guidelines of the profession.

2. Know personal preferences regarding boundaries in relationships with families and understand how a family's sense of boundaries might affect us.

3. Consider the preferences of families and what will help them feel safe and engaged.

4. Discuss issues of boundaries with families as necessary to certain situations.

When working with families, we may find ourselves operating from our personal experiences with our own family. This is particularly likely when we are working with more challeng-

ing families. As we meet a new child and family, typically the first thing we notice on our own emotional level is whether or not this family is receptive to us (i.e., are their boundaries open or closed?). When we encounter a family that is similar to our own family, we may react to the family in the same way we would react to personal family members, whether positively or negatively. Encountering a family that is different from our own may cause us to be judgmental because the family is not displaying what we consider to be appropriate emotions, actions, or relationships.

It is often from our personal lens that our passion for working with children with special needs and their families arises. Our passion and commitment are great resources and strengths that we bring into our professional relationships. As professionals, we can adjust for the bias our lens brings to our work by recognizing that from time to time our lens will interfere in our relationships with families, and by becoming aware of our own reactivity. When we are judgmental about or critical of families, we are reactive to their system dynamics and not likely to do our best work. Although complete neutrality is impossible, it is vital to know our own value system and work to separate our values when they conflict with others. It is from this place of recognition that we can move to collaborative work with others.

Experiences of Families Who Have Children with Special Needs

Whether a child was born with a disability or developed it at a later age, families typically experience very powerful emotions and worries upon learning of the disability. The process families go through has been likened to a grief response (Marshak & Prezant, 2006; Perryman, 2005; Williams, 2001) with overwhelming feelings of fear, loss, anger, and sadness. Families fear the present and future as they face all the unknowns about their child's health and well-being. Families lose the assumed reality of a healthy, typical child who grows into a healthy, typical adult. Anger and sadness often are the only possible emotions to feel as parents and siblings face their own helplessness. In addition to grief responses, it is normal for families to feel shock, denial, anxiety, guilt, depression, and possibly hope and new meaning (Williams, 2001).

Siblings are particularly vulnerable when their role in the family changes to one that requires them to take on responsibility beyond their years (Robinson & Robinson, 1965). After the initial shock and adaptation of the family to the child's special needs, siblings may feel and express jealousy (either verbally or physically) regarding the attention their sibling receives, and/or they may try to be perfect to cause less stress for their parents. Siblings grieve as well; how they express that grief is what distinguishes them from the adults in the family. The following vignette demonstrates the complex feelings family members of children with disabilities experience.

Ben and Alex

As a family, we have been challenged to identify with and accept two children with disabilities in our beautiful family of five. Our struggle began early on when our first son, Ben, at age 2, wasn't communicating like other children his age. Ironically, our first struggle was with friends and family who wanted Ben to be just fine and normal. They would tell us, "He is a boy, and boys develop slower,"' or "He isn't talking because you meet all of his needs," or "He will talk eventually." No one wanted to face the frightening truth that we were living with.

My son was diagnosed with developmental delays. Ironically, one of the reasons Ben's disability was difficult for people to see was because he was so happy and easy going. This is a problem that plagues Ben still. Even now people have difficulty seeing the disability because he is so well liked. By age 3, he had picked up the name "Happy Ben." This has actually been a hurdle to receiving appropriate diagnoses and intervention.

My everyday life seemed to be much like those bad dreams where you are trying to scream and nothing can come out and no one can hear you. The

scream was that there was something wrong with my beautiful boy, while all around me I was being accused of overreacting.

Finally, when Ben was 3½, we were able to get him evaluated. To my horror as well as my relief, my first born, who carries all the dreams and hopes and expectations of young parents, was diagnosed with speech and motor difficulties. To say that the experience of deep relief and nightmarish fear hitting at the same time was surreal would be an understatement. Still, I felt like no one was listening to me, except for one person, my sister, Angela. Angela is also struggling with her firstborn, who is only 5 months older than Ben, and the label of autism is on her radar. Both of us were crying on the phone, taking turns comforting each other. For us, denial, anger, bargaining, and depression were not something you read about in a book, but they were emotions that hit us all at once.

After Ben's diagnosis, we began intervention with speech therapy three times a week and occupational therapy two times a week. At this point, I was still struggling as a mom who noticed that, at 4½, Ben just didn't play like other kids. Again, no one else seemed to see it, except for me and my husband. We live daily with the fact that our son cannot identify letters; that at 5 years old, he can't fully run; that he can't write his name; and that he just can't do so many things that he should be able to do.

My nightmare continued when my second son, Alex, started showing signs that were of concern. Later, he was identified with speech delay and motor difficulties.

I worried that this must be my fault. I am the mom. I am with them all the time. If only I had stimulated them more. We paint, we play with mud, we draw, we walk, we talk, we read, but it feels like it's not enough. If only I had done things differently. The guilt overwhelms me.

When Ben was in kindergarten, his teacher called me and requested that we talk about Ben. He is unable to follow directions like the other kids. My feelings of relief and grief were back—relief that someone else saw the problem, and grief that it was true. At that point, things became worse. Teachers in the next few years did not listen to me about Ben's disabilities. It was as if I was screaming again, but no one was listening. The five-page paper that I wrote about the issue with diagnosis and suggestions was politely filed, not to see the light of day. "Yes, Mrs. Findley, thank you for coming in," I was told.

Now I have two sons, 5 and 2½, who cannot communicate effectively. Ben cannot follow two-step instructions, and Alex has daily emotional outbursts. Alex screams if a drop of juice falls on his chest. A pea on the floor that he has not touched but that is in his path has the ability to cause my sweet toddler to start screaming. His sensory issues control our every moment together. Now, I have two sons in therapy. I have two sons who are not considered so-called normal. As the issue becomes evident in our extended family, his grandparents express denial and shame. It is too hard to connect to their grandsons, so they give up. There are even others who deny and reject, blaming us as we already do.

As Ben gets further into the school system, my nightmare is now my reality. I no longer just try to be the loving mother, but a fierce lioness. I have to fight for my son with teachers, psychologists, and administrators who collectively either want to label my son with autism or want to take any diagnosis away and label him as perfectly normal. Ben has had teachers who see his difficulties and help him in amazing, creative, self-sacrificing ways. This eases my nightmare, and I don't feel as alone in my worry and grief.

I have moments of hope. There are moments when I remember that my son is perfect, and the systems and demands he encounters aren't. There are moments when I can imagine our family having a good life that isn't defined by "normal." There are moments when I remember my beautiful boys, their love for me, and my love for them. And then there are moments when a pea turns up on the floor.

Collaborative Care as a Best Practice

In the U.S. major culture, most interventions, such as medical, psychological, and educational, were historically based on a receivership model (e.g., the physician heals the patient, the teacher lectures the student, the counselor advises the client). Within this framework, the professional is active and the consumer is passive. The professional is the expert and is the only person able to improve a person's life. In contrast to the re-

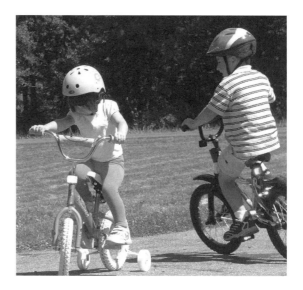

ceivership model, collaborative health care arose to provide a complete, systemic care system to patients and their families, and it is based on the assumption that everyone involved in a health care relationship is acting on others (McDaniel, Hepworth, & Doherty, 1992). This version of care, also known as the collaborative resource approach, is very useful when it comes to supporting children with special needs and their families (Ho & Keiley, 2003). A collaborative approach can assist families in accepting their child's diagnosis, intervention, and future.

If we consider the triangle of care to be professionals, child, and family, clearly there are multiple avenues of action and potential. Professionals act and affect each other's intervention plans, the child, and the family. Family members act and have an impact on each other, the child, and the professionals. Within the professional corner of the triangle, providers typically work together via a variety of communication techniques, including meetings. When professionals work in isolation from each other, intervention plans and practices may contrast in ways that cause more problems for children and their families. When we work together, sharing plans, discussing challenges, and identifying strengths in the child, family, and ourselves, the potential for improvement and increased support to the child and family is more likely to be realized. Collaborative care also helps professionals be more aware of how their personal lens is playing out in their relationships with families. As we hear perspectives from other professionals, we have additional information to consider that does not contain the bias of our own perspectives. This is especially important when we are struggling with a particular family.

The collaborative health care model suggests that expertise exists in each corner. Professionals derive expertise from their education, skills, experience, and person. The child is an expert on himself or herself. Families have expertise regarding how they function, feel, what they know about their child, and what does and does not work in their family. Added to this process is the family's perspective and experience, including what they report to the professional about the child during private family time, the relationships between the family members and the child, and the dynamics of the family system as it pertains to the child's growth.

Cross culturally, there are varying rules and practicalities that dictate who participates in the collaborative team and who teaches and works with children. When we enter a family's system, it is helpful to figure out who the teacher is so that we can coach the person most likely to be working with the child. For example, the single parent of a child with severe developmental disabilities may work 70 hours per week to cover survival needs, and it is the older sibling, grandmother, aunt, or uncle who is caring for the child most frequently and helping him or her with exercises and getting to appointments. It becomes our challenge to respect the role of the parent, while at the same time including the person or other people who are most able to support the child's development.

Every family has its own dynamics that dictate how they operate, and these dynamics typically will determine the involvement of families in services. The model of collaborative care assumes that all three partners (i.e., professional, child, family) actively participate to the extent that they can in the improved well-being of the child, and that all partners have valuable expertise to contribute.

To achieve best practices in a collaborative care relationship, the following guidelines are recommended by Raver (2005):

1. View parents and/or caregivers as potential partners and experts in the intervention of their child. Encourage their participation at a level that is most meaningful.

2. Focus on building trusting, consistent relationships with the family, child, and other professionals involved in the care relationship.

3. Communicate sensitively, honestly, and often with the family, child, and service delivery members.

4. Provide emotional support and practical suggestions.

5. Demonstrate patience as parents take time to make decisions about their child's care.

6. Check-in with the family and child about their concerns.

7. Trust that by collaboratively teaming, other team members may be able to access information or help the family when we cannot.

The Family as Context

The family is the natural context for teaching infants and children. Every child is born into a family, and our first relationships and experiences of the world are viewed through the lens of our family. Families are made up of individuals who share a past and a future, with numerous generations being bound by biological, legal, or historical means (Carter & McGoldrick, 2004). With the addition of new members, families change over time.

Whether a child is with his or her biological, foster, or adoptive family, the child is inherently affected by and affects the family. It is in the family that we see the primary dynamics—those relationships that, to a large extent, form who we are and how we relate to others. These primary dynamics are passed down from generation to generation (Bowen, 1978). It is in the family that children gather their strength and their security. It is within the family that children's very survival rests.

Because of these factors, children and infants and those people who care for and love them can be most easily reached, affected, and helped in their families. It is our closest relationships that lend safety wherever we are. It is also in the family that we find those most able, on a daily basis, to implement care plans, such as the individualized family service plan (IFSP) and the individualized education program (IEP). Turnbull and Summers describe this altered perspective well.

> Let's pause to consider what would happen if we had a Copernican Revolution in the field of disability. Visualize the concept: the family is the center of the universe and the service delivery system is one of many planets revolving around it. Now visualize the service delivery system at the center and the family in orbit around it...we would move from an emphasis on parent involvement (i.e., parents participating in the program) to family support (i.e., programs providing a range of support services to families). (1985, p. 12)

A family-based practice operates from the philosophy of identifying strengths of the child and family. Service delivery professionals work to support the child's development, build strengths, and lessen stress of family members through a collaborative relationship that respects family needs for balance and offers supports and resources (Raver, 2005). Teaching children in the presence of their families enhances potential learning, as the following vignette demonstrates.

The Family as a Team

When my son was 2 years old, he began receiving speech therapy. My husband or I attended almost every session, three times per week. We asked for and received suggestions from his speech therapist that supported our son's speech development. Our speech therapist said at every review that our active support was a big part of his success. My son is now 5, and he has graduated from speech therapy. We worked together as a team—me, my husband, our son, and the speech therapist—to help him move through his speech delay and gain mastery. It is in the family that children live every day. Every single morning our son had the opportunity to work on words and retrieval as we offered him choices first. Later, when we began asking him what he wanted, we learned to give him time for his retrieval efforts to improve. We learned to speak slowly and deliberately and to wait patiently

through his stuttering instead of offering words to help him. If we had not been seen as integral to the team working with our son, we would not have been taught to do these things. If our speech therapist had not valued our contributions as parents, we would not have been included. We would have continued to encounter our frustration, as well as his, with his difficulty in saying what he wanted. Our dynamic would have impeded his efforts at speaking, and his progress would have been much slower.

It is through a collaborative team approach that professionals, families, and parents can best work toward a common goal.

Contemporary Families

It is important to be aware of the makeup of today's families. There is a temptation to use the nuclear family, which is defined as a heterosexual married couple with biological children, as the form for family and to judge and/or compare every other family against this form. This is not the only, or predominant, form of family life. Keep in mind that although many families determine membership by marriage or blood, many identify other significant people as members. Diversity across families is the norm (e.g., single parent [male or female], blended and remarried families, gay/lesbian couples with children, multigenerational extended families, families of brothers and/or sisters or aunts and nieces, unmarried partners).

What are the facts about contemporary families?

- In 2003, 26% of all U.S. households consisted of just one person compared with 17 percent in 1970 (McFalls, Jr., 2003). The majority of single-person households are made up of adult women.

- Less than 25% of all households are nuclear families (Schmitt, 2001).

- The majority of two-parent households are dual earners; in families with children under 6 years of age, more than half of the mothers work, and almost all fathers work (Roehling & Moen, 2003).

- First marriages are occurring later in life than ever before. The average age of marriage is 27 years for men and 25 years for women. Divorces occur in approximately 45% of married couples (Carter & McGoldrick, 2004; Walsh, 2003).

- Twenty percent of children live in remarried families, and within 1 year of divorce, half of the fathers have virtually lost contact with their children (Carter & McGoldrick, 2004).

- Three quarters of welfare recipients leave welfare within 2 years, but instability of jobs and lack of child care often force their return. Only 15% stay on welfare for 5 consecutive years. The majority of welfare recipients are Caucasian (Carter & McGoldrick, 2004).

- As of 2006, the United States population was as follows (U.S. Census Bureau, 2006):

  White alone (including people of Middle Eastern background): 73.9%, or 221.3 million

  Black or African American alone: 12.4%, or 37.1 million

  Asian alone: 4.4%, or 13.1 million

  American Indian or Alaska Native alone: 0.8%, or 2.4 million

  Native Hawaiian or other Pacific Islander alone: 0.14%, or 0.43 million

  Some other race alone: 6.3%, or 19.0 million

  Two or more races: 2.0%, or 6.1 million

In families with children with special needs, additional stressors are layered on the relationships of spouses, siblings, and the parent–child relationship. These include

- Financial burdens of medical bills not covered by insurance, lack of health insurance prediagnosis, and continual battling for reimbursement of expenses

- Loss of income due to caring for a child or the costs of hiring specialized care providers

- Emotional strain of sometimes chronic grief, sadness, and anger

- Adjusting to the life families now have versus the life they dreamed of

- Diversity of experience within each family as spouses, siblings, and the child process the effects of the delay

- Extended family members' opinions, input, and respective stress

- Change in friendships due to new demands

- Concerns regarding the stability of the couple's relationship as it faces increased strain, required changes, and sacrifice

Although research is contradictory regarding the effects of child disability on divorce rates (Eddy & Walker, 1999; Hodapp & Krasner, 1994; Mauldon, 1992), it is clear that significant strain and stress are added to family systems and relationships when a child has special needs.

Family Roles

The recognized roles in families consist of grandparent, parent, sibling, child, grandchild, and spouse. Parents are expected to discipline their children; children are expected to respect their parents and grandparents; siblings are expected to work out socialization skills; grandparents are expected to guide and provide elder wisdom; and spouses are expected to work together in managing family life. Five essential roles for effective family functioning have been identified by researchers over time:

1. Provision of resources to ensure that all family members have survival needs of food, shelter, and clothing

2. Provision of comfort, love, nurturance, and reassurance within families

3. Life skill development, including physical, emotional, educational, and social, of family members

4. Maintenance and management of the family system through leadership, decision making, finances, and boundaries among family and others

5. The sexual partnering of couples

As recently as 2000, men and women have expressed high levels of egalitarian expectations for marriage (Botkin, Weeks, & Morris, 2000). They rate marital equality as very important in their own marriages, including gay and lesbian relationships (Carrington, 1999; Rosenbluth, Steil, & Whitcomb, 1998). Some families are moving toward more liberal gender socialization for children, and fathers are more involved in raising children than in previous generations. Attitudes are changing with time regarding roles in families, but behavior lags behind. In heterosexual relationships, women who are employed carry close to 80% of the household chores and child care (Fraenkel, 2003). Women are the primary caregivers of ill and elderly family members (Walsh, 2003) and provide the emotional and organizational work in families. Rosenbluth et al. (1998) found that despite attitudes of egalitarianism, less than 28% of the couples in their research actually shared household tasks. Carrington (1999) found this to be true in gay and lesbian couples studied as well.

According to Cohen and Petrescu-Prahova (2006), the majority of American children with disabilities live in families in which the care of the children is primarily done by women. Children with disabilities are more likely to live in single-parent families, especially with only their mothers, and those not living in their biological families are more likely to live in women-led households.

Additional factors to consider are that poor child health may be a factor in mothers getting divorced or living singly (Mauldon, 1992), and mothers in urban settings are not likely to be involved with the father of the child in poor health 1 year after its birth (Reichman et al., 2004). These findings minimally suggest that professionals are much more likely to be providing care to children of single-parent families. Over a decade ago according to Hanson, Heims, Julian, and Sussman (1995), single mothers of children with disabilities were often younger and had less education and lower incomes than those mothers who have partners—and such situations still hold in 2008. As first-time motherhood age moves into later years, however, these findings may not accurately represent the families that professionals

now encounter. We need to be aware of underlying assumptions in our culture about who should take care of children with disabilities (women) and their defining characteristics, such as low income and young, which typically indicates lacking in resources. Although these findings are discouraging, they also carry hope. A potential exists with the involvement of fathers and their growing desire to be more active parents.

Implicitly, roles may become assigned as family members begin to do things to meet a need and take on that role. In families with healthy functioning roles, distribution of roles is balanced to help avoid any one member being overwhelmed all the time. Some roles are decided day to day; others are decided and followed long-term. The following supports to helping families develop healthy roles are imperative:

- Encourage clear roles that are identifiable and agreed on (flexibility is necessary to ensure family health).

- Encourage fair role allocation to prevent resentment and burnout.

- Demonstrate responsibility when carrying out roles in the family to build cohesion in family units.

Families with clear, flexible roles can handle crises, stressors, and unexpected demands much more easily than families with vague, less fluid roles.

When family members are faced with a new diagnosis for their child, anxiety and stress grow as they move through the process of adjusting to new demands, grieving the loss of the child they expected, and in some cases worrying about the very survival of their child. In effective families, role sharing allows the family to deviate from their usual patterns when encountering transitions or stressors. Individuals in the family demonstrate willingness to learn new abilities to take care of family needs.

Life Cycle Changes

All families experience change and transition as the ages of their members change. The idea of family life stages has organized our thinking regarding families for many decades. Individuals go through fairly predictable patterns that have remained constant (i.e., birth, infancy, childhood, adolescence, young adulthood, maturity, senescence, and death). Although illness, accidents, and other unexpected events can interrupt or delay these stages, they are the typical sequence. For families, typical life cycle stages are harder to define due to overlapping of events that have an impact on the family, culture, and ethnicity variables, as well as the vast increase in types of family makeup. Life cycle events and culture vastly affect and complicate life cycle stages in families. With the greater configurations of families today, a broader perspective regarding development and normalcy is necessary when attempting to understand families in life cycle stages (Carter & McGoldrick, 2004). We need to remember that healthy functioning is a potential within a variety of family arrangements.

When we see a family, we are seeing a snapshot (i.e., observing the system at a moment in time) that defines that particular moment and its relationships, stages, subsystems, roles, boundaries, closeness, and distance. The family system is not the same in the previous snapshot, nor will it be the same in a future one. We never see the entire family; however, they are all there in the room—generations of elders; the absent members due to geography, estrangement, or death; those who cannot attend because of their age or ability; those who are blaming parents for their child's disability; and grandparents, aunts, or uncles who carried the same weight for a child of their own. Yet, the family's shared history, present and future, forever keeps them connected (Carter & McGoldrick, 2004).

Table 4.1 presents the stages of the life cycle. Although the stages of the life cycle are rather arbitrary breakdowns, they can serve as markers for what families may typically go through (Carter & McGoldrick, 2004). Using a life cycle perspective can help families remove themselves from the difficulty of the moment. That is, families who are struggling with their child's disability will not be struggling (at all or in the same way) in the future, and families can be reminded of easier moments in the past. Using the life cycle stage provides professionals with a flexible yardstick that defines the typical issues families face

Table 4.1. Life cycle stages

Stage	Goals	Changes
Unattached adult	Identify relationship and professional goals	Achieve separation from family of origin physically and emotionally; develop intimate relationships with peers and significant other; establish career
Couple	Establish unit that is physically and emotionally separate from family of origin	Commit to new relationship; re-arrange relationship with family of origin and peers
Child	Adjust to new member(s) and loss of freedom; extra responsibility	Parenting roles established; extended family relationship and roles change; emotionally grieving
Adolescent	Adjust to child's burgeoning independence; letting go of childhood	Adolescent moving in and out of the system; parents focus/refocus on career; grandparent needs
Launching of young adult	Complete adjustment to member's entrances and exits in family system; meet older generation's new needs; couple's maintenance of their relationship	Grandparent needs and death; parental unit's retirement and health needs; coping with death of eldest generation

and can help families remember and anticipate easier moments in life.

In the typical life stage, most family theorists start with the single young adult who is formulating goals, both relationally and professionally. Next comes the physical relationship of two people, often followed by the birth of children. The children's stages of life then preoccupy the family through adolescence until they leave the family, which is sometimes accompanied by parents having to care for their parents. The later years of parents include watching their children enter adulthood, relationships, and have their own families.

With each life cycle transition, key relational changes must happen. For the single adult with a disability, the goal the adult and his or her parents have may not be physical and emotional separation. The goal must be adjusted according to the demands of the disability. Although typical single adult changes are realized through developing intimate relationships with peers and significant others, establishing a career or work life, as well as seeing oneself as distinct (but not necessarily separate) from one's family, the adult with a significant delay and his or her family must modify their life cycle goals. The parents are not necessarily back to their pre-child relationship, and school has ended for their adult child. They must face what comes next.

When two adults commit to each other, the joining of families occurs. Marriage is often the celebration of this commitment, but some heterosexual and most gay and lesbian couples commit in ways that indicate a committed relationship without marriage. The primary relationship goal at this stage is commitment to a new life together, which necessitates the rearrangement of relationships with extended family and peers. With the first new child, a couple creates a new generation of family members. The couple must adjust to this new person, learn how to be a parent, and extend family relationships to include parenting and grandparenting roles (as well as aunts, uncles, siblings, and cousins). When a couple has a child with serious health issues, disabilities, or both, this process takes on the strain of extra demands and services for the child, grieving, and often anger regarding the loss of freedom and the dream of a typical family. They may also experience sadness, grief, fear, and hopelessness for their child who must face threats to his or her health and/or development.

As children grow, the family faces new challenges. Expectations regarding development must be adjusted to the child's actual abilities, and this must be done publicly when the child goes to school. The family may grieve and hurt as they allow outsiders to enter their family system to provide services and watch their child with special needs face debilitating delays and health problems.

The typical process of an adolescent becoming more independent must be tempered by his or her ability to separate. An increase in family boundaries must gradually occur for adolescents to gain more independence and prepare for adulthood. The emotions that accompany that transition may be very typical; however, frustration on the part of the child with disabilities and his or her parents may add to the strain of this stage because their feelings are accompanied by the actual likelihood of achieving developmental milestones.

The parents' ability to focus or refocus on career and midlife issues and address the needs of their own parents may be impaired. As the parents age, fears regarding the well-being of their child with disabilities may grow.

Other events usually happen during the life cycle that offset these transitions as well. The loss of income in two-person households that occurs when one person must become a full-time caregiver may cause changes in living arrangements and will most certainly affect the relationships of family members. Single parenting due to divorce or the death of one parent has an impact on the life cycle. Remarriage requires flexibility in family relations with new members and renegotiated roles. The raising of children by grandparents, aunts, uncles, or foster parents due to parental inability creates both opportunities for strengths and challenges. Childhood illness and death place intense stress on family systems at any point during the life cycle.

Family Systems

Although the makeup of families is significantly varied, systems tend to be predictable. It is helpful to consider family systems with the Circumplex Model (Olson, 2000). This model focuses on three dimensions of family life: cohesion, flexibility, and communication. More than 250 studies using the Family Adaptability and Cohesion Evaluation Scales (FACES) as the measure have shown this model to be viable in guiding work with families (Olson, 2000).

Looking more closely at this model, cohesion measures the togetherness in families. It is defined as "the emotional bonding that family members have toward one another" (Olson, 2000, p. 145). This dimension considers how families balance separateness and togetherness. Cohesion covers a continuum of four levels: disengaged, separated, connected, and enmeshed. Families that exist in the extremes of cohesion—disengaged or enmeshed—tend to have more difficulty with individual and relationship development. One of the more important aspects of cohesion is boundaries. Boundaries tell us how open or closed families are to nonfamily members.

Some families have very thick boundaries that allow only a few people into their system. Nonfamily members who are allowed in have been deemed worthy of that right. Other families have boundaries that are open, which allow easy access to anyone who wants entrance. In these two extremes, we see how families regulate the entries into and exits from their systems. When we encounter rigid boundaries, we must ask permission to enter and tread very carefully. Outsiders earn the right to enter closed systems by showing family members openness and empathy as professional services are offered. Once we are offered complete access, the family is demonstrating their trust, and our entrances and exits may be less regulated.

Excessively loose boundaries may indicate a more disengaged cohesion style. Professionals who encounter families operating from this perspective do not experience difficulty entering the system. Instead, they may feel inappropriately exposed to the system and suspect a lack of caring or investment from family members. To work within this kind of system, professionals need to assert appropriate boundaries, both to protect the relationship with the family and to model appropriate cohesion. The professional can also look for moments of family members demonstrating appropriate togetherness and emphasize these moments within the intervention plan with concrete examples.

Flexibility is the second circumplex model characteristic that defines the capability within the family to change its leadership, roles, and system rules as needed (Olson, 2000). This area focuses on how families balance stability with change. The four levels range from rigid to structured to flexible to chaotic. As with cohesion, the

extremes of flexibility are less functional for family and individual development.

Roles and leadership reflect the flexibility in families. Rigidly flexible families will show less pliable roles and autocratic leadership. Families like this find new demands and required change very difficult because they are unable to shift individual roles easily to meet new needs. The process of change happens autocratically. Best practice in this kind of system involves connecting with the identified leader of the family. Once this connection is established, the system may demonstrate more acceptance of change through intervention plans. Validating the feelings of individual members about the situation can be helpful to a certain extent, followed with praising every effort made by the family to adjust to the new demands in their system and suggesting small ways that the family can adjust.

In chaotically flexible families, roles are typically unclear, shift to different family members, and leadership happens erratically. In chaotically flexible families, the process of engaging members in tasks may prove difficult. To work within this system, keeping suggestions small and concrete can help families achieve success. Also, problem solving with the family about how and when they will implement their part of the treatment plan is helpful.

Communication is the third and facilitating dimension of the circumplex model (Olson, 2000). Communication is the way in which movement occurs in terms of cohesion and flexibility. These skills include listening, speaking, self-disclosure, clarity, tracking, and the expression of respect and regard (Olson, 2000). Balanced systems tend to demonstrate good communication styles, whereas unbalanced systems tend to demonstrate poor communication styles. The most powerful way professionals can affect communication in the systems they encounter is by modeling good communication styles. By empathically listening, clearly communicating, and demonstrating respect and positive regard, professionals communicate positively to families and demonstrate the power of relationships. When encountering communication styles that are disrespectful or strained, professionals can best support the family by slowing down the communication process, which helps individuals be better heard and understood; writing down salient points for the family to reconsider again later; and encouraging and supporting the times that family members show healthy communications. It is not helpful to judge or criticize family members regarding their styles of communication. These approaches most likely result in a family emotionally distancing themselves from professionals and disregarding professional suggestions.

Embedded within the circumplex model is the assumption that families can and will change to adapt to developmental needs and situational stress (Olson, 2000). This is a very important point for professionals to keep in mind when a family first encounters new needs that cause stress. Within the ebb and flow of life, the family system is going to be in a different place regarding these three areas of functioning (i.e., cohesion, flexibility, and communication) at different times, and at different stages they may be more open to change than at others. Most importantly, professionals support families and create strong, healthy, collaborative relationships by meeting them where they are emotionally regarding their children. This perspective requires setting aside professional agendas for a time (this, of course, excludes emergent health care) in order to consider with the family their perceptions, concerns, and needs. Furthermore, professionals help them meet their needs and allow them to experience the grief, anger, sadness, hopelessness, bargaining, denial, and worry that is ever present with having a child with special needs. In addition, we, as professionals, can continue our support of families by modeling good communication, healthy boundaries, respectful caring, and validating appropriate changes in family roles and problem solving. Intervention planning through this model also helps families achieve more balanced cohesion and flexibility. These dimensions can be added into intervention plans with the addition of a counselor and/or marriage and family therapist or social worker to the intervention team. Treatment planning that incorporates this aspect into family life can help families adjust to new needs required by their children with disabilities.

Stressors and Resiliency

Much of this chapter has emphasized the need for professionals to see the uniqueness of each family and to help families identify their strengths and resiliencies. Resiliency within family systems may be defined in terms of the ways in which families continue to function after facing crises and how they then recover from such crises and respective demands (McCubbin & McCubbin, 1988). Historically, the origins of resiliency in families emerged from longitudinal research on resiliency in children. These studies have suggested the critical importance of the family system in fostering resilience in children. In particular, Cohler (1987) proposed that there is a complex interaction among the protective factors within the child, the family, and the social context. Accordingly, this construct offers many foci for identifying resiliency when working with families.

Although it has become clear that the family is the central protective factor for individuals with disabilities, it has been only since the 1990s that research has identified some of the qualities within the family that actually facilitate resiliency. Specifically, at least three types of factors have been cited as benefiting families in crisis: 1) family protective factors, which can affect their abilities to continue in the face of crisis; 2) family recovery factors, which, when combined with protective factors, can uniquely help family members in recovering from crisis; and 3) general family resiliency factors, which can help fam-

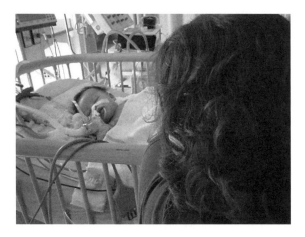

ilies endure and adapt to the new needs resulting from crisis (McCubbin, McCubbin, Thompson, Han, & Allen, 1997). As professionals who support the families we work with, we can look for these unique dimensions that help them get through stressors and the unique factors that surface as they recover from stressful situations. We can help them find something special that families experience and learn about themselves and that glues them together as they weather crises. Moreover, in discussions with families, professionals should attempt to identify these strengths and consider ways in which to enhance the family relationships and healthy behaviors.

Families with children who have special needs are more likely to face more stressors because of the health problems, disabilities, or other challenges. McCubbin (1995) found that for families with preschool and school-age children, religious programs, community support, and the sense of coherence of fitting into the larger community of which they felt a part were the most important protective resiliency factors. For families with adolescents, their status, income, mutual support from the family and spouse, family cohesiveness and bonding, and fitting into the larger community of which they feel a part were the most important protective factors.

When faced with crises, families initially tend to react with the protective factors already in existence in their systems. As time passes, they recover from the crises and events, which subsequently become part of the histories of their systems (McCubbin et al., 1997). Accordingly, critical family recovery factors include

- Family integration: how well adult members work to keep the family together and maintain an optimistic outlook

- Family support and esteem-building: how adult family members garner support from outside the family system (e.g., community, peers) and how able they are to develop their self-esteem and confidence in handling crises

- Family recreation and organization: the extent to which families value and participate in recreational activities that are known to be positively associated with resiliency of children and the family's positive emphasis on

structure (e.g., rules, organization, procedures)

- Optimism and mastery: the family's ability to maintain a sense of order and optimism, which have been correlated with greater improvements in the health of their children

General resiliency factors that we as professionals should look for, emphasize, and provide strategies for, if missing, are the following:

- Affirmation of communication when problem solving

- Accessible spiritual support

- Flexibility

- Truthfulness, both within the system and between the family and service providers

- Hope

- Family hardiness, shown by families that demonstrate an ability to work together

- Protection of family time and routine

- Social support

- Physical and emotional health and well-being of family members

The most powerful interventions we can offer to families of special needs children open the windows into their inherent strengths. By emphasizing these resiliencies, we reveal to families the fact that we see hope and strengths within their systems.

Child Development

Children are found within the preceding frameworks of family systems, life cycles, and roles. Children develop within the context of their most intimate relationships. Bowlby (1988) first identified and investigated these attachment bonds, which are most easily influenced when we are very young (i.e., from infancy to young childhood). Attachment is that quality that bonds and glues us to each other and creates dependency, reliability, and emotional closeness. Babies and children learn more at these times in their lives than at any other; this is in part due to the attachment relationships they have, including anxiety, security, and detachment.

The literature shows four noteworthy trains of thought regarding child development. These theories are individualistic in nature and focus primarily on the changes within the child. These developmental changes may be delayed or affected by environmental chaos, which is high noise, high traffic, high crowding, and little structure (Wachs & Corapci, 2003), or genetic issues (within the biology of the child).

In addition, consideration of environment and/or context have been salient pieces of the puzzle in understanding theoretical underpinnings of child development. Budwig (2003) suggested that historically we have viewed context as a situational factor. Alternatively, he indicated that "context" and "environment" should be seen as having interactive qualities and constitute "a negotiated process that involves very subtle interpretations . . . that draw in part on symbolic forms" (p. 104). In other words, we have historically seen context as something static upon which we layer objects and events. In fact, context and environment are dynamic and are integral to the interactions with objects and people.

Locke's Behavioral Theory (Meisels & Shonkoff, 2000) is perhaps the oldest framework of child development. It is based on the premise that children are centrally influenced by their environment. He viewed the child as a blank slate upon which people, places, and experiences write.

Rousseau posed a theory of maturationism. This suggests that children go through predetermined growth patterns that are essential for nurturing and play-focused development and growth (Shonkoff & Meisels, 2000).

Piaget is one of the most accepted theorists regarding child development. His constructivist theory suggests that environment writes on the child; biology plays a predetermined part in children's development; the act of play contributes greatly to development and maturation; and, ultimately, the construct of a child's intellect is derived from the interaction of the environment and play (Shonkoff & Meisels, 2000).

Vygotsky (1934) elaborated on Piaget's constructivist theory by emphasizing that children learn through the dialogues that they have with others, both of their own ages and older; that

knowledge, tasks, and skills provide transitions between stages; and, ultimately, that children actively construct their own knowledge. Therefore, this socially constructed knowledge is the vehicle for development.

Although there are some limitations to Piaget's constructivist theory stages, they do offer insight into what one looks for in assessing the development of young children. Inevitably, limitations apply across cultures and over time. Given these limitations when using the stages as guideposts in working with children, Piaget (1972) offered four stages to explain development from birth to adulthood. They include 1) the sensorimotor period from birth through 2 years, 2) the preoperational period from 2 years through 8 years, 3) the concrete operational stage from 8 years to 12 years, and 4) the formal operational stage from 12 years to adulthood. Transitions between stages occur over time, and, thus, the end points of stages are merely approximate. In the discussion that follows, we will be most concerned with the first three stages.

During the first 2 years of life, the cognitive development of babies and toddlers is formed by their physical senses and motor activities. For example, an infant's random movement, such as waving his or her hands in the air, eventually results in bringing hands to midline and contact and exploration with hands to the mouth. The baby subsequently repeats this random movement until this becomes a deliberate and repeated action with a cognitive milestone achieved. In the family system, those caring for the baby notice this accomplishment and respond with great enthusiasm and pleasure. The baby experiences this emotion from the caregiver, and the internal cognitive shift is supported by the emotional experience. Thus, the role of experience is significant in development and transitions (Lockman, 2003). This kind of process continues as the baby grows and develops until he or she begins to transition to the preoperational period.

Typically between the ages of 2 years and 3 years, children become increasingly able to use symbolic information, thus utilizing one object to represent another. This is a critical step toward abstract thinking. A 28-month-old toddler wants

Mommy every night before bed, but if Mommy is not home for bedtime, Daddy may offer the toddler Mommy's watch. The toddler readily accepts this object as a representation of Mommy and is content and able to sleep. This ability to substitute certain things for others grows and matures from 3 years to 8 years.

To fully consider how children develop, Gardner's (1983) work on "intelligences" can enhance our understanding and more completely guide us in identifying strengths in children cross culturally. Specifically, Gardner proposed that humans have multiple intelligences, consisting of the following:

- Linguistic intelligence: found in the kinds of words first uttered, how quickly and well the skill is mastered, and how children reflect the language of their caregivers and siblings

- Musical intelligence: reflected in the imitation of singing and rhythms until accepted songs of the culture take precedence

- Logico-mathematical intelligence: evident in learning by rote in the preoperational stage and followed by conceptual understanding in the concrete operational stage

- Spatial intelligence: reflected in the ways in which children orient themselves to their environment (e.g., the size and distance of things; imagining an object when it is not immediately visible)

- Bodily-kinesthetic intelligence: expressed through how children handle things with their bodies and control their movement

- Intrapersonal and interpersonal intelligences: understanding oneself and others based on the bond developed between infant and mother

By including these aspects of development, we can better appreciate child development as capacities rather than merely stage achievements. These dynamics are evident in studies of Japanese mothers, who are known to spend more time with infants; before their babies are 2 years of age, the mothers rarely leave them. This approach has a great impact on attachment and creates a potentially more intense and singularly focused relationship, which subsequently affects child development. In contrast, we know that chaotic attachment leads to delayed development; well-attached children are more likely to develop on time or early.

In a study by Lewis (1986), research indicated that Japanese mothers and teachers motivated toddlers very differently in developing interests and special talents very early in life (around 2–3 years). Specifically, mothers engaged in musical activities, but then denied their children access to the respective instruments. Gradually, their children were permitted to use the instruments occasionally with a few minutes of lessons. Later, the lessons were stopped before the children lost interest, which then encouraged the children to maintain interest in subsequent musical lessons. This approach is very different from child-driven interests and motivations seen in the United States. The eventual research findings of Lewis, based on these two approaches to child development across cultures, revealed that Japanese children seem to be further developed, at least temporarily. Indeed, these findings raise questions about how motivation is conceptualized cross-culturally and its ultimate impact on child development.

Similarly, another example of cultural influence is seen in the accepted mode of peer discipline in Japanese schools (Lewis, 1986). Teachers are less likely to step into conflict situations among children, which appears to enhance self- and peer reliance and turn resolution into everyone's problem.

It is clear that culture, ethnicity, and individual care practices greatly affect child development. According to New, "Significant differences exist in caregiving patterns and priorities throughout childhood, variations associated with cultural belief systems as well as environmental restraints" (1994, p. 70); cultural variation in the socialization of young children is evident in many studies on peer relationships (Corsaro & Eder, 1990). These variations suggest that western world theories of child development may not always be entirely applicable and a central need exists for flexibility in working with diverse populations of families and young children.

Conclusion

Professionals who work with children with disabilities inevitably encounter significantly complex issues and relationships. To prepare ourselves with the best possible strategies and tools, it is imperative that we understand child development, understand ourselves, and include family members as part of collaborative, family-centered, strength-based approaches. By including and valuing family members, professionals have additional allies when encountering challenging social issues, school systems, and agency rules.

As we interact with families, it is helpful to hold with some degree of tentativeness our knowledge about child development, family systems theories, life cycles and roles, and our specialized education. Such flexibility allows us to use what we know appropriately while refraining from imposing assumptions from our training onto the individuals and families with whom we work. As we relationally join with children and families, we can provide best care for them and ourselves by attending to our personal lens. Our lenses inevitably influence our care relationships with children and families, negatively or positively. Collaborative, family-centered care is most successful when it includes families, children, and diverse professionals who view everyone as experts with valuable contributions and who identify the strengths and resiliencies within the system.

When families are stressed, professionals need to accept the realities of where families are rather than try to move them into places that are more comfortable for the professionals. It is only by meeting the families where they are that professionals can build trust and respect in their relationships. Furthermore, professionals need to build on family priorities. This approach involves asking families and children (if possible) what is important to them, discussing what the professionals see and hope for, and only then building care plans that incorporate all. Discussing functional, concrete outcomes offers families specific objectives to look forward to and work toward.

Educating a family about their child's behavior and disabilities can have a significant impact on the family system with regard to how members respond to the child. Inviting the child and family to educate us about their habits, preferences, strengths, and struggles will help us better tailor our intervention plans and recommendations. Finally, sharing information clearly and in multiple ways (verbal and written) that are free of jargon communicates to the family our commitment to understanding the needs of their child. To conclude, authors Marshak and Prezant (2006) offer a comprehensive list of things that we should do when working with families.

- Listen to and respect parent input.

- Share expertise and information.

- Collaborate and communicate.

- Follow through consistently in our work.

In conclusion, the professional behaviors that parents have found to be most problematic include poor performance on the job, underestimation of children, and refusals to make accommodations. Quite simply, the inclusion of family in supportive services is the most central key to guiding children and those who love them on their life path. By including family, professionals demonstrate respect for the immediate world where children live and mobilize the very people most likely and able to continue the support needed to help children reach their growth potentials.

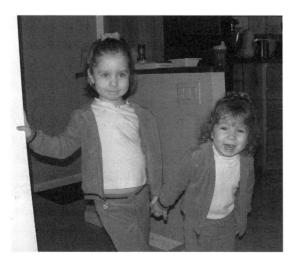

REFERENCES

Botkin, D.R., Weeks, M., & Morris, J.E. (2000). Changing marriage role expectations: 1961–1996. *Sex Roles, 42*(9–10), 933–942.

Bowen, M. (1978). *Family therapy in clinical practice.* New York: Jason Aronsen.

Bowlby, J. (1988). *A secure base: Parent–child attachment and healthy human development.* New York: Basic Books.

Budwig, N. (2003). Context and the dynamic construal of meaning in early childhood. In C. Raeff & J.B. Benson (Eds.), *Social and cognitive development in the context of individual, social, and cultural processes* (pp. 103–130). New York: Routledge.

Carrington, C. (1999). *No place like home: Relationships and family life among lesbians and gay men.* Chicago: The University of Chicago Press.

Carter, B., & McGoldrick, M. (2004). *The expanded family life cycle.* New York: Pearson.

Cohen, P.N., & Petrescu-Prahova, M. (2006). Gendered living arrangements among children with disabilities: Evidence from the 2000 census. *Journal of Marriage and Family, 68*, 630–638.

Cohler, B.J. (1987). Adversity, resilience, and the study of lives. In E.J. Anthony & B.J. Cohler (Eds.), *The invulnerable child* (pp. 363–408). New York: Guilford Press.

Corsaro, W.A., & Eder, D. (1990). Children's peer cultures. *Annual Review of Sociology, 16*, 197–220.

Eddy, L.L., & Walker, A.J. (1999). The impact of children with chronic health problems on marriage. *Journal of Family Nursing, 5*(1), 10–32.

Fraenkel, P. (2003). Contemporary two-parent families: Navigating work and family challenges. In F. Walsh (Ed.), *Normal family processes* (3rd ed., pp. 121–152). New York: Guilford Press.

Gardner, H. (1983). *Frames of mind: The theory of multiple intelligences.* New York: Basic Books.

Hanson, S.M.H., Heims, M.L., Julian, D.J., & Sussman, M.B. (1995). Single parent families: Present and future perspectives. In S.M.H. Hanson (Ed.), *Single parent-families: Diversity, myths and realities* (pp. 1–26). Binghamton, NY: Haworth Press.

Ho, K.M., & Keiley, M.K. (2003). Dealing with denial: A systems approach for family professionals working with parents of individuals with multiple disabilities. *The Family Journal, 13*(3), 239–247.

Hodapp, R.M., & Krasner, D.V. (1994). Families of children with disabilities: Findings from a national sample of 8th grade students. *Exceptionality, 5*(2), 71–81.

Lockman, J. (2003). Object manipulation in context. In C. Raeff & J.B. Benson (Eds.), *Social and cognitive development in the context of individual, social, and cultural processes* (pp. 149–167). New York: Routledge.

Lewis, C. (1986). Children's social development in Japan: Research directions. In H. Stevenson, H. Azuma, & K. Hakuta (Eds.), *Child development and education in Japan* (pp. 186–200). New York: W.H. Freeman.

Marshak, C.E., & Prezant, F.P. (2006). *Married with special needs children: A couple's guide to keeping connected.* Bethesda, MD: Woodbine House.

Mauldon, J. (1992). Children's risks of experiencing divorce and remarriage: Do disabled children destabilize marriages? *Population Studies, 46*, 349–362.

McCubbin, H.I. (1995). Resiliency in African American families: Military families in foreign environments. In H.I. McCubbin, E.A. Thompson, A.I. Thompson, & J. Futrell (Eds.), *Resiliency in ethnic minority families: African American families* (pp. 67–97). Thousand Oaks, CA: Sage Publications.

McCubbin, H.I., & McCubbin, M.A. (1988). Typologies of resilient families: Emerging roles of social class and ethnicity. *Family Relations, 37*, 247–254.

McCubbin, H.I., McCubbin, M.A., Thompson, A.I., Han, S., & Allen, C.T. (1997). *Families under stress: What makes them resilient?* Washington, DC: American Association of Family and Consumer Sciences Commemorative Lecture.

McDaniel, S.H., Hepworth, J., & Doherty, W. (1992). *Medical family therapy.* New York: Basic Books.

McFalls, Jr., J.A. (2003). *What's a household? What's a family?* Retrieved March 18, 2008, from http://www.prb.org/Articles/2003/WhatsaHousehold-WhatsaFamily.aspx

Meisels, S.J., & Shonkoff, J.P. (2000). Early childhood intervention: A continuing evolution. In J.P. Shonkoff & S.J. Meisels (Eds.), *Handbook of early childhood intervention* (2nd ed., pp. 3–31). New York: Cambridge University Press.

Nelson, L.G.L., Summers, J.A., & Turnbull, A.P. (2004). Boundaries in family–professional relationships. *Remedial and Special Education, 25*(3), 153–165.

New, R.S. (1994). Culture, child development & developmentally appropriate practices. In B. Mallory & R. New (Eds.), *Diversity and developmentally appropriate practices* (pp. 65–83). New York: Teachers College Press.

Olson, D.H. (2000). Circumplex model of family systems. In A. Carr (Ed.), *Empirical approaches to family assessment* [Special issue]. *Journal of Family Therapy, 22*(2), 144–167.

Perryman, H. (2005). Parental reaction to the disabled child. *Family Court Review, 43*(4), 596–606.

Piaget, J. (1972). *Psychology of intelligence.* Totowa, NJ: Littlefield, Adams & Co.

Raver, S.A. (2005). Using family-based practices for young children with special needs in preschool programs. *Childhood Education, 82*(1), 9–13.

Reichman, N.E., Corman, H., & Noonan, K. (2004). Effects of child's health on parents' relationship status. *Demography, 41*, 569–584.

Robinson, H., & Robinson, N.M. (1965). *The mentally retarded child.* New York: McGraw-Hill.

Roehling, P.V., & Moen, P. (2003). *Sloan Work and Family Research Network encyclopedia: Dual-earner couples.* Retrieved April 17, 2008, from http://wfnetwork.bc.edu/encyclopedia_template.php?id=229

Rosenbluth, S.C., Steil, J.M., & Whitcomb, J.H. (1998). Marital inequality: What does it mean? *Journal of Family Issues, 19*(3), 227–244.

Schmitt, E. (2001, May 15). For the first time, nuclear families drop below 25% of households. *The New York Times,* pp. A1, A41.

Turnbull, A.P., & Summers, J.A. (1985). *From parent involvement to family support: Evaluation to revolution.* Paper presented at the Down Syndrome State of the Art Conference, Boston.

U.S. Census Bureau. (2006). *2006 American Community Survey data profile highlights.* Retrieved April 21, 2008, from http://factfinder.census.gov/servlet/ACSSAFFFacts?_submenuld=factsheet_0&_sse=on

Vygotsky, L.S. (1934). *Thought and language.* Cambridge, MA: The MIT Press.

Wachs, T.D., & Corapci, F. (2003). Environmental chaos, development and parenting across cultures. In C. Raeff & J. Benson (Eds.), *Social and cognitive development in the context of individual, social and cultural processes* (pp. 54–83). New York: Routledge.

Walsh, F. (2003). *Normal family processes: Growing diversity and complexity.* New York: Guilford Press.

Williams, M. (2001). *Raising a child with a disability.* Address at the 2001 BYU Families Under Fire Conference, Provo, UT.

SECTION **II**

Early Problems
and Developmental Courses

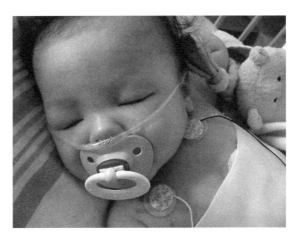

CHAPTER 5

Neonatal Neurology

Marilyn A. Fisher

At the conclusion of this chapter, the reader will

* *Understand the typical development of the neurological system*

* *Understand atypical development of the neurological system and name a few etiologies for atypical neurological development*

* *Be familiar with the management of a variety of types of dysfunction of the neonatal neurological system*

This chapter provides information regarding the typical development of the brain and central nervous system, in addition to information about the neurological examination of the newborn. It also describes aspects of atypical brain development and abnormalities in brain and nervous system function due to particular insults and disease processes.

Prenatal Brain Development

Weeks 3–8 of gestation are referred to as the embryonic period. During the embryonic period, the human embryo forms the brain and other organs (organogenesis). During this time, the embryo transforms sequentially from a flat, three-layer disk to a curved cylinder and then to an embryo with a head, brain, eyes, ears, nose, heart, and limbs.

The brain develops its external form during the embryonic period. Formation of the structures of the brain and nervous system, an event known as neurulation, starts in the third week. The neural plate, neural folds, neural crest, and neural tube form during the embryonic period. Figure 5.1 shows how the neural tube, which ultimately gives rise to the brain and spinal cord, is

created by the folding of the embryonic neural plate into the neural groove; the neural groove then closes to form the neural tube (on day 25 at the cranial end and on day 27 at the posterior end) (Moore, 1988).

Microscopically, the cells in the forebrain differentiate, collect, and migrate, which gives rise to the cells of the brain, spinal cord, and motor and sensory nerves, including sensory cells of the eyes, ears, and nose. Grossly, the transformation process is complex as the forebrain (front part of the neural tube) folds down toward the forming heart, creating a more rounded head, which begins to show human characteristics. During this crucial embryonic period, if the embryo is exposed to conditions or agents that cause atypical development (teratogens), major congenital malformations may result. Teratogens that may adversely affect the developing brain include toxins, such as certain drugs, alcohol, and radiation; infections with certain viruses; and nutritional problems, including deficiency of folic acid. Brain malformations may also be caused by genetic (chromosomal) abnormalities. In addition, they may be caused by multifactorial inheritance or a genetic predisposition to develop a certain malformation, which, when combined with often undetermined other factors (e.g., folic acid defi-

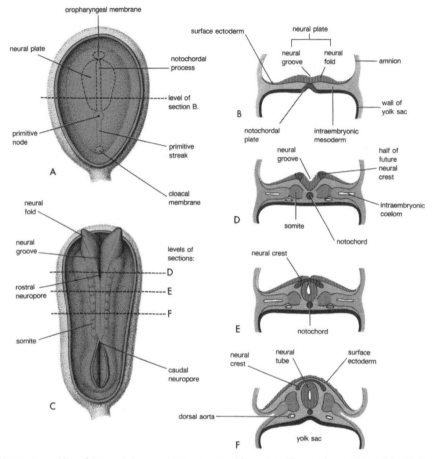

Figure 5.1.   Folding of the neural plate into the neural tube and formation of the neural crest. A) Dorsal (back) view of a flat, three-layer 18-day embryo. B) Transverse section of an 18-day embryo showing the early invagination of the neural plate portion of the surface ectoderm into the neural groove. C) Dorsal view of a 22-day embryo. The neural tube has fused in the middle of the embryo at the level of the somites, but remains open at either end. D) Transverse section of a 22-day embryo at the level of plane D (as indicated by the dotted line labeled D on the diagram C). The neural groove has deepened. Some of the neuroectodermal neural plate cells are destined to become the neural tube; some are destined to become neural crest cells. E and F) Transverse section of a 22-day embryo at the level of planes E and F respectively (as indicated by the dotted lines labeled E and F on diagram C). The neural plate cells have become distinct and separate from the surface ectoderm. Some neural plate cells have migrated into the mesoderm to form the neural tube—the primordium of the central nervous system. Some neural plate cells have migrated into the mesoderm to form the neural crest, which will ultimately form spinal ganglia, autonomic ganglia, cranial nerve ganglia, peripheral nerve sheaths, meninges covering the central nervous system, bones, cartilage, and ligaments of the orofacial region. (This figure appeared in Moore, K.L., Persaud, T.V.N., & Shiota, K. [1994]. *Color atlas of clinical embryology* [p. 17]. Philadelphia: W.B. Saunders; Copyright © 2008 Elsevier; reprinted by permission.)

ciency) above a certain threshold, may cause the malformation.

Weeks 9–38 of gestation are referred to as the fetal period. During the fetal period, there is growth of organs that have already formed. Some organs (e.g., the heart and limbs) already have fairly complete development by the end of the embryonic period. All that remains to be done during the fetal period is further growth

and differentiation. Most organs are generally not susceptible to malformations after the embryonic period, even if they are exposed to teratogens during the fetal period, because they have already formed. Even though it has already attained its gross form during the embryonic period, however, the brain is still undergoing important microscopic developmental changes during the fetal period (which will continue for several years after birth as well). Therefore, even during the fetal and neonatal period, the brain remains vulnerable to damage.

During the fetal period, the first important change occurring within the brain is neuronal proliferation (Volpe, 2000), which increases the number of brain cells. By 20–24 weeks of gestation, the human cerebral cortex has its full number of neurons. Brain blood vessel growth is especially active during the time of neuronal proliferation. A growing blood vessel network is required to provide the necessary blood flow to a brain of increasing mass. One type of neuronal proliferation involves the brain cells replicating their DNA, dividing, and spreading out within the brain. This occurs from 2 to 4 months of gestation. The other type of neuronal proliferation occurs from 5 months of gestation to beyond a year after birth. This second type involves multiplication of glial cells. The glial cell proliferation is responsible for the next important microscopic event in fetal brain development, which is migration. Millions of nerve cells migrate from locations in and around the brain's ventricles (collections of cerebral spinal fluid) to sites within the central nervous system. Migration occurs into a variety of brain locations, including the cerebral cortex (the area of the brain responsible for higher thought processes). Peak neural migration activity occurs from 3 to 5 months of gestation. Organization of brain cells occurs between 5 months of gestation and many years after birth. During this lengthy process, brain cells are established, differentiated, and oriented with respect to each other; connections (synapses) are established between cells; and elimination of unnecessary synapses and nerve tissue occurs.

The final phase of the important fetal brain developmental changes is myelination. Myelin is a material composed of alternating fats and proteins. It forms a membrane around the nerve cells that is necessary for the cells to function correctly. During the late fetal period and into the first 8 postnatal months, in response to various growth factors and hormones, myelin is laid down on spinal cord and other nerves. Myelination begins in the peripheral nerves far away from the brain, and starts in motor nerves (which send messages

controlling movement) before sensory nerves. Then myelination occurs in the central sensory area, followed by the sensory motor areas. At approximately 20 weeks of gestation, nerve fibers develop a whitish appearance due to the deposition of myelin on them. Nerve fibers become functional at about the same time that they become myelinated. Therefore, it is believed that a fetus does not perceive pain or sensation until approximately 20 weeks of gestation because its sensory fibers leading to the brain are not myelinated until that time. Finally, myelination begins within the brain in areas associated with higher neurological function. This myelination within the brain starts late in fetal life and progresses even into adult life, with the most rapid myelination occurring within the first 8 months after birth. Exposure to teratogens during the fetal or neonatal period is less likely to cause gross brain malformation than exposure to teratogens during the embryonic period. However, the developing brain is exceedingly sensitive to damage during the time of all of these developmental changes, even after delivery of the infant.

Postnatal Brain Development

After birth, the brain maturation that began during fetal life continues. There is further organization, myelination, and growth of the brain. Fatty acids are important for the proper myelination and development of the brain, both before and after birth. The quantity and types of fatty acids found in the mother's diet are reflected in the quantity and proportions of these substances found in the mother's breast milk (Xiang et al., 2005). The long chain polyunsaturated fatty acid, docosahexaenoic acid (DHA), ingested in foods by the mother during gestation and by the infant after birth, is deposited in developing brain tissue and in the developing retina. DHA is deposited in increasing quantities in the brain from approximately 20 weeks of gestation until at least 24 months after a full-term delivery. DHA has been found by some researchers to be associated with improved infant neurodevelopment and vision (Jensen et al., 2005) and may be associated with improved memory and learning in young children (Heinemann & Bauer, 2006). This development occurs because DHA is concentrated in the phospholipid bilayer within the biologically active brain and retinal neural membrane, making it important in neuronal and eye function. DHA stores in the brain also help to protect the brain from damage when it experiences low levels of oxygen and poor blood flow (Yavin, 2006).

The presence of another long chain polyunsaturated fatty acid, arachidonic acid (ARA), helps to protect DHA from conversion to prostaglandins (other fatty acids that dilate blood vessels, but may lead to low blood pressure) and to leukotrienes (which may cause tissue inflammation) after poor oxygen or blood flow to the brain. An embryonic or fetal brain deprived of the fatty acid linolenic acid during maternal dietary manipulation will also develop low levels of DHA (Green, Kamensky, & Yavin, 1997). It will also develop a decreased number of brain cells and a decreased thickness of the cerebral cortex of the brain (the center of higher brain function) (Coti Bertrand, O'Kusky, & Innis, 2006), which potentially increases the risk of poor neurodevelopmental outcome.

Adequate levels of DHA help keep the body's serotonin levels adequate as well. Sufficient serotonin levels may help prevent attention-deficit/hyperactivity disorder (ADHD), depression, and Alzheimer's disease. Rats genetically predisposed to Alzheimer's disease have improved memory when given a high DHA diet compared with those high-risk rats with a low DHA diet (Hashimoto, Hossain, Agdul, & Shido, 2005). The low levels of fetal DHA caused by restriction of fatty acids in the maternal diet can lead to a drop in brain phosphatidylserine. This drop in phosphatidylserine can then decrease levels of neurotransmitters (Tam & Innis, 2006) that help the brain and nerve cells communicate with each other. Phosphatidylserine deficiency increases the rate of brain cell death. DHA and arachidonic acid (ARA) are both important within the nervous system. Neither can be synthesized by mammals. Instead, in order to have proper brain development, DHA and arachidonic acid, or their precursors, must be consumed in the diet. Due to this recent positive information about DHA and ARA, since 2002, all infant formula companies in the United States have been adding DHA and ARA to their formulas to make them more similar to breast milk. Preterm infant formulas also have DHA and ARA added to them. Preterm infants fed formula supplemented with ARA from fungal oils and DHA from algal (algae) oils grew better than preterm infants fed a standard formula unsupplemented with DHA or ARA and better than preterm infants fed a formula supplemented with ARA from fungal oils and DHA from fish oils (Clandinin et al., 2005). However, preterm infants fed formula supplemented with ARA from fungal oils and DHA from either fish or algal oils had better neurodevelopmental outcomes than those fed the unsupplemented formula.

DHA is also present in flaxseed, flaxseed oil, walnuts, walnut oil, canola oil, oily fish (e.g., salmon), and foods to which DHA has been added. Ocean-raised salmon are able to synthesize DHA because they have a special gene that allows them to do so. Scientists are working to introduce this gene into other types of fish to enhance their DHA levels, which will give humans other fish options to increase dietary DHA intake (Alimuddin, Yoshizaki, Kiron, Satoh, & Taekuchi, 2005). Most fish, however, contain DHA due to the fact that they consume microalgae that produce DHA.

Nervous System Teratogens

Exposure to various conditions can affect the developing nervous system. These are described in the following subsections.

Toxic Substances

A variety of drugs has been associated with teratogenic effects and/or malformations on the developing brain. These include alcohol, a variety of anticonvulsant drugs, isotretinoin, and cocaine. The effect that each of these teratogens has on the developing fetus is dependent on the quantity of the drug taken, pattern of usage, and timing of exposure during gestation.

Alcohol Both prenatal and postnatal exposure to alcohol decrease levels of brain DHA as well as phosphatidylserine. This condition is associated with abnormal, premature death of brain cells. It is this decrease in these substances that is thought to cause the effects of fetal alcohol syndrome (FAS). With FAS, abnormalities in every stage of brain development may be seen. FAS is associated with both pre- and postnatal global growth deficiency. The head and brain are too small (microcephaly); intellectual disabilities usually occur; and hyperactivity and behavioral disturbances may also be present. These do not improve significantly, even though the home environment may be optimized. Those affected may have distinctive facial features, especially a thin, curvy upper lip; a long philtrum in the midline between the nose and the upper lip; and small eyes (see Figure 5.2). They may also have heart malformations, especially ventriculoseptal defect.

Anticonvulsant Medications Several anticonvulsant drugs that pregnant woman may take to control seizures have been implicated in fetal brain malformations. Drugs in the hydantoin family (phenytoin), as well as phenobarbital, primidone, and carbamazepine have been associated with multiple fetal malformations, including atypical facial appearance, nail defects, microcephaly, and intellectual disabilities (Figure 5.3).

Trimethadione and paramethadione have been associated with microcephaly; intellectual disabilities; atypical facial appearance; and malformations of the heart, genitourinary structures, trachea, and esophagus. Valproic acid has been associated with spina bifida, minor abnormalities of the face, bony defects of the arms and legs, and heart defects. When a woman who uses anticonvulsant medications is contemplating becoming pregnant, she and her physicians need to select her medications carefully, ideally before conception.

Isotretinoin Isotretinoin (a vitamin A analogue) is used as a treatment for severe acne. At least one third of users of isotretinoin are females 13–19 years of age who might not recognize the

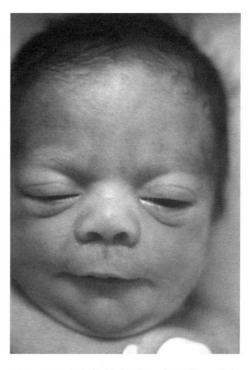

Figure 5.3. Facies in fetal hydantoin syndrome. (From Clark, D.A. [2000]. *Atlas of neonatology* [p. 27]. Philadelphia: W.B. Saunders; reprinted by permission.)

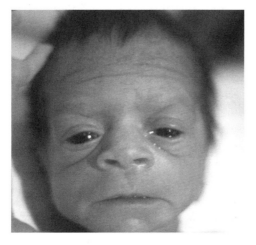

Figure 5.2. Fetal alcohol syndrome facies in premature neonate. Long, flat philtrum; thin upper lip; short palpebral fissures. (From Clark, D.A., private collection; reprinted by permission.)

early stages of pregnancy when the drug is exerting its major teratogenic effects. Whether used by mouth or applied directly to affected skin, it causes fetuses to have malformed or absent ears, severe heart malformations, small brains, hydrocephalus, and intellectual disabilities. These fetuses have a 25% chance of being miscarried. Because approximately 36% of fetuses exposed to isotretinoin through maternal usage during the 1st trimester have serious malformations or death, the prescribing physician and the drug manufacturer generally require that the woman about to receive the drug sign a contract that states that she will not become pregnant while she is being treated with the drug.

Cocaine   Cocaine has also been described as a teratogen on the developing fetal brain. It has been blamed for microcephaly, brain and eye malformations relating to neuronal migration problems, and abnormal neuronal proliferation and differentiation. In addition, the development of neuronal circuitry may be disordered. Infants exposed to cocaine in utero have a higher chance of having tremors, a high-pitched cry, irritability, and so forth. Some infants exposed to cocaine seem to have normal neurodevelopment; others have neurobehavioral and motor (movement) abnormalities.

Although cocaine is responsible for some brain malformations due to atypical initial development of the brain under cocaine's influence, some brain problems related to cocaine exposure occur because of cocaine-mediated destruction of previously normally formed brain tissue. Cocaine is a potent constrictor of blood vessels. When blood vessels in the fetus's brain (and other organs) constrict, there is poor blood flow to the tissue downstream, which causes sick or dying cells. In addition, it has been postulated that cocaine-mediated poor blood flow from the placenta to the fetus causes extremely low levels of oxygen in the fetus, impairing the fetus's ability to control blood flow to its brain. Subsequent sudden increases in blood pressure due to stress may set up the fetus for bleeding within the brain. This bleeding within brain tissue may destroy brain cells.

Metabolic Defects

Mothers with poorly controlled phenylketonuria (PKU) have extremely high blood levels of phenylalanine, a naturally occurring chemical found in only small quantities in people without this metabolic defect. When an embryo or fetus is exposed to high levels of phenylalanine because of elevated maternal levels, that embryo or fetus is at high risk for being miscarried, or, if he or she survives, for developing microcephaly, intellectual disabilities, intrauterine growth restriction, and congenital heart defects. Therefore, an embryo or fetus may be severely affected by the mother's high phenylalanine levels without actually having the metabolic defect.

Environmental Effects

Several different environmental exposures may have adverse effects on the developing embryonic or fetal brain. Maternal hyperthermia (high body temperature), due to either fever or hot tub use during the first trimester, is associated with neural tube defects, small brain, and small eyes. Maternal exposure to mercury, a heavy metal, is associated with intellectual disabilities, small brain, vision problems, and cerebral palsy. Maternal exposure to another heavy metal, lead, is also associated with intellectual disabilities and ADHD. Ionizing radiation in doses exceeding 10 rads (i.e., radiation absorbed dose), especially during the first trimester, is associated with small brain and intellectual disabilities. Higher dose radiation, more than 100 rads, has been associated with the development of multiple malformations of the fetus, including hydrocephalus and eye abnormalities. An average routine x-ray exposes the patient to approximately 0.02 rads; exposure to 500 average x-rays would give a cumulative dose of 10 rads. It is unlikely that a pregnant woman in the first trimester will be exposed to 500 x-rays.

Infections

Exposure to certain viruses during gestation may cause brain malformations and dysfunction. Several of these viruses and their effects are described here.

Cytomegalovirus   Fetal infection with cytomegalovirus (CMV), a member of the herpes virus family, usually occurs during a first-time maternal infection when the mother initially has no antibodies against the virus to help her and her fetus combat the infection. The effect of congenital CMV infection on the fetal brain includes small brain, blindness, optic atrophy (lack of development of the nerve that sends visual messages to the brain), other eye problems, seizures, and progressive hearing loss.

Varicella   Congenital varicella (chickenpox), another member of the herpes virus family, may be transmitted to the fetus during a first-time maternal chickenpox infection. If infected during the first 20 weeks of gestation, a fetus can be born with a variety of brain, eye, and other malformations, including intellectual disabilities.

Herpes Simplex Virus   Herpes simplex virus, if acquired across the placenta during fetal life, may also cause the fetus to be growth restricted, have a small brain that may have calcifications within it, have necrosis and absorption of the cerebral cortex (hydranencephaly), and have eye disease. As with cytomegalovirus and varicella, transplacental herpes infection of the fetus usually occurs as a result of a first-time maternal infection, but on rare occasions can follow a recurrent maternal infection.

Rubella   When a mother contracts rubella (known as 3-day measles) during the first 8 weeks of gestation, there is a 90% chance that the disease will be transmitted to her vulnerable fetus. Rubella may cause the fetus to have a small brain, intellectual disabilities, eye problems, hearing loss, and congenital cardiac defects, as well as many other defects.

Toxoplasmosis   Congenital infection with *Toxoplasma gondii* (toxoplasmosis), a protozoa parasite, may lead to intellectual disabilities, vision impairment, small brain, seizures, and deafness due to the fact that the parasite disrupts forming or already formed neurological tissue. Cats are a frequent source of toxoplasmosis infection. They get the infection by consuming infected small rodents or uncooked meats and then shedding the parasite in their feces. Therefore, pregnant women can avoid infection by not changing cat litter pans and refraining from gardening and by washing their hands carefully after such activities if they cannot be avoided.

Neurological Examination

Specific features are included in the neurological examinations of fetuses and newborns. These processes are explained next.

Evaluation of the Fetus

Even during fetal life, a baby exhibits various types of movements (e.g., startle reflex, postures, sucking, swallowing, yawning, stretching, heart rate reactivity, eye movements, chest wall movements similar to breathing) that indicate distinct states of consciousness. A fetus's neurological intactness, as well as its general health, may be suggested by observation of these behaviors. In addition, it is generally believed that a fetus that has normal activity will have a longer umbilical cord than a fetus that does not have normal activity. A fetus with normal activity will also have a higher chance of becoming positioned with its head down than one with activity that is below normal.

Physicians may employ testing to determine the health of a fetus. For instance, the nonstress test observes for normal acceleration of the fetal heart rate in response to spontaneous fetal movement or a vibratory or audiological stimulus (i.e., the fetal heart rate should rise when the baby is stimulated or excited). Conversely, a contraction stress test observes to ensure that there is no drop in the fetal heart rate in response to a uterine contraction, which could indicate poor blood flow to the fetus from the placenta. A normal contraction stress test would show a stable, reactive fetal heart rate. The biophysical profile (see Table 5.1) is an observation of several fetal measures to determine the well-being of the fetus. Most of these measures are carried out by observation of the fetal neurological state. Normal fetal heart rate reactivity to stimuli; normal gross body move-

Table 5.1. Biophysical profile used to determine the well-being of the fetus.

Biophysical variable	Normal (Score = 2)	Abnormal (Score = 0)
Fetal breathing movements	One or more episode(s) ≥ 20 seconds within 30 minutes	Absent, or no episode of ≥ 20 seconds within 30 minutes
Gross body movements	Two or more discrete body or limb movements within 30 minutes	Fewer than two episodes of body or limb movements within 30 minutes
Fetal tone	One or more episode(s) of active extension with return to flexion of fetal limb(s) or trunk	Slow extension with return to partial flexion, movement of limb while in full extension, partially open hand, or absent fetal movement
Fetal heart rate	Two or more episodes of acceleration of ≥ 15 bpm of > 15 seconds associated with fetal movement within 20 minutes	Fewer than two episodes of acceleration or acceleration of FHR or acceleration of < 15 bpm within 20 minutes
Amniotic fluid volume	One or more pocket(s) of amniotic fluid measuring ≥ 2 cm in vertical axis	No pocket of amniotic fluid, or largest pocket measuring < 2 cm in vertical axis

Source: Manning, Morrison, Harman, Lange, & Menticoglou (1987).

Key: FHR = fetal heart rate; bpm = beats per minute; cm = centimeter.

ments and fetal tone (assessed by observing flexing and extending of the limbs rather than limp body tone); normal breathing-like chest wall movements; and normal volume of the amniotic fluid are all important measures in determining fetal health and neurological intactness. Normal amniotic fluid volume indicates that the fetus has been receiving enough blood flow from the uterus and placenta to have adequate blood pressure and oxygenation with subsequent good kidney function. Fetal urine makes up the majority of amniotic fluid volume. Therefore, a fetus with chronically good utero-placental blood flow and a normally formed urinary tract would be expected to have adequate amounts of amniotic fluid. Too little amniotic fluid (oligohydramnios) could result from an absence of the fetal kidneys, an abnormal or obstructed urinary tract, or prolonged poor utero-placental blood flow to the fetus. Long-standing oligohydramnios may be associated with fetal lungs that are too small (pulmonary hypoplasia) due to chronic com-

pression of the fetal chest by the maternal tissues without the normal buffer of amniotic fluid as the fetus is trying to grow.

Normal amniotic fluid volume also indicates that the fetus has been swallowing amniotic fluid. The swallowing of amniotic fluid requires a brain with enough capacity to cause the fetus to swallow. The liquid of swallowed amniotic fluid is absorbed by the fetal gastrointestinal tract, passes via the blood back to the placenta and to the mother where it is eliminated from her body. Swallowing of amniotic fluid also requires a normal, not obstructed, upper gastrointestinal tract. In the absence of adequate fetal swallowing, excess amniotic fluid accumulates (polyhydramnios), causing excess uterine stretching and increasing the risk for preterm labor. Normal parameters for these assessments vary with gestational age.

Evaluation of the Newborn

The neurological exam of the newborn baby looks at several different measures.

General Evaluation   A general evaluation of the baby includes an estimation of gestational age. Because babies become capable of performing different activities at different stages of development, it is important to know their gestational age to determine what activities they can be reasonably expected to perform. For instance, an average 2-month-old baby should be able to bring his or her hands together in mid-line. However, if that baby were born 2 months prematurely, one would not expect him or her to bring hands together in mid-line until 4 months after birth (to allow for a correction for prematurity).

General evaluation of the newborn also includes an assessment of head size and shape. A head that is excessively large or small may indicate problems with the underlying brain. Assessment for any external facial or head malformations or asymmetry may reveal risk factors for underlying brain problems as well. Overall, measurement of a neonate's level of alertness is probably the most sensitive assessment of all of his or her neurological functions because it depends on the function of several different levels of the nervous system.

Mental Status   Neurological evaluation of the newborn includes an assessment of the neonate's level of alertness. The observer will note whether the baby is excessively lethargic and unresponsive to external stimuli or whether he or she is irritable and unable to be soothed. Typically, babies pass between periods of deep sleep to quiet wakefulness to awake and/or crying. Full-term babies have a greater frequency, duration, and quality of wakefulness than premature babies.

Cranial Nerves   Neurological evaluation of the newborn includes assessment of cranial nerve function. Assessment of the second cranial nerve controlling vision reveals that, by 26 weeks of gestation, the infant blinks in response to bright light, even if the eyelids are still fused. By 32 weeks, the infant squeezes his or her eyelids shut in the presence of bright light. Beginning at 32 weeks, infants begin to demonstrate visual fixation and tracking in which they will watch a red ball as it is moved around in front of them. By 34 weeks, 90% of infants will consistently demonstrate visual fixation and tracking skills.

The pupillary constrictive reflex response to light, mediated by the third cranial nerve, begins to appear at 30 weeks of gestation and is consistently present at 32–35 weeks of gestation. Extraocular movements (controlled by cranial nerves 3, 4, and 6) are sometimes assessed via spinning the baby or pouring cold water into one ear and watching for the presence or absence of nystagmus (eye flickering) and eye deviation in an effort to determine the extent of any neurological abnormality. The fifth cranial nerve allows a baby to have sensation of the face and provides innervation to the swallowing and chewing muscles. The seventh cranial nerve also provides facial movement. Sucking and swallowing muscles receive their innervation by a combination of cranial nerves 5, 7, 9, 10, and 12. The twelfth nerve controls tongue movement. Hearing is controlled through the eighth cranial nerve. Neck movement, using the sternocleidomastoid muscles, occurs through the eleventh cranial nerve. The sensation of smell occurs via the first cranial nerve. The sensation of taste is mediated through the seventh and ninth cranial nerves.

Obviously, assessment of some of the cranial nerve functions (e.g., assessment of the sensations of taste and smell) is difficult to perform in a neonate. Nevertheless, during feeding, an infant may use these nerves to locate and identify his mother. Functions of other cranial nerves can be more readily evaluated in the neonate.

Assessment of specific cranial nerve function is helpful in determining the location of a particular lesion or area of damage. The most common cranial nerve injury seen in the neonate is that associated with compression of the underlying facial nerve, cranial nerve 7, causing weakness on that side of the face (see the Peripheral Nerve Injury section later in this chapter; see Figure 5.4).

Motor Function   The newborn evaluation includes an assessment of motor function. The following sections describe features of typical and atypical motor function.

Typical Motor Function   In addition to assessing the function of the cranial nerves, the neurological exam of the neonate also assesses motor function. It is important to assess the symmetry, quality, and quantity of the infant's spontaneous movements. Muscle tone and posture are evaluated by observing the baby's movements or resistance to movement while subjected to a series of passive manipulations of the baby's position. These findings may be affected by gestational age

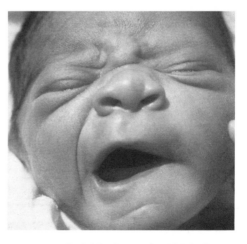

Figure 5.4. Left-sided facial nerve palsy with lack of expression on left side of the face. (From Clark, D.A. [2000]. *Atlas of neonatology* [p. 138]. Philadelphia: W.B. Saunders; reprinted by permission.)

and level of alertness. The exam may look at the baby's power and primitive reflexes. One test frequently done assesses the baby's ability to hold his or her head for several seconds in the same plane as the rest of his or her body (see Figure 5.5).

Deep tendon reflexes may be assessed by sharply percussing (tapping with fingertip or a reflex hammer) over specific tendons. The knee jerk is just one of the tendon reflexes able to be elicited in the newborn.

Atypical Motor Function   Hypertonia (excessive muscle tightness) may be seen after intrauterine or extrauterine brain injury (often due to low oxygen levels and/or poor blood flow to the brain) with a resultant cerebral palsy. The stiffness, or hypertonia, often takes weeks to months to develop. When hypertonia is associated with cerebral palsy, the legs tend to be more severely affected than the arms. Stiffness of the muscles may be helped with the use of physical therapy and muscle stretching exercises. In more severe cases, a surgical procedure can be done to loosen the contractures. This procedure is most commonly performed on the Achilles tendon of the ankle.

Generalized hypotonia and localized weakness are relatively common motor abnormalities in neonates with disorders of the nervous system. Generalized hypotonia may also be due to muscular dysfunction or problems at the junction of the nerves and the muscle. Eliciting the pattern of the weakness using the neurological examination is important in determining the level of the neurological abnormality. For instance, specific weakness of the arm may indicate a brachial plexus nerve root injury. Flaccid weakness of all extremities, perhaps involving the muscles of respiration, may indicate a systemic disorder (see the Hypotonia section later in this chapter).

Primary Neonatal Reflexes   Several primary neonatal reflexes are elicited in the newborn during a neurological evaluation. The Moro reflex (see Figure 5.6), elicited best by suddenly dropping the baby's head backward, is characterized by spreading the arms and hands wide (abduction), followed by flexing the arms toward midline (adduction) as if embracing his mother. This reflex has been described as a self-protective reflex. With sudden loss of stability, the embracing movements of the infant's arms seem to be an attempt to grab onto his mother to prevent being dropped. Attempting to elicit a neonate's Moro reflex may uncover abnormalities of the central nervous system or localized nerve disease.

Movements similar to walking are called the placing and stepping reflexes. These can be elicited by holding the neonate so that the sole of his foot contacts a flat surface (see Figure 5.7).

The tonic neck response, also called Fencer's reflex, causes the baby's arm to extend on the side to which the head is turned. The arm on the side toward which the head is not turned bends up at the shoulder and elbow, as if the baby is fencing. Finding abnormalities on this exam may suggest cerebral disease, such as cerebral palsy.

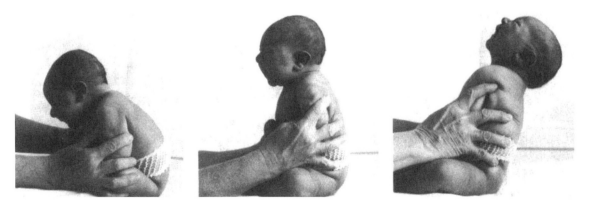

Figure 5.5.   Demonstration of proper tone of the neck muscles. (From Amiel-Tison, C., & Davis, S.W. [1987]. Newborn neurologic examination. In A.M. Rudolph, J.I.E. Hoffman, & S. Axelrod [Eds.], *Pediatrics* [p. 126]. Norwalk, CT: Appleton & Lange; Copyright © 2008 The McGraw-Hill Companies; reprinted by permission.)

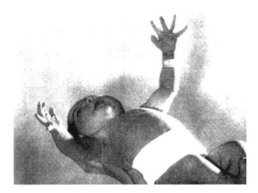

Figure 5.6. Moro reflex, abduction phase. (From Egan, D.F., Illingworth, R.S., & Mac Keith, R.C. [1971]. Developmental screening 0–5 years. *Clinics in Developmental Medicine, 30,* 47. London: Spastics International Medical Publications; reprinted by permission.)

The Palmar grasp reflex causes a neonate to curl his fingers around an object placed in his palm (see Figure 5.8). This reflex appears at 28 weeks of gestation and is strong enough at 37 weeks of gestation to allow the neonate's upper torso to be pulled up from his bed as he holds onto the fingers of an examiner. Abnormal findings on examining the Palmar grasp may suggest either peripheral nerve or cerebral disease. These primitive neonatal reflexes fade away after the first several months of life. With the exception of the Moro reflex, the evolutionary significance of the primitive neonatal reflexes is not entirely clear.

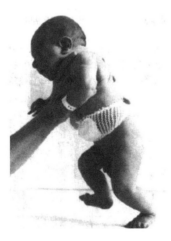

Figure 5.7. Placing and stepping reflexes. (From Amiel-Tison, C., & Davis, S.W. [1987]. Newborn neurologic examination. In A.M. Rudolph, J.I.E. Hoffman, & S. Axelrod [Eds.], *Pediatrics* [p. 126]. Norwalk, CT: Appleton & Lange; Copyright © 2008 The McGraw-Hill Companies, Inc.; reprinted by permission.)

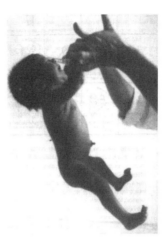

Figure 5.8. Palmar grasp reflex. (From Amiel-Tison, C., & Davis, S.W. [1987]. Newborn neurologic examination. In A.M. Rudolph, J.I.E. Hoffman, & S. Axelrod [Eds.], *Pediatrics* [p. 126]. Norwalk, CT: Appleton & Lange; Copyright © 2008 The McGraw-Hill Companies, Inc.; reprinted by permission.)

Sensory Capabilities   Sensory capabilities of a neonate may be demonstrated by his or her ability to respond to the pain of a pin prick, for instance. In response to pain, a full-term baby will pull his or her extremity away from, or turn the face away from, the source of the pain. This response is known as withdrawal. The infant may also exhibit universally recognizable facial movements in response to pain, such as a grimace. In addition, he or she may cry in response to pain. Although extremely premature babies in the intensive care unit may be too weak to respond to pain by withdrawing from pain or by crying aloud, they may exhibit grimacing, fist clenching, toe curling or extension, fast heartbeat, and high blood pressure. Health care professionals in the intensive care unit watch for these more subtle signs of pain and treat accordingly.

In the past, physicians believed that infants were incapable of experiencing pain because their nervous systems were not yet fully developed. Consequently, painful procedures were performed on them without supplying adequate analgesia. Although it is true that their nervous systems are still maturing, it has been shown that even extremely premature infants can discriminate between touch and pain. After experiencing tactile touching, even extremely premature infants may become more alert and begin to move spontaneously. After experiencing pain, they may attempt to cry and withdraw from the source of the pain (Bartocci, Berquist, Lagercrantz, & Anand, 2006; Saint-Anne Dargassies, 1966). Therefore, today, health care professionals take great care to treat pain in neonates with appropriate analgesia.

In brief review, the neurological exam can be helpful in predicting a baby's long-term neurodevelopmental outcome. One single isolated abnormal finding during a neonatal neurodevelopmental examination is not highly predictive of neurological dysfunction. However, if sequential neurological exams repeatedly reveal the same abnormal findings, or if multiple abnormal findings are detected during the same neurological examination, there is a higher risk that the infant may have permanent neurological disability. The Collaborative Perinatal Project of the National Institutes of Health (Nelson & Ellenberg, 1979) showed that infants with abnormalities of tone in the limbs, trunk, or neck were 12–15 times more likely than infants without those abnormalities to develop cerebral palsy. Infants with decreased spontaneous activity level for more than 1 day had a 19-time higher risk of cerebral palsy. Infants with poor sucking ability had a 14-time increased risk. Of premature infants who proceed to develop cerebral palsy, 80% had an abnormal neurological examination at the time of discharge from the neonatal intensive care unit (Allen & Capute, 1989). This means that up to 20% of premature babies with a completely normal neurological exam at the time of discharge from the neonatal intensive care unit were ultimately diagnosed with cerebral palsy. Repeated assessments over time are important in monitoring these babies at risk. Early intervention can help to maximize function.

Nervous System Impairment _____

Nervous system impairment can take various forms. These are described in the following subsections.

Hypotonia

Disorders causing hypotonia are relatively common in the neonate. They range from disorders of the cerebral cortex of the brain (asphyxia [see the Perinatal Asphyxia section later in this chapter]), intracranial hemorrhage (see the Intracranial Hemorrhage section later in this chapter), infection, metabolic and toxic causes, and muscular disorders to disorders at the level of the peripheral nerve (see the Peripheral Nerve Injury section later in this chapter). A work-up to determine the etiology of a neonate's hypotonia may include an electromyogram, nerve conduction velocity, imaging of the brain, muscle biopsy, and examination of his parents, as well as specific blood tests. The enzyme creatine phosphokinase may be elevated in the bloodstream of infants affected by certain muscle diseases, such as Duchenne muscular dystrophy. Levels of the enzyme serum glutamic-oxaloacetic transaminase (SGOT) may be elevated in hypotonic infants affected by disorders having liver involvement, such as Pompe glycogen storage disease (deficiency of acid alpha-glucosidase). Disorders of the lower motor neuron are the most frequent cause of hypotonia or weakness in the neonate.

Werdnig-Hoffman Disease / Spinal Muscular Atrophy Type I   Werdnig-Hoffman disease/ Spinal Muscular Atrophy Type I is the most common disease of the lower motor neuron. Patients have flaccid weakness of all extremities, some weakness of the respiratory muscles, and, initially, less weakness of the facial muscles and the muscles supplied by the cranial nerves. This disorder is inherited in an autosomal recessive manner (i.e., if each parent is an asymptomatic carrier, statistically each new fetus has a 25% chance of developing the disease and 50% of the offspring will be carriers of the disease). The genetic passage of the disease has been determined to be an abnormality on the 5th chromosome.

Fetuses with this disease may have decreased fetal movements, weakness with consequent respiratory distress at birth, total lack of reflexes, poor suck and swallow strength, occasional muscle fasciculations (i.e., muscular twitching involving the simultaneous contraction of contiguous groups of muscle fibers), and muscle atrophy. Contractures of the wrist and/or ankle joints due to lack of movement of these joints may develop over time or in utero. When joint contractures occur in utero, it is known as arthrogryposis multiplex congenita. Findings of arthrogryposis are not specific to Werdnig-Hoffman disease, but they may occur due to many different disorders of the brain, nerves, muscles, neuromuscular junction, and joints affecting the developing fetus.

Patients with Werdnig-Hoffman disease have normal sphincter and sensory function. The clinical course is progressive deterioration, with 60% of patients dying within the first year of life. The earlier the age of onset of disease, the earlier the patients may be expected to die. The cause of death usually stems from respiratory complications, such as repeated aspiration pneumonias, inability to clear tracheal secretions, or an inability to breathe effectively.

Congenital Myasthenia
Global generalized weakness or hypotonia throughout the entire body, usually including the cranial nerves, may indicate a problem with the neuromuscular junction, as seen in one of the congenital myasthenia syndromes. At the neuromuscular junction, the nerve ending is supposed to send a chemical called acetylcholine to be received by the acetylcholine receptors of the muscle, which, in turn, makes the muscle contract as the nerve is directing it to do. When that chemical reaction at the meeting of the nerve ending and the muscle does not occur properly as a result of defects in the synthesis of acetylcholine, or, more commonly, insufficient acetylcholine receptors at the muscle end of the neuromuscular junction, the muscle does not receive the message and, therefore, cannot respond or cannot respond as forcefully as intended. In the case of transient neonatal myasthenia gravis, infants acquire, transplacentally, antibodies from their myasthenic mothers against acetylcholine receptors at the muscle end of the neuromuscular junction. Treatment may be carried out with anticholinesterase medications. The mean duration of the neonatal transient myasthenia gravis syndrome is 18 days.

Congenital Myotonic Dystrophy
Congenital myotonic dystrophy (Figure 5.9) is almost always inherited from the mother. It is a muscle disorder that causes the neonate's muscles to be excessively weak. The earlier the disorder presents in life and the more severely affected the mother is, the more severely the baby will be affected. Offspring become more severely affected as the disease is passed down through the generations. The disorder is often apparent at birth, causing such weakness of the respiratory muscles that ventilatory support may be needed. In addition, the neonate's muscles involved in feeding may be so weak that nutrition may need to be supplemented via feeding tube. While in utero, the affected fetus may be too weak to move his extremities and may develop contractures (arthrogryposis) of his joints. The fetus may also be too weak to swallow in utero, developing excessive amounts of amniotic fluid, the volume of which should be decreased by normal fetal swallowing. During the first 2–3 months after birth, infants may develop improved muscle strength. Facial weakness and a tent-shaped upper lip may persist. Infants unable to take adequate nutrition by mouth or to breathe unassisted have a high mortality rate. Weakness of the heart muscle (cardiomyopathy) may also be a cause of neonatal death. Survivors often have poor gastric and intestinal motility, which causes problems with digestion, even if the patient is able to take his feedings by mouth. Survivors also have orthopedic problems stemming from their arthrogryposis.

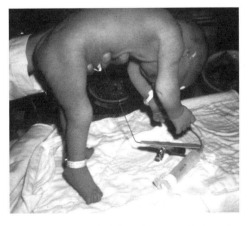

Figure 5.9. Hypotonic infant with myotonic dystrophy. (From Clark, D.A., private collection; reprinted by permission.)

Unfortunately, nearly all survivors with congenital myotonic dystrophy have intellectual disabilities with IQ scores in the 50–65 range (severely challenged to challenged). In view of the poor outcome for critically ill neonates diagnosed with congenital myotonic dystrophy, a determination needs to be made as to whether it is in the neonate's best interest to provide ongoing life sustaining treatment. Diagnosis of this disorder is made by muscle biopsy. Electromyography (EMG) may support the diagnosis by showing myotonic electrical discharges emanating from the percussed muscle. Genetic counseling is imperative for families of these neonates. Transmitted in an autosomal dominant fashion from an affected mother's abnormal 19th chromosome, there is a 50% chance of each of her fetuses being affected. Occasionally, mothers are unaware of their diagnosis. The diagnosis may be suspected in the mother if she has a long, thin face due to atrophy of the temporalis and masseter muscles, a straight smile, drooping of the eyelids (ptosis), and is unable to open her hand and/or eyelids after closing her fist and/or eyes tightly for several seconds (myotonia).

Excessive magnesium levels in the blood as well as treatment with the aminoglycoside class of antibiotics (e.g., gentamicin), especially in babies with a propensity to hypotonia (i.e., myotonic dystrophy), can cause transient weakness due to poor function at the neuromuscular junction.

Perinatal Asphyxia

Perinatal asphyxia may cause temporary or permanent dysfunction of the fetal or newborn brain. Asphyxia is the condition that occurs as a result of low levels of oxygen, high levels of carbon dioxide, poor perfusion (blood flow), and/or abnormally low pH (acidosis) in the blood of the fetus or newborn. The term asphyxia refers to organ damage that occurs anywhere within the body of the fetus or newborn due to abnormalities in these parameters. Often as asphyxia is occurring, the body will attempt to send adequate amounts of blood flow to the brain at the expense of blood flow to less vital organs. Therefore, an asphyxiated baby with brain dysfunction also

may be expected to have at least temporary dysfunction of the intestines and kidneys. Sometimes, however, the severity of the asphyxia is such that even the brain cannot be spared. In this situation, the subsequent brain damage is called hypoxic-ischemic encephalopathy (HIE).

Timing of Asphyxia   Although it is sometimes assumed that all neonatal asphyxia occurs during the delivery process, this is not true. Asphyxia can occur while the fetus is still within the uterus before any labor begins. If the mother herself suffers from low oxygen levels in the blood as a result of cardiac or lung problems or if she has severe anemia, she will not be able to send enough oxygen to her fetus. Red blood cells carry oxygen to the tissues; if there are not enough red blood cells in the mother's circulation, not enough oxygen will be delivered to her fetus. If there is a problem with the placenta, such as abruptio placenta (premature separation of the placenta from the uterine wall) or placenta previa (placenta growing over the cervical opening), which causes inadequate fetal carbon dioxide elimination and/or inadequate oxygenation, then the fetus will be at risk. If the mother is unable to send enough blood to her side of the placenta due to low maternal blood pressure, severe maternal hypertension with blood vessel constriction, or excessively strong and prolonged uterine contractions, then the fetus will not get enough oxygen and will have inadequate carbon dioxide elimination. If this problem goes on in a relatively mild manner for several weeks, it may manifest by poor fetal growth without acute asphyxia.

If the poor fetal growth is reflected in poor growth of the head and brain, there is an increased neurodevelopmental risk to that infant. The fetus also will not get enough oxygen or gas exchanging ability if the umbilical cord circulation is impaired by the cord being compressed between the baby's head and a maternal pelvic bone, twisted around body parts of the baby, or prolapsed through an open cervix with the baby's head compressing it or by having a true tight knot in the cord.

If the fetus itself has poor oxygen delivery to its organs due to severe fetal anemia, then the fetus is at risk for asphyxia. Furthermore, if the fetus has extremely low blood pressure because of infection or bleeding, then it will not have adequate perfusion to its organs and will also be at risk for asphyxia. After birth, if the baby has severe cardiac or pulmonary problems or cannot adjust to the extrauterine environment, he or she may experience poor oxygen delivery or suboptimal blood flow to the organs, increasing his or her risk for asphyxia. Both the seriousness of the perfusion and oxygenation abnormalities, as well as the length of time that a fetus is exposed to poor perfusion and low oxygen levels, may be correlated with the degree of severity of the neonate's asphyxia.

Historical Aspects of Asphyxia   Not recognizing that cerebral palsy might be associated with asphyxia occurring before labor or after delivery, physicians since the 1800s blamed the delivery process as the sole etiology of cerebral palsy. However, they observed that cerebral palsy would occur despite intermittent auscultation of (listening to) the fetal heart rate by the physicians. In the 1960s, ability to assess the fetus during labor via fetal scalp blood sampling or continuous monitoring of the fetal heart rate using Doppler (ultrasound) technology was expected to decrease significantly the incidence of cerebral palsy, birth asphyxia, and fetal and/or neonatal death during or after labor. However, the use of continuous fetal heart rate monitoring, using Doppler technology, has not significantly decreased the incidence of cerebral palsy. Cerebral palsy occurs in 1–2 babies out of 1,000 births (Freeman & Nelson, 1988; Naeye, Peters, Bartholomew, & Landis, 1989). Cerebral palsy linked to fetal asphyxia occurs only 1–2 times in 10,000 births. Only 9% of cases of cerebral palsy have been linked to intrapartum events (MacDonald, 1997), and more than 80% of children with cerebral palsy had no evidence of intrapartum or perinatal asphyxia (Blair & Stanley, 1988). This is because most asphyxia occurs independently of the labor process.

In most cases, the factor responsible for the cerebral palsy or brain injury is not able to be identified (Kuban & Leviton, 1994). Doppler assessment of umbilical cord arterial blood flow velocity has the potential to identify those fetuses at increased risk for cerebral palsy, asphyxia, and in utero death due to rising blood pressure in the placenta because of placental pathology. Doppler technology, however, cannot be expected to identify brain damage. Once risk factors are identified, the pregnant woman and her physicians must balance the risks of premature elective delivery with the risks of continuing poor intrauterine blood flow.

Severity of Asphyxia   Researchers have divided asphyxia (or more precisely, HIE) into three categories. Mild HIE may show up initially as brain dysfunction (e.g., excessive irritability; uncoordinated suck, swallow, or breathing; excessive sleepiness), which is sometimes not recognized by the neonate's caregivers. A mildly asphyxiated neonate's initial hyperirritability may be misinterpreted by caregivers as indicative that the baby is just hungry and that everything is all right. It may be the inability to take in substantial amounts of milk that draw attention to the caregivers that something is not right with the baby. Babies with mild HIE do not have seizures as a result of their insult. An electroencephalogram (EEG) to measure brain wave activity will not show seizure activity, but may show some abnormalities of baseline brainwave activity. These abnormalities of the EEG are temporary; in the case of mild HIE, they last less than 14 days. By 14 days of age, the mildly asphyxiated baby has a completely normal neurological examination and EEG. Babies with mild HIE have a good likelihood of ultimately becoming neurodevelopmentally normal.

Babies with severe HIE typically have poor Apgar scores, which are assessed at birth in order to record neonatal health. Researchers (Nelson & Ellenberg, 1981) have noted that babies with Apgar scores that are persistently low (0–3 out of 10 possible) at 20 minutes after birth have a 100% chance of either being permanently severely neurologically damaged or dying within the first year of life. Severe HIE often presents with obtundation or coma, or as initial hyperirritability (related to cerebral edema, brain swelling), which subsides into lethargy, obtundation, and coma when the cerebral edema goes away. Babies with severe HIE may have seizures, and they may lack the normal primitive neonatal reflexes. Seizures may be apparent on the EEG; abnormalities of baseline brainwaves, including a burst-suppression pattern, may also be apparent. Persistence of these findings is extremely worrisome, as they are poor prognostic indicators.

The most severely abnormal EEG would be isoelectric, with no brainwaves whatsoever. Such an isoelectric EEG may be used to help the physicians confirm their clinical suspicions of brain death. If, over the course of many hours, a severely asphyxiated infant exhibits no self-preserving reflexes (e.g., no eye blinking, no withdrawal from painful stimuli), no spontaneous movements, no attempt to breathe even when his carbon dioxide level is elevated in his bloodstream, physicians may entertain the diagnosis of brain death. In the unfortunate situation where brain death is confirmed, the physicians would discuss the diagnosis of brain death with the baby's family. After brain death, the brain's role in regulating heart rate and blood pressure is lacking. Such a patient's heart rate and blood pressure would slowly drop to 0, even if the patient remained on mechanical ventilation (the respirator). Therefore, after a diagnosis of brain death is made and the family is notified, plans are made to remove the patient from the ventilator because further efforts to make the baby survive or to have a typical life would be futile. Many families choose to be present to hold their babies when they are removed from the ventilator. The hospital staff is available to assist families through this difficult time.

Moderate HIE represents a middle ground between mild and severe HIE. These infants often initially present with decreased spontaneous movements and hypotonia or with hyperirritability. Some of these babies will have seizures; some will not. Many will have some improvement in their initially abnormal neurological exam but still will be left with some permanent disabilities.

For full-term neonates with asphyxia, the mortality rate is about 10%; for premature babies with asphyxia, the mortality rate is 30% (Volpe, 2000).

Clinical Findings   Immediately following asphyxia affecting the brain, a baby may have hypertonia and hyperirritability, or hypotonia, stupor, and coma. He or she may have seizures, breath-holding spells, and/or inability to breathe regularly on his or her own. During the next day or two, some of the abnormal findings may actually worsen as a result of brain swelling related to the asphyxia, then begin to resolve. Whether the baby's neurological exam eventually becomes normal depends on the severity of the asphyxial insult he or she has sustained. Long-term neurological disorders affecting these babies may include intellectual disabilities, spastic quadriparesis (cerebral palsy), seizures, choreoathetoid (involuntary writhing) movements, and ataxia (inability to walk or balance).

When infants with severe HIE survive, they may require daily medications to help to prevent seizures. They also may have an inability to suck and swallow or to coordinate these activities with breathing. Therefore, to provide these infants with adequate nutrition, once their intestines recover from the asphyxial event, they may require nutrition (pumped breast milk or formula) to be fed to them through feeding tubes. Initially, a small, flexible plastic tube can be inserted through the nose or mouth into the stomach through which the infant can be fed. If the patient demonstrates a long-term inability to feed by mouth, a feeding gastrostomy tube (g-tube) can be inserted by the surgeons into the stomach through a nick in the abdominal wall. The g-tube, compared to the tube that enters the stomach through the nose or mouth, has the advantages that it does not often fall out (but if it does fall out, it requires a health care professional to replace it), and it is hidden under clothing.

In addition to having feeding difficulties, babies with severe HIE may have difficulty swallowing their own secretions, as well as difficulty with gastroesophageal reflux when stomach contents are regurgitated up into the mouth. Medications and a surgical procedure, called a fundoplication, to tighten up the connection between the esophagus (swallowing tube) and the stomach can help with this problem. However, despite this, infants with severe HIE are at increased risk of having recurring aspiration pneumonias due to breathing secretions into their lungs. This is a significant cause of shortened lifespan in these babies.

Seizures

There are several kinds of seizures. This section describes the presentation and causes of various types.

Clinical Presentation   Neonatal seizures are a result of abnormal electrical activity emanating from the brain. Neonatal seizures may be manifested by rhythmic, slow, relatively intense jerking movements of the extremities or by movements that are much more subtle. Seizures may involve rowing movements of the arms; bicycling movements of the legs; prolonged extension or stretching out of one or more extremities; neck extension and turning of the head in one direction; lip-smacking; tongue-thrusting (which could be misinterpreted as signs that the baby is hungry); eyelid twitching or fluttering; horizontal jerking of the eyes to one side; nonsynchronized twitching of body parts; cessation of breathing (apnea); or autonomic changes (e.g., an abnormal drop in or rise of heart rate or blood pressure).

An important distinguishing feature between seizures and other neonatal behaviors is that seizures cannot be stopped or extinguished by other people. For instance, during a seizure, touching, cradling, or rubbing a baby will not cause the seizure to cease. If a neonate who is having some unusual behaviors is touched and the behaviors stop, those behaviors likely were not a result of seizures. Similarly, seizures cannot be elicited by other people. Startling a baby with a sudden loud noise or sudden touch may cause him or her to exhibit a Moro startle reflex, to alter level of arousal, or even to show some temporary jittery movements; however, being startled cannot cause a neonate to have a seizure.

When a neonate is suspected of having seizures, an EEG is typically performed to verify this suspicion. An EEG measures brain wave activity by utilizing electrodes and wires that are temporarily glued to the baby's scalp. However, an EEG can actually miss detecting the seizure in progress if the seizure does not occur during the period of the time that the EEG is being performed. An EEG may also miss a seizure that occurs during the performance of the EEG if the abnormal brain waves occur in the center of the brain but do not move all the way to the outside of the brain where the EEG electrodes are positioned. Even if electrical seizure activity is not seen on EEG in a baby who has seizures, the EEG may still be useful. In cases where the seizure's electrical activity does not reach the peripherally placed EEG electrodes or when the seizure occurred before the EEG was begun, some localized evidence of cerebral irritability may still be evident in the electrical waveforms. Also, the baseline brainwave activity may be abnormal, which indicates some cerebral disturbance (e.g., HIE) that can make a baby vulnerable to seizures.

When a baby is suspected of having seizures, the brain is often imaged using ultrasound, computed tomography (CT scan), or magnetic resonance imaging (MRI). The purpose of the imaging study is to help to determine the reason for the seizures. Likewise, when a baby is suspected of having a seizure, various blood tests are drawn to help to determine the etiology of the seizure.

Etiologies of Seizures   Neonatal seizures may have many potential etiologies and, as noted previously, the medical work-up is performed to determine the reason for the seizure. Once the reason for the seizure is known, health care professionals have a better chance of successfully stopping the seizures. Unlike larger pediatric patients, neonates do not have seizures due to fever (febrile seizures), and the etiology of their seizures rarely is determined to be idiopathic epilepsy. Most commonly, the etiology of their seizures is an acute insult to the central nervous system, such as asphyxial injury or infection.

Hypoxic-Ischemic Encephalopathy   Approximately 50%–60% of neonatal seizures are caused by hypoxic-ischemic encephalopathy (HIE), which is usually secondary to perinatal asphyxia (see the Perinatal Asphyxia section in this chapter). Typically, the seizures occur in the first

24 hours after birth. Frequently, the neonate will appear extremely irritable or lethargic before the onset of HIE-associated seizures. About one fifth of neonates with seizures due to HIE will have cerebral infarction recognized on brain imaging studies. Seizures also can be caused by cerebral infarction without there being any global asphyxial event (see the Stroke section later in this chapter).

Meningoencephalitis   A neonate with seizures may have a fever or, more commonly, a low body temperature as a result of meningoencephalitis (infection and inflammation of the brain and surrounding membranes). In this situation, meningoencephalitis causes both the seizures and the abnormal body temperature; the abnormal temperature is not the cause of the seizures. Meningoencephalitis can also be a cause of seizures or abnormal neurological activity without an abnormal body temperature. Meningoencephalitis can be due to a variety of bacteria or viruses.

Hypoglycemia   Hypoglycemia (low blood sugar) can cause the brain to have a deficit of sugar or energy, which can lead to seizures. Prior to actually developing seizures, a hypoglycemic baby may be limp, unresponsive, jittery, or sweaty. Ironically, seizure activity further depletes the brain of its energy stores and precipitates more seizures. Treatment of hypoglycemic seizures with anticonvulsant medications is not effective. Instead, correction of the low blood sugar will cause the seizure to stop.

Low blood sugar may be seen in infants of diabetic women. In this situation, if the mother had chronically high blood sugar levels, the baby would have been exposed to high sugar levels crossing from the mother to the baby via the placenta. The baby would have responded by making a large amount of insulin in an attempt to get his blood sugar down toward normal and to store the sugar energy in the form of fat. Once birth occurs, however, the baby is suddenly removed from his high sugar source. The infant cannot suddenly turn off his or her insulin production, and his or her high insulin levels cause his or her blood sugar to drop down to danger-

ously low levels. Generally, physicians consider a blood sugar level lower than 40 milligrams per deciliter (mg/dl) to be risky in a full-term neonate; lower than 35 mg/dl is considered risky in a premature neonate. Treatment for neonatal hypoglycemia involves getting additional glucose into the baby. This may be done through oral or tube feedings, intravenous fluids containing a moderate concentration of glucose through a peripheral IV, and/or intravenous fluids containing a high glucose concentration through an umbilical venous catheter or other central line.

Hyponatremia   Hyponatremia (low sodium levels in the blood, less than approximately 130 milliequivalent per liter) can lead to seizures. Similar to the case with low glucose levels, treatment of seizures due to hyponatremia with anticonvulsant medications is not effective at stopping seizures. Instead, treatment of the low blood sodium will stop the seizures. Babies may develop severely low sodium levels for a few reasons. If the baby consumes too much water compared to the amount of sodium that he or she takes in, his or her blood sodium will become diluted by free water, causing the sodium level in the blood to drop. This happens most commonly when the baby's formula is being mixed with water in the wrong concentration, which can cause water intoxication. A baby may also have a condition known as syndrome of inappropriate antidiuretic hormone (SIADH) causing his or her body to excrete water inappropriately. In this situation, a baby's blood sodium level drops because it becomes diluted with too much water. In congenital adrenal hyperplasia, a baby may waste excess sodium in the urine while retaining excess potassium. The high blood potassium may cause abnormal rhythms of the heart, and the low blood sodium may cause seizures. Congenital adrenal hyperplasia also may be associated with incomplete differentiation of the genitalia.

Hypocalcemia   Hypocalcemia (low blood calcium levels that are generally below 8 mg/dl) can cause seizures. Before actually developing seizures due to hypocalcemia, babies may have twitching, jitteriness, and abnormal heart rhythms.

Treatment of hypocalcemic seizures with anticonvulsants is likely to be ineffective. Instead, treatment should be directed at correcting the low calcium level. Low calcium levels may occur in babies who have high phosphorus levels (kidney disease, excessively early consumption of cow milk), in infants of diabetic mothers, small-for-gestational age babies, and babies with a poorly functioning parathyroid gland. Those babies with hypoparathyroidism also may have a poorly formed thymus gland and abnormalities of the heart and their great vessels associated with a gene deletion on the 22nd chromosome (known as DiGeorge syndrome).

Hypomagnesemia   Occasionally, low magnesium levels are associated with seizures. Magnesium levels may be low as a result of either the mother or the neonate wasting magnesium in the urine.

Narcotic Withdrawal   When a pregnant woman chronically receives narcotics, both she and her fetus become dependent on these medications. When the baby is born, he or she is suddenly removed from the narcotic source. Within 24–72 hours after birth, infants may show signs of narcotic withdrawal syndrome. They may have frantic sucking, overeating, excess irritability, prolonged crying, sweating, fast heart rate, vomiting, diarrhea, and seizures. Treatment for neonatal narcotic withdrawal syndrome includes providing a dark, quiet environment with minimal external stimuli and swaddling. Some physicians treat seizures due to narcotic withdrawal with anticonvulsants, but such seizures (as well as the other clinical findings of narcotic withdrawal) respond well to a regular regimen of slowly decreasing doses of the narcotic.

Stroke   Strokes (cerebral infarctions) may cause seizures in a neonate or may cause a more subtle focal neurological deficit, such as poor movement of one hand. If the neurological deficit is minor, the fact that the patient had a stroke may not be immediately recognized. Strokes are relatively rare in the neonate. When they do occur, they may be associated with poor cerebral blood flow occurring during an event that also caused HIE (discussed in a previous section of this chapter). They may also occur as a consequence of cerebral arterial occlusion that is caused by an embolus (blood clot) that breaks loose from another location, such as the placenta, or a thrombus that forms in the cerebral blood vessel. When such an event occurs, physicians may decide to do laboratory studies to determine if the baby has excessive and inappropriate clotting of the blood. This diagnosis is important to make in order to prevent future strokes or clotting within blood vessels that supply blood to important organs. Because the excess clotting disorder (hypercoagulability) may run in families and may have health implications with regards to other family members, doctors may need permission from parents to do genetic studies on the baby. If a genetically mediated hypercoagulability is identified, the family may be invited to discuss this with a genetic counselor or doctor.

Strokes also may occur because blood that was supposed to perfuse a particular region of the brain never reaches that area due to hemorrhaging of one of the blood vessels leading to that area. This is called a hemorrhagic infarction or hemorrhagic stroke.

Treatment for stroke includes supporting the neonate's cardiorespiratory status, supporting his blood volume and blood pressure, and working to prevent further strokes by diagnosing the cause of the stroke and anticoagulating the blood (in the case of hypercoagulability) or correcting any deficient clotting factors (in the case of a hemorrhagic stroke).

Intracranial Hemorrhage   Bleeding within the skull can have many different causes. It may or may not lead to seizures, and it may or may not lead to permanent or temporary neurological disability. Outcome may depend on which area of the brain is affected by the bleeding, the extent of the bleeding, and how much adjacent brain has been poorly perfused during the hemorrhagic event. Whenever any type of intracranial bleeding occurs, attention must be directed to whether the baby has the expected ability to clot his or her blood. If the infant's blood does not clot correctly, he or she may have one of various types of bleeding disorders, such as a low plate-let count, hemophilia, or disseminated intravascular coagulation (blood clots forming and using up circulating clotting factors in inappropriate locations). Transfusion of clotting factors may help to bring the hemorrhaging under control.

Furthermore, all forms of hemorrhage may be increased in infants who have vitamin K-deficient hemorrhagic disease of the newborn. In these cases, the baby's prothrombin activity in the blood is decreased, which sets him or her up for bleeding. Vitamin K levels in the newborn are generally low, especially from the second to seventh day of life. Hemorrhagic disease of the newborn occurs most frequently on these days in infants who do not receive a vitamin K_1 injection into the muscle around the time of delivery. Oral vitamin K_3 is potentially dangerous as it causes hemolytic anemia, which could lead to jaundice, kernicterus, and brain damage. Therefore, the safe and effective injectable vitamin K_1 is administered to neonates around the time of birth (Aballi & de Lamerens, 1962).

Subarachnoid hemorrhage may be related to a traumatic delivery, a hypoxic-ischemic event, or a premature delivery. Some subarachnoid hemorrhages are extremely minor and present with only minimal signs or are asymptomatic. Some present with seizures in an otherwise healthy appearing baby, usually on the second day of life. Rarely, a subarachnoid hemorrhage will present with massive intracranial blood loss shortly after birth with a catastrophic progression to death. Diagnosis of subarachnoid hemorrhage is best performed by CT scan or MRI, which also will help to ensure that the hemorrhage did not originate from some other intracranial location. Outcome varies with the severity of the hemorrhage. Patients with minimal to no signs generally do very well. Those with seizures as a complication of subarachnoid hemorrhage ultimately have a normal neurodevelopmental follow-up 90% of the time (Volpe, 2000). Those with catastrophic subarachnoid hemorrhage either die or are left with serious permanent neurological deficits.

Subdural hemorrhage is the least common of the neonatal varieties of intracranial hemorrhage. It occurs most commonly after traumatic deliveries in both full-term and premature neonates. Therefore, it is most likely to occur if the baby is large compared to the birth canal; the maternal pelvis is rigid (first-time mother or older mother); labor is not long enough to allow the pelvis to dilate maximally; labor is too long (subjecting the fetal head to prolonged repetitive compressions); malpresentation of the fetus occurs; the skull is very compliant (as with premature neonates); or extraction of the fetus requires forceps, vacuum, or rotational procedures. Similar to other types of intracranial hemorrhage, subdural hemorrhages may have minimal or no clinical signs (e.g., hyperalertness, apneas, irritability), moderate signs (e.g., focal neurological signs, seizures), and severe or lethal syndromes. Diagnosis is made by CT scan or MRI. Posthemorrhagic hydrocephalus may occur, and some patients may need a neurosurgical procedure in which a ventriculoperitoneal drainage shunt is inserted. Outcomes are variable.

Intraventricular hemorrhage (IVH) is most common in the premature infant. The more premature the infant, the more frequent and the more severe the intraventricular hemorrhage (see Figure 5.10).

The fetal brain has a rich supply of immature and fragile blood vessels that course along its surface and dive down into the brain tissue. These blood vessels are vulnerable to asphyxia and to fluctuations in blood pressure. They are prone to leaking and bleeding, which usually start in the region of the subependymal germinal

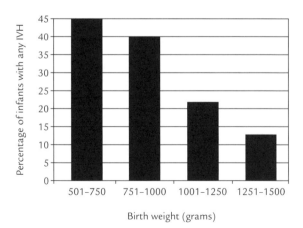

Figure 5.10. Incidence of intraventricular hemorrhage (IVH) as a function of birth weight. (*Sources:* Fanaroff et al., 1995; Hack et al., 1991; & Sheth, 1998).

matrix. Intraventricular hemorrhages have been grouped into four categories. Grade 1 IVH refers to hemorrhaging that has occurred only along the surface of the brain in the area of the subependymal germinal matrix. Grade 2 IVH refers to hemorrhaging that has broken through the subependymal germinal matrix into the spinal fluid-filled lakes within the brain (i.e., the lateral ventricles). Grade 3 IVH refers to hemorrhaging that has not only entered the lateral ventricles, but has filled the ventricles with blood and, therefore, distended them. Grade 4 IVH occurs when the hemorrhaging has also invaded and destroyed the brain tissue. This is believed to be a result of a hemorrhagic infarction (i.e., hemorrhagic stroke), caused by the lower grade hemorrhaging. When blood is not being delivered to brain tissue downstream from a lower grade IVH, a hemorrhagic stroke can occur in the poorly perfused brain tissue.

Outcomes following IVH are generally more favorable with the lower grade IVH (Grades 1 and 2) than the higher grade ones (Grades 3 and 4). However, any baby with IVH may be at risk for neurodevelopmental complications. There are a few reasons for this. Hemorrhage in the subependymal germinal matrix can lead to destruction of glial precursor cells whose job is to migrate into the still developing brain tissue and provide further brain development. Loss of blood from important brain blood vessels means that the vulnerable brain is not getting appropriate amounts of blood supply in downstream regions. Therefore, localized regions of poorly perfused, poorly oxygenated brain tissue may develop. Blood clots within the ventricles may both stimulate the production of excessive amounts of cerebrospinal fluid (CSF) and block the reabsorption of CSF. Over time, the irritating effect of the blood clot may cause permanent scarring that obstructs CSF flow and absorption. Ultimately, too much CSF may accumulate, causing posthemorrhagic hydrocephalus. The skull bones of a baby will eventually fuse and cause the skull to, essentially, become a closed box. If the swelling of the ventricles within the skull is sufficient to cause concern that there will be excessive pressure within the closed skull and pressure on the brain that impairs its blood flow, the patient may

require surgical placement of a drainage tube called a ventriculoperitoneal shunt.

Development of IVH in a full-term baby is relatively uncommon. When a full-term baby does develop an IVH, a history of a traumatic delivery or asphyxia should be sought. However 25% of full-term babies with IVH have no history of trauma or asphyxia. As described previously, full-term babies with intracranial hemorrhaging should generally have an investigation of their ability to clot because clotting disorders may predispose toward intracranial hemorrhage. The lack of IVH in premature babies or in full-term babies does not necessarily mean that the baby's brain will function normally.

An abnormal connection of cerebral arteries to cerebral veins, known as an arteriovenous malformation, may result in hemorrhage (a bleeding arteriovenous malformation) within the brain. Although intracranial hemorrhage is the most common way that these blood vessel malformations present, even without hemorrhage, these patients may have seizures, signs of high-output congestive heart failure due to inefficient delivery of blood to the brain, hydrocephalus, and neurological dysfunction. The physician may hear a murmur, called a bruit, when listening over the scalp with a stethoscope. Treatment is surgical.

Developmental Brain Defects   Sometimes an error occurs during early embryonic or fetal brain development that results in a brain that has abnormal anatomy and/or function. Babies with this problem have a high risk for seizures. Unfortunately, the seizures are not easily controlled with antiseizure medications, and we cannot correct the underlying condition. In addition to seizures, these patients will not have typical neurodevelopmental outcome because the brain is not formed properly.

Inborn Errors of Metabolism   When a baby with a congenital inability to metabolize nutrients is in utero, the mother's placenta eliminates the toxic metabolites from fetal circulation. The infant will, therefore, appear asymptomatic at birth. However, within the first several days of life, as the infant ingests milk that he or she is unable to properly metabolize, the toxic metabolites will build up in his or her circulation. These toxic metabolites include ammonia and excessive quantities of certain amino acids from the improper metabolism of proteins in his or her diet; organic acids due to improper metabolism of carbohydrates or proteins in his or her diet; and organic acids, fatty acids, and/or ammonia due to improper metabolism of fatty acids in the mitochondria or peroxisomes of the cells. Excessive quantities of certain amino acids, organic acids, or ammonia can lead to neurodevelopmental abnormalities, including seizures, acidosis, and death. Treatment for these conditions is complicated and incomplete. It involves restriction of whatever component of milk is unable to be metabolized, occasionally dialysis to remove the offending toxins, and a variety of partially effective medications. These infants are at extremely high risk for long-term neurodevelopmental complications and death due to their metabolic disorder.

Hyperbilirubinemia   Bilirubin arises from breaking down red blood cells. High bilirubin levels in the blood may occur as a result of blood group incompatibility or the formation of abnormal red blood cells in the baby, with excessive breakdown of these cells. High bilirubin levels can also occur because of poor feeding or poor stooling, dehydration, prematurity, and breakdown of red blood cells in the baby's skin (bruising) or within a body compartment. Excess of bilirubin causes jaundice, a yellow coloring of the skin and eyes. Severe jaundice can cause bilirubin to pass from the bloodstream into the brain, causing seizures, neurodevelopmental delay, and deafness. Neurological effects of the hyperbilirubinemia can be temporary (acute bilirubin encephalopathy) or permanent (kernicterus). Acutely, seizures due to hyperbilirubinemia may be managed by anticonvulsant medications as well as exchange transfusion to decrease the level of the bilirubin. If seizures persist after the bilirubin has been controlled, chronic treatment with anticonvulsants may be necessary.

Fifth Day Fits (Benign Idiopathic Neonatal Seizures)   Some infants develop a flurry of seizure activity on approximately the fifth day of

life. Between seizures, their neurological exam seems normal. The fact that the seizures have occurred is generally surprising because there is no medical history of asphyxia or other common causes of neonatal seizures. The EEG confirms seizure activity; however, the medical work-up for the etiology yields no results. The seizures generally disappear before 15 days of age and never recur. Providing their respiratory function is supported during the seizures, these infants generally grow up to be neurologically typical (Clancy, 1997).

Benign Neonatal Familial Seizures   As with Fifth Day Fits, benign neonatal familial seizures are considered benign because the seizures are generally mild, easily controlled, do not limit the quality of life nor shorten the length of life, and are not associated with neurological disability. EEG confirms seizure activity. Benign neonatal familial seizures are genetically transmitted in an autosomal dominant fashion that is linked to either the long arm of the 20th or the 8th chromosome. The affected gene causes an abnormal production of an acetylcholine receptor in the maturing brain. Usually, this seizure disorder disappears with maturity; however, such babies may be at increased risk for febrile seizures of childhood and for epilepsy in later life (Clancy, 1997).

Pyridoxine Dependency   When one of the B vitamins (vitamin B_6), pyridoxine, does not bind to the glutamic acid decarboxylase apoprotein properly, not enough gamma-aminobutyric acid (GABA) and too much glutamate are present in the cerebrospinal fluid. GABA's role is to inhibit excitatory neurotransmitters such as glutamate. Without enough GABA and with too much glutamate, seizures can occur that are refractory to standard anticonvulsant medications. Supplementing pyridoxine levels should help to stop the seizures as well as to arrest the brain abnormalities that may occur due to exposure to excess glutamate levels. Maternal placental function does not help to correct this problem, unlike many of the other metabolic reasons for neonatal seizures. Therefore, babies with pyridoxine dependency may have seizures within the first hours after birth or even while in utero.

Benign Neonatal Sleep Myoclonus   Some babies may have repetitive and usually symmetric jerking of the extremities that occurs only during sleep. These myoclonic jerks are not associated with an abnormal EEG and resolve spontaneously within a couple of months. Although they appear to be similar to a seizure, they are actually not seizures. These babies are expected to be neurologically typical.

Treatment of Seizures   Treatment for neonatal seizures is supportive (i.e., maintenance of adequate respiratory, cardiologic, and metabolic function) with a correction of any underlying defect if possible and the consideration of treatment with a variety of anticonvulsants (e.g., phenobarbital, phenytoin, lorzepam, levetiracetam). The choices of anticonvulsant medications are more narrow for treatment of neonatal seizures than for treatment of adult seizures as a result of the availability of less scientific data on the use of these drugs in neonates.

Apneas

Breath-holding spells in neonates are called apneas. Apneas must be differentiated from periodic breathing when a baby breathes regularly and then has a pause in breathing for less than 20 seconds. During this pause, there are no signs or symptoms, the baby's skin color does not become blue (cyanosis), and his or her heart rate does not drop to low levels. The more premature a baby is, the higher the chances of periodic breathing. Even some full-term babies may have periodic breathing. Periodic breathing has no symptoms, and it is not dangerous. Periodic breathing is due to an imbalance between, and immaturity of, the peripheral and central chemoreceptors of ventilatory drive. Periodic breathing requires no treatment. Babies will outgrow their tendencies for periodic breathing, and their prognosis is excellent.

Apneas of prematurity are more significant than periodic breathing. Similar to periodic breathing, the more immature a baby is, the higher the chance that he or she will have apneas of prematurity. In addition, the more immature the baby, the more severe the apneas of prematurity. During episodes of apneas of prematurity, an infant's skin may exhibit cyanosis and his heart rate may drop to low levels. There is an increased neurodevelopmental risk in babies with significant apneas of prematurity. Babies with apneas of prematurity have a decreased breathing response to high levels of carbon dioxide in the bloodstream, which they are supposed to exhale out of their bodies.

The etiology of apneas of prematurity may be an immature central nervous system (the brain not sending the impulse to breathe regularly) and/or a weak, fatigued diaphragm (breathing muscle) in 40% of the cases. The etiology is airway obstruction due to an immature, floppy airway in 10% of the cases. A combination of these reasons causes 50% of the cases of apneas of prematurity.

While in the neonatal intensive care unit, babies at risk for apneas of prematurity are generally monitored with a cardiorespiratory monitor, which will detect an apnea of prematurity if it occurs. When the monitor sets off its alarm, it notifies the health care professional to evaluate the patient and to end the apnea event. If the apneic baby does not resume breathing spontaneously, he or she can generally be successfully treated with only tactile stimulation (touching the baby or rubbing his or her back). Sometimes apneas of prematurity may require more aggressive intervention, such as tactile stimulation with oxygen administration or even a few supplemental breaths using a face mask.

Apneas of prematurity is a diagnosis of exclusion (i.e., when a baby has multiple apneas, the health care providers will consider other, more serious reasons for the apneas). Some of the more common diagnoses that may initially masquerade as apneas of prematurity include infection, gastroesophageal reflux, anemia, intracranial hemorrhage, and seizures.

Apneas of prematurity may be treated with caffeine citrate by the health care professional. Caffeine helps to increase the baby's sensitivity to high blood levels of carbon dioxide and may decrease the ventilatory depression following episodes of low blood oxygen levels. Caffeine may also decrease diaphragm muscle fatigue. Because caffeine is very slowly eliminated from the body, babies usually are maintained on the cardiorespiratory monitor for several days after stopping caffeine to ensure that the apneas of prematurity do not recur in the absence of the caffeine.

Apneas of prematurity have also been treated with nasal continuous positive airway pressure (NCPAP) in which air flows from wide nasal cannulae into the baby's nose under some pressure. Treatment with NCPAP may stimulate the pulmonary stretch receptors, and, therefore, stimulate the brain to initiate more regular breathing efforts. Treatment with NCPAP may also help to keep the upper airway open to prevent apneas of prematurity caused by airway obstruction and may improve the efficiency of ventilation so that the baby's respiratory muscles do not fatigue as quickly.

With the development of increasing maturity of the brain and strength of the respiratory musculature, apneas of prematurity generally spontaneously resolve by 32–34 weeks of corrected gestational age.

Peripheral Nerve Injury

Stretching or tearing injuries to peripheral nerves may occur in neonates and are most often associated with difficult deliveries. The two types of common peripheral nerve injuries in neonates are facial nerve and brachial plexus injuries.

Facial Nerve Injury   Facial nerve injury is the most common peripheral nerve injury in the neonate, with an incidence of approximately 7 per 1,000 births. The facial nerve (cranial nerve 7) passes under the zygomatic arch (cheekbone). If the labor and/or delivery process causes hemorrhage and/or edema in or around the facial nerve, a weakness of the muscles supplied by the nerve may result. It is believed that facial nerve injury is caused by pressure exerted by the maternal sacral promontory (tailbone) on the side of the fetal face during labor and delivery. Facial nerve palsy likewise may be related to a difficult mid-forceps delivery, but only rarely to low or outlet forceps application. Permanent, severe congenital facial nerve palsy seems to be most often related to intrauterine position of the baby against his mother's sacral bones.

A baby with facial nerve palsy will have weakness of the upper and lower facial muscles (see Figure 5.4). The baby will have decreased facial expression on the affected side and will be unable to close his or her eye tightly, wrinkle the eyebrow, raise the corner of his or her mouth, or open his or her mouth widely to create a crying face. While feeding, he or she may dribble milk from the corner of the mouth on the affected side. Fortunately, the weakness occurring with facial nerve injury is usually temporary and resolves when the hemorrhage and/or edema (swelling) into the nerve sheath resolves. Most facial nerve palsies resolve spontaneously within 1–3 weeks. Only rarely will an affected infant have a residual deficit several months later.

There is no specific treatment for facial nerve palsy. Supportive measures to protect the eye from corneal injury if eyelid closure is ineffective include the use of artificial tears and/or temporarily taping the eyelid shut.

Brachial Plexus Injury   Brachial plexus injury occurs 0.5–2 times per 1,000 births. It is most common in full-term infants, especially large babies (i.e., babies with broad shoulders that do not pass easily through the maternal pelvis), babies with evidence of fetal distress, and babies born to mothers with an abnormal labor and delivery. This injury generally comes about by traction being applied to the head (during head first deliveries) or to the shoulders (during breech deliveries), so that the head and shoulder are stretched away from each other.

The brachial plexus is a bundle of nerves that originate from cervical (neck) spinal segments 5, 6, 7, 8 (C-5, C-6, C-7, C-8), and thoracic (chest) segment 1 (T-1). These nerves supply the arm on that side. Stretching or tearing of the higher of these nerves (C-5 and C-6) causes a Duchenne-Erb's brachial plexus palsy and results in weakness or paralysis of the upper arm. There may also be some minor deficits in sensation, but this is difficult to evaluate in the neonate. The Moro reflex will be asymmetric with the affected side being limp or weak. The infant will hold the affected arm close to his chest with the elbow straight and internally rotated so that the palm of his hand points behind him. The wrist will be flexed, and the grasp reflex preserved. If the injury also involves spinal cervical segment 3 and/or 4 (C-3, C-4) above the brachial plexus, there will be poor movement of the diaphragm on that side, which puts the baby at risk for respiratory compromise. Diaphragmatic paresis is associated with Duchenne-Erb's palsy about 6% of the time.

When the injury involves only the lower nerve roots, C-7, C-8, and T-1, the forearm and hand will be affected. This is called Klumpke palsy. The wrist and fingers may be flexed, and the baby will not have any voluntary hand movement. The grasp reflex is absent, but the deep tendon reflexes are present. When T-1 is affected, the baby may have eyelid droop on that side and persistent constriction of the pupil of the eye (Horner syndrome). If the nerve injury does not heal, the iris of the affected eye eventually may have a deficit in pigment formation and remain unpigmented (blue).

More common than Klumpke lower nerve palsy but less common than Duchenne-Erb's upper nerve palsy is the total brachial plexus palsy. In this situation, both paralysis and sensory deficit are most severe and extend from the fingers to the shoulder on the affected side. All reflexes are absent. Radiological or clinical evaluation of diaphragmatic function should be carried out in patients with Duchenne-Erb's or total brachial plexus palsy.

Long-term prognosis for peripheral nerve injury of the brachial plexus depends on the extent and severity of the lesion. Infants with initial mild weakness of only upper nerve roots (C-5, C-6) have the best chance for typical outcome. Complete spontaneous recovery of most brachial plexus palsies has been reported in 50%–80% of patients. Clinical improvement within 2–4 weeks after birth is a favorable prognostic indicator. Infants destined to have complete, or nearly complete, recovery usually attain that recovery by 6 months of age. Infants with total brachial plexus injury have the worst outcome, with only about 15% of them spontaneously recovering typical function.

After brachial plexus injury, x-ray studies may be indicated to look for injury to the clavicle (collar bone), upper humerus (long bone of the upper arm), shoulder joint, and cervical (neck) spine.

Treatment involves initial partial immobilization of the affected limb to avoid any additional trauma. Physical therapy should be delayed for 7–10 days after the injury due to the development of painful posttraumatic neuritis. Later, physical therapy includes gentle, passive range of motion of joints of the shoulder, elbow, wrist, and hands to prevent joint contractures. Pain may be controlled with acetaminophen and gentle massage. Occasional splinting of the wrist and hand into a position of function may be useful to prevent joint contractures. Evaluation by the orthopedic surgeon to investigate any bone or joint abnormalities may be useful if the infant is not making much progress.

When affected infants have exhibited no recovery by 3 months of age, evaluation by the neurosurgeon may be helpful. Removal of scar tissue involving the nerve and surgical correction of torn nerves are some of the procedures sometimes offered by neurosurgeons for this condition.

Malformations of the Central Nervous System

Malformations of the central nervous system can have serious effects. Particular types of malformations are described next.

Anencephaly The most severe of the neural tube defects, anencephaly (see Figure 5.11), is caused by a failure of the primitive neural tube to

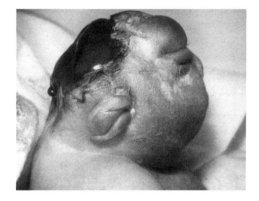

Figure 5.11. Anencephaly. (From Clark, D.A. [2000]. *Atlas of neonatology* [p. 126]. Philadelphia: W.B. Saunders; reprinted by permission.)

close at the level of the anterior neuropore at the most cephalad (head) portion of the neural tube. Anencephaly may be associated with craniorachischisis, which is failure of the neural tube to fuse in its more caudal (toward the tailbone) locations as well. The neural tube should be completely closed by the 28th day of embryonic life. Anencephaly is a lethal malformation in which the skull bones are absent, and the tissue within the base of the open skull consists of disorganized nerve cells. There is no significant amount of cerebral cortex. The nerve tissue that is present is exposed to the environment, causing heat, fluid, and electrolyte loss into the environment and thus subjecting the child's open nervous tissue to trauma and infection. This condition is not surgically correctable and infants with anencephaly generally die within several days after birth as a result of environmental effects on the open neural tube defect and/or apnea and due to the malfunctioning brain stem.

Anencephaly and other open fetal defects (see the discussion of meningomyelocele) may be detected by in utero ultrasound, elevation of alpha-fetoprotein (AFP) in amniotic fluid, or elevation of alpha-fetoprotein in maternal serum. Once a fetus has been diagnosed with anencephaly, many families opt for termination of the pregnancy.

Once a family has had one fetus or child affected by any type of neural tube defect, the recurrence rate for subsequent offspring is approximately 2%–5% (Laurence, 1981). Supplementation of the maternal diet with folate before conception may help to lessen the frequency of occurrence of all types of neural tube defects, including anencephaly.

Meningomyelocele   Also known as spina bifida, meningomyelocele (see Figure 5.12) is caused by a defect in the closure of the neural tube, generally in its caudal (lower) location. Meningomyelocele may be noted on fetal ultrasound, and it may be suspected by the detection of the fetal serum protein, alpha-fetoprotein. Elevated AFP levels in the amniotic fluid and in the maternal serum may originate from an open (not skin-covered) meningomyelocele. In England in 1970, meningomyelocele and other neural tube

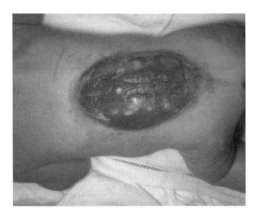

Figure 5.12. Meningomyelocele. (From Clark, D.A., private collection; reprinted by permission.)

defects occurred in 4.5 of 1,000 live births. By 1991, the occurrence rate had dropped to 0.18 of 1,000 live births (Seller, 1994). Between these two dates, two main interventions occurred that may account for the decrease. The advent of ultrasonography to detect fetal defects gave families information about their fetuses early enough that some elected to terminate the pregnancies. The use of maternal dietary periconceptional folate supplementation from at least 1 month before conception until the third month of pregnancy also was believed to have a significant role in the lower occurrence rate of neural tube defects. Folate is an important co-factor for DNA synthesis and is important in neural tube closure. Dietary folate supplementation is believed to prevent 60% of neural tube defects (MRC Vitamin Study Research Group, 1991).

Arnold-Chiari malformation is present in nearly all children with meningomyelocele. Arnold-Chiari malformation consists of elongation of the lower part of the brain stem and downward displacement of the cerebellum. The posterior fossa (back part) of the skull is shallow and crowds the brain stem, cerebellum, and fourth ventricle filled with cerebrospinal fluid, which causes herniation of cerebellar tissue into the spinal canal of the neck. As a result of the pressure on the fourth ventricle, obstruction of cerebrospinal flow to the subarachnoid space at the level of the foramen magnum occurs and leads to hydrocephalus in about 40% of the newborns with meningomyelocele. At birth, there may be increased intracranial pressure due to the Arnold-Chiari malformation, but there may be no signs of hydrocephalus initially because decompression of excess cerebrospinal fluid may occur through the open meningomyelocele into the amniotic sac. Only after surgical closure of meningomyelocele may signs of hydrocephalus ensue.

Management of meningomyelocele includes protecting the open neural tube defect from trauma, infection, and the loss of heat and fluid. This can be accomplished by placement of warm, moist, sterile pads over the lesion at the time of birth, then covering the area with a sterile plastic bag until surgical closure of the lesion is accomplished. Care should be taken to avoid trauma to the area. The sterile pads should be kept moist, as dry pads will cling to the moist neural tissue when being changed. The baby should be positioned so as not to lie directly on his lesion.

After surgical closure is accomplished, evaluation for hydrocephalus should be done. CT scan, MRI, and ultrasound all have been used for quantitation of cerebrospinal fluid volume within the ventricles over time. If hydrocephalus is present, surgical placement of a ventriculoperitoneal shunt is indicated.

Depending on the level of the meningomyelocele on the spine, affected children may have weakness or paralysis of the lower limbs; orthopedic problems, including hip dislocations; difficulty with stooling; and urinary retention. When urinary retention is present, evaluations (e.g., ultrasound, voiding cystourethrogram) may be done to determine whether hydronephrosis (i.e., excess urine collection within the kidneys) and/or vesicoureteral reflux backward from the bladder to the kidneys is present. When hydronephrosis and/or vesicoureteral reflux occur, the child is at increased risk for urinary tract infection and may benefit from daily oral antibiotic prophylaxis against infection. When urinary retention is present, it is common for the urology physician to prescribe intermittent catheterizations of the bladder every 3–4 hours to allow the urine to drain.

A long-term multidisciplinary approach is required when managing the medical and developmental needs of a child with meningomyelocele. Generally, this team includes a primary care pediatrician, a neurodevelopmentalist and/or neurologist, a urologist, an orthopedist, an occupational and/or physical therapist, and a social worker.

Hydrocephalus   Hydrocephalus refers to dilation or swelling of the cerebrospinal fluid filled ventricles within the brain. This may lead to enlargement of the head and/or bulging of the head at the anterior fontanelle (soft spot) (see Figure 5.13).

Aqueductal Stenosis   Aqueductal stenosis is the malformation responsible for the development of hydrocephalus in one third of infants with hydrocephalus apparent at birth. Some newborns with aqueductal stenosis may have no other brain malformations, but many have associated intellectual disabilities and/or brain dysfunction. One variety of aqueductal stenosis is genetically inherited in an X-linked fashion (occurring almost exclusively in males) and associated with flexion deformity of the thumbs, agenesis of the corpus callosum, and intellectual disabilities. Mean IQ scores for surviving children with aqueductal stenosis is about 70. Some patients die before they are able to have their IQs tested. Surgical management and placement of a ventriculoperitoneal shunt does not cure the defects in formation nor improve the function of the brain.

Arnold-Chiari Malformation   Nearly one third of children with hydrocephalus apparent at birth have co-existing Arnold-Chiari malformation associated with meningomyelocele. Mean IQ scores for children with meningomyelocele,

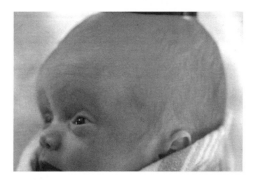

Figure 5.13.   Hydrocephalus. (From Clark, D.A., private collection; reprinted by permission.)

Arnold-Chiari malformation, and hydrocephalus is 108 (i.e., average IQ).

Dandy-Walker Malformation   Dandy-Walker malformation is responsible for 5%–10% of cases of hydrocephalus apparent at birth. Anatomically, these children have an extremely dilated, cystic fourth ventricle, absence of the cerebellar vermis, and dilation of the lateral and third ventricles. Many cases also have agenesis of the corpus callosum, defects in neuronal migration, and a variety of other brain defects.

Surgical management to control hydrocephalus involves placing a ventriculoperitoneal shunt to generally drain both the contiguous lateral and third ventricles as well as the cystic fourth ventricle. Surgical management does not cure the defects in formation nor function of the brain. Outcome is not favorable, with nearly 40% of newborns dying and 75% of survivors having intellectual disabilities. Mean IQ scores for surviving children with Dandy-Walker malformation are 45 (severely compromised).

Intrauterine Infection   Intrauterine infection may cause hydrocephalus at birth. Infection with cytomegalovirus (CMV) or the protozoa *Toxoplasma gondii* are the most likely infectious agents to cause congenital hydrocephalus. CMV is acquired by 25%–75% of children in child care settings and then brought home to family members, including non-immune women carrying vulnerable fetuses in the first and second trimester. Maternal infection may be asymptomatic or may present as a systemic illness with fever, malaise, and other symptoms. The virus then passes across the placenta from maternal circulation to fetal circulation. Gaining access to the developing fetal central nervous system, the virus causes inflammation, tissue destruction, neuronal migration disorders, and microcephaly caused by a decrease in the number of brain cells. Cerebral calcifications, chorioretinitis of the eye, progressive hearing loss, and hydrocephalus may occur.

For fetuses that are infected with CMV and have obvious neurological abnormalities, including hydrocephalus, about 95% have intellectual disabilities, cerebral palsy, deafness, seizures, and/or result in death. The mean IQ for infected, neurologically affected survivors is approximately 50–70. Treatment for CMV is suboptimal and involves long-term treatment with antiviral agents, such as acyclovir and gancyclovir. Use of these agents has been associated with modest improvement in some of the systemic findings of the disease (e.g., hypotonia, large liver) and may slow progression of hearing loss.

Treatment of hydrocephalus in children with CMV with placement of a ventriculoperitoneal shunt simply ameliorates the hydrocephalus without treating the underlying infectious disorder or central nervous system dysfunction.

Toxoplasmosis   Toxoplasmosis may also cause the development of hydrocephalus, which is apparent at birth. The *Toxoplasma gondii* parasite may be ingested by a pregnant woman in uncooked meat or may reach a pregnant woman through the feces of a house cat that consumes raw meat. Once the pregnant woman becomes infected, the organism proliferates within her blood stream, infects the placenta, and crosses the placenta to the fetal circulation. It is more common for a fetus to become infected in the third trimester than during the first or second trimester, but when infection does occur in the first or second trimester, the fetus's vulnerable developing central nervous system is at significant risk. Toxoplasmosis may cause tissue inflammation and destruction of the immature fetal nervous system, especially in the aqueductal location, which often leads to aqueductal stenosis and subsequent hydrocephalus. Systemic findings are similar to those with CMV infection.

When diagnosed during pregnancy, treatment of an infected mother–fetus pair with spiramycin, pyrimethamine, sulfadiazine, and folinic acid may have a significantly beneficial effect on the severity of the fetal infection. After birth, treatment of the infected neonate with pyrimethamine, sulfadiazine, and folinic acid has halted progressive injury of the central nervous system and may allow for some reversal of injury. Mean IQ for survivors of congenital toxoplasmosis is 89.

When hydrocephalus is present, surgical placement of a ventriculoperitoneal shunt may ameliorate the hydrocephalus, but it does not address the infectious problem or the damage already caused to the baby's brain.

Vein of Galen Malformation   Vein of Galen malformation also may cause hydrocephalus. In this condition, cerebral arteries shunt blood into a normally transient blood vessel that supplies the vein of Galen. This blood vessel dilates with cerebral blood in an aneurysmal fashion, stealing blood away from other areas of the brain. Cerebral infarctions, hemorrhagic lesions, and an intracranial mass effect may occur. The effect of the massive aneurysmal dilation may compress the aqueduct, causing hydrocephalus. In addition, these infants may have a cranial bruit (i.e., murmur) heard over the back of the head and may have severe high-output congestive heart failure because the heart does not have access to enough blood to pump efficiently to the body. Previously lethal in more than 80% of the cases, current management of vein of Galen malformation with arterial embolization of the arteries feeding the problematic vein or embolization of the vein itself using fluoroscopic or ultrasound guided catheters has led to the survival of two thirds of the children, with nearly half of the infants being neurologically typical at the time of follow-up.

Posthemorrhagic Hydrocephalus   Following an intraventricular hemorrhage, there is risk for hydrocephalus to occur. The more severe the hemorrhage, the higher the likelihood of development of hydrocephalus. The presence of blood within the ventricles may act as an irritant, causing excess production of cerebrospinal fluid. In addition, if the blood clot or any ensuing fibrous tissue obstructs the normal flow of cerebrospinal fluid, there will be an overaccumulation of fluid within the ventricles. When posthemorrhagic hydrocephalus develops, serial measurements of ventricular volume are done. Sometimes there is a temporary ventricular dilatation that resolves. Other times, the ventricles continue to accumulate excessive volume.

Therapy for Hydrocephalus   The mainstay of therapy for significant hydrocephalus is surgical placement of a ventriculoperitoneal shunt. This is a soft, sterile plastic tube placed into a distended ventricle of the brain. The other

end of the tube is tunneled under the skin and drains the extra cerebrospinal fluid into the sterile space of the abdomen, the peritoneum. When hydrocephalus occurs early in life, before the skull bones fuse to form a closed cranial compartment, the neonate's head can expand to contain a very large volume of cerebrospinal fluid. After the skull bones fuse, however, development of worsening hydrocephalus will cause the excess cerebrospinal fluid to compress the brain tissue. This development of high pressure within the skull causes poor blood delivery to the brain and adds to the risk of brain damage.

Holoprosencephaly   Failure of proper early embryonic development of the left and right cerebral hemispheres that leads to partially formed left and right hemispheres or to a cerebral cortex with one single large anterior ventricle and absence of the interhemispheric fissure is known as holoprosencephaly (see Figure 5.14). Holoprosencephaly may be associated with trisomy 13, a lethal chromosomal defect. Holoprosencephaly also may occur in the absence of a genetic abnor-

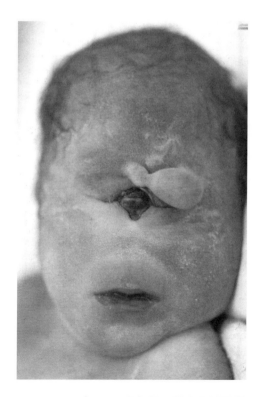

Figure 5.14.   Holoprosencephaly. (From Clark, D.A. [2000]. *Atlas of neonatology* [p. 127]. Philadelphia: W.B. Saunders; reprinted by permission.)

mality. Mid-line facial defects, such as a mid-line flattened single nostril, cleft palate, hypotelorism (eyes placed abnormally close together), or cyclopia (a single mid-line eye), are frequently associated with holoprosencephaly.

The rare child who survives is left with severe intellectual disabilities, motor deficits, and high risk for seizures due to this major brain malformation. As a result of malformation or dysfunction of the pituitary gland located in the mid-line of the brain, these children also may have hormonal problems, such as diabetes insipidus.

Conclusion

This chapter has presented information regarding the typical development of the brain and central nervous system, as well as information regarding the normal neurological examination of the newborn. It also has described aspects of atypical brain development, as well as abnormalities in brain and nervous system function due to certain insults and disease processes. The abnormalities presented here are among the more common occurring in the neonate. Many other developmental complications and abnormalities of the central nervous system may affect the newborn. These can include a variety of conditions characterized by disordered growth of brain tissue (i.e., the nerve cells or the nerve cells and supportive tissue). Developmental outcome will vary in each individual circumstance, depending on the severity and location of the lesion within the brain.

The brain and nervous system compromise a wonderfully complex network that integrates all of our bodily functions and development. Unfortunately, once serious impairment has taken place as a result of atypical development or injury, there often is little that can be done to correct the abnormality. The severity of a brain malformation or the magnitude, timing, and duration of an insult to the brain and/or neurological system and the location within the nervous system of the abnormality will have a significant impact in determining the severity of residual dysfunction. Medical and, in some instances, surgical intervention may be used to improve the well-being and developmental outcome of a young

child with a neurological disability. Ongoing work with children and their families in the form of early intervention (e.g., physical, occupational, and speech therapy; appropriate cognitive challenges; education), as well as careful periodic assessment of the progress of the child, will be critical to determine the degree of developmental disability and the nature of continuing intervention strategies to be employed to minimize the impact of such disabilities and to maximize the potential of the young child at risk.

REFERENCES

Aballi, A., & de Lamerens, S. (1962). Coagulation changes in the neonatal period and in early infancy. *Pediatric Clinics of North America, 9*, 785–817.

Alimuddin, Yoshizaki, G., Kiron, V., Satoh, S., & Taekuchi, T. (2005). Enhancement of EPA and DHA biosynthesis by over-expression of masu salmon delta6-desaturase-like gene in zebrafish. *Transgenic Research, 14*(2), 159–165.

Allen, M.C., & Capute, A.J. (1989). Neonatal neurodevelopmental examination as a predictor of neuromotor outcome in premature infants. *Pediatrics, 83*, 498–506.

Amiel-Tison, C., & Davis, S.W. (1987). Newborn neurologic examination. In A.M. Rudolph, J.I.E. Hoffman, & S. Axelrod (Eds.), *Pediatrics* (p. 126). Norwalk, CT: Appleton & Lange.

Bartocci, M., Berquist, L.L., Lagercrantz, H., & Anand, K.J. (2006). Pain activates cortical areas in the preterm newborn brain. *Pain, 122*(1–2), 109–117.

Blair, E., & Stanley, F.J. (1988). Intrapartum asphyxia: A rare cause of cerebral palsy. *Paediatrics, 112*, 515–519.

Clancy, R.R. (1997). The management of neonatal seizures. In D.K. Stevenson & P. Sunshine (Eds.), *Fetal and neonatal brain injury: Mechanisms, management, and the risks of practice* (2nd ed., p. 449). New York: Oxford University Press.

Clandinin, M.R., VanAerde, J.E., Merkel, K.L., Harris, C.L., Springer, M.A., Hansen, J.W., et al. (2005). Growth and development of preterm infants fed infant formulas containing docosahexaenoic acid and arachidonic acid. *The Journal of Pediatrics, 146*(4), 461–468.

Clark, D.A. (2000). *Atlas of neonatology.* Philadelphia: W.B. Saunders.

Coti Bertrand, P., O'Kusky, J.R., & Innis, S.M. (2006). Maternal dietary (n-3) fatty acid deficiency alters neurogenesis in the embryonic rat brain. *The Journal of Nutrition, 136*(6), 1570–1575.

Dubowitz, V. (1978). *Muscle disorders in childhood.* Philadelphia: W.B. Saunders.

Egan, D.F., Illingworth, R.S., & Mac Keith, R.C. (1971). Developmental screening 0–5 years. *Clinics in Developmental Medicine, 30*, 47. London: Spastics International Medical Publications.

Fanaroff, A.A., Wright, L.L., Stevenson, D.K., Shankaran, S., Donovan, E.F., Stoll, B.J., et al. (1995). Very-low-birth-weight outcomes of the National Institute of Child Health and Human Development Neonatal Research Network, May 1991 through December 1992. *American Journal of Obstetrics and Gynecology, 173*, 1423–1431.

Freeman, J.M., & Nelson, K.B. (1988). Intrapartum asphyxia and cerebral palsy. *Pediatrics, 82*(2), 240–249.

Green, P., Kamensky, B., & Yavin, E. (1997). Replenishment of docosahexaenoate acid in n-3 fatty acid-deficient fetal rats by intraamniotic ethyl-docosahexaenoate administration. *Journal of Neuroscience Research, 48*(3), 264–272.

Hack, M., Horbar, J.D., Malloy, M.H., Tyson, J.E., Wright, E., & Wright, L. (1991). Very low birth weight outcomes of the National Institute of Child Health and Human Development Neonatal Network. *Pediatrics, 87*, 587–597.

Hashimoto, M., Hossain, S., Agdul, H., & Shido, O. (2005). Docosahexaenoic acid-induced amelioration on impairment of memory learning in amyloid ß-infused rats relates to the decreases of amyloid ß and cholesterol levels in detergent-insoluble membrane fractions. *Biochimica et Biophysica Acta (BBA)—Molecular and Cell Biology of Lipids, 1738*(1–3), 91–98.

Heinemann, K.M., & Bauer, J.E. (2006). Docosahexaenoic acid and neurologic development in animals. *Journal of the American Veterinary Medical Association, 228*(5), 700–705.

Jensen, C.L., Voigt, R.G., Prager, T.C., Zou, Y.L., Fraley, J.K., Rozelle, J.C., et al. (2005). Effects of maternal docosahexaenoic acid intake on visual function and neurodevelopment in breastfed term infants. *The American Journal of Clinical Nutrition, 82*(1), 125–132.

Kuban, K.C.K., & Leviton, A. (1994). The epidemiology of cerebral palsy. *The New England Journal of Medicine, 330*, 188–195.

Laurence, K.M. (1981). Recurrence risk of neural tube defects (letter). *Journal of Medical Genetics, 18*(4), 322–323.

MacDonald, D. (1997). The use of intrapartum fetal heart rate monitoring to reduce perinatal asphyxia in the term infant. In D.K. Stevenson & P. Sunshine (Eds.), *Fetal and neonatal brain injury: Mechanisms, management, and the risks of practice* (2nd ed., p. 176). New York: Oxford University Press.

Manning, F.A., Morrison, I., Harman, C.R., Lange, I.R., & Menticoglou, S. (1987). Fetal assessment based on fetal biophysical profile scoring: Experience in 19,221 referred high-risk pregnancies. *American Journal of Obstetrics and Gynecology, 157*, 880.

Moore, K.L. (1988). *The developing human. Clinically oriented embryology* (4th ed., pp. 65–73). Philadelphia: W.B. Saunders.

Moore, K.L., Persaud, T.V.N., & Shiota, K. (1994). *Color atlas of clinical embryology* (p. 17). Philadelphia: W.B. Saunders.

MRC Vitamin Study Research Group. (1991). Prevention of neural tube defects: Results of the Medical Research Council Vitamin Study. *Lancet, 338*(8760), 131–137.

Naeye, R.L., Peters, E.C., Bartholomew, M., & Landis, J.R. (1989). Origins of cerebral palsy. *American Journal of Diseases of Children, 143*, 1154–1161.

Nelson, K.B., & Ellenberg, J.H. (1979). Neonatal signs as predictors of cerebral palsy. *Pediatrics, 64*, 225–232.

Nelson, K.B., & Ellenberg, J.H. (1981). Apgar scores as predictors of chronic neurologic disability. *Pediatrics, 68*(1), 36–44.

Saint-Anne Dargassies, S. (1966). Neurological maturation of the premature infant of 28–41 weeks' gestational age. In F. Falkner (Ed.), *Human development*. Philadelphia: W.B. Saunders.

Seller, M.J. (1994). Risks in spina bifida. *Developmental Medicine and Child Neurology, 36*(11), 1021–1025.

Sheth, R.D. (1998). Trends in incidence and severity of intraventricular hemorrhage. *Journal of Child Neurology, 13*(6), 261–264.

Tam, O., & Innis, S.M. (2006). Dietary polyunsaturated fatty acids in gestation alter fetal cortical phospholipids, fatty acids and phosphatidylserine synthesis. *Developmental Neuroscience, 28*(3), 222–229.

Volpe, J.J. (2000). *Neurology of the newborn* (4th ed.). Philadelphia: W.B. Saunders.

Xiang, M., Harbige, L.S., & Zetterstrom, R. (2005). Long-chain polyunsaturated fatty acids in Chinese and Swedish mothers: Diet, breast milk and infant growth. *Acta Paediatrica, 94*(11), 1543–1549.

Yavin, E. (2006). Versatile roles of docosahexaenoic acid in the prenatal brain: From pro- and anti-oxidant features to regulation of gene expression. *Prostaglandins, Leukotrienes and Essential Fatty Acids, 75*(3), 203–211.

CHAPTER 6

Performance Assessment

NEW CONNECTIONS AND FUTURE PERSPECTIVES

Gail L. Ensher

At the conclusion of this chapter, the reader will

- *Understand the differences between developmental outcomes of extremely premature and moderately premature infants*

- *Understand the importance of developmental follow-up of premature infants*

- *Be knowledgeable about developmental markers of concern in infants, toddlers, and preschool children*

- *Be familiar with new trends in assessing infants and young children with disabilities and at developmental risk*

- *Be familiar with qualities of best practice in assessing infants and young children*

This chapter addresses the issue of developmental outcomes, focusing on the importance of developmental follow-up. It covers current procedures for follow-up, as well as best practice issues for assessment of young children with disabilities.

The Need for Follow-Up within the Context of Developmental Outcome

Key findings from the Centers for Disease Control and Prevention (CDC) and National Center for Health Statistics (2007) reveal the following data on trends in the United States regarding birth rate, rates of prematurity, birth rates for teenagers, childbearing by women in their 30s and 40s, and birth rates by race and ethnicity.

- A preliminary estimate of births in 2005 was 4,140,419, an increase of 1% from the statistics of 2004.

- Births rose for Hispanic, American Indian or Alaska Native, Asian or Pacific Islander, and non-Hispanic black women, but declined slightly for non-Hispanic white women.

- The preterm birth rate rose from 12.5% to 12.7% for 2004–2005. The percentage of infants delivered at less than 37 weeks of gestation has risen 20% since 1990 (from 10.6 %). Preterm rates rose significantly for non-Hispanic white (11.7 % for 2005), non-Hispanic black (18.4%), and Hispanic (12.1%) infants between 2004 and 2005. Rates for non-Hispanic white and Hispanic births have been rising for more than a decade, increasing 38% for non-Hispanic white and 10% for Hispanic infants since 1990. The preterm rate for black infants declined modestly during the 1990s, but has been on the rise since the year 2000.

- The proportion of all infants born very preterm (less than 32 weeks of gestation) rose slightly between 2004 and 2005 (from 2.01% to 2.03%). Late preterm births (34–36 weeks) increased more markedly from 8.9% to 9.1% for the same period.

- All measures of childbearing by unmarried women increased to record levels in the United States in 2005. These statistics were evident despite a decline in birth rate for teenagers of 2% in 2005, which fell to 40.4 births per 1,000 women age 15–19 years, a 35% drop compared with the most recent peak in 1991.

With marked technological advances and individualized developmental care in neonatal intensive care units, both survival rates and developmental outcomes of preterm infants have improved dramatically. Browne wrote,

> Thanks to improvements in medical and technological intervention, infants born at 23–26 weeks, who usually weigh between 500 and 750 grams, have a 40%–60% chance of survival. Babies born at 27–28 weeks (about 750–1,000 grams) have approximately an 85% chance of survival. . . . As the pregnancy goes on, survival rates increase dramatically, so that almost all infants born at 34 weeks or later survive. Unfortunately, survival alone does not ensure a premature baby's health or typical development. Premature infants continue to face a significant risk of severe neurodevelopmental problems, including major, permanent neurosensory impairments; cognitive and language delays; motor deficits; neurobehavioral and socioemotional problems; and learning disabilities. . . . Rates among preemies of permanent neurosensory deficits such as cerebral palsy, mental retardation, and hearing or visual impairments have not decreased substantially in recent years. (2003, pp. 5–6)

In light of what we now know about medical and developmental outcome, follow-up of premature and otherwise compromised newborns continues to be a critical component to best practice of early identification and intervention. It is well-documented that infants and young children change dramatically as they develop during the first months of life, the toddler years, and the preschool years. Furthermore, although some children may have experienced high-risk medical histories or been exposed to a continuum of adverse environmental events, it still remains a difficult task to predict future performance and learning outcomes. For instance, it is not uncommon for children to demonstrate sleeper effects in which they may appear to be functioning within typical ranges at one point, but then reveal problematic development later.

Clearly, as noted by Browne (2003), extremely low birth weights of less than 1,000 grams and gestations of 23–28 weeks place infants at much greater risk for later developmental and behavior problems (Als, Butler, Kosta, & McAnulty, 2005; Anderson, Doyle, & Victorian Infant Collaborative Study Group, 2004; Aylward, 2002; Hack et al., 2004; Hoekstra, Ferrara, Couser, Payne, & Connett, 2004; Horbar et al., 2002; O'Shea, 2002; Vohr et al., 2000). Bennett (1999) has indicated that the major neurodevelopmental problems associated with prematurity continue to surface as cerebral palsy (in particular, spastic diplegia), intellectual disabilities, sensorineural hearing loss, and visual impairment as a result of retinopathy of prematurity (ROP) and myopia. Such problems usually are evident by 2 years of age, and are two to five times more frequently seen in extremely low birth weight infants versus full-term infants. At the same time, it is important to acknowledge that development is not a uniform process. Not infrequently, young children with significant birth histories may do surprisingly well if given the benefit of enriched home environments, whereas those with much less severe medical histories ultimately have significant behavioral and academic difficulties for a number of reasons. In addition, children born between 32 and 37 weeks of gestation, as a result of various environmental, genetic, or neurological factors, may present a range of other learning, attention, or less severe pervasive developmental disorders once they begin school that place them at risk for achieving academic success. Accordingly, Bennett wrote:

> Although major disabling sequelae are by far the easiest to quantify and report, a large and persuasive body of long-term follow-up studies clearly indicates that a broad spectrum of cognitive, behavioral, and other minor neurodevelopmental and neurobehavioral sequelae are substantially more

prevalent in surviving LBW, premature infants. These morbidities become increasingly apparent in a variety of clinical manifestations with increasing age, particularly during the first 6 years of life. These early, often subtle, developmental and behavioral delays and differences are not necessarily outgrown but frequently portend future school dysfunction and may therefore become major impediments to normal academic and social progress. Collectively, these problems often are referred to as the "new morbidity" of prematurity, reflecting their more insidious nature and more intense scrutiny in recent years. (1999, p. 1487)

Prematurity in combination with less advantageous home environments is especially noteworthy and may be devastating in terms of later school performance.

Although recent environmental changes in neonatal intensive care units in the United States have had a positive impact on the development of preterm newborns, infants born at earlier gestational ages (i.e., at or less than 32 weeks) and/or lower birth weights (less than 1,000 grams) overall look very different from preterm babies delivered closer to full term and weighing more than 1,500 grams. Not unlike their full-term counterparts, preterm infants demonstrate well-documented variability in their patterns of neuromotor development, temperament, social and/or behavioral interactions, and the acquisition of other early milestones. However, neonates born prior to 32 weeks gestation often are hypotonic initially, with an extended persistence of asymmetries and newborn reflexes, such as the startle response or Moro reflex up to 6 months of age. Yet, milestones such as rolling over and reaching, which typically are evident between 3 and 4 months, may be delayed well beyond the 5th or 6th month, and independent sitting may not be seen in some infants until the 8th, 9th, or 10th month.

Extremely low birth weight infants tend to be much less responsive in terms of their interactions; for example, parents and caregivers frequently report their baby shutting down, avoiding eye contact, and being very difficult to soothe. Although full-term babies begin to develop genuine social smiles in response to the primary individuals in their families within the first 2 months of life, it may be well into the 4th

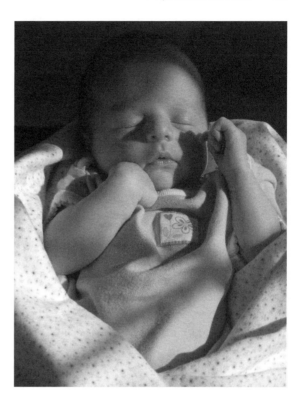

month before parents of some preterm infants are able to elicit such mutually satisfying interactions. Similarly, feeding by bottle or breast for the extremely low birth weight or early-for-dates newborn may be a slow and somewhat painstaking process for parents who are understandably concerned about weight gain and nutrition after hospital discharge. The sucking response does not develop until the 32nd week of gestation, and, therefore, in micropreterm (i.e., infants weighing less than 800 grams) newborns sucking and eating by mouth may continue to be an issue. Furthermore, these extremely low birth weight babies may seem to catch up in some developmental areas during the course of the first 18 months of life, but then display delays in other domains (e.g., receptive and expressive language) that need to be addressed.

Although there have been numerous debates about corrected or adjusted age, it is clear that for extended periods of time, extremely low birth weight infants continue to manifest significant delays beyond what is expected within the ranges of typical development. Consequently, careful periodic follow-up and developmental surveillance during the first 5–8 years among se-

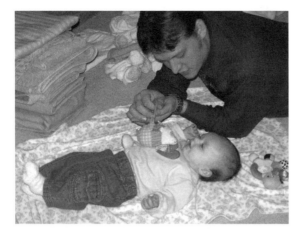

verely preterm children are a critical component of best practice in early childhood.

Infants born between 34 and 37 weeks are less worrisome in terms of their developmental outcomes (Bennett, 1999). Similar to the growth and development of more severely preterm neonates, outcomes for these moderately premature babies are influenced by many biological and environmental considerations. However, typically, initial delays are not as significant or long lasting, although longer term prognoses tend to be somewhat conflicting. Given the nature of development, often more subtle learning and behavioral concerns may not become issues until young children enter school when academic skills and concepts call upon more complex processing abilities. Thus, although follow-up efforts should not be so overzealous as to become self-fulfilling prophecies, it is important to be vigilant so that problems can be addressed as early as possible. Relative to the domain of language development, for example, Ensher and Clark wrote:

> The point at which an early intervention program should be initiated is a difficult clinical judgment. Professionals should not overreact, and certainly if a toddler is beginning to use even a few familiar words appropriately at about 20 months, there is justification for cautious expectations that the child will achieve a normal range of performance by 3 years. Such hopes probably are warranted if delays are uncomplicated by symptoms of excessive drooling, feeding difficulties, tongue thrusting, hearing impairment, or other obvious abnormalities. On the other hand, if a child appears frustrated in not being able to communicate, does not appear to

understand what is said, and lacks a minimal level of intelligible expressive language of a few words, assistance before age 3 is indicated. There are, of course, differing points of view on these issues, some professionals taking a conservative approach and merely waiting. We differ with this position because language is so crucial to later learning and school performance. If the cooperation of parents can be enlisted in the face of early developmental lags, problems frequently can be ameliorated or at least greatly minimized. We have seen dramatic changes in young children born at risk, given the benefit of formal programming and family support. (1994, p. 74)

Parents as Partners in the Assessment Process

Recent developments in early childhood assessment have emphasized the importance of parents and primary caregivers as partners in the evaluation of their young children (Ensher et al., 2007; Linder, 1993; Meisels, 2001; Meisels, Dombro, Marsden, & Weston, 2004; Provence, Erikson, Vater, & Palmeri, 1995; Turnbull, Turnbull, Erwin, & Soodak, 2006). For several reasons, this has been a new central perspective in the field of early childhood special education and developmental follow-up. Too often, families have been left on the fringes of assessment and only consulted at the end of the process after results have been discussed and final recommendations generated.

Although it seems to be a cliché, families do know their children best. They are invaluable reporters who can validate observations and results of the evaluation, confirming whether or not child behavior noted by team members is representative of typical daily routines and best performance. This dimension of assessment is essential in light of the fact that infants and young children often are seen initially in unnatural and unfamiliar environments outside of their own homes, schools, or educational settings and with unfamiliar people. Temperament, language, and a child's social-emotional behaviors are especially susceptible to such changes in the environment. For example, despite the abilities of very experienced professionals, it is not unusual for teams to spend a significant amount of time on a visit with a very quiet child only to observe that child beginning to interact playfully and communicatively with a familiar caregiver just as they are preparing to leave the home or are walking down a school hallway to an exit. In the absence of the parent or primary caregiver, such behaviors may not be revealed until a much later point, if at all. Parent perspectives need to be affirmed and placed at the heart of the evaluation of their young children in terms of both validation of the information gathered and recognition of priorities they share for the future development of their sons or daughters.

Additional factors need to be taken into consideration in the evaluation of young children. In Chapter 1, we discussed the growing diversity of different ethnic groups, cultures, and income levels across the United States. In the face of these demographic changes, professionals often find themselves in situations where they are challenged to evaluate children outside their own home-based cultures and historical points of view (Ensher et al., 2007; Hanson & Lynch, 2004). Respectively, issues on both sides of the evaluation may be encountered as follows:

• Families may have culture-specific views of disability and children with special needs (Lynch & Hanson, 2004). In response, professionals must be knowledgeable about this diversity of perspectives because they likely will affect the building of future relationships with individual family members.

• Families from different ethnic and cultural backgrounds may not share our views and beliefs about the importance of early intervention. In response, professionals must be respectful of such differences in the name of helpfulness and service.

• Families may have priorities and goals for their children that vary a great deal from those identified by professionals. In response, professionals need to start where families are, begin with family goals, and work toward mutual objectives on behalf of the child.

• Families easily can become lost in the terminology and jargon of testing results. In response, professionals need to use simple language, may need to utilize the services of interpreters to avoid confusion and miscommunication, and must be willing to explain in multiple ways for understanding.

• Professionals must be able to differentiate language differences from communication disorders in young children where English is not the primary spoken language at home. Not infrequently, differences have been mistakenly identified as disorders (Ensher et al., 2007). Professionals need to take the time to sort out the distinctions between difference and disorder in terms of the child's primary spoken language.

• Finally, families challenged by poverty may be particularly distrustful of the system as a result of painful prior experiences. As always, it is important for professionals to focus on the strengths of the family, listen, and bring to the table a positive and nonjudgmental approach that will open doors to communication and interaction.

Each of these issues underscores the importance of authentic relationship building early in the assessment process and the need for shared decision making (Turnbull et al., 2006). In the absence of this kind of trust and reciprocity, any intervention and programming on behalf of the child will likely be less than fully realized.

Beyond Eligibility: Linking Assessment to Intervention

Translated into best practice, assessment and early intervention with young children should be seamless and ongoing processes. To accomplish this goal, several pathways need to be explored, including consideration of the assessment instruments used, flexibility of administration, the settings or environments where evaluations take place, scheduling, persons who participate in the initial and annual review evaluations, and

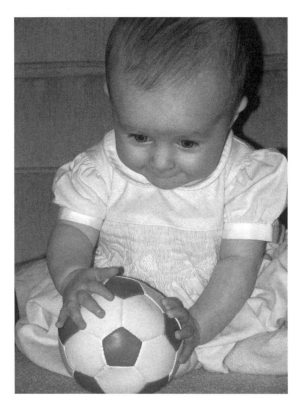

ways in which assessment information then is infused into strategies for programming and family intervention. In combination, all of these elements move far beyond the more limited parameters of establishing initial eligibility for services, which historically has been the primary focus in the evaluation arena.

In all of its phases, evaluation of young children is complex and consists of multiple steps that need to be individualized for families and children. Unfortunately, this often has not been the case. Professionals frequently have selected instruments with which they are most familiar and comfortable, and one blueprint of assessments, schedules, people, and settings then becomes the template for all. Although such routines are favorable in the interest of professional time and decision making, they too often are not tailored to the everyday commitments and responsibilities that families face. Furthermore, and equally important, they may not represent best practices in terms of children and the determination of their optimal performance.

With principles of best practice in mind, evaluation processes linked to intervention and

programming consist of several stages. At a minimum, these include planning, evaluation, and a final stage of postassessment. Although these phases are uniform in some respects, the ways in which they are carried out should vary from family to family.

Planning

The planning phase establishes the context for the child's and family's evaluation. During this time, the team meets and reviews reasons for the referral, previous reports, and any other available pertinent information. Professional roles are assigned for speaking with the family, and additional special considerations, such as the need for interpreters or translators, are addressed. Paperwork may be sent to the family in advance of the first meeting; however, this information always should be reviewed when team members and the family sit together face to face. It is not unusual for teams to discover that initial reasons for referral on paper constitute only part of the complexity of problems, which are later revealed during the evaluation.

The roles of the individuals who will speak with the family in person, work with the child, and carry out observations are designated during this initial phase. An arena approach for assessing the child also may be used. In this case, one individual whose discipline most addresses the child's primary area of challenge is selected to serve as the main facilitator or examiner, whereas other members of the team observe. For preschool children, family members should be included in the plans for the assessment and asked to sit next to the child or actually participate in aspects of the evaluation as needed and appropriate. For older children, kindergarten through 8 years, the format may vary. As part of the planning stage for this age group, families are less likely to be considered part of the actual assessment process, although if English as a second language is an issue, they should be present and a translator should be available to the child.

During the planning phase, the team will need to make decisions about the number of people physically present during the actual evaluation and other aspects of the assessment. For instance, some children are easily distracted and limiting the number of team members will be an important consideration for helping the child to focus on tasks and activities at hand. In addition, depending on the child's areas of need, particular specialists in the areas of speech-language development, physical and occupational therapy, pediatrics, as well as psychologists and teachers may need to see the child on a more individual basis or in group settings. Accordingly, plans for these various scenarios should be adapted for the child. If families are not physically present with the child during the evaluation, it is advantageous to make provisions for them to observe sessions with a team member so that the process of evaluation can be described and any questions answered.

Another important aspect of planning is the selection of appropriate data-gathering instruments. Decisions about such measures will depend on several considerations including the chronological or adjusted age of the child; areas of suspected delay; anticipated behavioral and performance challenges during the assessment; utility for recording family information; the breadth of developmental, functional, and learning areas covered by the instruments; and the flexibility and adaptability of instruments in various settings and situations. As McLean (2004) pointed out, historically "psychometric traditions" (i.e., using norm referenced evaluation instruments) have dominated the field of assessment of children with disabilities. More recently, however, recognition of the centrality of family-centered practice, the need for collaboration among team members, the importance of natural environments (McLean, 2004), and the relevance of measures for programming have greatly influenced precedence of the past. Attention to the latter concern among early childhood special educators, in particular, has increased the use of curriculum- and criterion-based measures.

Finally, settings and scheduling for the assessment need to be determined during the planning phase. For families and very young children, there are no substitutes for home visits where social history information can be verified and initial contact made to begin to establish re-lationships. If the child is attending a preschool program, kindergarten, or the primary grades, visits to these settings will also need to be set up for the team and decisions made as to who will be making these visits. In addition, the team will need to confirm a schedule of visits for the administration of the child-focused developmental and performance-based measures. This approach to serial assessment for the initial evaluation realistically provides for information gathering in a variety of settings with different people and offers a broader, more ecological picture of the child within the context of his or her family over time, rather than basing decisions on single opportunity sessions.

In summary, Bagnato, Neisworth, and Munson described the multiple purposes of assessment as follows:

> The various assessment procedures and the purposes they address (i.e., screening/identification, comprehensive assessment/curriculum referencing, program planning/intervention, progress monitoring/program evaluation) should all be included and be connected to one another. Each procedure/purpose in this sequence serves as a prerequisite for the one it precedes, and, as the sequence proceeds, it becomes increasingly fine-focused: Screening provides only a gross estimate of a child's status; children are assigned to one of two categories—those with problems that merit further examination and those without problems. Comprehensive assessment yields a finer, more detailed analysis. This level of assessment provides direction and items for tying assessment measures to curricula and for planning programs. Next, program planning guides the actual day-to-day content and methods of a program. Because planning is attached to comprehensive assessment, professionals are able to design goals and objectives that are feasible for use in a given program. Finally, a child's progress and a program's efficacy are evaluated on the basis of whether and to what extent developmental and behavioral goals are achieved. To summarize, multiple-purpose assessment may be used to assess a child's development, place that child in an appropriate setting, plan a program, monitor the child's progress, and evaluate the program impact. (1997, pp. 21–22)

The authors went on to say, "Proponents of authentic assessments for children with special needs advocate the design of individualized as-

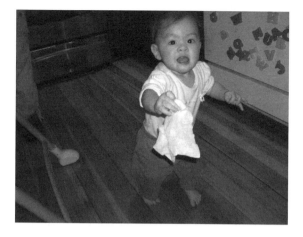

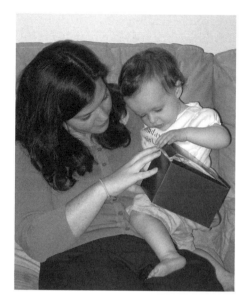

sessment strategies that receive high marks for being performance based, authentic, and connected to instruction" (1997, p. 27).

Evaluation

Sometimes it is just as instructive to learn what we should do by observing the consequences of what not to do (as demonstrated in the following vignette) when spending time with families and evaluating young children.

Some weeks ago I happened to meet a graduate student, Shaen, who was enrolled in a clinical course on assessment of young children. He stopped to chat for a few minutes, concerned about what he had observed earlier in the week during an evaluation of a child who had been referred to an excellent preschool local program. He noted that the young child of approximately 4 years of age had been separated from his mother for a psychological evaluation. The child had not appeared troubled by this separation; however, his mother had been left in an empty hallway by herself for more than an hour. Prior to the school-based session, she had been concerned about her son's possible delays and impending diagnosis. By the time various team members had returned to speak with her, she was on the verge of tears.

Even the best programs make unfortunate decisions in this less than perfect world, but professionals always need to be mindful of the fact

that the child must be seen within the context of the family, who should not be left on the sidelines. Under optimal conditions, assessment of their young children is stressful for parents and caregivers. Thus, in the interests of all concerned, it is important to make every effort to assess within natural contexts. The best information will be gathered from the family and while working with the child.

The evaluation phase includes data collection along two dimensions. One involves the family as the reporter and caregiver of their child. The second entails the use of diverse measures and strategies for determining the child's challenges and strengths in various developmental and learning areas of behavior and performance. These areas of evaluation will depend largely on the age and performance levels of the child referred. For the family, team members should be sensitive to a number of questions across all age levels during the assessment processes including:

- What are the caregivers' or parents' main concerns about their child?

- What are the caregivers' or parents' priorities for their family and child?

- What educational supports and resources would make life easier for the family?

- If the family and child have been involved in an educational program, what services have they been receiving and are the parents satisfied? Have there been any concerns relating to transition to subsequent programs?

- If the child participates in an educational program, are there differences in behavior that have been noted between home and school? If so, what are they?

- If English is a second language for the family and child, has this difference in communication and culture been an issue or concern for either the family or for the child?

A thorough family and child social history is the first step in the evaluation process and should precede any formal assessment of the child. Although one person of the team usually takes the lead in interacting with the caregivers or parents, other members of the team should feel free to join in the discussion and take notes during this stage of the evaluation. Often families have made valuable observations during the course of daily living and interacting with their child; they may not have a name for the behaviors that they have seen, but it is likely that they can describe in detail the challenges and strengths.

The next part of the evaluation—actual interaction with the child—needs to be carried out in different settings, with different people, and with different strategies for gathering data over a brief period of time. This approach to serial assessment should help the team to determine the following:

- Differences in the child's patterns of interaction with familiar (i.e., family members) and unfamiliar persons

- Levels of assistance that facilitate the child's learning and positive behavior

- Developmental and instructional areas that are strengths for the child

- Developmental and instructional areas that are more challenging for the child

- Settings that are conducive to the child's best performance and learning (e.g., unstructured versus less structured)

- Quality of the child's responses to various play and instructional activities

- Strategies for communicating (e.g., augmentative systems versus verbal expressive language)

With very young children, often developmental areas overlap and clearly defined distinctions are difficult to make. Thus, information that is descriptive and that relates directly to instructional purposes is extremely helpful. In addition, norm-referenced measures are much less reliable with children of very young ages in which temperament, sensory issues, and the nature of the behavior sampled, among others, have a major impact on performance and testing results (McLean, Wolery, & Bailey, Jr., 2004; Salvia, Ysseldyke, & Bolt, 2007). Often, identifying primary areas of challenge and strength for infants and young children can be facilitated by examining clusters of items and activities across measures; observed behaviors that are confirmed by parent report; areas of development that are more resistant to change over time versus areas of greater growth; areas where the child's behavior changes during the course of assessment and the child requires more effort; and, finally, the child's processing abilities with different kinds of stimuli and information. Furthermore, teams should always be mindful of the fact that even when young children display multiple areas of delay, they likewise have domains of relative strength that are important to define for programming. Clinically astute student assessment teams with multiple disciplines can sort out these complex puzzles with infants and young children as they work in partnership with families.

Children ages 5–9 years are more stable in their profiles of performance and, with appropriate assessment modifications, learning and behavior can be sampled more authentically with a variety of strategies that focus on prereadiness and academic content. Among the numerous data collection possibilities, there are appropriate norm-referenced instruments, curriculum- and criterion-based instruments, teacher- and clinician-made assessments, parent report, direct classroom and home observations, and student portfolios (Salvia, Ysseldyke, & Bolt, 2007). A detailed discussion of the myriad strategies and instruments that are available and ever expanding is beyond the scope of this text; however, teams responsible for evaluating children in kindergarten, first, and second grade and/or children between the ages of 5 and 9 years need to keep in mind the following guidelines when selecting assessments.

- Strategies need to be sensitive to diverse cultures and children who are learning English as a second language.

- Strategies should be connected directly to educational programming.

- Strategies must include parent or caregiver priorities.

- Strategies should include a variety of measures across content and behavioral domains targeted to answer questions of learning and performance.

- Strategies must include adequate adaptations for the child so that they are valid in terms of the content and behavior sampled.

- Assessment information needs to be reliable across multiple observers, team members, and parents.

Assessment of young children is a complex task, at best, and controversies concerning how best to evaluate students for initial eligibility purposes undoubtedly always will exist. As Salvia, Ysseldyke, and Bolt (2007) point out, children may be eligible for special education in one state, but not in another. Ultimately, best practices will be achieved when we are able to determine educational needs of a given child, to the extent possible, within the context of the regular curriculum. Assessment is a given in today's standards-based system of accountability, and children with special needs are a part of that system. To deny certain populations of children opportunities afforded their peers is exclusionary. However, new visions of the assessment process must be focused more centrally on concepts of optimal performance and growth rather than the traditional deficit-oriented models. Finding those fine lines between eligibility guidelines, diagnosis, and longer term services that are flexible and

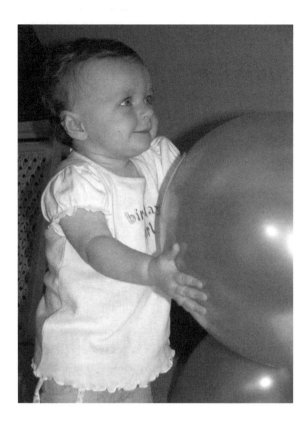

open to change is a charge that all educators share on behalf of young children and their families.

Postassesment

The postevaluation phase subsequently is focused on conferencing among members of the assessment team and parents and on developing recommendations that are based on respective state guidelines. These legislative requirements, established at the federal level, vary by age, by lead funding agency, and by state-stipulated bases for eligibility. For example, the term *infant or toddler with a disability*

(A) means an individual under 3 years of age who needs early intervention services because the individual: (i) is experiencing developmental delays, as measured by appropriate diagnostic instruments and procedures in one or more of the areas of cognitive development, physical development, communication development, social or emotional development, and adaptive development; or (ii) has a diagnosed physical or mental condition which has a high probability of resulting in developmental delay; and

(B) may also include, at a state's discretion, at-risk infants and toddlers. The term "at-risk infant or toddler" means an individual under 3 years of age who would be at risk of experiencing a substantial developmental delay if early intervention services were not provided to the individual. (Shackelford, 2005, pp. 1–15)

Eligibility for the preschool and primary age child (3–9 years), however, is defined as follows by categories of disability:

(A) The term "child with disability" means a child (i) with mental retardation, hearing impairments (including deafness), speech or language impairments, visual impairments (including blindness), serious emotional disturbance (hereinafter referred to as "emotional disturbance"), orthopedic impairments, autism, traumatic brain injury, other health impairments, or specific learning disabilities; and (ii) who, by reason thereof, needs special education and related services. (B) Child aged 3 through 9— The term "child with a disability" for a child aged 3 through 9 may, at the discretion of the State and the local educational agency, include a child (i) experiencing developmental delays, as defined by the State and as measured by appropriate diagnostic instruments and procedures, in one or more of the following areas: physical development, cognitive development, communication development, social or emotional development, or adaptive development; and (ii) who, by reason thereof, needs special education and related services. (Muller & Markowitz, 2004, p. 87)

Respectively, for infants and toddlers from birth through 2 years who qualify for services, initial plans subject to periodic review are spelled out in the form of individualized family service plans (IFSPs). Likewise, for young children between the ages of 3 and 9 years who qualify for services, initial plans periodically revisited are developed as individualized education programs (IEPs).

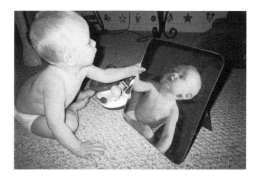

Decisions as to whether children qualify for services and the respective generation of plans for future programming are made jointly among team members that represent various disciplines. In the spirit of best practice, these decisions should be accomplished in partnership with families who ultimately are most responsible for carrying out these recommendations in collaboration with future service providers. The time of day for services, the place where they occur (home, child care, and/or school), the number of visits by professionals, the nature of the classroom environment (e.g., inclusive or least restrictive), the need for one-to-one program aides, participation in community programs, family support services, and further developmental and neurological evaluations are just a part of several dimensions that may be important for families and their young children. Bailey (2004) has described this partnership in the decision-making process as follows:

The family assessment process has as its ultimate goal the identification of family resources, priorities, and concerns so that early intervention and preschool programs can be tailored to individual family needs and desires for services. In striving to achieve this goal, the strategies by which family assessment information is gathered ought to foster a trusting relationship between parents and professionals and help families feel confident in their roles as team members and parents. Ample research suggests that programs are not providing the full array of family services, that parents want such services (DeGangi, Royeen, & Wietlisbach, 1992; Mahoney, O'Sullivan, & Dennebaum, 1990), and that parents are frustrated when services are provided in a way that ignores the other demands of family life or fails to consider how intervention efforts fit into family routines and environments (Brotherson & Goldstein, 1992). Family assessment can identify the kinds of services or resources parents want so that programs can become more responsive. . . . The key is for families to be involved in the assessment and planning process, and for them to feel that their opinions have been valued and their concerns heard. (pp. 196–197)

Postconference meetings are only part of the initial evaluation phase. If a child qualifies for services, assessment across developmental and performance areas then becomes an ongoing process of annual updates of child progress. This process, conducted with multiple disciplines, thus becomes the companion basis for program change and development. In summary, most effective evaluations are coupled with counterpart intervention strategies.

The Need to See Children and Families in Their Natural Environments

Funding, convenience of scheduling, time limitations, centrality of location, age of the child, and family preference are a few of the factors that affect decisions about evaluation sites. As young children move from infancy into the preschool years and then to kindergarten and the early primary grades, both families and professionals traditionally have selected settings for assessment that are situated in school-based locations. Although such decisions may be more appropriate for older students, there is no substitute for seeing young children in natural situations of home, in larger groups with age-appropriate peers, and in individual one-to-one events. For instance, it is important for future programming to know how children interact with various family members, how well children are able to focus and attend in smaller versus larger groups, how children relate to their peers versus adults, and how children relate to familiar and unfamiliar persons. Such information can be garnered only by seeing chil-

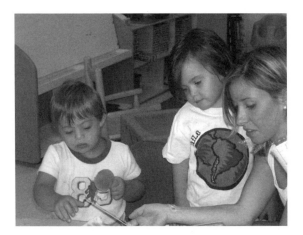

dren across multiple, authentic situations and settings. Furthermore, if children are learning English as a second language, time and familiar settings will offer professionals an advantage toward establishing comfort levels for both young children and their families.

In an insightful article entitled *Fusing Assessment and Intervention: Changing Parents' and Providers' Views of Young Children*, Meisels elaborated on new visions for the assessment of young children as follows:

> Several features or criteria that are common to performance assessment are potentially of great value to the assessment of very young children with special needs. . . . including 1) documenting children's daily activities as well as their initiative and creativity; 2) providing an integrated means to evaluate the quality of children's performance and behavior; 3) reflecting an individualized approach to intervention; 4) evaluating those elements of learning and development that most conventional assessments do not capture; 5) utilizing the information acquired in the intervention to further elaborate the evaluative picture of the children that is emerging from the assessment; and 6) focusing the caregiver's attention and activity away from the typical content of test-taking and onto the learning of the child and the environment in which intervention is taking place. (2001, p. 6)

In the closing discussion to this article, Meisels wrote:

> A final implication of this dynamic view of assessment is that our interventions as well as our assessments must be multi-dimensional. We will learn very little about a child's skills, approaches to learning, areas of strength, or areas of weakness if the intervention model in use is narrow and one-dimensional. If our goal is to create a responsive, performance-based system of assessment and intervention that has beneficial effects on development, then it is critical that the interventions and the assessments reflect common values based on knowledge of optimal child and family functioning. . . . Assessments today must include active participation of the child's family, information about the broad context in which the child and family live, varied methods of collecting assessment data, and intervention-relevant applications of assessment data. Only in this way can we expect assessments to advance our goal of helping all children and families reach their potential—the highest stakes goal of all. (2001, p. 10)

Fading Models

Ensher and Clark (1994) echo similar themes in their discussion of assessing infants and preschool children within a family context. Referencing traditions of the past, they likewise advocate new visions that depart from the historically dominant approaches of evaluating young children and their families. They wrote:

> In recent years, much research on infant and preschool assessment has concentrated on more natural approaches, whereas developmental evaluation in pediatrics and education has continued to rely heavily on standardized, traditional practices. Frequently, the screening and assessment of young children have been based on brief visits, with parent and child in strange situations, with unfamiliar professionals, under sometimes strained and difficult circumstances. The net result has been a less than optimal response from caregiver and child. Moreover, formal assessment has historically almost always involved standardized instruments, sometimes informal measures, and rarely systematic data-based observations. Ideally, best practice in evaluation combines all three techniques, and this strategy is now receiving greater recognition in the various fields of developmental and child psychology, as well as in the clinical-educational disciplines.
>
> It is important to identify and describe a child's characteristics in relation to those including the substantial basic information that is most closely related to the planning and implementation process; e.g., the quality of responses.
>
> Unfortunately, with few exceptions, traditional approaches to infant and preschool evaluation have assumed a unidimensional rather than a problem-solving model of behavior and learning. For instance, while many norm-referenced tests and scales have included diverse items for motor, language, cognitive, and behavioral development, rarely do they provide tasks for observation within the context of varying situations of social interaction with familiar and unfamiliar persons, the use of familiar and unfamiliar materials, and the use of alternative testing procedures and modalities for response. Moreover, parallel information about home and school environments that might confirm or invalidate test findings and expand on test results with the soliciting of caregiver input has seldom been pursued, because of the exclusive adoption of more traditional practice and intelligence testing. Experience and expertise with vulnerable and developmentally disabled young populations consistently show strong evidence that all of the variables we have discussed deeply affect the quality of responsiveness of such children and that, without planned variability and a more natural setting for assessment, many youngsters are severely penalized. (pp. 210–213)

Conclusion

In conclusion, we would like to emphasize the following in terms of best practices in assessing young children with disabilities:

- All aspects of evaluation in the early years must reflect interactions of child, family, professional, and setting.

- Methodology and process need to be guided less by individual preference, availability, and ideology and more by an understanding of immediate problems and dynamics.

- In the least, measures should include means toward assessing child endurance, temperament, various dimensions of play, attention-gaining and self-calming abilities, responsiveness to new tasks and unfamiliar situations, unstructured discovery and spontaneous activity, levels of frustration, and primary modes of communication.

- Finally strategies need to embrace the goal of achieving a more natural, integrated, and flexible approach to evaluation.

REFERENCES

Als, H., Butler, S., Kosta, S., & McAnulty, G. (2005). The assessment of preterm infants' behavior (APIB): Furthering the understanding and measurement of neurodevelopmental competence in preterm and full-term infants. *Mental Retardation and Developmental Disabilities Research Reviews, 11,* 94–102.

Anderson, P.J., Doyle, L.W., & Victorian Infant Collaborative Study Group. (2004). Executive functioning in school-aged children who were born very preterm or with extremely low birth weight in the 1990s. *Pediatrics, 114,* 50–57.

Aylward, G.P. (2002). Cognitive and neuropsychological outcomes: More than IQ scores. *Mental Retardation and Developmental Disabilities Research Reviews, 8,* 234–240.

Bagnato, S.J., Neisworth, J.T., & Munson, S.M. (1997). *LINKing assessment and early intervention: An au-*

thentic curriculum-based approach. Baltimore: Paul H. Brookes Publishing Co.

Bailey, D.B., Jr. (2004). Assessing family resources, priorities, and concerns. In M. McLean, M. Wolery, & D.B. Bailey, Jr., *Assessing infants and preschoolers with special needs* (3rd ed., pp. 172–203. Upper Saddle River, NJ: Prentice Hall.

Bennett, F.C. (1999). Developmental outcome. In G.B. Avery, M.A. Fletcher, & M.G. MacDonald (Eds.), *Neonatology: Pathophysiology & management of the newborn* (5th ed., pp. 1479–1497). Philadelphia: Lippincott Williams & Wilkins.

Browne, J.V. (2003). New perspectives on premature infants and their parents. *Zero to Three, November*, 4–12.

Centers for Disease Control and Prevention (CDC)/ National Center for Health Statistics. (2007). *Births: Preliminary data for 2005*. Retrieved on August 15, 2007 from http://www.cdc.gov/nchs/products/pubs/pubd/hestats/prelimbirths05/prelimbirths05.htm

Ensher, G.L., Bobish, T.P., Gardner, E.F., Reinson, C.L., Bryden, D.A., & Foertsch, D.J. (2007). *Partners in play: Assessing infants and toddlers in natural contexts*. Clifton Park, NY: Thomson Delmar Learning.

Ensher, G.L., & Clark, D.A. (1994). *Newborns at risk: Medical care and psychoeducational intervention* (2nd ed.). Gaithersburg, MD: Aspen Publishers.

Hack, M., Youngstrom, E.A., Cartar, L., Schluchter, M., Taylor, H.G., Flannery, D., Klein, N., & Borawski, E. (2004). Behavioral outcomes and evidence of psychopathology among very low birth weight infants at age 20 years. *Pediatrics, 114*, 932–940.

Hanson, E.W., & Lynch, M.J. (2004). Family diversity, assessment, and cultural competence. In M. McLean, M. Wolery, & D.B. Bailey, Jr., *Assessing infants and preschoolers with special needs* (3rd ed., pp. 71–99). Upper Saddle River, NJ: Prentice Hall.

Hoekstra, R.E., Ferrara, T.B., Couser, R.J., Payne, N.R., & Connett, J.E. (2004). Survival and long-term neurodevelopmental outcome of extremely premature infants born at 23–26 weeks' gestational age at a tertiary center. *Pediatrics, 113*, 1–6.

Horbar, J.D., Badger, G.J., Carpenter, J.H., Fanaroff, A.A., Kilpatrick, S., LaCorte, M., Phibbs, R., & Soll, R.F. (2002). Trends in mortality and morbidity for very low birth weight infants, 1991–1999. *Pediatrics, 110*, 143–151.

Linder, T.W. (1993). *Transdisciplinary Play-Based Assessment (TPBA): A functional approach to working with young children* (Rev. ed.). Baltimore: Paul H. Brookes Publishing Co.

Lynch, E.W., & Hanson, M.J. (Eds.). (2004). *Developing cross-cultural competence: A guide for working with children and their families* (3rd ed.). Baltimore: Paul H. Brookes Publishing Co.

McLean, M. (2004). Assessment and its importance in early intervention/early childhood special education. In M. McLean, M. Wolery, & D.B. Bailey, Jr., *Assessing infants and preschoolers with special needs* (3rd ed., pp. 1–21). Upper Saddle River, NJ: Prentice Hall.

McLean, M., Wolery, M., & Bailey, D.B., Jr. (2004). *Assessing infants and preschoolers with special needs* (3rd ed.). Upper Saddle River, NJ: Prentice Hall.

Meisels, S.J. (2001). Fusing assessment and intervention: Changing parents' and providers' views of young children. *Zero to Three*, February/March, 4–10.

Meisels, S.J., Dombro, A.L., Marsden, D.B., & Weston, D.R. (2004). *The ounce scale*. New York: Pearson/ Early Learning.

Muller, E., & Markowitz, J. (2004). *Disability categories: State terminology, definitions & eligibility criteria.* Alexandria, VA: Project FORUM, National Association of State Directors of Special Education (NASDSE).

O'Shea, T.M. (2002). Cerebral palsy in very preterm infants: New epidemiological insights. *Mental Retardation and Developmental Disabilities Research Reviews, 8*, 135–145.

Provence, S., Erikson, J., Vater, S., & Palmeri, S. (1995). *Infant-toddler developmental assessment*. Itasca, IL: Riverside.

Salvia, J., Ysseldyke, J.E., & Bolt, S. (2007). *Assessment in special and inclusive education*. Boston: Houghton Mifflin.

Shackelford, J. (2005). State and jurisdictional eligibility definitions for infants and toddlers with disabilities under IDEA. *NECTAC Notes, 18*, 1–15.

Turnbull, A., Turnbull, R., Erwin, E., & Soodak, L. (2006). *Families, professionals, and exceptionality: Positive outcomes through partnerships and trust* (5th ed.). Upper Saddle River, NJ: Prentice Hall.

Vohr, B.R., Wright, L.L., Dusick, A.M., Mele, L., Verter, J., Steichen, J.J., et al. (2000). Neurodevelopmental and functional outcomes of extremely low birth weight infants in the National Institute of Child Health and Human Development Neonatal Research Network, 1993–1994. *Pediatrics, 105*, 1216–1226.

CHAPTER 7

Autism Spectrum Disorders in Young Children

NEW PARADIGMS

Ellen B. Barnes, Janet O'Flynn, and Lori Saile

At the conclusion of this chapter, the reader will

- *Understand primary markers of autism in young children*

- *Understand current research and theories about the causes of autism in young children*

- *Understand some primary cognitive and psychosocial challenges of young children with autism*

- *Understand contemporary educational strategies and interventions used in working with young children with autism*

- *Understand challenges confronting families of young children with autism*

First recognized as a syndrome by Leo Kanner in 1943, the identification of children with autism has been rising steadily ever since. Most recent studies suggest that as many as 1 in 150 people carry a diagnosis of autism (Centers for Disease Control and Prevention [CDC], 2008). This number is substantially more than earlier estimates of 2–5 per 100,000. Although this may be due, in part, to better screening and diagnosis, there is nonetheless a growing public awareness of the importance of developing better understanding of the causes of autism, the needs of individuals with autism and their families, and the best approaches to teaching and supporting individuals with autism.

What Is Autism?

Autism is considered a spectrum disorder because it involves a cluster of several characteristics that can occur in various patterns and intensities.

Individuals with autism display characteristics in different ways and to different degrees. The signs of autism appear early in life (i.e., by definition before a child is 3 years old), although diagnosis may happen at a later age. Many parents of children with autism report noticing differences in the ways their children interact and respond in infancy compared with other infants. Others believe that their child's development was completely normal for the first 1–2 years, but followed by a rapid loss of skills. Regardless of the age of onset, the effects of autism are lifelong. Although individuals with autism may develop better skills for functioning and interacting in the world, the learning characteristics that lead to a diagnosis of autism do not go away. There is no cure for autism.

The *Diagnostic and Statistical Manual of Mental Disorders, Fourth Edition, Text Revision* (*DSM-IV-TR*; American Psychiatric Association [APA], 2000), provides the official definition used in diagnosing individuals with autism disorders. This diagnostic manual clusters autism and related disabilities under the umbrella of pervasive developmental disorders, which indicates that the characteristics of autism affect multiple areas of development simultaneously. Another commonly used term for disabilities that fall under this diagnostic umbrella is autism spectrum disorders (ASDs). Diagnoses subsumed under this umbrella have changed over time. At present, they include autism, Asperger syndrome, childhood disintegrative disorder (CDD), Rett syndrome, and pervasive developmental disorder-not otherwise specified (PDD-NOS). In this definition, individuals with ASDs are identified as demonstrating delays or differences in three areas of development: reciprocal social interaction skills, communication skills, and repetitive and/or stereotyped interests and behavior. The Individuals with Disabilities Education Improvement Act (IDEA) of 2004 (PL108-446), as well as the writings of individuals with autism, implicate a fourth developmental area of difficulties considered sensory processing. These areas of need overlap and, in many cases, the impact of delays or differences in one area can be seen as partially creating or explaining a delay or difference in another area, as indicated in Figure 7.1 (i.e., sensory/motor processing, cognitive style/ development, social interaction/social emotional development, interests and routines, and com-

munication). Accordingly, certain behaviors and learning styles can mask or overshadow others, often making it difficult to sort out the primary area of challenge.

What Causes Autism?

The causes of autism are not yet clearly established or understood. Autism appears to be a neurologically based disorder, and autopsy studies have revealed differences in the brains of individuals with autism as compared with those without the disorder (Bauman & Kemper, 2006). However, there also may be genetic and environmental factors that have an impact on the development of autistic characteristics. Rett syndrome is the only ASD for which scientists have identified a gene clearly responsible; however, families that have one child with an ASD are statistically far more likely to have another child with autism than other families in the general population. This observation suggests the possibility of a genetic component for susceptibility to autism.

No specific environmental factors contributing to the development of autism have been noted. Yet, the rapid rise in prevalence of autism in recent years has led to speculation about the possibility of an environmental contributor. In addition, many parents report that their children were developing typically until about the time of their measles, mumps, and Rubella (MMR) vac-

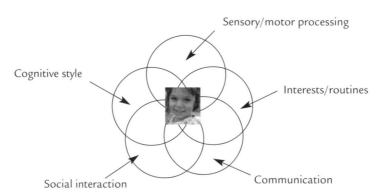

Figure 7.1.   A framework for understanding the interface among developmental domains in children with autism.

cinations, and then they showed a rapid loss of skills and development of autistic characteristics. There is a large group of parents who feel strongly that the vaccine, or a component of it, is the cause of their children's autism. Although current studies have failed to establish a definitive, causal relationship between the MMR vaccine and autism, the concern remains for many families (Verstraeten et al., 2003).

Since the late 1990s, research in the field of neurobiology has offered new explanations of early social functioning and the disorders that have been associated with autism. Mirror neurons, which fire in tandem with one's own motor actions and fire alone when watching motor actions of another person, allow us to imitate the motions of others without conscious effort. They are part of our development of empathy; that is, by their action we feel the same experience as another person feels. Research since the start of the new millennium suggests that in autism the mirror neuron system may be dysfunctional (Ramachandran & Oberman, 2006; Rizzolatti, Fogassi, & Gallese, 2006). A disorder of that system has important implications for impaired development of social interaction and the acquisition of language and communication. It is hoped that such research eventually may point to earlier diagnosis, psychological and pharmacological therapies, and earlier intervention. Clearly, however, there is a need for further studies before a definitive cause for autism can be identified. Because it is a syndrome and varies so much from person to person, it is possible that there are multiple causes.

Sensory and Motor Challenges

Individuals with ASDs have sensory and motor challenges. This section details their presentation and source, as well as various interventions used to address these challenges.

What Do We See?

Sensory integration is a normal part of human development. A. Jean Ayres, the pioneer in development of this theory base, first defined sensory integration or sensory processing disorders (Ayres, 2005). Ayres wrote,

> Our senses give us information about the physical conditions of our body and the environment around us. Sensations flow into the brain like streams flowing into a lake. Countless bits of sensory information enter our brain at every moment, not only from our eyes and ears but from every place in our body. We have a special sense that detects the pull of gravity and the movements of our body in relation to the earth. (2005, p. 5)

Sensory development in people with autism is significantly different from the typical patterns of sensory development. Many children with autism show unusual reactions to a variety of sensory inputs, including vision, the auditory system, smell, taste, and touch. These differences may involve sensitivity to stimulation, selectivity or focus, and timing of responses. When children are hypersensitive, they may avoid tactile contact, be irritated or particular about clothing or foods, cover their eyes or ears in response to bright light or loud noises, or gag in reaction to everyday smells. Ordinary sensory experiences may be painful. Other children with autism are unusually hyposensitive (i.e., unusually underresponsive) to a variety of sensory input. For example, they may seem not to feel pain as quickly as their peers, may bite or hit themselves, or may not appear to hear their names being called or notice people in their environment. They may seem oblivious to extreme temperatures, and they may seek items to smell or mouth. Many children on the autism spectrum show fluctuat-

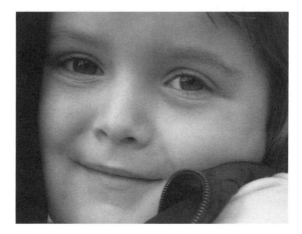

ing responses to sensory input, and, in addition, they may be overselective or underselective in their attention and more or less rapid in their responses to stimulation. Such differences go a long way toward explaining the behavior of people with autism, who are often seen as displaying acute sensitivity and overstimulation (Gillingham, 1998).

Two sensory systems that are fundamental to the development of sensory integration are hidden: the vestibular and proprioceptive systems. The vestibular system gives information about movement, gravity, and balance (through the inner ear), and the proprioceptive system gives information about the body's position in space (through muscles and joints). Many children with autism show unusual responses to motion. Children who are underreactive to movement may crave certain motions. For example, they may love to spin themselves, to watch spinning objects, to run and jump, or crash and bump their way through their environment. They may have severe difficulty with motor coordination, roaming without purpose or effective motor actions. Children who are overreactive to movement may stay still to the point where they appear to be passive and immobile much of the time. They may startle when picked up or rocked, show gravitational insecurity, or resist any attempt to move their feet off of the floor. They may show fear when they have to close their eyes. Children with difficulty processing proprioceptive input may appear clumsy, easily fatigued, and have problems grading their movements or changing positions in response to an activity.

A third system that is basic to our sense of self is the tactile system. Although we consider touch to be one of the five senses, we often do not consider its role in the development of body awareness and motor skill. The sensory receptors for light touch are at the base of the hairs on our skin. They initially have an alerting or alarming function, warning us of anything thin or sharp (e.g., an insect's tiny feet) before it can injure our skin. As we mature, light touch becomes integrated with other sensory information and then gives us fine discrimination ability, especially in

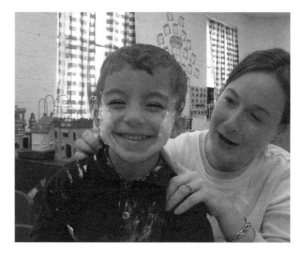

our fingertips and mouth. The sensory receptors for deep pressure are under the skin like a layer of little pillows. When they are pressed, they have a calming and organizing function, which gives information about where we are touched and how hard, as well as reassuring us emotionally that we are safe. When the elements of the touch system are balanced and when they match up well with information coming in from joints and muscles, we are able to move our bodies securely without having to pay specific attention to the elements of that movement. These systems together are considered the somatosensory systems (from somato, meaning body, and sensory).

A child who is overresponsive to tactile input may appear defensive, passive, and withdrawn, or, conversely, he or she may appear ready to fight off physical contact at the least provocation. A child who is underresponsive to tactile input will not have a secure body image. He or she may appear oblivious to his or her surroundings, or, conversely, he or she may appear to be craving and seeking out more intense sensation than most children can tolerate. Such a scenario is reflected in the following vignette by Tito Rajarshi Mukhopadhyay (as cited in Biklen):

The feeling of pain escaped me. I remember once touching a table fan and getting a shock. It was not "painful" but a new sensation for me. And I had tried to check it again by touching it once again to feel my hands. (2005, p. 137)

Motor planning is the process of deciding what our bodies have to do and then doing it. This process includes conceptualizing, planning, initiating, sequencing, and executing actions. This is the complex integration of sensory feedback and processing, memory and cognitive skills, motor initiation, and executing and adjusting movements. Breakdowns can occur at any point in this sequence (Anzalone & Williamson, 2000). Children on the autism spectrum with motor dyspraxia (which may include severe difficulties with speech) may have difficulty initiating motor actions; stopping, starting, and changing movements; manipulating objects; and avoiding perseverative behaviors. They may exhibit slumped posture and a fear of transitions from one activity to the next, and they may require adult support to sequence fine and gross motor actions (e.g., select and explore a toy). First person accounts by individuals with autism offer an extraordinary look into the reality of having autism. These accounts describe a variety of sensory experiences. One of the strongest themes is the lack of sensation of body awareness; that is, the basic subconscious knowledge of where one's body is, what it is doing, and what it can be relied on to do next:

> It took me many years to realize that I have a body. I think that it is not because of my preoccupation with other thoughts. I was totally aware of sounds and colors, which my senses picked up for me. I was, as if watching from a distant moon without actually being any part of everything. So the feeling that I have a body never occurred to me. Even to this day sometimes I feel that I am walking without legs. (Mukhopadhyay, as cited in Biklen, 2005, p. 137)

One area of great practical significance for children with autism is the mutual influence of sensory processing differences and behavior of children. Children with differences in sensory processing may be driven to behave in ways that are out of synchronization with the children and adults in their immediate environment. The most obvious and stereotypical behaviors of flapping or spinning are actions developed by children to help regulate their state of alertness by predict-

able visual, proprioceptive, and vestibular input. With time, the behaviors become habitual, happen without conscious awareness, and cease to be voluntary. The term self-stimulation may or may not be appropriate, depending on the meaning it is intended to convey. If it implies that the child is trying to get to a playful, distracted state instead of paying attention, the term is erroneous. However, if it implies that the child is seeking to eliminate distraction and focus the mind, in the same way that stimulants have that effect on children with attention-deficit/hyperactivity disorder (ADHD), it may be an accurate term. It is also true that children with autism voluntarily may behave in nonrepetitive, episodic ways that affect their sensory processing. The child who runs away or screams to drown out another person's words may be behaving in this way to avoid an unpleasant experience that he or she remembers from the past. The behavior in this case is voluntary, but it is not intended to disturb or alienate others; it seems necessary to the child at the time.

What Is the Source of Sensory and Motor Challenges?

As noted previously, neurobiological research is rapidly identifying brain structures that develop differently in autism. Identification of these structures does not necessarily mean that abnormal structures have caused autism; these structures may mean, instead, that when a child has autism, the brain develops in an unusual way. Cause and effect must be carefully studied in the years ahead. Nevertheless, the structures that show differences are strongly correlated with sensory processing. To begin with, the brain itself is oversized in children with autism. During the normal process of fetal development and infancy, the brain overproduces neurons. They migrate from the inner part of the brain to the outer cortex. Those that connect into active circuits become stronger, whereas those that do not connect wither away. By the age of 2 years, the child's brain should have experienced a great deal of pruning away of inefficient redundant neurons. The brain of a child with autism remains larger and heavier, leading to the hypothesis that there has been an error in the pruning process. The effect is not yet well understood, but the assumption can be made that having too many inefficient neurons produces neurological confusion (Bauman & Kemper, 2007).

In terms of more specific structures, neuron-anatomic differences have been found in the cerebellum and limbic system of people with autism. The cerebellum is a primary processor of balance and movement. It has a well-established role in motor coordination. Since the late 1990s, research has revealed that it is also a massive filter for incoming sensory information in all modalities. It contains a unique kind of nerve cell, the Purkinje fiber, which is shaped like a shrub above with one root below. The bushy Purkinje branch-like structures take in reams of sensations and reduce them, within the span of one cell, to one sensation (i.e., just one axonal impulse that is relayed to the rest of the nervous system). The cerebellum has been found to be smaller than normal in 80% of people with autism and to be larger than normal in the other 20% (Bauman, 2007). Many children with autism show an unusual attraction to spinning themselves and to watching spinning objects. Spinning stimulates the cerebellum to become more active. Both of these unusual responses of hyper- and hyposensitivity in all sensory modes could result from faulty operation (allowing too much sensation or too little) of this filter for sensation.

Another important area of neurobiological difference is in the limbic system, which is the primary center for both emotion and memory. Research has shown differences between the limbic system of people with autism and neurotypical individuals (Bauman, 2007). People with autism experience extremes of fear or desire (cravings) that probably originate from mapping of events to emotions in a highly irregular way. Triggers for emotional attachment may seem trivial to an observer, but they are meaningful and important to the person experiencing them. For instance, one adult with autism may carry an object with her, even though she is cognitively aware that this strong attachment makes her look different.

What Are the Goals of Intervention?

There are three main goals for intervention in the area of sensory and motor challenges. These include redefining and reframing a child's behavior, creating a sensory diet to modify the environment and provide coping strategies, and reorganizing the sensory system to function at a higher developmental level. It is important to make a clear distinction between the intention to enhance the development of competence and the intention to provide a cure. An analogy to the usefulness of therapy for a child with cerebral palsy may be helpful. Occupational, physical, and speech therapies are important in guiding the development of a child with cerebral palsy, but they are not thought of as a cure for cerebral palsy. In the same way, use of sensory integration strategies by therapists, teachers, and parents in the rehabilitation of children with autism should not be thought of as a cure for autism.

Sensory integration (SI) intervention for a person with autism can be significant in reducing bodily distractions and in enhancing motor efficacy (Eide, 2003). Sensory integration therapy or intervention can be defined as follows (Kurtz, 2007, p. 575):

> Sensory integration (SI) refers both to a theory and a model for therapy that has evolved since its introduction by A. Jean Ayres in the 1960s (Ayres, 1972; Bundy et al., 2002; Schaaf & Miller, 2005). It was originally developed to address the sensory processing, perceptual, and motor impairments of children with learning disabilities or other forms of developmental disability, but is now applied to children with a wide range of disabilities (Roley, Blanche, & Schaaf, 2001).

Relief from pain and freedom to move voluntarily are worthy goals of treatment. Intervention can allow the person to join the social environment and interact with the educational and work environment in a way that enhances connection and function. The timeline for efficacy of SI treatment was thought for some years to end in early childhood. It is now considered appropriate to incorporate SI approaches into daily life throughout the lifespan of a person with autism (Eide, 2003).

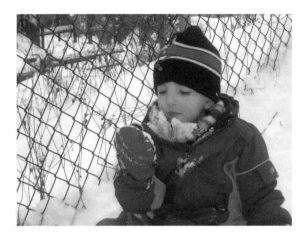

the *Test of Sensory Functions in Infants* (DeGangi & Greenspan, 1989) and the *DeGangi-Berk Test of Sensory Integration (3 to 5 years)* (Berk & DeGangi, 1983) are still useful evaluation tools for direct observation.

Observation questions to ask during this evaluation phase include:

- What type of stimulation is the child seeking?

- What type of stimulation is the child avoiding?

- How is the child affected by touch, movement, sounds, smells, and sights?

- When is the child most alert?

Sensory and motor differences in autism can be addressed most directly by application of sensory integration theory in three ways. The first avenue involves a redefining or reframing of behavior by teachers, parents, and perhaps the children themselves. Teachers and parents who used to think of a child's constant motion or strong aversion to sounds or touch as oppositional can come to see such behavior as an understandable response in light of what the child is experiencing. Children can begin, at an early age, to understand their own behavior and can become a part of its solution.

An increasing number of excellent books, audiotapes, and videos are now available for teachers, parents, and children that describe the sensory experience of people with autism, as well as explaining sensory integration. Such general information provides a good context for understanding an individual child's behavior, but it is not a substitute for individual evaluation and consultation. Parents can work directly with therapists who are able to evaluate specific sensory processing patterns for individual children, and who also can recommend resources to increase understanding. Evaluation tools for infants and young children include questionnaires, such as the *Sensory Profile* (Dunn, 1999) and *Infant/Toddler Sensory Profile* (Dunn, 2002); tests, such as the *Miller Assessment for Preschoolers (MAP)* (Miller, 1982) and *Function and Participation Scales* (Miller, 2006); and clinical observations by therapists who have obtained specialty certification in this area. For infants and very young children,

The second major way that SI theory can be applied is by allowing modification of the environment to reduce or eliminate unpleasant stimuli and to introduce or support existing positive coping strategies. These two strategies are embodied in the idea of making a sensory diet for the child to follow each day (Wilbarger, 1984, 1995). A sensory diet refers to the right balance of experiences during a day to nourish the child's sensory systems and to prevent overfeeding sensations. It is specifically tailored for the child through the collaboration of the teacher and parent, with input from the child when feasible. Understanding the kinds of sensations that are considered calming and the ones that are considered alerting is necessary for this planning process (Kranowitz, 1998). For instance, imagine an appropriate sensory diet for a child who needs additional vestibular input but has difficulty handling auditory input. The day could begin with having the child do 100 jumps on a mini trampoline to increase alertness in the morning. The parent could choose to drive the child to school rather than send him or her on the bus if the noise level on the bus is too high. At school, the child could immediately help the teacher take the chairs down off the desks to incorporate heavy work (which is always organizing) into the sensory diet. At the end of the day, after school, the child might need to sit in a rocking chair (for the calming effect of the rhythmic forward and back motion) and listen to a favorite piece of music, at a low volume, to restore calm and relaxation.

Two books that help parents design sensory diets to meet their children's needs are *The Out-Of-Sync Child: Recognizing and Coping with Sensory Integration Dysfunction* (Kranowitz, 1998, 2005) and *The Out-of-Sync Child Has Fun: Activities for Kids with Sensory Integration Dysfunction* (Kranowitz, 2003). Teachers can find help for creating sensory diets during the school day in *Answers to Questions Teachers Ask About Sensory Integration, Second Edition* (Kranowitz, Szklut, Balzer-Martin, Haber, & Sava, 2001); *Building Bridges Through Sensory Integration, Second Edition* (Yack, Sutton, & Aquilla, 2002); and *How Does Your Engine Run: A Leader's Guide to the Alert Program for Self-Regulation* (Williams & Shellenberger, 2002). Teachers and parents may also find the 25th anniversary edition of *Sensory Integration and the Child* (Ayres, 2005) to be accessible and helpful. This book by Dr. Ayres has recently been reissued with additional, supplemental commentary and information.

Several daily strategies might also prove to be useful and effective interventions. These might include planning an appropriate home and school sensory diet that gives a child with autism a foundation of security. Children do not enjoy the feeling of being out of control; therefore, a daily routine that supports alerting and calming at appropriate times allows a child to be at his or her best for learning and interacting. The purpose of a sensory diet is to expand the length of time every day during which the child is available for interaction with other people and with the environment. With time and discussions about what the child seems to be experiencing, the child learns to recognize his or her own level of alertness. In time, a child may learn to advocate for him- or herself and make activity choices that enhance self-regulation (Williams & Shellenberger, 2002).

The third application of SI theory might entail sensory integrative therapy to enhance development. The goal of direct SI therapy is to support an increasing range of sensory interactions that are acceptable to the child in order to facilitate reorganization of the sensory and motor systems for a higher level of function. Direct sensory integration therapy requires use of suspended equipment, such as a swing (over a floor mat for protection) and balls or bolsters, to set up play situations that provide the "just right challenge" for the child's increasing mastery of the environment. It also requires a therapist, usually an occupational therapist, but sometimes a physical therapist or a speech-language clinician with specialized training and experience, to conduct therapy sessions with maximum benefit to the child. It begins with an evaluation, based on parent and teacher questionnaires (see evaluation questions noted earlier in this chapter); classroom observation (and preferably home observation as well); and direct interaction.

Additional information from the evaluation includes persistence of immature reflexes; response to somatosensory input; response to visual, auditory, and oral input; preferred motor patterns for looking and moving; bilateral motor coordination; and balance. The child's sensory processing will be analyzed for overall patterns of response that show low or high threshold for awareness of sensory stimuli and for active or passive modes of responding to stimuli (Dunn, 1999). This information provides a starting place for therapeutic intervention.

Direct SI therapy often is initially prescribed for a period of 3–6 months. After that time, progress is reevaluated and further therapy may extend for up to 2 or more years. Frequency may be one to three times per week. Each session may be about an hour long. Some therapy clinics provide a one-way mirror so that parents can watch the therapy session without being observed. The hour is filled with active play.

An SI session early in the course of therapy may begin with the therapist acknowledging the activity that the child is interested in by engaging in the activity with him or her. Playfully, the therapist then adds sensory input that is known to be acceptable to the child. When the child interacts with that acceptable sensory input, indicating that it should continue, the therapist begins to introduce complexity (e.g., a challenge at the just right level, which is not too hard but not so easy that it is boring). Strategies that make the session productive for the child with autism include acknowledging every instance of communicative intent, giving play activities or games a name to enhance memory, and supplying pretend narratives. Sessions should end with functional tasks, even if the task is only to organize and put away play materials.

An SI session later in the course of therapy may begin with a greeting routine. The child may eagerly initiate a familiar play routine, and then the therapist engages in that routine and offers choices for elaboration that the child directs. The therapist uses his or her familiarity with the child's sensory processing and motor skills to conduct the session like a piece of music, with an introduction, an elaboration, variations on a theme, perhaps a grand finale, but always with a postlude of calming and reorganizing to make the transition back to functional tasks. During this latter transition, the child may be thinking about activities for the next time or drawing a picture of how the swing and tunnel were set up so that it can be reproduced again. The child can put away equipment. Progress can be mutually acknowledged, and perhaps the child will be congratulated for having managed to come in and wait his or her turn without being disruptive or can be celebrated for getting shoes on independently.

During the course of therapy, the therapist can use the sensory integration knowledge base, not just to help adjust the child's alertness level, but also to facilitate more rapid sensorimotor progress toward neurological maturity. For instance, if a child's ability to coordinate eyes and hands for catching a ball is limited, the child will benefit from play in the prone or quadruped (a four-point position or on hands and knees) position, such as propelling him- or herself on a scooter board between bean bag targets, which uses muscle resistance to inhibit reflexes that interfere with eye–hand coordination. If the child is afraid of having his or her feet off the floor (i.e., gravitational insecurity), SI play begins in contact with the floor with added weight to activate the proprioceptive system, which helps modulate vestibular input (Ayres, 2005). One more powerful intervention that is frequently appropriate for children with autism is the Wilbarger Deep Pressure Treatment Protocol, also known as brushing and joint compressions (Wilbarger,

1984; Wilbarger & Wilbarger, 1991). As Yack, Sutton, and Aquilla (2004) explained,

The Wilbarger Protocol is a specific, professionally guided treatment regime designed to reduce sensory defensiveness. The Wilbarger Protocol has the origins in sensory integration theory, and it has evolved through clinical use. It involves deep touch pressure throughout the day. (p. 1)

Special Challenges for the Therapist in Working with People with Autism

SI offers just one tool box (albeit a generously overflowing one) to people with autism and their caregivers. The person using the tools needs an open mind and the time to observe both difficulties and successes that already exist before the tools can be used most productively. There is some element of trial and error, especially in the first few sessions to determine ways in which the child's responses will be most productive. It is also true that SI work with a person with autism may be mentally and physically challenging to the therapist. This is most true when the child's dyspraxia, or difficulty in motor planning, causes him or her to show little or no interest in motor play. In such situations, a therapist may need to open another tool box to supplement the SI approach (e.g., the motor prompting approach that is usually used with adults with Parkinson's disease).

Autism is known to be marked by dyspraxia or deficits in motor planning. Motor planning difficulty means being unable to perform a new or unfamiliar action. The normal process of motor planning has several stages, any or all of which can break down. For example, the child may have difficulty with ideation (i.e., having an idea of how to move). If, for example, a child with autism is brought into the room with an unfamiliar piece of play equipment, such as a tricycle, and ignores it or interacts with it in an idiosyncratic way, such as turning it over and spinning the wheels, he or she is displaying difficulty with ideation. Furthermore, it is possible that watching a demonstration will not elicit imitation, probably because autism may affect the mirror neuron system, as discussed previously. In addition, verbal instructions may not lead the

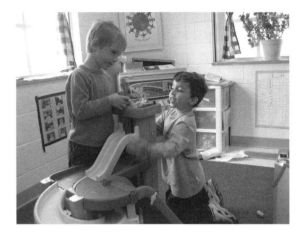

child to sit on or ride a tricycle as a result of difficulty with auditory processing. Often, the most likely way to introduce the child to the intended play purpose of the tricycle is to place him or her on the seat, place his or her feet on the pedals, and begin slowly pushing it. At that point, the second stage of motor planning may cause the child problems; namely, managing the placement of body parts and sequencing motions in the absence of reliable feedback from the body (somatosensory input). The child needs to feel the resistance in first one foot on its pedal and then the other in a repeating sequence; and at the same time the child needs to inhibit motion in the trunk so that he or she can remain balanced on the seat. The lack of contact with the floor, and the moving environment, may trigger a feeling of falling, which also needs to be inhibited. Lack of a purpose in moving away from the caregiver, without a destination, may make each stage of this motion less and less rewarding.

Finally, the third stage of motor planning is motor execution, which is physical skill and coordination. Autism affects the development of motor skill, even for familiar tasks; therefore, skill in unfamiliar tasks is that much more challenged. It may not be possible for the child to shift his or her weight rhythmically from one leg to the other, as needed for pedaling, or steering may be so poor that the tricycle cannot travel straight ahead. It is in the work on motor execution that more physical prompting may be needed. The intermittent presence of fluid and coordinated movement in other parts of the

child's life makes it harder to understand this lack of movement in unfamiliar tasks. A person with autism appears not to be motivated to move or even to be passively resistant to the agendas of caregivers (Donnellan, & Leary, 1994).

Children who first benefited from SI therapy were then described as having minimal brain dysfunction. Usually they had awkwardness associated with soft neurological signs and learning disabilities (Ayres, 2005). They were more likely to show a wide variety of movements, even though the movements were awkward and unskilled, and were less likely to show the limited repertoire of stereotyped pacing or rocking associated with autism. Therapists working with children with autism, using the SI frame of reference, have always paid careful attention to the effects of sensory hyper- and hyposensitivity in designing play that would free the child to increase his or her repertoire. That approach has been fruitful. Therapists need to stretch that frame again slightly, enough to consider that the motor actions are limited equally by primary motor deficits in the basal ganglia and cerebellum. Brain research on autism increasingly supports the hypothesis that the neurobiological processes that govern starting, stopping, sustaining, timing, and speed are physically impaired, just as in Parkinson's disease or Tourette syndrome. Therapy approaches that support those more purely motor functions must be incorporated into SI therapy as well. Strategies such as using drum beats to facilitate timing of responses, touch cues to assist in initiating and stopping motion, visualization and internal verbal scripts for cueing, and rhythmic motion on a step aerobics machine or trampoline to prepare the motor system to initiate motion may be helpful additions to therapy with children with autism.

Cognitive and Learning Style

This section explores the cognitive and learning style of people with ASDs. Although individuals with ASDs vary in ability level, they tend to share certain features in this area. The interventions discussed later in this section address these features.

What Do We See?

Children with autism demonstrate varying levels of cognitive ability. Until the late 1990s, intellectual disabilities were considered likely in children with autism, reportedly occurring in up to 75% of these individuals (APA, 2000). As technological and practical advances in the use of augmentative and alternative communication systems have allowed more and more people with autism to express their knowledge and ideas, there is growing recognition that this is not an accurate statistic. Some may appear to have mental disabilities, particularly at younger ages, as they are unable to follow basic directions or complete basic tasks. Others, once they have a reliable means of self-expression, may seem to have average or above average cognitive abilities. Still others may show uneven patterns of cognitive development, with well-developed and sometimes even advanced skills in one area and weak skills in another area. Still others may demonstrate remarkable knowledge about topics of particular interest to them.

Many young children with autism seem to have relatively well-developed rote memory and seem to demonstrate pre-academic skills, such as color, shape, letter, and/or number recognition. In some instances, skills such as counting or labeling letters and/or arranging them in alphabetical order emerge before other, more functional communication skills. Some individuals with autism are hyperlexic, which means that they develop the ability to read at very young ages and without formal teaching. However, children with autism may have difficulty when asked to apply these rote skills to real life problem-solving situations or have trouble with demonstrating the same skill in a variety of situations. Often, a specific cue or environmental circumstances are necessary to elicit the skill.

Children with autism also show variable attending skills, and they may appear highly distractible. In addition, they may become hyperfocused on certain things, such as a spinning fan or a favorite toy, and appear oblivious to other things happening in their environment. In some instances, parents first seek help for their children because they are concerned about their hearing as they do not respond when their names are called or turn toward familiar sounds in the environment. However, these same children may be hyperaware of certain sounds, such as the crinkling of the wrapper on a favorite food, even when it is rooms away. Some may be fascinated with input from one modality, such as the visual stimulus of watching shifting light and shadows, but relatively unresponsive to information in another modality, such as speech.

Children with autism are often described as being highly rigid and dependent on specific routines and sequences, and as becoming very upset when these routines are altered. In addition, the play of young children with autism may be quite repetitive and frequently is based on manipulation of objects rather than imaginative play. They may be interested in lining up toy cars or in turning them over and spinning their wheels, but not in using them to enact taking a trip to a particular location. They may not appear interested in toys, but may show great fascination with observing repetitive actions, such as shaking a string or sifting small objects through their fingers. Initially, imitation of adult and peer play models may be limited as well. Finally, these children can be very literal, struggling to understand idioms, jokes, sarcasm, and other abstract ideas.

What Is the Source of Cognitive Challenges?

Because the cognitive profiles of individuals with autism are so variable, it is difficult to make generalizations; however, there are some similarities in cognitive style that can be seen across people with autism. These similarities have to do with attention to environmental stimuli and information, the ways that information is perceived, and with how information is processed.

As mentioned previously, attending skills in children with autism often fluctuate. On the one hand, they can be difficult to engage, with problems in joint attention and distractibility. On the other hand, they can become hyperfocused on items or topics of interest to them and have a hard time shifting their attention to other stimuli. This tendency may be related to difficulties with sensory processing that make it challenging to sort out the mass of information coming in from their senses at any given time. It is possible that overfocusing on familiar stimuli or ideas may help to block out other confusing, anxiety-producing, or overwhelming input. In addition, some individuals with autism may have difficulty interpreting what is most relevant, for instance, to a social situation.

As discussed in the section on sensory processing, some individuals with autism have trouble perceiving information from certain senses. At times, perceptions may be distorted, as in sounds being perceived as much louder, softer, or garbled; and it may be difficult to feel one's own body and where it is in space. Some individuals report mono-channel processing, meaning that they are able to focus on and process information from only one sensory channel at a time. Thus, if they are asked to focus visually on someone's face, they may have problems with auditory processing what that person is saying. Even when children understand what is going on in their environment and what is being asked of them, motor planning challenges may interfere with their ability to respond behaviorally in a way that demonstrates their understanding. Many describe instances of knowing what they need to do but not being able to make their bodies respond appropriately.

Some children may focus on visual stimuli, such as letters and words, because, in contrast with movement or speech that once executed disappears, visual stimuli are nontransient. A visual cue remains in place for a child to take time to process and to check back with as needed. This may be why so many young children with autism respond better to pictures and even written language than to verbal cues.

In terms of processing, many people with autism appear to learn holistically by taking in chunks of information at one time. Rote memory and memory for details can be strong, but also cued through association. For example, a particular song played or article of clothing worn by a parent or teacher when the child learned a new skill might elicit that skill at another time, even when it seems out of context. Temple Grandin (1995) has described her cognitive process as

"thinking in pictures" (p. 19). Although most people have memories stored under verbal labels, Grandin described seeing a series of images in her head, each of which cues another image, thus moving through images until she has retrieved the concept she sought.

> Unlike those of most people, my thoughts move from video-like, specific images to generalization and concepts. For example, my concept of dogs is inextricably linked to every dog I've ever known. It's as if I have a card catalogue of dogs I have seen, complete with pictures, which continually grows as I add more examples to my video library. If I think about Great Danes, the first memory that pops into my head is Dansk, the Great Dane owned by the headmaster at my high school. The next Great Dane I visualize is Helga, who was Dansk's replacement. The next is my aunt's dog in Arizona, and my final image comes from an advertisement for Fitwell seat covers that featured that kind of dog. My memories usually appear in my imagination in chronological order, and the images I visualize are always specific. There is no generic, generalized Great Dane. (1995, pp. 27–28)

This associational thinking may explain why it is often hard for individuals with autism to generalize skills from one setting to the next, because they may be dependent on specific environmental cues to call up the memory of a particular skill.

Many individuals with autism are concrete and literal thinkers. They do well with rote memorization of specific, unchanging facts, but have difficulty making connections between ideas or thinking abstractly. This explains why social interactions, which involve abstraction and nuances, often may be troublesome to decipher. Jokes, idioms, and sarcasm likewise may be challenging for people with autism to interpret.

What Are the Goals of Intervention?

Cognitive goals for children with autism are not unlike those for all children—to develop a range of skills that can be functionally applied to expand thinking and solve problems. Because many individuals with autism have shared that they were capable of understanding so much more than they were able to demonstrate at a young age, it is important to presume competence and to offer children exposure to a range of age-appropriate content with support to demonstrate their skills. Skills may be developed in rote ways, but it is important to work on generalizing these to a variety of situations and applications. Because children with autism tend to be rote learners, it is essential to teach thinking and problem-solving skills that promote flexibility and application of skills. Consideration of the specific learning styles of these children will be important in meeting these goals.

What Are Some Useful Interventions?

It is useful to task analyze skills to be taught into smaller steps and to provide for lots of practice and repetition. Cognitive skill practice can be built into daily routines so that familiarity and repetition can increase the likelihood of success. Once a child is successful with a particular skill, it is important to work on generalizing that skill by varying task formats, settings, and/or cues that are used to elicit the skill. Whenever possible, teaching the child functional skills in real-life situations will minimize the need for generalization later.

Visual strategies are particularly beneficial in helping a child with autism to focus on what is relevant to organize his or her responses. These offer a nontransient stimulus that the child can return to as needed, allowing the child time to process the information. Visual supports include objects, pictures, and/or written words. The abilities of children to respond to print cues at a young age often are surprising. Print supports can include written sequences or schedules for daily or novel tasks, labels to identify where things can be found, and cues and reminders about how to handle a situation. Hodgdon offers wonderful, practical, hands-on examples of visual supports in her books, *Visual Strategies for Solving Behavior Problems in Autism: Practical Supports for Home and School* (1995) and *Solving Behavior Problems in Autism: Improving Communication with Visual Strategies* (1999).

It is important to consider teaching children in multiple modalities in light of their individual

learning style strengths. Most classrooms and traditional instruction are strongly language based and, although continuing to expose children to oral language is important, auditory learning frequently is more challenging for children with autism. Pairing verbal instruction with other modalities can help. For skills involving a great deal of language, such as listening to a story, visual cues (e.g., pictures, props to act out various scenarios) may make information more engaging and accessible to the child. Some children are responsive to the use of an animated and enthusiastic tone to gain their attention; others who are easily overstimulated may respond better to quieter and calmer approaches. Hands-on activities may help to hold a child's interest, as well as allowing a child with limited verbal skills a way to participate and demonstrate his or her knowledge. Some children enjoy music, and singing can be another way to elicit skills that they have more difficulty demonstrating verbally. Others are more kinesthetic learners, developing and demonstrating new skills best through sensory and movement-based activities. For children with motor planning difficulties, hand-over-hand support initially may help children learn motor patterns to complete tasks. To promote indepen-

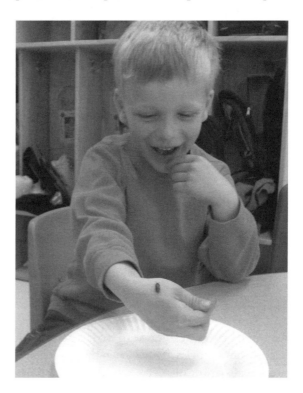

dence, care should be taken to fade this support as soon as children are successful. Varying levels of support may be needed at different times.

Finally, incorporating the child's special interests into the content to be taught can maximize engagement and motivation. Although a reasonable long-term goal might be to expand children's interests and abilities to work on another's agenda, meeting children where they are within activities that are motivating to them is an important way to support social engagement and build meaningful relationships, as well as to increase task performance. Particularly with young children, it is helpful to use a light, playful, and curious tone when working to stretch their engagement in problem-solving tasks.

Communication

There are variations in the communication abilities of children with ASDs. This section discusses the range of communication skills across these individuals, as well as related interventions.

What Do We See?

Although many indicate a desire and willingness to interact with others, the communication abilities of children with autism vary widely. Some are nonverbal or have limited verbal skills. These children may rely on context, body language, vocalizations, facial expressions, physical orientation and moving toward the object or location desired, eye gaze, touch, gestures, tears and tantrums, and other nonsymbolic forms of communication to convey their intents. Therefore, their success with communication is highly dependent on their communication partner's knowledge of them and ability to read their intent. They also may use sign language, picture or letter choice boards, and/or other augmentative and alternative communication systems to communicate.

Other children use echoed speech—repeating words or phrases they hear others use—but generate little spontaneous language of their own. This echolalia may be immediate, with repetition of a word or phrase just after hearing an expression, or it may be delayed, with words, phrases, or even entire scripts that have been heard repeated hours or even days later. Echoed speech some-

times is interactive and intended to communicate a message or initiate and extend an interaction; or it may be noninteractive and not directed toward a listener or intended as communication. For some children who use echoed speech interactively, it may be an avenue toward more spontaneous speech that gradually emerges over time.

Some children have relatively age-appropriate oral language skills, but demonstrate difficulty with pragmatic skills or the rules of using language for social interaction. They may use limited eye contact and/or have challenges with the understanding or use of facial expression, body language, and gestures. Some children also have differences in their voice quality, tone, rhythm, or volume of speech and are described as speaking in a flat tone of voice, whereas others have a sing-song quality to their speech. Furthermore, some struggle with participating smoothly in the rhythmic, give-and-take nature of conversation, having difficulty with skills such as initiating a conversation, turn-taking, maintaining a topic, and reading cues of others in conversation. In addition, they may have limited or repetitive conversational topics and need longer processing time to respond.

In terms of their receptive language skills (i.e., the ability to understand what has been said), children with autism vary widely. These skills may range from being significantly delayed to being age-appropriate and beyond. Furthermore, understanding for a particular child may fluctuate from situation to situation.

What Are the Sources of Communication Challenges?

Many nonverbal people with autism who develop a functional means of open-ended communication describe their inability to speak as rooted in motor challenges. Lucy Blackman, a woman with autism who communicates primarily through typing, described her efforts at speech by explaining, "This often happens. I believe I have spoken but only in my brain not in my throat. In fact, I often make a sound I believe to be a word, but it has no form" (Blackman, as cited in Biklen, 2005, p. 148).

The motor planning process for speech is extremely complex, involving conceptualizing what one wishes to say, breaking that message down into component speech sounds, sending neural messages to the speech sound articulators to form a sound, and sequencing sounds together to form words. For one whose motor planning skills are challenged, speech production can be extremely difficult. These same individuals likewise may have difficulty with other movement skills related to communication, such as forming gestures or signs or even accurately pointing to choices on a communication device.

Children who use echoed speech may be using this strategy as a means for learning language. The memorization and repetition of phrases or even whole scripts may reflect a holistic learning style in which language is learned first in chunks and then broken down into its component parts. Echoed speech thus plays a role in learning linguistic functions and structures. This is particularly true when echoed speech is used functionally and interactively to convey a message, even though its connection to the context may be difficult to decipher or its form may be slightly removed from the situation. When some individuals with autism use echoed speech repetitively, in noncommunicative ways, it may be used to self-regulate (e.g., blocking out an overwhelming sensory environment). In some cases, such expressions are involuntary responses to stress or anxiety. Close observation is necessary to determine whether echoed speech is being used with communicative intent or noncommunicatively.

Some challenges with pragmatic skills, as well as variability in receptive language skills, relate to difficulties in sorting out the sensory environment. As noted previously, some people with autism describe their sensory processing as mono-channel, meaning that they can attend to and process information from only one sensory channel at a time. These individuals say that if they are forced to make eye contact with a communication partner, they have a hard time listening to what is being said. Still others experience sensory distortions that make it difficult for them to make out and comprehend spoken language. Other challenges with pragmatic skills are connected to problems with understanding the abstract rules of social engagement.

What Are the Goals of Intervention?

"The Communication Imperative," conceived by Robert Williams (1991) noted that "every person, regardless of the severity of his or her disability, has the *right* to communicate. Everyone has the *ability* to communicate. Everyone should be given the *chance, technology, respect,* and *encouragement* to do so" (p. 543). For individuals with autism, the challenge lies in determining the best means to support communication. The goal for all children should be meaningful, spontaneously accessed, and open-ended communication, whether it is through speech or through other means. For those who use echoed speech to interact, the goal would be to use scaffolded cues and supports to shape that speech to be more functional and spontaneous and to serve a range of communicative intent. If echoed speech is not used interactively, and/or functional oral communication is not developing, augmentative and alternative communication systems may need to be developed.

When choosing an augmentative or alternative communication system for children with limited oral language skills, it is important to consider what they may want to say, the situations in which they want to communicate, and to whom they want to direct their message. Ultimately, no one should be dependent on the adults in their world (i.e., those who program appropriate communication choices into their devices, select appropriate times to provide access

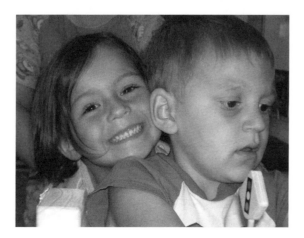

to devices, or who are knowledgeable about designated communication systems). Although adult-programmed communication choices and other supports may be an important step along the way, all should keep in mind the long-term goal of open-ended and spontaneous communication opportunities anywhere and with anyone. Toward this end, when a child is using unique or idiosyncratic means of communicating, another important goal might be to teach peers, family members, and teaching staff to understand the child's communication system.

What Are Some Useful Interventions?

In supporting the development of a communication system for children, it is crucial first to look at ways in which they are already communicating. Likely they are communicating some things effectively to well-known communication partners. Looking at how they are doing so offers useful clues as to the most effective system for them. These early communication strategies possibly can be shaped into more conventional and effective means. Thus, the role of the teacher or therapist is first not to teach communication but to find it, listen to it, and build sharing and understanding between the person with autism and others in his or her world.

Speech and language texts and resources offer multiple common sense strategies for expanding a child's verbal language, including modeling and expansion, commenting, expectant waiting, various levels of prompts, and ways to manipulate the environment to create a need for and elicit communication. Rydell and Prizant (1995) have done excellent work around assessing the functions of echoed speech and shaping and expanding it into more effective and spontaneous expressions. They argue that echoed speech initially should be encouraged as legitimate communication for a variety of purposes and within a variety of contexts. As echoed speech is understood, responded to, expanded, and shaped, it will gradually be replaced by more spontaneous utterances. Rydell and Prizant suggest both indirect and direct intervention strategies, such as the following:

Indirect Intervention Strategies

- Increase communication among all participants regarding assessment results and intervention strategies.
- Modify the environment to increase predictability and consistency, while reducing highly confusing and arousing situations.
- Simplify language input to match the child's level of linguistic processing.
- Vary adult verbal interaction styles to reduce cognitive, social, and communicative demands and promote a variety of pragmatic functions.
- For early language users, model conventional and relevant utterances that can be easily borrowed and eventually converted into more sophisticated forms.

Direct Intervention Strategies

- Acknowledge and appropriately respond to echoic utterances that are used for instrumental, cognitive, and social purposes.
- Model conventional and appropriate utterances to promote specific communicative functions.
- Provide systematic modifications that serve to reduce, replace, or expand constituent parts of the echoed phrase to promote increased linguistic processing and creativity.
- AAC (augmentative and alternative communication) may be considered to augment verbal productions or replace challenging verbal behaviors. (1995, p. 124)

For children who are not developing spoken language or who are unable to communicate without frustration, augmentative and alternative communication systems may be needed. It is important to note here that augmentative systems have not been found to interfere with the development of communication, but in fact enhance these systems. Thus, providing a child with an augmentative communication system does not decrease the likelihood that he or she will talk. In developing an augmentative system, consideration needs to be given to the communication and motor skills that the child is already demonstrating. A child who is able to imitate fine motor movements may do well with sign language. Although this communication system relies on listeners who are familiar with sign language, it is a system that is always available. In addition, use of sign language provides a visual cue and also may support receptive understanding, even among children who rely on a different means to communicate expressively. For those with more extensive motor planning challenges, communication that involves pointing to a choice of messages—such as communication boards, the Picture Exchange Communication System (PECS; http://www.pecs.com/whatispecs.htm), and computerized devices with voice output—should be considered. Some individuals may need physical and emotional support or facilitation in order to access communication choices effectively. This method called facilitated communication was developed in Australia by Crossley and was brought to the United States by Biklen (1993). The physical support provided by a facilitator may include assistance with isolating the index finger for pointing; stabilizing the arm to overcome tremor; a touch of the forearm, elbow, or shoulder to help the person initiate pointing; and/or pulling back on the arm or wrist to help the person slow down and focus. Emotional support may involve providing encouragement, reassurance, and a feeling of safety, as well as treating the individual as a person who has an important message to contribute. The idea is never to guide the person to a particular selection, but to support and encourage him or her to move toward his or her own choice. With practice and improved confidence, many individuals who begin to use facilitated communication later move toward independence in pointing to choices or typing to communicate.

In terms of receptive understanding of language, the literature of Hodgdon (1995, 1999) offers a range of models and ideas for visual supports and other strategies for becoming a better communicator. In particular, she has noted the importance of

1. Getting on the child's level
2. Establishing and maintaining attention
3. Preparing the child for what you are going to communicate
4. Using gestures and body language meaningfully
5. Supporting communication visually
6. Speaking slowly and clearly
7. Limiting verbalization
8. Including wait time in interactions
9. Guiding or prompting the child to respond if needed after waiting
10. Staying with an interaction until a desired response is reached

Social Interaction

Impairment in the area of social interaction is often considered a defining feature of autism. The following discussion explores manifestations of this challenge and interventions to address it.

What Do We See?

Social engagement challenges frequently are mentioned as a primary characteristic of children with autism. Infants and toddlers with autism often seem less aware of the people in their environment and less engaged with their caregivers, as well as not seeking comfort when hurt. Approaches to others may be awkward (e.g., backing into a parent's lap or hugging legs from behind). Cuddling, typically welcomed, may seem aversive to those with hypersensitive tactile systems. They may ignore peers or actively avoid contact (which causes them to be perceived as being "in their own world"). When they do interact, they may be out-of-sync, showing delayed responses to the words or actions of others. Efforts to initiate are awkward and focused only on their own agenda. Direct eye contact can be infrequent. A child may appear to look past another person, use a fleeting sideways glance, or when others are watching, may look away. Lack of initiation in social situations can be the norm. The pragmatics of social interaction, such as how to read the cues of others and engage in turn-taking in play and conversation, often are not evident. There may not be age-appropriate reactions in social situations. For example, children may react to peers as if they are threatening, but not appear anxious around strangers. Children with autism may seem to prefer to be alone rather than following the lead of other children, and to play with toys in a stereotypic, unimaginative way. Yet, it is important to remember that what we see does not always accurately reflect what is happening receptively for an individual. Adults and peers may find it challenging to decipher the intent of a child's facial expressions and gestures. Moreover, although the child with autism may appear not to be listening, it may be clear later that he or she took in the content of the interaction.

What Are the Sources of Social Challenges?

The sensory elements of social interactions have a heavy impact on a child's ability to attend and respond. In addition, the language-based nature of most social encounters can be confusing for children who have difficulty processing nonverbal behavior, facial expression, and abstract verbal communication. Social rules are flexible, not literal, and many children with autism seek concrete, explicit, and predictable social routines. For example, Barron (Grandin & Barron) wrote,

> I spent most of my first five years pretty much living in a vacuum of my own devising. I did many repetitive, stereotypical and often destructive and anti-social behaviors because I sought to find relief and security from the constant fear I felt....I developed a tunnel-vision approach toward processing information....It was so much easier for me to fixate on an individual carpet fiber, even if it meant missing everything else going on around me, simply because such an activity made my world seem less overwhelming. The problem with going through my early years like this was that I was missing experiences that I needed in order to develop the social skills I so desperately wanted. (2005, pp. 61–62)

Some authors (e.g., Howlin, Baron-Cohen, & Hadwin, 1999) describe children with autism as missing "a theory of mind," or the capacity for empathy to understand the feelings and perspectives of others. (This is a characteristic now being examined through research on mirror neurons as described earlier in this chapter.) Individuals with autism have indicated that social misunderstanding is a shared problem. As they have difficulty understanding the perspective of those who are neurotypical, we also are "blind" or oblivious to the experiences of the person with autism (Smukler, 2005). Williams (2003) talked about the high level of "exposure anxiety" that

she has felt in social situations. She also described herself as functioning most effectively one channel at a time, which only allows her to listen to someone's words if she does not look at the person or make eye contact. Similarly, Rubin wrote,

> I have found in my experience that it is very hard for an autistic person to initiate relations with others. This does not mean that we do not desire communication. . . . Instead our social rules are not socially acceptable. . . . My inability to look at someone when speaking to him or her does not mean that I am avoiding the person as many presume. Sometimes, eye contact literally is painful for me to achieve. (Biklen, 2005, p. 88)

What Are the Goals of Intervention?

The main goal of intervention is that young children will develop spontaneous, joyful relationships, first with primary caregivers (parents) and later with peers, as they move past infancy into toddler and preschool age. The elements of these relationships include becoming comfortable in the proximity of others, finding pleasure in the emotional reactions of others, observing and imitating the actions of others, playing first in a parallel and then cooperative fashion, and initiating and responding to the initiations of others. Greenspan and Wieder (1998) described the first four developmental milestones related to social interaction as:

1. Shared attention and regulation

2. Engagement and relating (with age-expected reciprocity)

3. Purposeful two-way communication

4. Symbolic thinking and social problem solving

Adult interactions can support the practice of these skills in young children with autism (see Schuler & Wolfberg, 2000, for example, for a discussion of the challenges and benefits of scaffolding peer play and socialization). Grandin and Barron offer great insights into the dilemmas of social relationships from the point of view of two individuals with autism. They list 10 unwritten rules of social relationships that every child on the autism spectrum needs to learn:

1. Rules are not absolute. They are situation-based and people-based.
2. Not everything is equally important in the grand scheme of things.
3. Everyone in the world makes mistakes; it doesn't have to ruin your day.
4. Honesty is different than diplomacy.
5. Being polite is appropriate in any situation.
6. Not everyone who is nice to me is my friend.
7. People act differently in public than they do in private.
8. Know when you are turning people off.
9. "Fitting in" is often tied to looking and sounding like you fit in.
10. People are responsible for their own behaviors. (2005, p. 119)

What Are Some Useful Interventions?

Many approaches help children develop the elements of social skills. In addition to providing a social climate that emphasizes engaging in reciprocal emotional interactions and identifying and labeling feelings, these include the following:

- *Developmental, Individual-Difference, Relationship-Based (DIR) Model/floor time*: One-to-one, intensive, playful, and interactive sessions that follow a child's interests, wooing him or her to engage emotionally and opening and closing circles of communication with the goal of linking emotions and intent with be-

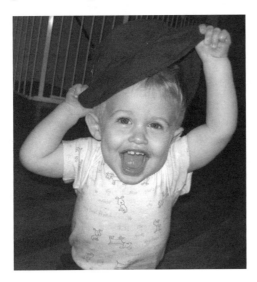

havior and eventually words (Greenspan & Weider, 1998)

- *Affection training:* A conscious focus on incorporating affectionate behaviors into typical preschool games, songs, and activities (McEvoy, Twardosz, & Bishop, 1990)

- *Paired play and/or integrated play groups:* Provision of supports in terms of play environments, materials, thematic scenarios and scripts, and flexible child-centered coaching of both children with autism and their typical peers (Fuge & Berry, 2004; Schuler & Wolfberg, 2000; Wolfberg, 2003)

- *Interest-based programming:* The use of a child's interests and/or obsessions to build social interactions, friendships, and self-esteem (Kluth, 2003; Leicestershire County Council & Fosse Health Trust, 1998)

- *Social Stories:* Writing Social Stories to describe a situation or skill that is difficult or a routine, special event, or a positive achievement (Social Stories include descriptive and factual sentences; perspective sentences that refer to the internal states or beliefs, usually of other people; directive sentences that gently suggest an appropriate response to a situation; and affirmative sentences that express a commonly held value within a particular culture) (Baker, 2001; Gray & White, 2002)

- *Skillstreaming (McGinnis & Goldstein, 1990):* Teaching social skills by task analyzing each one into sequential steps, role-playing the skill, documenting the steps, and posting them as cues to support their generalization

- *Inclusive programming:* Offering opportunities for incidental teaching of social and play skills with classmates who model, initiate, and maintain interaction (Kluth, 2003; Schwartz, Billingsley, & McBride, 1998; Strain, McGee, & Kohler, 2001)

Initiation skills can be encouraged by incorporating into a child's play routine strategies that require interaction. In these scenarios, the adult has control of the materials, plays hide and seek, offers parts rather than all of the required pieces, and makes purposeful mistakes (Cardon, 2007). Adults working with young students in groups can support positive relationships by modeling prosocial skills; using books that have themes about age-appropriate social issues; including diversity awareness and community building activities in preschool and school experiences; providing opportunities for peer buddies in playgroups, as well as cooperative learning approaches in classrooms; and identifying and celebrating positive interactions.

Individuals with autism express that they want to be valued for who they are and for their uniqueness. Adult efforts to model an appreciation of each child's special gifts make a strong statement to both the individuals with autism and their peers. It is helpful to talk with typical peers and siblings about the way that autism has manifested itself in an individual's learning style and needs and to suggest ways to communicate and relate.

Behavior and Routines

Children with ASDs tend to demonstrate certain behaviors. These are described next, along with interventions to help address problem behavior.

What Do We See?

Children with autism often seek predictability and rules. When faced with change and novel situations, they can easily become anxious, distractible, distraught, and exhibit mood swings

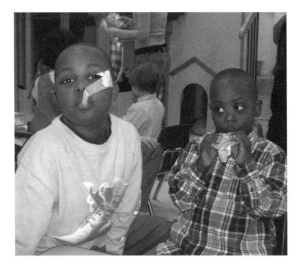

and intense reactions. In environments that are loud, chaotic, and require close contact with uncomfortable materials or people, they can be overwhelmed. These states may present themselves as impulsive, uninhibited behavior; tantrums; withdrawal or flight; stereotypic, obsessive actions; inflexible adherence to rituals and routines; and attempts to control the situation. Some children may attempt to injure themselves or others. Each child's pattern of actions is unique, and adults need to decode the source of a particular behavior. It is important to remember that young children with autism demonstrate the behaviors of children their age. Thus, when a 2-year-old child bites a peer or a 3-year-old child demands his or her choice of snack or refuses to share, this is typical behavior for the age and not a symptom of autism.

What Are the Sources of Behavioral Challenges?

Behavior is a function of a person interacting with his or her environment. The physical and sensory setting and the demands and expectations of the adults and peers have a major impact on the inner states and sensory sensitivities of the child. For example, a highly stimulating environment (e.g., a trip to a busy grocery store, a birthday party, a noisy classroom) or unexpected and unexplained change in routine can lead to distress and tantrums. The behavior seen by others communicates something about the child's state and serves a variety of purposes for the child with autism, such as play, protection, control, escape, self-regulation, and organizing patterns.

Behavior can become a habitual response to gain a particular effect—that is, a response that works and, therefore, is rewarded. For instance, many preschoolers protest the interruption of a favorite activity, and when adults back off from a request to avoid a conflict, the child's protest works. He or she learns an effective strategy to have needs met. Such adult attention can reinforce inappropriate behaviors.

Positive behavioral supports begin by asking "why" and seeking to connect challenging behaviors with the child's temperament, sensory system, language deficits, anxiety, or low tolerance for change. Behavior is influenced also by illness, allergies, side effects of medication, hunger, sleeplessness, and fatigue. It is important to rule out and/or address these conditions in the problem-solving process. Developmental issues, family circumstances, and cultural expectations are factors as well. The demands in an environment have an impact on the behavior of the child, including confusing and unclear instructions, unpredictable schedules, activities that are too difficult or too easy, limited opportunities to communicate, and inadequate assistance. As adults try to understand the source of challenging behavior, they can see how a change in the setting, the structure of an activity, or the behavior of the adults or peers may alter the behavior of the child with autism.

What Is the Goal of Intervention?

The goal of intervention is the creation of strategies to help children cope with their environment and have their needs met so that they can be safe, regulated, and communicative. When their senses are overloaded, they need strategies to calm themselves. When they are anxious, angry, or upset, they need to learn effective ways to make their feelings known, see a problem in a different way (reframe it), develop internal controls, handle transitions, become more flexible, and act in a way that takes into account the impact of their actions on others. Children should feel empowered to make motivating choices (not overpowered) and grow to become independent. Ideally, behavior changes should be independent of adult cues but embedded in environmental demands, peer models, and the learned and applied problem-solving strategies of the student. Hodgdon explains that

> We need to remember that our students with special needs are human beings. They are children with body systems that are not working totally correctly. They handle life in ways that make sense to them. They use the skills they have to use. They behave in the ways they know to accomplish their purposes. That is behavior. Sometimes the behavior they use is considered appropriate and acceptable. At other times their behavior is unsatisfactory. It needs to be changed. When it needs to be changed,

we usually need to do something to help it to change. (1999, p. 38)

What Are Some Useful Interventions?

Planning interventions for a child's behavior involves engaging in a team-based, problem-solving process and a functional behavioral assessment (Janney & Snell, 2008; O'Neill et al., 1997) that fulfills several purposes. These include

- Identifying when the behavior occurs and does not occur

- Making good guesses about the most likely function of the behavior for the child

- Brainstorming ways to change the antecedents for the behavior to prevent it, teaching new and more appropriate behaviors to fulfill the same function, and developing positive strategies when the behavior of concern does occur

Functional assessment looks at the environment as well as the person, and at the adults as well as the child. The focus is on teaching desirable behaviors, not punishing challenging ones. Prevention should be the primary intervention. Moreover, there are some basic principles for guiding a positive approach to behavior. They are each discussed in the following sections.

Effective Interventions Occur within Relationships.   It takes time and effort to build a trusting relationship, and this process begins with respect, empathy, mutual affection, and regard. As adults live and work with young children with autism, they will get to know them as unique individuals and foster engagement and joy in their interactions. When children become familiar with those around them and develop trust, they are more willing to try new things, stretch themselves and take risks, and respond to redirection and limit setting by adults.

All Children Benefit from Predictable Structure and Rehearsal.   Children can be supported by organizing the environment and the schedule so that they understand the use of space and time and can anticipate the expectations of a particular activity. Routines are so important! When children have learned the routines for different parts of the day, whether it be dinnertime at home or snack time at school, they can confidently participate. Routines can be about interactions. A child can learn how everyone is greeted in the morning ("High five!") as when entering the classroom or how the "Hello Song" at circle time is the same every day. Cues about transitions, supported by visual schedules, for example, help children move from one activity and set of expectations to another without distress. Strategies for what to do when you have to wait are helpful to all young children. One-to-one rehearsal of actions that are part of the routines of the day can aid in a child's comfort and ability to participate more independently.

Supports Need to Take into Account a Child's Learning Style, Sensory Sensitivities, and Interests.   As described earlier in this chapter, many individuals with autism are strong visual learners. Providing nontransient, visual cues is one of the most significant interventions adults can offer (Hodgdon, 1999). Schedules of the day, rules and expectations for particular areas of the room or activities, and if-then consequences expressed in visuals can help children know what to do, when to do it, as well as what not to do (expressing guidelines positively rather than as negatives is most effective). Using visuals for limited choices in many situations can reduce the anxiety of a distraught preschooler who feels his life is out of his control. Children also benefit from musical cues to help them transition through the day, as well as many opportunities for movement. It is important that adults are respectful of a child's preferences and not force participation in an activity that the child clearly perceives as unpleasant; expanding a child's tolerance occurs over time and with thoughtful exposure. As is the case for all preschoolers, teachers need to decrease waiting time. Finally, embedding a child's strong interests into an experience can be motivating and allow him or her to tolerate something that under other circumstances might produce a distraught reaction, as reflected in the words of a parent describing her journey from diagnosis to acceptance.

My son has always needed his world to make sense. His innate drive to bring order out of chaos is awesome. When he was young we didn't always understand what his intense interest in things like road maps, street signs, and big industrial storage tanks was all about, but slowly we realized this is not a game of trivia: he was working on unlocking the secrets of how the world is ordered, how categories are formed and connections made. Viewing his interests in this way was productive for him and for us. (Amos, as cited in Autism National Committee, 1999)

Learning Appropriate Ways to Handle Stress Is an Important Skill for Teachers to Develop in Young Children.   Knowing that a situation is difficult for a child with autism means considering what to teach that will allow him or her to manage him- or herself. With young children, begin with identifying feelings (in self and others) by using games, role play, and children's books (Buron, 2006; Jaffe & Gardner, 2006). Being aware of one's own arousal state, that is, is your body running on high, low, or just right? (Williams & Shellenberger, 2002), is the first step to regulating oneself independently. Reframing perceptions (cognitive restructuring) can allow a child to tolerate circumstances that were previously difficult; for example, for the child who needs to always get it right, lessons about how it is okay to make a mistake become critical. Knowing that everyone is faced with situations that are stressful, the goals are to learn how to become calm, exercise self-control, and request a break from a situation. Acknowledge and help a child feel good about the progress he or she is making toward gaining control in stressful situations. In addition to addressing sensory issues through preventive approaches, strategies described earlier, such as Social Stories (Gray, 2000), self-management strategies (Myles & Southwick, 1999), and Skillstreaming (McGinnis & Goldstein, 1990) are essential tools to support children in handling stress.

Some Behaviors Are More Important to Pursue than Others.   Pick your battles by choosing carefully. There are priority levels for problem behaviors (Janney & Snell, 2008). Distracting behaviors may be annoying (e.g., echolalia, hand flapping), but they do not cause any harm. Disruptive behaviors, such as running out of the room or loud crying, may be unsafe or interfere with learning or participation. Destructive behaviors are threatening to the health or safety of the child or the group. Focus on those issues that are high priority, knowing that in the hundreds of decisions made every day, one cannot make everything a crisis. Remember that the needs of the individual have to be weighed against the needs of the group and that sometimes the short-term pain is chosen over the long-term gain. If an upset can be avoided by redirection or using humor to reduce the tension, by all means do so.

Teaching Positive Alternatives Rather than Saying No Is Imperative for Young Children. Often adults assume that children know what is expected of them, and yet adults with autism tell us that those expectations too frequently were and still are a mystery. The more specific adults can be about positive behaviors, the more likely they will be understood and incorporated. For example, teach an alternative way to get a peer's attention (e.g., tap her on the shoulder, say her name) or ask for help when stressed. If a child is yelling to get a drink, teach the sign. If she continually asks to go to the gym, provide and redirect her to a personal schedule with the symbol for the events of the day in sequence. Instituting an activity that is incompatible with a negative behavior is a helpful approach as well (e.g., it is difficult to bite yourself or a friend if you are chewing gum). Create a rich pattern of opportunities for a child to be successful and then respond in a reinforcing way. If the problem behavior is ineffective (i.e., it does not get the child what he or she wants) and the alternative behavior is effective, the alternative is more likely to be used. As much as possible, consequences should be natural (i.e., sensibly related to the behavior). For example, if juice is intentionally dumped on the floor, then it must be cleaned up and there is nothing more to drink. In teaching alternative behaviors, provide opportunities for the child to generalize the new skills to different environments, adults, and peers.

In a Crisis, the Attitude and the Posture of the Adults Matter Most. When a child with autism is out of control, adults need to be calm,

matter-of-fact, and supportive. Eliminate seductive objects, relocate the students and others to prevent harm and reduce an audience, talk less, give the child time, remove unnecessary demands, and provide an option for a graceful exit. Assess whether or not the behavior at the time is under the child's control. A gentle teaching approach (McGee & Menolascino, 1991) interrupts the chain of negative behavior by using humor or a stimulus change, and once calm, it ignores the negative actions and redirects the child to a neutral or positive behavior.

In his book, *Learning to Listen: Positive Approaches and People with Difficult Behavior*, Lovett (1996) reminds us that we should always ask "If I were in this person's shoes, how would I feel? What would I need? How would I want to be treated?" Often adults escalate power struggles with students because they themselves feel threatened and impotent to change a child's difficult behavior. Stressed children produce stress in their teachers and parents. Being reflective about one's own values and teaching is so important. Adults, similar to children with autism, frequently continue to use the same strategies over and over, even when they are not working. If an approach is not working, change it. Parents and teachers should use the opportunity to problem solve together. In difficult times, hold onto a sense of humor, to the joy that is each child, and remember the progress that is being made with the student.

Autism and the Family

When a child receives the diagnosis of an ASD, his or her whole family is often affected. The following discussion explores the impact on families and ways to help families reach certain goals.

What Is the Impact of Autism on Families?

Parents are seldom prepared for the news that their child has autism. Differences between typically developing children and those with ASDs can be discerned by the age of 2 years (Landa & Garrett-Mayer, 2006). The developmental red flags include poor eye contact; reduced responsive smiling; diminished babbling; and difficulty with language, play, and initiating or sustaining social interaction. Parents describe having concerns about the development of their children in infancy, but families frequently are told by physicians to give it time, and that the language, attention, or social skills will catch up. Although there is hope that this is true, the lingering worries are there and intensify as the months pass. Some have described that even though the evaluation process and the announcement of its result were painful, it also was a relief to connect a name to their child's behaviors (Gray, 2003; Nissenbaum, Tollefson, & Reese, 2002). There is evidence that mothers experience a greater toll on their emotional well-being than do fathers (Gray, 2003). Marital difficulties can result from the different ways that two parents handle the diagnosis, ensuing decisions, and life changes (Greenspan & Wieder, 1998). This is the first step of a lifelong journey of understanding the unique needs of their son or daughter, making choices about interventions, developing routines that help the family get through each day, finding ways to balance their own emotional ups and downs, and seeking a positive attitude about the future possibilities. Many of these emotions are echoed in the words of this parent:

> My son was diagnosed with autism when he was three years old. The news was devastating. I thought I had lost him. All I really understood was that this was incurable. My only context for autism was the movie *Rainman*. Like other parents with children on the autism spectrum, I wanted someone to blame. And I wanted to fix him. There are many therapies out there. I would spare no expense to help him overcome this terrible condition. And I found that there was no shortage of people out there prepared to take every dime I could spend to help me relieve my guilt for creating an imperfect child. . . . Eventually over time, by trial and error, we would try different strategies, and keep the things that worked and throw away the ones that didn't. Most importantly, my son's inclusive preschool helped me to look past the diagnosis and see my child again. I had never lost him. He was always there. It was me who had the problem. I had loved him for who he was before he was diagnosed. Afterwards, while I was trying to "fix" him, I could only see the label. I felt locked out of his world. The teachers . . . taught me to see him again

as the complex, intelligent, talented child he is. (Parent, personal communication)

The stressors in a family with a young child with autism are many (Marcus, 1984), including the following:

- The unrelieved daily care of their child

- Obtaining good assessments that lead to program recommendations

- Inadequate educational and support services

- The neglect of the personal needs of the parents

- Balancing attention to all family members, including the siblings

- Episodic difficult behavior of their child and the fear that the behavior will recur

- Feelings of inadequacy and helplessness

- Their child's (and often the family's) limited social relationships

- Perceptions of extended family, neighbors, school personnel, and the public

Taking an individual with autism out into the community can be a source of stress for parents. People may stare, make comments, or fail to understand any mishaps or behavior that may occur. As a result of these experiences, families often feel uncomfortable taking their child to the homes of friends and relatives. This makes holidays an especially difficult time. Parents of children with autism may experience a sense of isolation from their friends, relatives, and community, as do many families of children with disabilities.

The lives of parents whose child receives an autism diagnosis will be dramatically changed as they learn about the disorder. They make connections with the world of special education and its procedures and professionals; and their energy, faith, and resilience as individuals and as a family are tested again and again (Koegel & LaZebnik, 2004). Parents do describe the positives that emerge out of having a child with autism, including personal growth, the development of advocacy skills, closer family relationships, and an appreciation of the small things in life, as described in the following statement.

This experience we did not choose, which we would have given anything to avoid, has made us different, has made us better. Through it we have learned the lesson of Sophocles and Shakespeare—that one grows by suffering. And that too is Jessy's gift. I write now what fifteen years past I would still not have thought possible to write: that if today I were given a choice, to accept the experience with everything it entails, or to refuse the bitter largesse, I would have to stretch out my hands—because out of it has come for all of us an unimagined life. And I will not change the last word of the story. It is still love. (Park, 1982, p. 320)

What Are the Goals for Families?

Professionals should have a number of goals in mind in their work with families of young children with autism.

1. Parents will become active participants in their child's programming. They will gain knowledge about development and the autism spectrum, as well as confidence and competence in their parenting. Dawson and Osterling (1997) found that when parents were involved in their child's program, they experienced a greater sense of relatedness with their child, an increase in their sense of competence and feeling of well-being, and a decrease in emotional stress. In addition, professionals and parents will work collaboratively as partners to create a program for the child.

2. Regular communication will occur between parents and professionals. Whether a child is receiving services at home or in a center-based program, parents will be kept up-to-date on the interventions being used and the progress being made by their child. Parents can share what is happening at home, share the strategies that are working for them, and request support to address particular goals and routines.

3. Parents will develop advocacy skills and learn how to access services (e.g., respite) in their community for their child and their family.

4. The network of relationships for parents will be expanded, including building on existing family and community supports and connecting with other parents.

5. Parents will embrace the joy of their child and find optimism in their life. Parents will discover, through the living of every day, that everything is not negative, as seen in the following family vignette. There are many positives to embrace and be gained.

I've learned to value collaboration and give up the illusion of control. Thanks to my son, I think I've become more laid-back in my approach to life, more appreciative, more attuned to the here and now. He gave me an advanced course on perspective, which keeps the complex landscape of our family life in balance. (Amos, as cited in Autism National Committee, 1999)

There are several major values that underlie a family-centered approach for parents of young children with autism. These include the following:

- The family-centered approach is grounded in a posture of respect for each parent and his or her life situation. Parents will engage if they believe that professionals are on their side and are not judging them but, rather, are trying to understand and accept them.

- A child's life is embedded within the family context: culture, priorities, parenting styles, support systems. Parents will engage if they experience professionals as being sensitive to their values and culture.

- Often the jargon of teachers and therapists gets in the way of effective communication about children and interventions. Parents will engage if what teachers and therapists say and do makes sense to them.

- Professionals need to treat their communication about children and parents with confidentiality. Parents will engage if they trust that their privacy will be protected.

- A collaborative approach has many benefits for the child. Parents know their child best and can share with teachers and therapists the strategies that they have found effective.

Parents will engage when they know their input is valued.

- It is critical to communicate acceptance and positive regard for every child. Parents will engage when they believe that professionals know and care about their child.

In addition, a supportive family-centered approach needs to

- *Empower parents to make choices:* Parents should be educated about the models that are available (their value base, the service delivery, timing, as well as other considerations) and be given an opportunity to choose what seems the best fit for their child and their family. Staff need to be mindful of their own values and acknowledge and respect that the family must choose what works for them.

- *Implement communication systems and concrete strategies:* Central to the program is the coordination of efforts between home and school. Arrange a communication system that is mutually acceptable (e.g., e-mail, notebook, telephone calls, observations, and/or team meetings). Help parents organize around their goals for students, using journals and workbooks (Abrams & Henriques, 2004), and incorporate their priorities into the goals and benchmarks of their child's plan. Staff should engage in joint problem-solving with parents and address home behavior management issues by helping structure daily routines, imbedding communication approaches into family life, and helping families gain access to community resources such as financial support and respite care that will reduce the stress at home. Listen to what the family says is helpful and what is not; pick up on between-the-lines concerns. Ask, "What can we do to help?" Address real issues by asking, "If you could change anything about your life, what would it be? When you lie awake at night worrying, what is it you worry about?" (McWilliam, 2003).

- *Celebrate progress:* Share with family members the positives that occur and be sure that communication addresses accomplishments, not just problems. Tell parents what they are

doing well, indicate appreciation of their contributions to the child's progress, and help them feel competent in their parenting role. Build on their long-term vision for the child and on the strengths of both the child and the family.

- *Create connections:* Many parents of children with special needs feel isolated, lonely, and afraid to reach out for help. Begin by inviting parents into the program to observe, participate, and share ideas. Allow time for social exchange and relationship-building. Offer activities for all members of the family, so that parents who normally are uncomfortable about accessing community events with their child can have a place to go where they feel safe and welcomed. Sponsor sibling groups appropriate to the age levels of the brothers or sisters. Facilitate contacts between parents, through one-to-one, parent-to-parent interaction; e-mail groups; and parent groups. In addition, share information about community-wide networks (e.g., the local chapter of the Autism Society of America), and pass on the names of books, journals, and web sites that educate and connect, including materials written by and for parents and by adults with autism.

- *Support parents in becoming advocates:* Offer opportunities for families to learn about the regulations within which services are provided and parents' rights within this process. Help families identify and articulately present what they think will best meet the needs of their son or daughter on the autism spectrum. Talk about building alliances with agencies and school staff. To ease transitions between service systems (e.g., early intervention to preschool, preschool to kindergarten), offer information, documentation of needs, the presence of service providers, service coordinators, and external advocates (including other parents) support family members through this process. Early childhood professionals will have contact with a child and family for a limited period of time; mothers, fathers, and grandparents will be responsible for supporting the child throughout life. Efforts to empower parents to work effectively with school and medical personnel and access community resources are an investment in the child's future.

- *Help parents manage their stress:* The neglect of personal, social, and physical needs is a major source of burnout for parents. Encourage families to utilize stress reduction techniques to manage each day: get sleep, let go of expectations to be the perfect family, reframe problems to see benefits, use positive self-talk, hit the "pause" button as needed, and see the humor in events. Remind parents to continue to see themselves as people, not only as parents of a child with autism, and to set aside time for themselves; for each other; for exercise; for music and artistic expression; and for vacations without guilt. In order to be the best mother or father, a parent needs to take care of him- or herself first.

Implications for Intervention and New Research

We would like to explore some thoughts about the implications for the treatment and education of young children with autism. This question has been at the center of much debate in the autism community, and a source of much confusion for parents who receive a diagnosis of autism for their child and who are attempting to determine the best course of action. There are several types of educational programs available, each with its own underlying values and beliefs about how children with autism learn best, and each with its own benefits and concerns. In general, well-publicized teaching approaches for students with autism tend to fall along a continuum, with behavioral approaches at one end and social-pragmatic approaches at the other. It is generally accepted that there is no one treatment or intervention that works well for all people with autism; thus, finding a match for the child and the family is an important goal.

Behavioral approaches draw heavily from the work of behavioral psychologists such as B.F. Skinner and the principles of operant conditioning. Desirable behavioral responses are seen as something best taught through modeling, prompting, and then reinforcing desirable acts. Undesirable behavioral responses are eliminated with various strategies, and behaviors are shaped into more desirable responses, which are then rewarded. These approaches typically follow a prescribed curriculum. Skills are carefully task-analyzed into small steps, which are often taught in isolation (to eliminate environmental distractions and/or conflicting stimuli), and careful data collection and analysis are used to determine mastery of skills and readiness for next steps.

After children have mastered basic skills in the curriculum sequence, incorporating the approach into a supported preschool program is recommended to encourage generalization. Some publicized approaches with a behavioral basis are Applied Behavior Analysis (ABA; an approach often used interchangeably or associated with behavior modification, behavior analysis, and positive behavior support), based on the work of Lovaas, and TEACHH (Treatment and Education of Autistic and related Communication-handicapped Children), a statewide program of service delivery for children with autism and their families in North Carolina. See Erba (2000) for further information on both of these approaches.

Social-pragmatic approaches are based on the belief that children learn and apply skills best within the natural environments where they will need to use them, eliminating concerns about generalization. Furthermore, they learn best through meaningful social engagement with others. Social-pragmatic strategies often begin by following the child's lead, starting with activities that are of natural interest, manipulating the environment to elicit interaction, and interacting in a style that the child will perceive as meaningful and rewarding. The communicative intent of a child's actions is considered and responded to, with attempts made, through modeling and scaffolded cues, to shape these actions into more conventional communicative and social skills, while maximizing current success. Positive social engagement and interaction are seen as central to development across multiple areas, and priority is placed on the child initiating and responding to environmental cues. Thus, although the curriculum considers a sequence of child development, it is individualized to address the child's unique learning profile and to build on success. A meaningful relationship with the child is at the core of these approaches, and their focus on developing skills within natural settings means that they most often involve elements of inclusion of the child with autism in classrooms and/or social environments with their peers without disabilities. Publicized educational models that use social-pragmatic approaches include the Developmental-Individual-Difference, Relationship-Based (DIR) Model and Floor Time strategies, developed by Greenspan and Wieder (1998), and the SCERTS® Model for supporting progress in Social Communication, Emotional Regulation, and Transactional Support (Prizant, Wetherby, Rubin, Laurent, & Rydell, 2006).

Some models combine elements of behavioral social-pragmatic approaches. In these models, skills are worked on within natural settings. Often children are the initiators of play/interaction, with teachers encouraged to follow their leads. Adults respond to communicative intents and reinforce any attempts at communication. The environment is engineered to increase the likelihood that a child will want and attempt to engage and communicate, and specific strategies are used to elicit and encourage communication. Some examples of these approaches are Incidental Teaching (McGee et al., 1999) and Pivotal Response Training (PRT; Koegel & Koegel, 2006; Koegel, Koegel, Harrower, & Carter, 1994). A number of programs combine components of multiple approaches.

Although a detailed examination of individual approaches is not practical for the scope of this chapter, Dawson and Osterling (1997) identified several common elements among approaches that report significant success. These include the following:

- Identification and services beginning as early in the child's life as possible

- Intensive levels of service (20–40 hours per week of active engagement in learning)

- Curriculum priorities including attending, imitating, comprehending and using language, playing, and interacting socially

- Highly supportive and intensive teaching environments

- A functional approach to problem behaviors

- High levels of family involvement

- Planned transitions to next settings (e.g., early intervention to preschool, preschool to kindergarten)

- Ongoing assessment and regular program adjustment

- Specialized instruction in settings where ongoing interactions with typically developing peers are possible

Regardless of the method or approach used, most comprehensive intervention programs for children with autism incorporate specific supports such as speech/language therapy and motor therapy (from occupational and/or physical therapists). Motor therapists work to address sensory needs and development, as well as specific motor skills. The specific types and amounts of therapy can vary, and are determined on the basis of a child's individual learning profile.

In addition to the previously noted strategies, educational programs should work to include children with autism in social and educational settings with their typically developing peers. One of the recognized characteristics of children with autism is their difficulties in generalizing skills from one setting to another. Given this tendency, it makes good sense to teach skills in settings where they will be needed. Similarly, because one of the core areas of need for children with autism is social interaction, it is important to provide opportunities for social interaction with peers who can be strong models and participants in the interaction. The presence of typically developing peer models allows for increased spontaneous learning opportunities, as well as potentially increasing motivation for engagement and interaction. Gillingham's (2000) work includes several examples of individuals with autism who showed remarkable progress, when moved from noninclusive to inclusive settings. Typically developing peers in inclusive settings also develop positive attitudes toward and strategies for successfully interacting with people who have widely varying abilities and needs. It is important, however, to note that successful inclusive settings include carefully planned modifications and supports, creating a balance of adapting the environment and interactions to meet the child's needs and supporting the child to increase his or her skills within that setting. Supports should be based on the previously discussed principles of effective early intervention. Staffing supports might include a special education teacher, speech, occupational and/or physical therapists, and paraprofessionals. The classroom environment, schedule, and activity formats may need to be adapted to address sensory, communication, cognitive, motor, and/or social needs, as well as specific teaching approaches. With skillful support, much of this intervention can happen within the classroom, so that the child is a fully included member of the educational community.

Finally, this chapter would not be complete without commentary on current alternative approaches to the treatment of young children with autism. A tour of the Internet can lead a parent or professional to hundreds of interventions for young children with autism that are described and supported by testimonials as well as research reports. Some approaches are substantiated with controlled trials, whereas the benefits of others are supported via anecdotal reports from families. Interventions that involve physiology include the following:

- Intravenous treatments (e.g., Secretin, chelation therapy)

- Diets and supplements (e.g., gluten-free/casein-free diets, antiyeast therapy megavitamins such as B_6 and the antioxidant amino acid supplement dimethyl glycine [DMG])

- Pharmacological treatments—often used for novel purposes (e.g., anticonvulsants, anti-anxiety drugs, antidepressants, stimulants)

- Specific sensory interventions (e.g., Irlen lenses, Wilbarger Protocol, squeeze machine,

auditory integration therapy, cranial-sacral therapy)

Examples of skill-based treatment programs include

- Cognitive behavior counseling

- Daily life therapy

- Music therapy

- Auditory integration therapy

- PECS

- Facilitated communication

To review some of these and other approaches, see the *Autism Treatment Guide* by Elizabeth Gerlach (2003).

Clearly, families and professionals always need to ask questions regarding any given approach. Some important ones to ask include the following:

- On what assumption is the approach based?

- Is the approach respectful of the child and family?

- Has the approach been validated scientifically?

- What training or credential is required to provide this treatment?

- How is the child assessed regarding this approach?

- What is the recommended frequency of the approach and how is it integrated into other treatments being utilized with a child?

- How and when will we know that it is working?

- What are the potential side effects?

- What are the potential costs and insurance coverage?

- Will the provider work with other primary care, teaching, and therapy staff?

Conclusion

In conclusion, everyone must be cautious about claims made by any approach and weigh the potential risks and side effects. Any intervention whose proponents maintain that it is a "cure" or appropriate for all children with autism should be suspect. Programs must meet the unique individual needs of children and their families, and be evaluated carefully in terms of the costs of dollars, time, and emotional energy for all concerned. In the words of Futterweit and Ruff,

No form of intervention is valuable for all children or parents, or at all times. Because development is an emergent rather than prescriptive process and depends on the confluence of many developing elements, unique needs cannot be met by prescribing the same intervention program for every child. Furthermore, interventions themselves need to be dynamic and changing, because no specific intervention will be valuable at all points in a given child's development. (1993, p. 166)

REFERENCES

Abrams, P., & Henriques, L. (2004). *The autism spectrum parent's daily helper: A workbook for you and your child.* Berkeley, CA: Ulysses.

American Psychiatric Association. (2000). *Diagnostic and statistical manual of mental disorders* (4th ed., text rev.). Washington, DC: Author.

Anzalone, M.E., & Williamson, G.G. (2000). Sensory processing and motor performance in autism spectrum disorders. In S.F. Warren & J. Reichle (Series Eds.) & A.M. Wetherby & B.M. Prizant (Vol. Eds.), *Communication and language intervention series: Vol. 9. Autism spectrum disorders: A transactional developmental perspective* (pp. 143–166). Baltimore: Paul H. Brookes Publishing Co.

Autism National Committee. (1999). *Through a parent's eyes: Mothers reflect on what they have learned about raising a child with Autism/PDD.* Retrieved August 13, 2007, from http://www.autcom.org/articles/ParentsEye.html

Ayres, A.J. (2005). *Sensory integration and the child* (25th anniversary ed.). Los Angeles: Western Psychological Services.

Baker, J. (2001). *The social skills picture book.* Arlington, TX: Future Horizons.

Bauman, M.L. (2007, January). Cerebellum and the brain stem in autism. Lecture presented during the course *Autistic Spectrum: The Bridge between Current Research in Neurology & Its Application to Clinical Practice.* (Available as published manual from Therapeutic Services, New York)

Bauman, M.L., & Kemper, T.L. (Eds.). (2006). *The neurobiology of autism.* Baltimore: Johns Hopkins Press.

Bauman, M.L., & Kemper, T.L. (2007, January). Neuropathology of autism spectrum disorders; What have we learned? Lecture presented during the course *Autistic Spectrum: The Bridge between Current Research in Neurology & Its Application to Clinical Practice.* (Available as published manual from Therapeutic Services, New York)

Berk, R.A., & DeGangi, G.A. (1983). *DeGangi-Berk Test of Sensory Integration.* Los Angeles: Western Psychological Services.

Biklen, D.P. (1993). *Communication unbound: How facilitated communication is challenging traditional views of autism and ability/disability.* New York: Teachers College Press.

Biklen, D.P. (Ed.). (2005). *Autism and the myth of the person alone.* New York: New York University Press.

Buron, K. (2006). *When my worries get too big! A relaxation book for children who live with anxiety.* Shawnee Mission, KS: Autism Asperger Publishing Co.

Cardon, T. (2007). *Initiations and interactions: Early intervention techniques for parents of children with autism spectrum disorders.* Shawnee Mission, KS: Autism Asperger Publishing Co.

Centers for Disease Control and Prevention. (2008, January 30). *Autism Information Center: Frequently asked questions: Prevalence.* Retrieved August 13, 2007, from http://www.cdc.gov/ncbddd/autism/faq_prevalence.htm

Dawson, G., & Osterling, J. (1997). Early intervention in autism: Effectiveness and common elements of current approaches. In M.J. Guralnick (Ed.), *The effectiveness of early intervention* (pp. 307–326). Baltimore: Paul H. Brookes Publishing Co.

DeGangi, G., & Greenspan, S. (1989). *Test of Sensory Functions in Infants.* Los Angeles: Western Psychological Services.

Donnellan, A., & Leary, M. (1994). *Movement differences and diversity in autism/mental retardation: Appreciating and accommodating people with communication and behavior challenges.* Madison, WI: DRI Press.

Dunn, W. (1999). *Sensory Profile.* San Antonio, TX: Harcourt Assessment.

Dunn, W. (2002). *Infant/Toddler Sensory Profile.* San Antonio, TX: Harcourt Assessment.

Eide, F.F. (2003). Sensory integration: Current concepts and practical implications. *Sensory Integration Special Interest Section Quarterly, 13,* 1–3.

Erba, H.W. (2000). Early intervention programs for children with autism: Conceptual frameworks for implementation. *American Journal of Orthopsychiatry, 70*(1), 82–94.

Fuge, G., & Berry, R. (2004). *Pathways to play! Combining sensory integration and integrated play groups.* Shawnee Mission, KS: Autism Asperger Publishing Co.

Futterweit, L., & Ruff, H. (1993). Principles of development: Implications for early intervention. *Journal of Applied Developmental Psychology, 2,* 153–173.

Gerlach, E. (2003). *The autism treatment guide.* Arlington, TX: Future Horizons.

Gillingham, G. (1998). *Autism: Handle with care.* Edmonton, Alberta, Canada: Tacit.

Gillingham, G. (2000). *Autism: A new understanding.* Edmonton, Alberta, Canada: Tacit.

Grandin, T. (1995). *Thinking in pictures.* New York: Vintage.

Grandin, T., & Barron, S. (2005). *Unwritten rules of social relationships.* Arlington, TX: Future Horizons.

Gray, C. (2000). *The new Social Story book.* Arlington, TX: Future Horizons.

Gray, C., & White, A.L. (2002). *My Social Stories book.* Philadelphia: Jessica Kingsley Publishers.

Gray, D. (2003). Gender and coping: The parents of children with high-functioning autism. *Social Science and Medicine, 56,* 631–642.

Greenspan, S., & Wieder, S. (1998). *The child with special needs.* New York: Perseus Books Group.

Hodgdon, L. (1995). *Visual strategies for solving behavior problems in autism: Practical supports for home and school.* Troy, MI: Quirk Roberts.

Hodgdon, L. (1999). *Solving behavior problems in autism: Improving communication with visual strategies.* Troy, MI: Quirk Roberts.

Howlin, P., Baron-Cohen, S., & Hadwin, J. (1999). *Teaching children with autism to mind-read.* New York: Wiley.

Individuals with Disabilities Education Improvement Act (IDEA) of 2004, PL 108-446, 20 U.S.C. §§ 1400 *et seq.*

Jaffe, A., & Gardner, L. (2006). *My book full of feelings: How to control and react to the size of your emotions.* Shawnee Mission, KS: Autism Asperger Publishing Co.

Janney, R., & Snell, M. (2008). *Teachers' guides to inclusive practices: Behavioral support* (2nd ed.). Baltimore: Paul H. Brookes Publishing Co.

Kluth, P. (2003). *"You're going to love this kid!" Teaching students with autism in the inclusive classroom.* Baltimore: Paul H. Brookes Publishing Co.

Koegel, R.L., & Koegel, L.K. (2006). *Pivotal Response Treatments for autism: Communication, social, and academic development.* Baltimore: Paul H. Brookes Publishing Co.

Koegel, L., Koegel, R., Harrower, J., & Carter, C. (1994). Pivotal response intervention. I: Overview of approach. *The Journal of The Association for Persons with Severe Handicaps, 24,* 174–185.

Koegel, L., & LaZebnik, C. (2004). *Overcoming autism: A state-of-the-art approach to reducing the symptoms of autism spectrum disorders.* New York: Viking Penguin.

Kranowitz, C.S. (1998). *The out-of-sync child: Recognizing and coping with sensory integration dysfunction.* New York: Perigee

Kranowitz, C.S. (2003). *The out-of-sync child has fun: Activities for kids with sensory integration dysfunction.* New York: Perigee.

Kranowitz, C.S. (2005). *The out-of-sync child: Recognizing and coping with sensory integration dysfunction* (Rev. ed.). New York: Perigee.

Kranowitz, C.S., Szklut, S., Balzer-Martin, L., Haber, E., & Sava, D.I. (2001). *Answers to questions teachers ask about sensory integration* (2nd ed.). Las Vegas: Sensory Resources.

Kurtz, L.A. (2007). Physical therapy and occupational therapy. In M.L. Batshaw, L. Pellegrino, & N.J. Roizen (Eds.), *Children with disabilities* (6th ed., pp. 571–579). Baltimore: Paul H. Brookes Publishing Co.

Landa, R., & Garrett-Mayer, E. (2006). Development in infants with autism spectrum disorders: A prospective study. *Journal of Child Psychology and Psychiatry and Allied Disciplines, 47*(6), 629–638.

Leicestershire County Council and Fosse Health Trust. (1998). *Autism: How to help your young child.* London: The National Autistic Society.

Lovett, H. (1996). *Learning to listen: Positive approaches and people with difficult behavior.* Baltimore: Paul H. Brookes Publishing Co.

Marcus, L. (1984). Coping with burnout. In E. Schopler & G. Mesibov (Eds.), *The effects of autism on the family* (pp. 311–326). New York: Plenum.

McEvoy, M.A., Twardosz, S., & Bishop, N. (1990). Affection activities: Procedures for encouraging young children with handicaps to interact with their peers. *Education and Treatment of Children, 13,* 159–167.

McGee, G., Morrier, M., & Daly, T. (1999). An incidental teaching approach to early intervention for toddlers with autism. *Journal of The Association for Persons with Severe Handicaps, 24,* 133–146.

McGee, J., & Menolascino, F. (1991). *Beyond gentle teaching: A non-aversive approach to helping those in need.* New York: Plenum.

McGinnis, E., & Goldstein, A. (1990). *Skillstreaming in early childhood: Teaching prosocial skills to the preschool and kindergarten child.* Champaign, IL: Research Press.

McKeon, T. (1994). *Soon will come the light.* Arlington, TX: Future Horizons.

McWilliam, R.A. (2003). Giving families a chance to talk so they can plan. *News Exchange, 8*(3), 4–6. Logan, UT: American Association for Home-Based Early Intervention.

Miller, L.J. (1982). *Miller Assessment of Preschoolers.* San Antonio, TX: Harcourt Assessment.

Miller, L.J. (2006). *Function and Participation Scales.* San Antonio, TX: Harcourt Assessment.

Myles, B.S., & Southwick, J. (1999). *Asperger syndrome and difficult moments.* Shawnee Mission, KS: Autism Asperger Publishing Co.

Nissenbaum, M., Tollefson, N., & Reese, R. (2002). The interpretive conference: Sharing a diagnosis of autism with families. *Focus on Autism and Other Disabilities, 17*(1), 30–43.

O'Neill, R.E., Horner, R.H., Albin, R.W., Sprague, J.R., Storey, K., & Newton, J.S. (1997). *Functional assessment and program development for problem behaviors.* Pacific Grove, CA: Brooks/Cole.

Park, C.C. (1982). *The siege* (with epilogue 15 years later). New York: Little, Brown.

Prizant, B.M., Wetherby, A.M., Rubin, E., Laurent A.C., & Rydell, P.J. (2006). *The SCERTS® Model: A comprehensive educational approach for children with autism spectrum disorders.* Baltimore: Paul H. Brookes Publishing Co.

Ramachandran, V.S., & Oberman, L M. (2006, November). Broken mirrors: A theory of autism. *Scientific American*, 62–69.

Rizzolatti, G., Fogassi, L., & Gallese, V. (2006, November). Mirrors in the mind. *Scientific American*, 54–61.

Rydell, P., & Prizant, B.M. (1995). Assessment and intervention strategies for children who use echolalia. In K.A. Quill, *Teaching children with autism* (pp. 105–132). New York: Delmar.

Schuler, A.L., & Wolfberg, P.J. (2000). Promoting peer play and socialization: The art of scaffolding. In S.F. Warren & J. Reichle (Series Eds.) & A.M. Wetherby & B.M. Prizant (Vol. Eds.), *Communication and language intervention series: Vol. 9. Autism spectrum disorders: A transactional developmental perspective* (pp. 251–277). Baltimore: Paul H. Brookes Publishing Co.

Schwartz, I., Billingsley, F., & McBride, B. (1998). Including children within inclusive preschools: Strategies that work. *Young Exceptional Children*, 2(1), 19–26.

Smukler, D. (2005). Unauthorized minds: How "Theory of Mind" theory misrepresents autism. *Mental Retardation, 43*(1), 11–24.

Strain, P.S., McGee, G.G., & Kohler, F.W. (2001). Inclusion of children with autism in early intervention environments: An examination of rationale, myths, and procedures. In M.J. Guralnick (Ed.), *Early childhood inclusion: Focus on change* (pp. 337–363). Baltimore: Paul H. Brookes Publishing Co.

Verstraeten, T., Davis, R.L., DeStefano, F., Lieu, T.A., Rhodes, P.H., Black, S.B., et al. (2003). Safety of thimerosal-containing vaccines: A two-phased study of computerized health maintenance organization databases. *Pediatrics, 112*(5), 1039–1048.

Wilbarger, J., & Wilbarger, P. (1991). *Sensory defensiveness in children aged 2–12.* Oak Park Heights, MN: PDP Products.

Wilbarger, P. (1984). Planning an adequate "sensory diet": Application of sensory processing theory during the first year of life. *Zero to Three Bulletin, 5*, 7–12.

Wilbarger, P. (1995). The sensory diet: Activity programs based on sensory processing theory. *Sensory Integration Special Interest Section Newsletter, 18*(2), 1–4.

Williams, D. (2003). *Exposure anxiety: The invisible cage.* Philadelphia: Jessica Kingsley Publishers.

Williams, M.S., & Shellenberger, S. (2002). *How does your engine run?: A leader's guide to the alert program for self-regulation.* Albuquerque, NM: Therapy Works.

Williams, R. (1991). Choices, communication, and control: A call for expanding them in the lives of people with severe disabilities. In L.H. Meyer, C.A. Peck, & L. Brown (Eds.), *Critical issues in the lives of people with severe disabilities* (pp. 543–544). Baltimore: Paul H. Brookes Publishing Co.

Wolfberg, P. (2003). *Peer play and the autism spectrum: The art of guiding children's socialization and imagination.* Shawnee Mission, KS: Autism Asperger Publishing Co.

Yack, E., Sutton, S., & Aquilla, P. (2002). *Building bridges through sensory integration* (2nd ed.). Las Vegas: Sensory Resources.

Yack, E., Sutton, S., & Aquilla, P. (2004, September–October). Ask the expert: The Wilbarger Protocol for sensory defensiveness. *Autism Asperger's Digest Magazine.* Retrieved on March 11, 2008, from http://www.thetherapyplace.net/newsletter/3_2.htm

CHAPTER 8

Sensory Processing Disorders

A TEACHER'S PERSPECTIVE

Toni S.P. Bell, Christy Cook Pica, and Janet O'Flynn

At the conclusion of this chapter, the reader will

- *Have a basic understanding of the neurobiological basis for sensory processing disorders*

- *Understand different types of sensory processing disorders*

- *Understand the motor, cognitive, language, and social-emotional challenges for young children and families as a result of sensory processing disorders*

- *Be knowledgeable about some contemporary early intervention therapies and strategies used to treat young children with sensory processing disorders*

Professionals will benefit from a general understanding of sensory processing disorders. This chapter provides the necessary neurobiological background for this understanding and explains the various types of sensory processing disorders. Readers are provided with an overview of current early intervention approaches for these disorders as well.

The Nervous System

As we move through our day, we are constantly processing information from our surroundings. This information helps us to perform everyday tasks and allows us to know how to interact with objects and people in our environments. Much of the information that we gather from our surroundings seems very evident to us, such as the smell of bacon in the morning, which signals that breakfast is ready. Other information that we gather is less overtly evident, such as feeling around in a drawer in the dark. The ability of our

hand to distinguish between a flashlight and a screwdriver seems so automatic that we do not think twice, for example, about the process of pattern recognition.

The process by which individuals gather information from their bodies and surroundings to help them function in their daily lives is called sensory processing. The most obvious way in which this information is gained is through the commonly known five senses of taste, smell, hearing, sight, and touch. Although these senses are very important in gaining sensory information, there are two additional senses of which most people are unaware—the proprioceptive and vestibular systems. The proprioceptive and vestibular senses operate automatically by sending information to the brain. The proprioceptive sense allows us to process information about our body position as to where and how our body is moving in space. This information is received through our muscles, ligaments, and joints. The vestibular sense allows us to process informa-

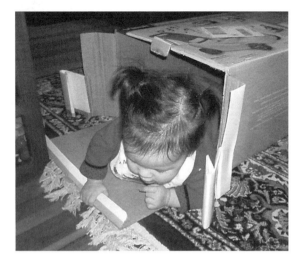

tion about gravity, movement, and balance, thus registering information about head motion in relation to the movement of objects around us (Smith & Gouze, 2004). This information is received through the inner ear, which is composed of the vestibular system and the cochlea (Batshaw, Pellegrino, & Roizen, 2007). Together, these two systems work to keep us oriented. They help to regulate our posture and muscle tone (Smith & Gouze, 2004).

The processing of the sensory information that we receive from our senses takes place in the central nervous system (CNS). As a sensation is presented, nerves in the peripheral nervous system register the information and activate the CNS (Williamson & Anzalone, 1997). Messages that we receive are transmitted through sensory neurons, which are found throughout our bodies. These neurons, which receive different impulses from our senses, help to activate functions through the central nervous and autonomic nervous systems, such as muscle movement, breathing, digestion, and sweat glands (Kranowitz, 1998). Some neurons convey messages that travel via the spinal cord, which then sends them to the brain, whereas others travel via the cranial nerves. The brain interprets and organizes these messages to execute cognitive and/or motor responses (Williamson & Anzalone, 1997). This process is the essence of sensory processing and reflects how the three complementary processes of sensory modulation, sensory discrimination, and motor planning work together to help us function in our daily lives.

Looking closer at the central nervous system, we are able to determine the different parts of the brain that have the greatest influence on sensory processing. The lower brain is thought to be the most primitive part of the brain and is acutely tuned into matters of survival and bodily maintenance (Smith & Gouze, 2004). This includes the brain stem and cerebellum, which are located at the base of the brain. The brain stem houses the 12 cranial nerves that control the functions of smell, vision, hearing, swallowing, articulation, facial expression, and breathing (Batshaw et al., 2007). From here, sensory information is gathered from the head and neck and relayed to the brain. Information from the body also passes through the brain stem on its ascending path. The other part of the lower brain is the cerebellum, which coordinates voluntary muscle activity (Batshaw et al., 2007). It is also important in the processing of proprioceptive and vestibular sensations with the coordination and timing of balance and movement.

The central section of the brain contains the limbic system. Within this section are basal ganglia that have an important role in working with the vestibular system and directing voluntary movement and balance (Batshaw et al., 2007). The hypothalamus is also located in this part of the brain and is responsible for coordinating the autonomic nervous system. This system helps to control the cardiovascular, digestive, endocrine, urinary, respiratory, and reproductive systems. In addition, it regulates our state of alertness or what is commonly known as our "fight or flight" response. The limbic system is also involved in

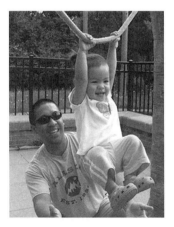

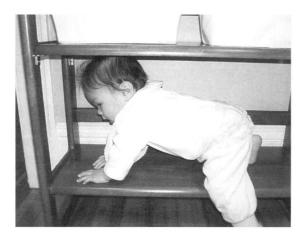

the regulation of emotions and motivation (Smith & Gouze, 2004).

The largest part of the brain, the cerebrum, is divided into two hemispheres. The left hemisphere is linked to more language-based, sequential cognitive functions, whereas the right hemisphere is linked to more visual-spatial, simultaneous cognitive functions. The cerebrum is the seat of consciousness and the center of cognitive functions, such as memory, learning, reasoning, judgment, and emotions. Information is transmitted between the two hemispheres through the corpus callosum.

Each hemisphere houses four major cortical lobes. First, the frontal lobe controls voluntary body movement and cognition. The next lobe is the parietal lobe, which integrates stimuli from all of the major senses, as well as the proprioceptive sense (pain and temperature) to give the whole picture (Kranowitz, 1998). Crossing over the top of these two lobes is the motor and sensory cortex. The sensory cortex is responsible for receiving tactile and proprioceptive sensations from the body, and the motor cortex sends messages to the muscles to direct movement and coordination.

The remaining two lobes, occipital and temporal, have more specific functions. The occipital lobe is primarily responsible for vision. Accordingly, visual tracts pass from the eyes through the deep parietal lobes to the occipital lobe. The temporal lobe is primarily responsible for communication, and more specifically for producing and comprehending speech and sensations. It also is very important for visual and auditory memory (Batshaw et al., 2007).

The background information described here reflects the complexity of the central nervous system and the many components working together to share information for appropriate processing and functioning. This complex system begins to develop from the moment of conception, and by 18 days of gestation the spine and neural plates are beginning to develop. The central nervous system continues to develop rapidly throughout the first 3 months of gestation at which point the brain structures are in place. For full-term newborns, the brain will have reached 90% of its final size by the age of 2 years. Throughout childhood and adolescence, the brain continues to grow and develop by making new synaptic connections and by thinning out those that are no longer needed (Smith & Gouze, 2004). This development creates the critical network of neural connections that allows us to process incoming sensory information, thus leading to better perception, attention, speech, memory, and abstract reasoning (Smith & Gouze, 2004).

Much of the information that we know today about sensory processing was initiated by the research of Dr. A. Jean Ayers in the mid-1960s. She felt that the organization, interpretation, and use of sensory information underlie all other aspects of human behavior (Smith & Gouze, 2004). She recognized that this processing system develops and is built on over time, much like building blocks. Accordingly, she broke down this development into four levels of integration (Kranowitz, 1998).

The first level of integration is the primary sensory system, which emerges by 2 months of

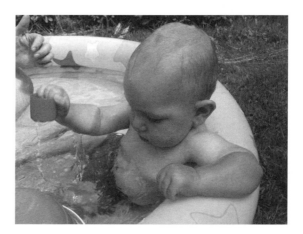

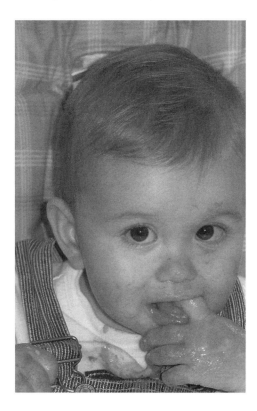

age. An infant receives sensory input into several systems, even before birth. For example, due to in utero stimulation (e.g., mother's voice, bowel sounds, placental sound of blood flow), hearing is well developed at birth, even in preterm infants (D.A. Clark, personal communication, May 2007). Through their tactile system, infants develop their sense of touch. A majority of this development is accomplished by mouthing objects. In addition, infants gain increasingly better control of their bodies through their movement, which helps to establish their proprioceptive and vestibular systems.

By 12 months of age, a child has reached the second level of integration, which is the perceptual-motor foundation level of development, and is beginning to have better body awareness and positioning. He or she also is starting to use both sides of the body in simultaneous, coordinated movements. This bilateral integration is important in moving objects from hand to hand, as well as crossing mid-line. At this level, children begin to display better postural and motor skills and abilities to control activity level, emotion, and attention.

The third level of development focuses on perceptual-motor skills, which are seen by the age of 3 years. Children now have better perception and cognitive understanding of information that they are receiving from their senses. Their hearing and sight have become more refined and precise, and they are better able to understand and communicate through expressive language. Through their greater understanding of spatial relationships and eye–hand coordination, fine and gross motor activities such as drawing and catching begin to develop.

The last level of development is academic readiness, which is achieved by 6 years of age. Children are capable of more abstract thought and reasoning that facilitate the acquisition of academic skills. They have more complex motor skills and tactile discrimination, and these skills lead to increased fine and gross motor control. Likewise, they have developed better visualization, discrimination, and increased social skills.

Although these developmental building blocks of sensory processing are logical, they are not uniform or consistent for everyone. As our brains develop, information that we receive is constantly changing the neural connections and patterns that shape our brains. As a consequence, our brains are uniquely formed, based on our own personal histories, which include our genetic influences, biological strengths and weaknesses, and positive and negative life experiences (Smith & Gouze, 2004). Of primary importance are environmental experiences that continue to exert a major impact on the acquisition of skills and abilities.

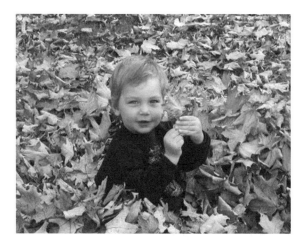

The fact that each brain forms uniquely, based on personal history, is supported by studies done with children in eastern Europe. Specifically, children who otherwise were healthy experienced significant developmental delays as a result of a lack of sensory stimulation. Moreover, Lin, Cermack, Coster, and Miller (2005) found that the longer children were institutionalized, the more severe their developmental and growth delays. The children also displayed eating problems, and social-behavioral, attention, and activity level difficulties. Lin and colleagues reported that institutionalized children received only 18% of the holding, rocking, and tactile input experienced by infants raised in a family, in addition to suffering nutritional deficiencies and potential environmental toxins, such as exposure to lead. In particular, their study confirmed that children institutionalized longer than 18 months showed greater difficulties in tactile, vestibular-proprioceptive, visual, auditory, and praxis functioning than those who were institutionalized for less than 6 months (Lin et al., 2005).

The next discussion focuses on young children for whom appropriate sensory processing difficulties are a chronic struggle in their daily lives. In her research during the 1970s, Dr. A. Jean Ayres used the term sensory integration dysfunction to describe behaviors related to specific difficulties with sensory processing. Specifically, she recognized that certain children experienced atypical social, emotional, motor, and functioning patterns of behavior in response to sensory stimuli (Miller, Cermack, Lane, Anzalone, &

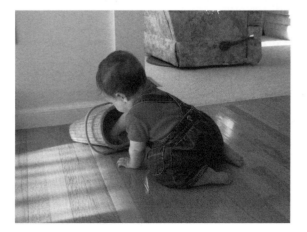

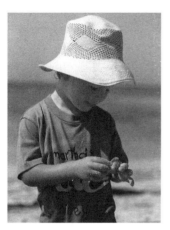

Koomar, 2004). Current literature refers to these conditions as sensory processing disorders (SPD) or disorders of sensory integration (DSI).

Sensory Processing Disorders

As typical children grow and develop, they learn how their senses work and learn to trust them. However, children with SPD do not take their senses for granted because they have learned that they cannot consistently depend upon them (Kranowitz, 2005). In particular, these children painfully find that their tactile, vestibular, and/or proprioceptive systems do not function efficiently, either separately or together, which directly affects their abilities to interact successfully with others and in and around their surroundings (Emmons & Anderson, 2005). Deficiencies in day-to-day functioning that result from instability of the nervous system can lead children with SPD to feel exhausted, terrified, or inept. Without intervention, they are at great risk for suffering deficits in their emotional, social, physical, and academic development (Kranowitz, 2005).

Suspected causes of SPD may include heredity, stressful prenatal conditions (especially drug or alcohol use), birth trauma, abuse and/or neglect, and other adverse environmental conditions. SPDs can coexist with a number of other disabilities, such as autism spectrum disorders, Down syndrome, fragile X syndrome, Prader-Willi syndrome, cerebral palsy, attention deficit-hyperactivity/disorder (ADHD), as well as very low birth weight (< 1,000 grams).

The results of a survey of incoming kindergarten children in a large school district in Colorado suggested that between 5% and 15% of all children (and adults) are affected by SPD. Moreover, it is estimated that SPDs affect between 40% and 85% of children with other disabilities (Miller, 2006).

SPD can be broken down into three classically occurring patterns for which terms may vary slightly. These include sensory modulation disorder (SMD), sensory-based motor disorder (SBMD), and sensory discrimination disorder (SDD). Each of these disorders and their respective subtypes are shown in Figure 8.1.

These patterns and their subtypes usually do not occur exclusively. Because our sensory systems are interconnected (Emmons & Anderson, 2005), these disorders can be related, and affected children may exhibit symptoms of more than one pattern or subtype. Figure 8.2 illustrates the incidence in which these disorders occur in isolation or in combination.

After examining the prevalence rates, we note that the majority of children, approximately 70%, who have been diagnosed with SPDs are affected by more than one pattern, with 43% exhibiting symptoms of two patterns and 27% showing symptoms of all three. Only 30% of children with SPDs are affected by just one pattern. Sensory modulation disorder is much more likely than the others to occur in isolation. Interestingly, however, the subtypes of SMD are also quite likely to overlap, with 59% occurring in combination (Miller, 2006).

Sensory Modulation Disorder

SMD can be seen in children who encounter difficulties with producing controlled responses appropriate for the intensity and nature of the sensory information received. In particular, children with these disorders have symptoms that fall into one or more of the following areas: sensory overresponsivity, sensory underresponsivity, and sensory seeking or craving (Miller, 2006).

Sensory Overresponsivity   Probably the most dramatic and disruptive of the SMDs is sensory overresponsivity (SOR). A child who is overresponsive reacts to sensory messages more intensely or more quickly, and often longer than children with normal sensory responsivity (Miller, 2006). Their defensiveness may include an aversion to certain touch sensations, tastes, sounds, textures, and/or movements. It is common for children with SOR to have extreme outbursts in reaction to sensory stimulation that might be

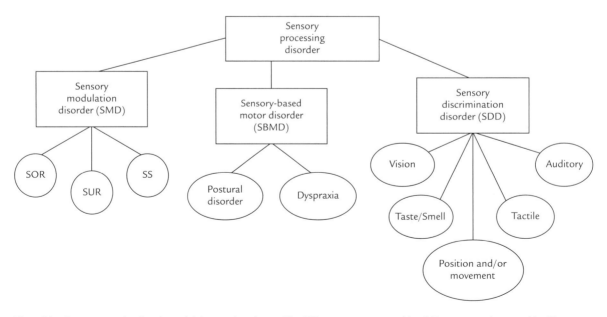

Figure 8.1.   Sensory processing disorders and their respective subtypes. (*Key:* SOR = sensory overresponsivity; SUR = sensory underresponsivity; SS = sensory seeking/craving.) (*Source:* Miller, 2006.)

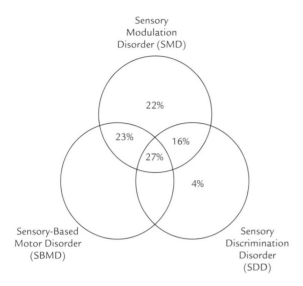

Sensory
Modulation
Disorder (SMD)

22%

23%   16%

27%

4%

Sensory-Based
Motor Disorder
(SBMD)

Sensory
Discrimination
Disorder
(SDD)

Figure 8.2. Incidences of sensory processing disorders in isolation and in combination. (*Source:* Miller, 2006.)

pleasant, slightly annoying, or completely unnoticeable to a typical child (Kranowitz, 2005).

A study carried out by the SPD Alpha Research Project in Denver, Colorado, indicated that children with SOR may have an ineffective autonomic nervous system. Their sympathetic nervous system seems to be overactive and inappropriately places them in a fight or flight survival mode. It then follows that the parasympathetic nervous system is underactive and does not sufficiently calm the children. When a child is surprised by unexpected stimuli, his or her body does not naturally return to homeostasis. In turn, because the child does not recover from the seemingly threatening experiences that occur throughout daily life, he or she is subject to meltdowns that result from sensory overload and the exhaustion of being perpetually in fight or flight mode (Miller, 2006).

This study also revealed that a child with SOR, compared with a typical child, is not able to habituate to nonthreatening stimuli. The nervous system continues to respond to familiar stimuli as if he or she were in danger, even when experience indicates that is not the case. This inability to habituate also affects the child's ability to filter out extraneous sensations, leaving him or her to address unimportant details consciously, rather than attending to things such as social cues or academic learning (Miller, 2006).

SOR usually affects more than one sense, although its influence often is more evident in one particular area. One of the most noticeable sensitivities that a child with SOR can have is tactile defensiveness. The nerve receptors for the tactile system are located under the skin and receive information about touch, pressure, pain, and temperature. A child with SOR responds defensively to these sensations because the central nervous system inefficiently processes this information. As a result, the child is likely to react with hostility to a light, friendly touch. The child may become agitated in response to kisses or light caresses or may refuse to wear certain textures of clothing or socks that have any seams or lumps. The child may be unable to sleep under typical sheets or blankets and may be overly sensitive to the temperature of bath water. Such children may also carry toys or objects to protect themselves from unwanted touch (Kranowitz, 2005; Miller, 2006).

Some tactile sensations that are pleasant, fun, or even unnoticeable to a typical child may be perceived as threatening and responded to accordingly. Feeling unsafe in one's daily life directly affects a child's emotional well-being. Unfortunately, because of their aversion to being touched by others, children with tactile defensiveness also may have trouble forming secure attachments that might help them to cope.

Another set of problems sometimes confronting a child with SOR is evident in the following account shared by the mother of a boy with auditory overresponsivity.

We could never sing around Tanner, not even "Happy Birthday." He cries intensely and incessantly at any sound. Sometimes his weeping from hearing sounds gets so loud and constant that he throws up. So our house and our family are very quiet. . . . Ever since Tanner was able to say any words, he has screamed, "Off! Off!" whenever we take him out. When we try to go to a store or a restaurant, he screams, "Off! Off!" like he wants me to "turn off" the store or "turn off" the restaurant the way I turn off the sound of the TV or radio. (DeWoody, as cited in Miller, 2006, p. 22)

A child with auditory defensiveness experiences sound more intensely than other children and perceives it to be threatening or overwhelming. A child with this disorder may have an excessively emotional reaction to sad music or may have a strong aversion to the sound of fire drills, police sirens, televisions, radios, or even the unpredictable playground noise at school, which causes him or her to feel insecure in his or her world (Miller, 2006).

A child with vestibular defensiveness also may be on uncertain ground in terms of emotional security; he or she feels alarmed by the slightest unexpected movement. The child may react with a fight or flight response if a teacher approaches to adjust the position of his or her chair gently. In addition, the linear movement that is involved in riding a bicycle, swinging on a swing, or riding in a car is not fun or soothing; rather, it may be overwhelming. The child may experience frequent car sickness or refuse to ride in a car. The rotary movement of a merry-go-round or a tire swing may be upsetting, and, in extreme cases, it may cause headaches or nausea. This aversion to movement may lead the child to miss out, not only on social activities, but also on the physical activity that is vital for the development of motor coordination, motor planning, and physical fitness (Kranowitz, 2005; Miller, 2006).

The vestibular system is closely linked to the proprioceptive system. A child who is overresponsive to proprioceptive input feels uncomfortable or anxious in response to the passive movement of his or her joints. He or she also may dislike physical activities, especially those that require weight-bearing positions. In addition,

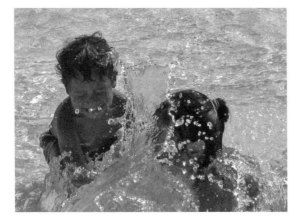

these children may be highly sensitive to smells and tastes (Emmons & Anderson, 2005).

Because a child with SOR often feels threatened and overwhelmed by the barrage of sensory information experienced daily, he or she is at considerable risk for emotional insecurity and low self-esteem. These problems, in turn, can affect both social and academic well-being and development. Interactions with family and classmates may be greatly affected by this disorder; in the struggle to "survive," these children may be very reactive, inflexible, and controlling (Kranowitz, 2005; Miller, 2006).

Sensory Underresponsivity   Unlike SOR, SMDs known as sensory underresponsivity (SUR) may not be overtly evident. Although symptoms can be just as devastating to the child, SUR is a more subtle condition. The following excerpt illustrates the delayed response a child with tactile underresponsivity might have to temperature or pain.

One evening when my son was three, he was playing in the living room while I was in the kitchen. . . . Jordan started to scream. . . . I raced to the living room but couldn't immediately see what was the matter.

Only after I got Jordan into better light did I understand. The inside of every finger on his right hand was red and blistering. . . . [W]e had to go to the emergency room, where doctors found second degree burns on Jordan's palm and fingers. It turned out that he had grabbed a light bulb and didn't let go of it right away. By the time the sense of heat reached him, it was already too late. (Fankhanel, in Miller, 2006, p. 21)

Similar to SOR, SUR may involve one or more of the external or internal senses, but a child with SUR encounters great difficulties in the arousal of these senses. His or her parasympathetic nervous system (autonomic nervous system includes parasympathetic and sympathetic systems) may be too active and cause the child to be excessively calm and relaxed. The child begins life as a seemingly easy baby—so easy that it is worrisome. Development moves along at a less than optimal pace because he or she frequently is uninterested in exploration. As the child grows older, he or she may lack motivation to learn to feed or dress him- or herself. These children respond slowly or with little intensity to stimulation and often become apathetic about school, sports, and social interactions. Their health may be affected because they prefer sedentary activities and seem unaware of hunger, hot or cold temperatures, pungent smells, or the need to use the restroom. Such children appear unalarmed by falls or minor injuries and have a high tolerance for pain. They may seem disconnected from themselves, unaware of when someone touches them, or feel the need to watch their own hands while using them.

Because a child with SUR requires much stimulation to arouse his or her system, he or she often struggles to complete schoolwork or to become involved in classroom activities. Unless the child is fortunate enough to find something at school of special interest to jump start his or her system, teachers may never observe the child's true abilities, and he or she is likely to be labeled as slow. In addition, as skills required for later grade levels become more complex, these children are apt to fall farther behind, having missed many prerequisite skills along the way (Miller, 2006).

Sensory-Seeking Disorders   A third form of SMD involves an insensitive nervous system. Yet the child with this disorder, known as sensory seeking, is highly motivated to meet his or her own sensory needs. The child seems to have an insatiable need for sensory stimulation. In a search to satisfy these cravings and to make sense of the environment, this child may crash into walls, bump into other people, engage in risky stunts, seek bright lights or colors, or enjoy hearing or producing loud noises. These children often run over other children and cause a commotion wherever they go. Because sensory seeking children often participate in high risk behaviors, which can be very disruptive and even dangerous for themselves and others, they usually receive a great deal of negative feedback. The con-

stant reprimands can make them feel as if they are somehow bad kids, and, most unfortunately, they may be labeled as such.

Sensory-Based Motor Disorder

Sensory-based motor disorder (SBMD) describes the second major group of SPD, which includes dyspraxia and postural disorder, both of which result from a dysfunction of the vestibular and proprioceptive systems (Miller, 2006).

Dyspraxia   Dyspraxia is a condition where sensory information is not easily translated into motor responses. Children with dyspraxia encounter difficulties with planning and executing physical movements, especially if tasks are unfamiliar or require a sequence of action. Dyspraxia can affect a child's gross motor, fine motor, and/or oral-motor functioning.

A child with gross motor dyspraxia is likely to have had trouble learning to crawl, walk, or run. As the child grows older, he or she will encounter problems keeping up with friends and performing the skills necessary for playground games. The multiple movements and sequences required for activities, such as dancing, karate, gymnastics, softball, or other childhood sports, may be beyond his or her capacity. Even riding a bike may seem to be an impossible task because it requires multiple steps of getting on a bike, balancing, pedaling, holding the handlebars, steering, and attending to obstacles.

Fine motor dyspraxia affects a child's ability to do things with fingers and hands. The child may struggle with self-care tasks, such as bathing, combing hair, or dressing. In school, he or she might have trouble playing with manipulatives, keeping a desk organized, completing multistep assignments, writing neatly, or coloring within the lines. These difficulties generally become evident at about 12 months of age when the child struggles to reach for, release, or hold small objects with his or her hands (Miller, 2006).

A child with oral-motor dyspraxia has difficulties using his or her mouth, tongue, and lips. As an infant, he or she has problems sucking, swallowing, and breathing while eating. Later there may be issues in terms of chewing. The child also may drool or have trouble coordinating his or her mouth, tongue, and lips to produce age-appropriate speech (Miller, 2006).

Dyspraxia sometimes affects a child in one or all of these areas, but usually one type will dominate. Children who suffer from dyspraxia are likely to have problems with self-esteem. They may feel frustrated because they frequently fail to do things that come so easily to their peers and may suffer some social rejection because of problems with poor personal care (Miller, 2006).

Postural Disorder   The second type of SBMD is classified as postural disorder. Postural disorders interfere with the ability to do many of the same things children with dyspraxia struggle to do, but for different reasons. In particular, the muscles of children with postural disorder receive insufficient input from the nerves that serve them, which results in low muscle tone (Kranowitz, 2005). As a result, these children appear limp and weak. They lack the strength to stand upright, support themselves while sitting at a desk, hang from a jungle gym, or stabilize themselves on a swing while pumping their legs. Such children may modify sitting positions on a chair or on the floor to avoid falling, possess little endurance, and tire easily.

Children with postural disorders also have trouble with bilateral coordination. Because their vestibular systems do not appropriately integrate sensory information from both sides of the body, they may have difficulty using both feet to jump or both hands to cut paper. They may be unable to cross mid-line, paint, or write across a page without switching hands midway. Children with these disorders are not likely to favor a dominant hand for writing or throwing, but change hands instead. Problems with crossing mid-line also may affect their ability to follow objects visually, causing them to blink and refocus when their eyes move from one side to the other (Kranowitz, 2005).

Sensory Discrimination Disorder

The last group of SPDs is characterized by challenges posed by trying to distinguish between sensory messages. This disorder can affect any of the external or internal senses and is called sensory discrimination disorder (SDD) (Kranowitz, 2005).

Tactile Discrimination   Children whose tactile sense is affected by SDD may be unable to discern what is in their hands without looking or to tell what is touching them or where they are being touched. They are likely to have trouble identifying objects according to shape, quality, or texture, and they may feel inclined to manipulate things to gain a sense of them. Such children may be unable to keep their desks organized or to distinguish between the items in it (Miller, 2006).

Visual Discrimination   A child whose vision is affected by sensory discrimination disorders encounters problems with distinguishing among shapes, colors, letters, or numbers and may be unable to separate an object from its background. He or she may be unable to space and organize writing on a page or play visual games, such as puzzles. The child may have trouble finding his or her way around and may not understand up–down, right–left, or spatial relationships (Kranowitz, 2005; Miller, 2006).

Auditory Discrimination   The life of children whose auditory systems are affected by SDD can be confusing because they have trouble differentiating between sounds. Background noise acts as interference because they cannot distinguish the sounds appropriately. Frequently, they need repetition or extra time to process instructions. They are likely to have delays in their receptive and expressive language skills because they are unable to differentiate the similarities and differences in spoken words (Kranowitz, 2005; Miller, 2006).

Problems with auditory discrimination can prevent a child from participating effectively in class activities and discussions, causing him or her to miss out on many learning experiences. Furthermore, because vestibular input can affect the functioning of the other senses, a child's unhappy experience may be due not only to the auditory discrimination problem, but also to the lack of vestibular input received on a given day (Brooks, 2006).

Vestibular Discrimination   When SDDs affect the vestibular system, a child experiences play and recreation much differently than a typical child because he or she does not feel secure in his or her relationship with gravity. The anec-

A Typical Child	A Child with Gravitational Insecurity
With his class, Jack, nine, goes for a hike up a little mountain. At one point, a thick vine hangs down from a branch. Jack takes a turn swinging on the vine, screaming "Tarzan!" Jack's efficient vestibular system permits him to enjoy exploring gravity as he swings and soars through the air.	The day his class goes hiking, Brad, nine, watches each step. He is grouchy, silent, and slow. He stands aloof while his classmates swing on a vine. When it's his turn, he takes the vine reluctantly. He can't move. The others cry, "Come on! What's your problem? It's fun!" Brad senses that if his feet leave the ground, he'll fall into the void. Saying, "I'm really not interested in this stupid game," he drops the vine and stalks away.

Figure 8.3.   How gravitational insecurity affects a child's behavior. (From THE OUT-OF-SYNC CHILD by Carol Kranowitz and Skylight Press, copyright © 1998, 2005 by Skylight Press and Carol Stock Kranowitz. Used by permission of Perigee Books, an imprint of Penguin Group [USA] Inc.)

dotes in Figure 8.3 compare the field trip experience of a typical child with that of a child whose vestibular sense is affected by SDD.

Children with a vestibular discrimination disorder feel vulnerable in the world. They exhibit unusual anxiety in reaction to falling or the prospect of falling. They do not enjoy experimenting with gravity and tend to refrain from jumping, swinging, doing somersaults, or engaging in similar large motor activities. Similar to children with SOR, they may surprise families, teachers, or classmates by reacting to being moved unexpectedly with a fight or flight response. As infants, they may have resisted being pushed in a stroller, rocked, or picked up.

Proprioceptive Discrimination   The quality of movement experienced by a child can be diminished if his or her proprioceptive system is affected by sensory discrimination disorders. Because the messages from the proprioceptive receptors allow the brain to know what the muscles and joints are doing, as well as where body parts are, unclear proprioceptive input can create some very distressing experiences. (The excerpt from an anecdotal notebook in Figure 8.4 illustrates the challenges faced daily by a child affected by SDD.)

In Figure 8.4, Paul inadvertently ran into objects because he was unaware of the position of his body in relationship to his surroundings. He was unable to gauge the amount of force needed, for example, to play with a toy or pick up and put down something. He had trouble playing sports because he had little awareness of his body position and the force required to catch or throw a ball. He walked and moved awkwardly, perhaps unconsciously pounding his

Behavior	Date, time	Circumstances
Walked into a telephone pole and required three stitches.	July 9 3:30 pm	Leaving ice cream parlor, he was paying attention to his cone, not to where he was going. So exasperating and frustrating!
Picked up Granny's china figurine; then, smashed it to smithereens when he set it down.	Aug. 2 8:00 pm	Maybe he was tired after long trip getting to Granny's, but even when he's rested he's clumsy. Granny's unhappiness worsened the situation. She wasn't angry at him, just sad; he was inconsolable.
Trying to play catch with a beach ball, he missed it every time.	Aug. 4 Noon	Paul either lunges at the ball at the wrong time or swats it away. His younger cousins are so mean and say, "Baby! Baby! Don't you even know how to catch a ball?"
At the restaurant, spilled his milk on the tablecloth and his good clothes.	Labor Day 6:30 pm	Sometimes Paul can't seem to manage getting milk into his mouth. Even though the waitress was a sweetheart, Paul was distraught.
Late for first day of fourth grade because he had a fit buttoning his new shirt.	Sept. 6 8:30 to 9:30 am	First he resisted wearing the shirt, and then buttoned it incorrectly, saying, "They made it wrong. I never do anything right." He works so hard to do the simplest things.

Figure 8.4.   Paul's problems (proprioceptive dysfunction). (From THE OUT-OF-SYNC CHILD by Carol Kranowitz and Skylight Press, copyright © 1998, 2005 by Skylight Press and Carol Stock Kranowitz. Used by permission of Perigee Books, an imprint of Penguin Group [USA] Inc.)

heels to gain more sensory information from the joints and muscles he was using. He likely sought out and enjoyed various jarring sensations because they offered him the extra proprioceptive input that he unconsciously craved (Kranowitz, 2005; Miller, 2006).

As children with SPDs struggle continuously to meet their daily challenges while dealing with various combinations of symptoms, they may begin to lose hope and feel like a failure. If they do not receive intervention, they are apt to fall behind in school and may develop a true learning disability (Kranowitz, 2005; Miller, 2006).

Early Intervention

There are various early intervention approaches for SPDs. These are discussed in the following sections.

Occupational Therapy

To safeguard the opportunity for children with SPDs to reach their potential, early intervention is essential. There are several types of therapy and intervention that can be beneficial. These include speech therapy, auditory training, physical therapy, nutritional therapy, adaptive physical education, and occupational therapy. According to much anecdotal data, occupational therapy has been shown to be a most effective means of intervention in treating young children with SPDs (Miller, 2006).

It is important for an occupational therapist working with children with SPDs to help them learn to play effectively. Out of necessity, therapy is built upon principles of sensory integration, offering these children opportunities to integrate fundamental sensory messages successfully. Because appropriate vestibular, proprioceptive, and tactile sensory input feels good and can help to calm, arouse, or organize a child's nervous system, the occupational therapist should use touch and movement experiences as the basis of intervention. Always careful to follow the child's lead, they would interface enjoyable and meaningful touch or movement experiences with tasks that help to develop skills and confidence that would then transfer to real-life situations (Brooks, 2006; Kranowitz, 2005; Miller, 2006).

One example of a movement experience that an occupational therapist might create includes two children moving back and forth on a tire swing through a sea of bubbles. Their task might be to use both hands to pop as many bubbles as possible (Miller, 2006). This activity would provide vestibular input and could help with tactile defensiveness, tactile discrimination, motor planning, bilateral coordination, and emotional security.

A child also might be given the task of using both hands to bat a ball suspended from the ceiling while lying prone on a gym mat. This task would offer vestibular input because of the tummy down, head up position, and likewise it would help to develop bilateral coordination, motor planning, muscle tone, and visual discrimination (Brooks, 2006; Kranowitz, 2005). Pulling or spinning a child on a scooter would offer vestibular input because of the brisk forward or rotary movement.

Another sensory integration technique that is well known is the Wilbarger Protocol (Wilbarger & Wilbarger, 1991). This technique involves tactile and proprioceptive input and is used to decrease sensory defensiveness in children with SPDs. This approach has been widely used with children with autism spectrum disorders and has produced compelling anecdotal results. The protocol entails only 3–5 minutes and is repeated approximately three times per day once the more intense initial stage has been accomplished. A soft surgical brush is used to provide deep pressure to the child by applying long, firm, up and down strokes on each of the arms, legs, and back. Gentle compressions are then applied to the joints in the fingers, wrists, shoulders, sternum, toes, ankles, knees, and hips. The brushing and bumps usually are pleasant for children and promote better attention and self-regulation, as well as less fear of touch or transitions. The results of this protocol are attributed to how it produces better communication between the peripheral and central nervous systems (Brooks, 2006; O-T Innovations, 2006).

A Balanced Sensory Diet

As discussed previously in this chapter, one of the goals of occupational therapists and educators working with young children is the improvement of their sensory diet and sensory input received throughout daily routines. The concept of a sensory diet was developed in the 1990s by the same occupational therapists who developed the Wilbarger Protocol (i.e., Julia and Patricia Wilbarger). Therapists make suggestions to parents or teachers to help them provide children with balanced sensory diets outside of therapy sessions at home and at school. In particular, vestibular, proprioceptive, and tactile sensory input can prepare the child by either calming or arousing his or her nervous system. Thus, children who are underresponsive may become more active and alert after spinning on a swing. Children with dyspraxia or postural disorder may become more coordinated and confident after experiencing the abrupt sensation of a teeter-totter repeatedly striking the ground (proprioceptive). Children who are overresponsive may be able to calm themselves and filter more sensations. Finally, children who are sensory seekers may be better able to resist bumping into classmates on the playground after experiencing heavy input (proprioceptive) (Miller, 2006).

At Home

Families can implement simple strategies at home to help their children experience balanced sensory diets. These diets should include activities that help the child's nervous system to become more alert, organized, and calm. For example, alerting activities might include taking a shower, eating crunchy foods, jumping on a trampoline, or bouncing on a therapy ball. Activities that help to organize sensory input and responses include eating chewy foods, pushing or pulling heavy things, and hanging by the arms from monkey bars. Calming activities might include sucking on foods, taking a bath, cuddling, getting bear hugs, receiving a back rub, and pushing against a wall or another person with different parts of the body (Kranowitz, 2005).

Parents can help their children develop their senses with fun activities at home. These activities are especially beneficial when siblings or friends are involved because they offer the child opportunities to interact successfully with peers. It is important to remember to follow the child's

lead and never to force a child to do something that he or she is not ready to do.

Activities that develop the vestibular sense include games in which the child's tummy is down and head is up. He or she might lie across a therapy ball and bat at a suspended ball (using both hands facilitates bilateral coordination) or rock back and forth while singing. Balancing challenges are beneficial as well and can be carried out with a t-stool, a therapy ball, a beach ball, a balance beam, or a teeter-totter. Sliding, swinging, or spinning are activities that offer a good deal of vestibular input. Riding vehicles that move forward also provide vestibular input while promoting motor coordination and planning as well (Kranowitz, 2005).

Other activities might focus on enjoyable ways to develop the proprioceptive system, including tasks or games that place pressure on joints or stretch muscles and provide ways to increase the tactile sense. In the latter case, water activities might involve games in which the child can rub many different textures of soaps and brushes on his or her skin; play in the sink with manipulatives, containers, and warm sudsy water; or paint with a paint brush and a bucket of water. Other sensory activities might include painting with finger paint, shaving cream, peanut butter, or paint mixed with sand. Science activities could include touching egg yolks, kneading bread dough, caressing animals, or describing things in a feely box. Parents also can play a people sandwich game with their child by using couch cushions for the bread and a washcloth to

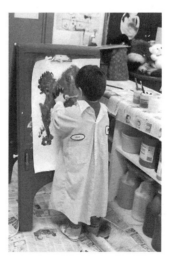

spread the pretend mustard and ketchup for deep touch enjoyment (Kranowitz, 2005).

To help their child develop their auditory system, parents should make sure that their communication is clear and simple, and use facial expressions, tone of voice, and gestures to clarify meaning. They need to model appropriate grammar and should frequently model the use of nouns, verbs, adjectives, prepositions, categories, names, time words, and feeling words. They should encourage their child to communicate with them by affirming and validating his or her ideas, feelings, and questions. They can help their child remember language by singing songs about everyday things and reading.

To help develop a child's visual system, parents can employ activities that are both visually interesting or challenging. Examples include experiences with shapes, numbers, or letters; using Play-Doh, finger paint, shaving cream, or string; putting together jigsaw puzzles, doing dot-to-dots, building with blocks, or copying designs onto a pegboard; or lying in supine in the grass to track birds, clouds, or planes in the sky (Kranowitz, 2005). Some of these activities also enhance fine motor skills.

Finally, a variety of activities can be used to develop motor planning and bilateral skills. To help a child who has difficulties with motor planning, a parent might engage a child in a jumping challenge in which the goal would be to jump a little farther each time. Likewise, the child might be encouraged to walk like different animals or to play Simon Says, Hokey Pokey, London Bridge, or Mother May I with his friends or siblings. To foster daily routines, parents can make a game of learning to get in and out of places, such as a cardboard box. To promote bilateral coordination, parents can create opportunities to use both hands to play sports, play games, or create art. For example, a child can practice batting at a ball while holding a bat, a broom, a rolling pin, or a cardboard tube with both hands. He or she can play tetherball with two hands, keep a balloon afloat with two hands, or use a rolling pin to roll dough or to smash crackers. In short, the home environment offers numerous opportunities for families to assist their young children with participating in and developing enjoyment from sensory-based experiences within the natural home environment.

Clinical Settings

Direct sensory integration therapy is provided in a clinical setting by an occupational therapist, physical therapist, or speech therapist who has received advanced clinical training. Therapists set up the clinic environment to provide a "just right challenge" to the child (i.e., a challenge that, through play, motivates the child to integrate varied inputs in order to form an adaptive response). Therapy is most commonly prescribed for 45- to 60-minute sessions one to three times per week, although other durations and frequencies are not unusual. Short- and long-term goals are written for an initial period of about 3–6 months. Progress is charted by the therapist, and parents are consulted frequently to allow close monitoring of functioning and developmental changes.

An intervention designed to join the vestibular and auditory systems to improve auditory processing and language skills is auditory integration training (AIT; Dejean & Freer, 2002). AIT is a technique developed by Alfred Tomatis, who emphasized that the ear is the root of many problems for those with difficulties in language, auditory processing, and sensory integration (Dejean & Freer, 2002). His AIT method focuses on the facilitation of effective listening through the use of an Electronic Ear (Dejean & Freer, 2002). By using sound stimulation, abilities to focus on certain sounds and ignore others are enhanced. The Electronic Ear also is intended to stimulate the

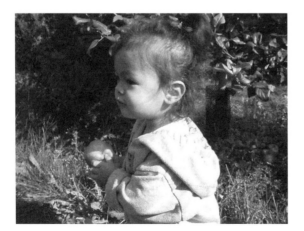

sounds heard by the child in-utero. As music (mostly Mozart or the mother's voice) is played, the Electronic Ear filters out the lower frequencies and allows the higher, more stimulating frequencies to be heard. This procedure thus allows the inner ear to reprogram itself, which leads to better processing and communication (Dejean & Freer, 2002).

The second form of AIT developed by Guy Berard, who first studied under Tomatis before moving on to create his own form of AIT, focuses on a different method of filtering sound. This form of AIT was designed to normalize hearing and the way that the brain processes auditory information, as well as reducing hypersensitivity (Edelson et al., 1999). The major difference in Berard's method is that it attempts to normalize hearing responses across all frequencies. As a child listens to music, the high and low frequencies are randomly deleted through the Ear's Education and Retraining System (EERS), therefore modulating what is being heard (Edelson et al., 1999; Rimland & Edelson, 1991).

Both of the methods described are intensive and carried out primarily in clinical settings. With the Tomatis method, the child may participate in 45–100 hours of listening during a 4-month period. Moreover, if the child has autism, this amount of time could be increased to 150–200 hours during a 6- to 12-month period (Rimland & Edelson, 1991). With the Berard method, the child participates in 20 listening sessions that are each 30 minutes in duration and are typically done twice a day for 10 days (with possible breaks in sessions, depending on the needs of the child). A second round of sessions can then be given after 6 months or more (Rimland & Edelson, 1991). Given that most of the evidence of success of the AIT methods is anecdotal with few unbiased scientific studies completed, continued research needs to be done to understand the genuine benefits of AIT for individuals with SPDs.

In the Classroom

Just as there are unique issues that develop at home for children and their families dealing with the effects of SPDs, there are additional issues and strategies that need to be addressed in the classroom. The classroom and school, in general, can be very overwhelming places for children with SPDs (Smith & Gouze, 2004). Open communication is fundamental for ensuring success. Teachers, parents, and additional professionals need to communicate with one another to maintain consistency and structure in all settings.

There are four key classroom strategies that teachers can use to help the child with SPDs be successful. The first is controlling the environment. The classroom is a very busy place, filled with things that are distracting to children with SPDs. Therefore, it is important to reduce sensory input as much as possible to prevent the child from going into sensory overload. Tactile distractions can be reduced easily by attending to the child's proximity to others. Providing the child with adequate personal space can help him or her feel more comfortable.

In addition, classrooms are full of visual distractions. Simply eliminating clutter and keeping items organized can help. Keeping papers and chalkboards clean and neat is important, and limiting the amount of information on each paper also helps children become and stay organized.

Auditory distractions can be reduced by covering hard surfaces with fabric and carpet. Teachers should pay close attention to where children are seated and any potentially distracting sounds near them.

Providing furniture that is the appropriate size and height helps maintain comfort and allows children to maintain focus. Another strategy often beneficial to encourage interest and attention is the use of a stability ball, which allows movement, or a cushion on a seat.

A second major area that teachers need to address is classroom management. This issue can be addressed by maintaining an organized room that has a visual schedule to provide children with a consistent routine. Transitions are especially difficult for some children; therefore, providing warnings of them and clearly explaining them is important. Using predictable sounds or motions to signify transitions is also beneficial. Moreover, young children need a lot of movement, which can be incorporated into transitions from one activity to another or through the use of breaks.

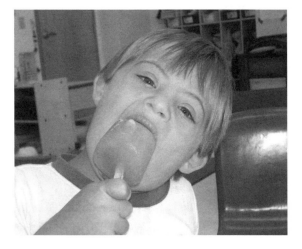

Teachers should be involved in helping children become better organized. Children need to be encouraged to learn actively through the use of all of their senses. Materials need to be interesting, relevant, and build on the natural sensory strengths and skills of children. Ample wait time is critical when teaching so that children have enough time to process information and respond. Likewise, an appropriate amount of time should be provided when asking questions to allow children opportunities to process what is being asked of them. Along with time, teachers should also make sure that instruction is simple and concise. Giving choices and providing response alternatives are also important for demonstrating respect and developing positive self-esteem.

The final area to be addressed in the classroom involves teachers adapting their own behavior. It is crucial that they emphasize the positive with all children. By maintaining a calm voice and demeanor, they can prevent children from becoming upset or anxious. It is vital to have realistic expectations of children and to offer both verbal and appropriate physical feedback. It is also essential that the teacher of children with SPDs implement all possible accommodations suggested by the occupational therapist. Even when sensory difficulties cannot be overcome, children receiving occupational therapy always can learn effective coping techniques that will improve their abilities to function and to achieve their fullest potential (Kranowitz, 2005; Miller, 2006)

It is evident that the problems that involve SPDs are extremely complex and are wide reaching. The brain's inability to process incoming sensory information can have enormous implications in terms of the abilities of children to develop and function appropriately. As research and awareness of SPDs grow, there is hope for the future of those affected to receive treatment so that their environments become much more approachable and enjoyable as they learn to process information more effectively.

The key to solving issues surrounding SPDs is early diagnosis and intervention. These lay the groundwork and increase the likelihood of future successes, thus preventing or minimizing secondary academic and social-emotional problems.

To start the process of early diagnosis and intervention, parents need to voice their concerns. Although knowledge and research about SPDs are becoming more prevalent, there are still many people who are naïve or skeptical because these disorders are not yet recognized in the *Diagnostic and Statistical Manual of Mental Disorders, Fourth Edition, Text Revision (DSM-IV-TR*; American Psychiatric Association, 2000). Therefore, parents must be advocates for their children. They need to pay close attention to the reactions of their children to touch, visual stimuli, movements, and sounds, as well as their emotional attachment and ability to self-regulate.

Pediatricians often are the first professionals in the lives of young children, and they are the first place that parents turn for advice. If there are concerns, physicians have the ability to make referrals to see other specialists for more complete evaluations. During the evaluation process, it is vital to maintain open communication between all parties involved. Parents need to be sure that they understand and agree with what is being discussed and considered. Maintaining good records and journaling about a child's behavior allows the evaluating team to achieve a more accurate view and assessment of what is going on in terms of the child's behavior and functioning.

Subsequently, a plan for intervention needs to meet the needs of children on at least three different levels (Williamson & Anzalone, 1997). First, intervention must help parents understand the behavior of their children and foster loving relationships. Second, the intervention needs to help in modifying the environment to ensure a good fit for children. This means that parents must look at the world as the child does through sensory lenses so that they truly understand the behaviors of their children. Finally, intervention needs to be designed specifically to meet the individual needs of children (Williamson & Anzalone, 1997). All children process sensory input differently. Pre-established protocols surely will fall short in meeting the needs of all children. Cues must be taken from the child. Finding the right balance of arousal, attention, affect, and action is fundamental to effective intervention and thus should lead to enhancement of functioning and performance for the whole child.

Progression of the Field

Looking ahead, the field of sensory integration is still fairly young. Dr. A. Jean Ayres was an occupational therapist with advanced studies in neuroscience and educational psychology who published her first clinical works for therapists in the 1960s (Ayres, 1965, 1966, 1969). She was a person of creativity and insight who saw possibilities for more sophisticated therapeutic approaches to children with learning disabilities. Dr. Ayres considered the soft neurological signs associated with learning disabilities to be clues about the kinds of sensory processing experienced by children. Sensory integration therapy was intended to be a refinement and elaboration within the field of pediatric occupational therapy.

Early research was designed to help formulate differential diagnoses within the domain of sensory integration (Ayres, 1972a, 1972c, 1977). Accordingly, the Southern California Sensory Integration Tests (SCSIT; Ayres, 1972b) provided a standardized evaluation instrument that allowed scored profiles of children with learning disabilities and associated sensory processing differences to be compared with profiles of typically developing children. Continued use of the SCSIT thus paved the way toward the development of a subsequent instrument with better reliability—the Sensory Integration and Praxis Tests (SIPT) pub-

lished in 1989. Unfortunately, Dr. Ayres died from cancer while she was still actively researching and publishing in the field of sensory integration.

Since the early 1990s, use of the sensory integration theory base has grown rapidly as a result of the fruitfulness of this approach. The popularity of parts of the theory, especially among parents, has drawn some criticism. Educators and medical researchers, as well as occupational therapists, have urged caution (Wilson & Kaplan, 1994; Wilson, Kaplan, Fellowes, Gruchy, & Faris, 1992) because sensory integration treatment has been undersupported, in large part by evidence-based research. In addition, a few studies were published that seemed to indicate that a sensory integration treatment approach was no better than a placebo in improving sensory processing. However, careful review of those studies revealed serious flaws (Vargas & Camilli, 1999). Most importantly, the treatments that were administered for purposes of the studies were minimal and not representative of actual practice.

Conclusion

In conclusion, it has taken time, but research is now being done that does bear up under collegial scrutiny. Studies are underway to verify that the conditions now being described as SPDs are in fact actual and distinct conditions (McIntosh, Miller, Shyu, & Hagerman, 1999; Miller et al., 1999; Schaaf, Miller, Seawell, & O'Keefe, 2003). Other studies are being done that compare the efficacy of actual sensory integration treatment, in all of its complexity, with perceptual motor training, social skills training, tutoring, and activity groups. This research is well designed and will yield important insights in shaping the path of this theory in the years ahead (Kimball et al., 2007; Miller, 2003).

For a thorough understanding of the field of sensory integration, the reader is referred to the textbook *Sensory Integration: Theory and Practice, Second Edition* (Bundy, Lane, & Murray, 2002), which is widely used in occupational therapy training. Chapter 1 of that text discusses the history of sensory integration research in detail. In addition for parent and teacher reference, more popular books, such as *The Out-of-Sync Child:*

Recognizing and Coping with Sensory Integration Dysfunction (Kranowitz, 1998, 2005), are recommended. In closing, the 25th anniversary edition of Dr. Ayres's own book for parents, *Sensory Integration and the Child* (Ayres, 2005), still gives the most thorough and clear presentation of SPD and sensory integration approaches. It has been updated with supplemental information, pictures, and commentary.

REFERENCES

American Psychiatric Association. (2000). *Diagnostic and statistical manual of mental disorders* (4th ed., text rev.). Washington, DC: Author.

Ayres, A.J. (1965). Patterns of perceptual-motor dysfunction in children: A factor analytic study. *Perceptual and Motor Skills, 20*, 335–368.

Ayres, A.J. (1966). Interrelationships among perceptual-motor functions in children. *American Journal of Occupational Therapy, 20*, 288–292.

Ayres, A.J. (1969). Deficits in sensory integration in educationally handicapped children. *Journal of Learning Disabilities, 2*, 160–168.

Ayres, A.J. (1972a). *Sensory integration and learning disorders.* Los Angeles: Western Psychological Services.

Ayres, A.J. (1972b). *Southern California Sensory Integration Tests manual.* Los Angeles: Western Psychological Services.

Ayres, A.J. (1972c). Types of sensory integrative dysfunction among disabled learners. *American Journal of Occupational Therapy, 26*, 13–18.

Ayres, A.J. (1977). Cluster analyses of measures of sensory integration. *American Journal of Occupational Therapy, 31*, 362–366.

Ayres, A.J. (1989). *Sensory integration and the child.* Los Angeles: Western Psychological Services.

Ayres, A.J. (revised and updated by the Pediatric Therapy Network). (2005). *Sensory integration and the child* (25th anniversary ed.). Los Angeles: Western Psychological Services.

Batshaw, M.L., Pellegrino, L., & Roizen, N.J. (Eds.). (2007). *Children with disabilities* (6th ed.). Baltimore: Paul H. Brookes Publishing Co.

Brooks, T. (2006, November 6). Unpublished interview with occupational therapist. Syracuse, NY: Elmcrest Early Childhood Center.

Bundy, A.C., Lane, S.J., & Murray, E.A. (2002). *Sensory integration: Theory and practice* (2nd ed.). Philadelphia: F.A. Davis.

Dejean, V., & Freer, A. (2002). *The Tomatis method of auditory stimulation—An overview.* Retrieved on November 16, 2006, from http://spectrumcenter.net/auditory.html

Edelson, S.M., Arin, D., Bauman, M., Lukas, S.E., Rudy, J.H., Sholar, M., et al. (1999). Auditory Integration Training: A double-blind study of behavioral and electrophysiological effects in people with autism. *Focus on Autism and Other Developmental Disabilities, 14*(2), 73–81.

Emmons, P.G., & Anderson, L.M (2005). *Understanding sensory dysfunction: Learning, development and sensory dysfunction in autism spectrum disorders, ADHD, learning disabilities and bipolar disorder.* Philadelphia: Jessica Kingsley Publishers.

Kimball, J.G., Lynch, K.M., Stewart, K.C., Williams, N.E., Thomas, M.A., & Atwood, K.D. (2007). Using salivary cortisol to measure the effects of Wilbarger protocol-based procedure on sympathetic arousal: A pilot study. *American Journal of Occupational Therapy, 61*, 406–413.

Kranowitz, C.S. (1998). *The out-of-sync child: Recognizing and coping with sensory integration dysfunction.* New York: Perigee.

Kranowitz, C.S. (2005). *The out-of-sync child: Recognizing and coping with sensory integration dysfunction* (2nd ed.). New York: Perigee.

Lin, S., Cermack, S., Coster, W., & Miller, L. (2005). The relation between length of institutionalization and sensory integration in children adopted from Eastern Europe. *American Journal of Occupational Therapy, 59*(2), 139–147.

McIntosh, D.N., Miller, L.J., Shyu, V., & Hagerman, R.J. (1999). Sensory modulation disruption, electrodermal responses, and functional behaviors. *Developmental Medicine and Child Neurology, 41*, 608–615.

Miller, L.J. (2003). Empirical evidence related to therapies for sensory processing impairments. *NASP Communique, 31*(5). Bethesda, MD: National Association of School Psychologists.

Miller, L.J. (2006). *Sensational kids: Hope and help for children with sensory processing disorder.* New York: Penguin Books.

Miller, L.J., Cermack, S., Lane, S., Anzalone, M., & Koomar, J. (2004). *Defining SPD and its subtypes: Position statement on terminology related to sensory integration dysfunction.* Retrieved on September 16, 2006, from http://www.sinetwork.org/aboutspd/defining.html

Miller, L.J., McIntosh, D.N., McGrath, J., Shyu, V., Lampe, M., Taylor, A.K., et al. (1999). Electrodermal responses to sensory stimuli in individuals with Fragile X syndrome. *American Journal of Medical Genetics, 83*, 268–279.

O-T Innovations. (2006). *O-T Innovations.com: Occupational Therapy Innovations.* Retrieved December 12, 2006, from http://www/otinnovations.com/content/view

Rimland, B., & Edelson, S.M. (1991). *Improving the auditory functioning of autistic persons: A comparison of* the Berard auditory training approach with the Tomatis audio-psycho-phonology approach. [ARI publ. No. 111]. San Diego: Autism Research Institute. Retrieved on December 7, 2006, from http://www .autismwebsite.com/ari/treatment/tomatis.htm

Schaaf, R.C., Miller, L.J., Seawell, D., & O'Keefe, S. (2003). Children with disturbances in sensory processing: A pilot study examining the role of the parasympathetic nervous system. *American Journal of Occupational Therapy, 57,* 442–449.

Smith, K.A., & Gouze, K.R. (2004). *The sensory sensitive child: Practical solutions for out-of-bound behavior.* New York: HarperCollins.

Wilbarger, J., & Wilbarger, P. (1991). *Sensory defensiveness in children aged 2–12.* Oak Park Heights, MN: PDP Products.

Williamson, G.G., & Anzalone, M. (1997). Sensory integration: A key component of the evaluation and treatment of young children with severe difficulties in relating and communicating. *Zero to Three Bulletin, 17*(5), 29–36.

Wilson, B.N., & Kaplan, B.J. (1994). Follow-up assessment of children receiving sensory integration treatment. *Occupational Therapy Journal of Research, 14,* 244–267.

Wilson, B.N., Kaplan, B.J., Fellowes, S., Gruchy, C., & Faris, P. (1992). The efficacy of sensory integration treatment compared to tutoring. *Physical and Occupational Therapy in Pediatrics, 12,* 1–36.

Vargas, S., & Camilli, G. (1999). A meta-analysis of research on sensory integration treatment. *American Journal of Occupational Therapy, 53,* 189–198.

CHAPTER 9

Respiratory Distress in Newborns

Upender K. Munshi, Michelle L. Eastman, and David A. Clark

At the conclusion of this chapter, the reader will

- *Be able to enumerate various stages of fetal lung development and their relevance to lung malformations or severity of lung immaturity*

- *Be able to define acute respiratory distress in newborns and the common diagnostic possibilities for its causation and principles of management*

- *Be able to describe chronic lung disease or bronchopulmonary dysplasia (BPD) and its implications for long-term developmental outcomes*

Respiratory distress is a common symptom requiring medical attention during the newborn period. With an increasing severity of respiratory distress, there may be less oxygen carried by the blood to the body tissues, known as hypoxia, and an accumulation of carbon dioxide due to less clearance from the lungs, which causes hypercarbia. The net effect of hypoxia and hypercarbia is an accumulation of acid products (lactic acid and carbonic acid, respectively) called acidosis, which, in severe cases, may lead to multiorgan damage, including injury to the central nervous system and risk for developmental delay. Respiratory distress can occur because of several underlying problems and may affect premature as well as full-term infants. With advances in medical technology and ventilatory support, the survival rates of most premature infants have improved; however, the number of very low birth weight babies surviving with chronic lung disease and developmental disabilities has increased. This situation poses significant challenges to the families of these babies and their medical care providers.

The underlying causes of acute respiratory distress may vary from mild, self-resolving problems to severe, life-threatening conditions. In broad terms, respiratory disorders affecting newborns can be divided into two categories: 1) transition disorders (which refer to problems that manifest at birth, in the delivery room, or within the first few hours of birth); and 2) post-transition disorders (which occur after successful transition to extra-uterine life is achieved, usually after the first 12–24 hours of life). The first category includes conditions such as transient tachypnea of the newborn, respiratory distress syndrome (RDS) due to prematurity, sepsis, meconium aspiration syndrome, and congenital malformations of the respiratory system (e.g., diaphragmatic hernia). The second category includes sepsis and/or pneumonia, duct-dependent congenital heart disease, inborn errors of metabolism, and aspiration pneumonia. Chronic lung disease of prematurity or bronchopulmonary dysplasia (BPD) is the condition that is seen in premature infants who initially present with acute RDS and then continue to require prolonged ventilatory support and/or oxygen therapy.

To understand the various disorders leading to respiratory distress during the newborn period and their medical management, this chapter reviews normal lung development (Ballard, 2004) and explains its relevance to various malformations of the respiratory system and severity of acute RDS.

Lung Development

Human fetal lung development can be defined in various phases at different gestational stages.

1. Embryonic phase (0–5 weeks): An initial lung bud arises from the foregut at 23–26 days after fertilization. This bud then divides into primary bronchi and forms the proximal part of the airway. Interference with development at this stage can result in conditions such as esophageal atresia with tracheoesophageal fistula. This congenital malformation is characterized by absence (atresia) of a segment of esophagus so that it ends as a blind pouch and the infant is unable to swallow anything down into the stomach. It is invariably accompanied by an abnormal communication (fistula) between the trachea and the lower end of esophagus, which is continuous with the stomach. Inability to swallow amniotic fluid before birth leads to an excessive accumulation of this fluid around the fetus, known as polyhydramnios, which may give the obstetrician a clue about this condition on prenatal ultrasound. After birth, the main danger is that of choking and aspiration of saliva. Infants with this condition need to be in a neonatal intensive care unit with pediatric surgery service.

2. Pseudoglandular phase (6–16 weeks): In this phase, the bronchial division continues to form conducting airways (bronchi and bronchioles) with epithelial-mesenchymal interaction (airway lining cells, derived from ectoderm, and lung parenchymal cells, derived from mesoderm layer of the primitive cell layers). All the structures are nonrespiratory, and gaseous exchange is not possible

throughout this phase. Bronchogenic cysts, congenital cystadenomatoid malformation (CCAM), and congenital lobar emphysema may result from abnormal development. CCAM is cystic abnormal lung tissue that does not function like lung tissue and, if large enough, may compromise the gaseous exchange and present with respiratory distress needing ventilatory support and eventual surgical treatment. Around 8–10 weeks of gestation, the diaphragm develops from the front as a septum between the heart and liver and progresses backward to separate the thoracic cavity from the abdominal cavity. Failure to close the last portion of the diaphragm, known as left Bochdalek foramen, before the bowel returns from yolk sac to abdominal cavity leads to a herniation of the bowel into the left hemithorax, which is called a congenital diaphragmatic hernia.

3. Canalicular phase (17–24 weeks): The continued branching of airways forms respiratory bronchioles that represent the first gas exchange structure within the tracheobronchial tree. During this phase, there is mesenchymal thinning, achieved by apoptosis (genetically programmed cell death) and development of pulmonary capillaries. By the end of this phase, respiration and, thus, survival are possible by gas-exchanging acini; however, the RDS is severe and adverse outcomes in terms of morbidity and mortality are very high.

4. Terminal sac phase (25–37 weeks): Primitive alveoli (saccules and subsaccules) develop during this phase, which increase the alveolar–blood barrier surface area and enhance the gaseous exchange capability. Severity of RDS and the outcomes improve markedly by the end of this phase.

5. Alveolar phase (38 weeks–3 years): Subsaccules form alveoli, and their proliferation and development continue throughout the newborn period to the first 2–3 years of life. This may explain the ongoing lung growth and the repair processes that help to resolve the chronic lung disease or BPD in growing premature babies, unlike the adult population with chronic lung diseases.

Finally, it is important to recognize that as the lungs are developing in structure, there are biochemical changes that take place simultaneously. Type II pneumocytes produce lipoproteins, which form a lining at the liquid air interface of mature alveoli in the full-term infant. This substance is called surfactant and is essential to keep the alveoli open and facilitate respiration (Avery & Merrit, 1991). Surfactant production starts by the end of the canalicular phase and continues to increase as gestation advances toward term.

Acute Respiratory Distress

Acute respiratory distress refers to difficulty in breathing that is manifested by a faster breathing rate (> 60 breaths per minute); chest wall retractions; flaring of external nares; grunting noise; and, in severe cases, a pale bluish hue of the skin on the face, chest, and lips (i.e., cyanosis). Because chest wall muscles, cartilage, and the rib cage of the newborn are not as strong as those of older children or adults, the chest wall and sternum appear to be drawn in during attempts at inspiration due to negative pressure created in the chest cavity by downward movement of the diaphragm. This is a cardinal finding in premature infants with surfactant deficiency. Knowing the time of the onset of respiratory distress may help in gaining a clue to its causation. Respiratory distress sometimes may be a problem related to organ systems other than the lungs.

Transition Disorders

At birth, there is a change from the intrauterine, placenta-dependent state to an entirely different extra-uterine environment of individual existence for the baby. It is amazing to see how this transition takes place so smoothly in the majority of newborns who adapt readily to their new outside world. However, some infants experience problems in this process of adaptation, which we refer to as transition disorders. These disorders begin to manifest at birth or within a few hours after birth and can occur as a result of various problems related to lungs, heart, blood vessels,

infections, congenital malformations, loss of blood, anemia (low hemoglobin), and even polycythemia (high hemoglobin). The common lung disorders related to transition include delayed clearance of fetal lung fluid or transient tachypnea of the newborn; lack of surfactant production in premature lungs, commonly known as RDS or hyaline membrane disease (HMD); and aspiration of material not normally present in airways, such as meconium, blood, or amniotic fluid. An infection acquired before birth may become evident as respiratory distress due to pneumonia at birth and is difficult to differentiate from the previously mentioned conditions by appearance alone. Other causes for respiratory distress at birth may be air leaks into the pleural cavity, mediastinum (the middle of the chest between two lungs), or pericardium (the thin-layered sac surrounding the heart). This may occur spontaneously or as a result of enthusiastic positive pressure ventilation given at the time of delivery. In addition, some congenital malformations of the respiratory system may cause respiratory distress immediately after birth (e.g., tracheoesophageal fistula, congenital diaphragmatic hernia, cystic lung lesions). Medications given to the mother during labor, such as opiate derivatives for pain or magnesium sulfate for treatment of hypertension or preterm labor, tend to cross the placenta and depress newborn respiratory effort immediately after birth. These babies require ventilatory support until they improve their own spontaneous breathing. Common causes of respiratory distress in the newborn are explained in greater detail in the following sections.

Fetal Lung Fluid

While in the uterus, the fetal lung is filled with fluid that is actively secreted by the lining of potential airways and air spaces. This fluid is referred to as fetal lung fluid and is not the same as amniotic fluid. It gradually extrudes out of the lungs by coming up the glottis and is added to the amniotic fluid pool in a one-way direction. Around the time of labor, there are certain hormonal changes in the mother and fetus that result in inhibition of lung fluid secretion and rapid absorption of remaining fluid in the airways (Jain & Eaton, 2006). These mechanisms work well for most newborns. If we listen to a newborn baby's chest at birth, we often hear coarse rales, which signify secretions in the airways that disappear within a matter of minutes as the airways are cleared of this excessive fluid. However, a few infants, particularly after elective cesarean sections (without labor), continue to have respiratory distress beyond the first few hours of life as a result of retained fetal lung fluid in the airways (Jain & Dudell, 2006). This condition is known as transient tachypnea of the newborn (TTN). Chest x-rays of infants with TNN show normal lung volumes and fluid in the fissure between the lobes of the right lung. Most infants with TTN require supplemental oxygen therapy with continuous positive pressure through nasal prongs, but there is seldom a need for endotracheal intubation with ventilatory support. As the name implies, the respiratory distress in transient tachypnea of the newborn begins to improve as early as 6–12 hours and subsides completely by 24–48 hours. Thus, a baby requiring ventilatory support beyond 24–48 hours suffers from problems other than TTN.

Respiratory Distress Syndrome

Surfactant deficiency syndrome or HMD of premature infants, mainly seen at less than 32 weeks of gestation, can occasionally affect term or near-term infants as well. It is caused by a lack of surfactant production due to immaturity of type II pneumocytes and relates to the late canalicular and early to middle terminal sac phases of lung development. Prenatal steroids given to mothers in preterm labor seem to have a beneficial effect for the baby in terms of lung maturation and surfactant production. Because air spaces are moist, there is an inherent tendency of the fluid molecules at the fluid–air interface to attract each other and collapse the air space. These molecules need surfactant to oppose this tendency and keep the air spaces open. Lack of surfactant causes progressive collapse of air spaces and decreases the surface area for exchange of oxygen and carbon dioxide. Respiratory distress manifests at birth

or within the first few hours and then worsens during the next 1–2 days. The result is injury of partially or completely collapsed air spaces and leaking of plasma proteins from the capillaries, which precipitate along the lining of air spaces and form hyaline membrane (which is the origin of the name—hyaline membrane disease). Most newborns with surfactant deficiency syndrome (see Figures 9.1 and 9.2) will need supplemental oxygen and some form of ventilatory support. In milder cases, positive pressure is exerted by snugly fitting nasal prongs, which deliver continuous positive airway pressure (CPAP). During this method of ventilatory support, breathing is done by the baby, and CPAP helps to supplement the baby's effort to keep the air spaces open and breathe comfortably. With increasing need of oxygen concentration and worsening of respiratory distress, CPAP alone may not be enough. From oral or nasal route, an endotracheal tube is placed in the mid-trachea (endotracheal intubation), and its end is connected to a ventilator. Positive pressure breaths are delivered by the ventilator to take over the work of breathing and open

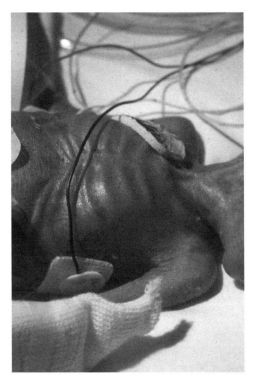

Figure 9.1. Intercostal retractions in a baby with respiratory distress syndrome. (From Clark, D.A., private collection; reprinted by permission.)

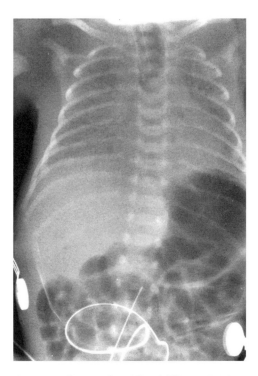

Figure 9.2. Chest x-ray shows bilateral diffuse opacity in lung fields consistent with respiratory distress syndrome due to surfactant deficiency in a premature infant. (From Clark, D.A., private collection; reprinted by permission.)

Table 9.1. Factors related to respiratory distress syndrome

Factors for increased risk	Factors for decreased risk
Acute fetal distress	Fetal growth restriction
Maternal diabetes	Prenatal corticosteroids
Multiple gestations	Toxemia of pregnancy
Perinatal asphyxia	
Prematurity	

From Clark, D.A. (1994). Respiratory distress. In G.L. Ensher & D.A. Clark, *Newborns at risk: Medical care and psychoeducational intervention* (2nd ed., p. 127). New York: Aspen; adapted by permission.

crease or prevent this chronic lung disease in preterm infants (Lindwall et al., 2005; Schreiber et al., 2003). Given the same degree of prematurity, there are certain factors that increase or decrease the risk of developing RDS (see Table 9.1).

Aspiration Syndromes

Amniotic fluid stained with meconium (i.e., the passage of newborn stools before birth) occurs in about 10%–15% of all deliveries. It is uncommon in premature deliveries less than 35 weeks but more common in postterm deliveries (41–42 weeks gestation). Only 1%–2% of neonates born with meconium-stained amniotic fluid develop meconium aspiration syndrome. Meconium has the mechanical effect of obstructing the airways and causing chemical irritation with inflammation and deactivation of surfactant (Clark, Neiman, Thompson, & Bredenberg, 1987). Pathophysiology of this disorder is further complicated by associated pulmonary arterial hypertension and hypoxic/ischemic injury to multiorgan systems (Munshi & Clark, 2002). *Hypoxic/ischemic injury* refers to injury due to lack of oxygen and blood flow; it affects various tissues of the body such as the brain, kidneys, heart, and lungs. In the lungs, blood vessels called pulmonary arteries tend to constrict due to hypoxia, which increases the blood pressure in them and thereby leads to an increase in the workload of the right side of the heart. Once the pressure in the pulmonary arteries exceeds that in the aorta (systemic pressure), there is shunting of deoxygenated (bluish-looking) blood from pulmonary to systemic circulation, which causes a bluish hue of the baby's skin and mucus membranes (cyanosis). It manifests at birth or within the first few hours as respiratory distress progressively wors-

up the collapsed air spaces so that effective gas exchange can take place. Today most ventilators have computer-backed sensors that can deliver synchronized ventilation, based on a baby's breathing effort.

The second most important reason for intubation is the administration of exogenous surfactant into the air spaces. Various surfactant preparations (Halliday, 2006; Pfister & Soll, 2005), mostly derived after purification from animal sources, are available in liquid form and are delivered to the lungs via an endotracheal tube. Prenatal steroid treatment of mothers in preterm labor, postnatal surfactant treatment, and the availability of newer-generation ventilators have revolutionized the management of this condition since the late 1980s. However, a significant number of extremely low birth weight babies (birth weights < 1,000 grams or < 2.2 pounds) still need prolonged ventilatory support and oxygen therapy and develop what is commonly referred to as chronic lung disease of prematurity or bronchopulmonary dysplasia. There is an ongoing effort to modify the ventilatory management to deens. It needs aggressive ventilatory management, including high-frequency ventilation and novel therapies such as inhaling nitric oxide or, in severe cases, invasive procedures such as extra corporeal membrane oxygenation (ECMO). In ECMO, a patient's blood is drawn through surgically placed catheters in the neck and made to pass into a machine outside the body, where gas exchange takes place through a synthetic membrane and is returned back to the patient.

Air Leak Syndromes ____

Following an aggressive resuscitation or sometimes spontaneously due to partially blocked airways acting as a ball valve, air can leak out of the distended air spaces and become trapped at various locations within the chest. This air is not available for the usual gas exchange and, if accumulated under pressure, it can compress the surrounding structures (i.e., lung tissue, heart, and blood vessels). This compression of tissues may interfere with the lung and/or heart function and cause life-threatening cardiorespiratory compromise if not recognized and relieved promptly. There are four types of air leaks. First, when air collects in the pleural cavity between the chest wall and the lungs, it is called a pneumothorax (see Figure 9.3). This is the most common type of air leak. About 5% of all newborn babies may

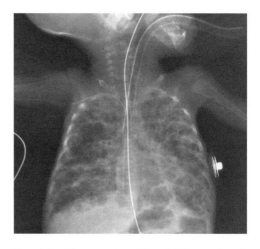

Figure 9.4.   Chest x-ray shows bilateral diffuse opacity and rounded lucent shadows of air in cystic lesions in a patient with bronchopulmonary dysplasia. (From Clark, D.A., private collection; reprinted by permission.)

have this type of air leak, but only 1% may develop respiratory distress. A small pneumothorax requires close monitoring, whereas large ones (particularly causing respiratory distress) require needle or chest tube drainage. The second type of air leak, pnuemomediastinum, occurs when air is trapped in the center of the chest around major blood vessels and airways. As more air accumulates, it may tract up toward the neck or reach the pericardium around the heart, causing the third type of air leak, a serious condition called pneumopericardium. Under tension, pneumopericardium does not permit adequate filling of the heart with blood, and, thus, dangerously lowers the cardiac output. Even with aggressive therapy, mortality or morbidity with this condition is very high (Carey, 1999; McIntosh, 1983).

Finally, a type of air leak that is found mainly in premature infants on ventilators with RDS, where small amounts of air escape at multiple places and traverse around the airways and blood vessels and form numerous tiny elongated cystic shadows on a chest x-ray, is called pulmonary interstitial emphysema (PIE). This condition often leads to prolonged ventilator support and development of chronic lung disease of prematurity (i.e., bronchopulmonary dysplasia) (see Figure 9.4).

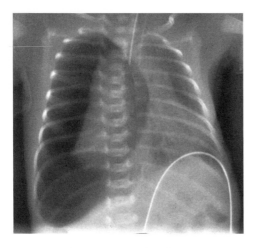

Figure 9.3.   Chest x-ray shows a large lucent shadow of air collection in the right lung field (pneumothorax) that has compressed the right lung tissue. (From Clark, D.A., private collection; reprinted by permission.)

Pulmonary Hemorrhage

Very low birth weight babies having severe respiratory distress, particularly those with patent ductus arteriosus (PDA) causing increased blood flow to the lungs, are at a high risk of pulmonary hemorrhage (Al Kharfy, 2004). Ductus arteriosus is normally patent during fetal life and tends to close in term and near-term infants within the first day or so after birth. It often remains open in very premature infants, causing extra blood shunting from the aorta to the pulmonary artery. It is often treated with medications, such as indomethacin or ibuprofen and, in a small number of babies who do not respond to medication, it is ligated surgically (Hermes-DeSantis & Clyman, 2006; Raval, Laughon, Bose, & Phillips, 2007). Blood loss due to pulmonary hemorrhage may cause shock and death despite aggressive intervention. Pulmonary hemorrhage manifests as fresh bleeding pouring out of the endotracheal tube that connects the baby to the ventilator and as sudden deterioration in the clinical status of the baby. Blood in the air spaces also deactivates surfactant, which further worsens the respiratory distress syndrome. Survivors are at risk of chronic lung disease of prematurity and developmental delays.

Neonatal Sepsis and Pneumonia Syndrome

Infection-causing organisms can reach the fetus along two pathways. One route is the mother's bloodstream where infection reaches the placenta and extends to the fetus via blood supply, which is called hematogenous spread. This spread, referred to as intrauterine infection, can occur at any time in the pregnancy, and it may pose a serious threat to the developing fetus and its growth. Such babies often are growth restricted; may have features of infection such as skin rashes, liver and spleen enlargement, jaundice, and cataracts; and may manifest respiratory distress. Common organisms include *Toxoplasma*, cytomegalovirus, rubella, herpes, HIV, and other infections (collectively referred to as TORCH). More com-

monly, infection from the maternal genital tract reaches the baby by ascending route just before or at delivery by exposure during passage. This is referred to as perinatal infection. Common organisms reflect maternal genital tract flora and include group B streptococcus, Klebsiella, E. coli, and herpes simplex virus. Although rare, some organisms can infect the fetus by either route, hematogenous or ascending (e.g., herpes simplex, HIV, hepatitis B virus).

Respiratory distress or apnea is a frequent symptom of perinatally acquired infections and can present as early as the delivery room and, thereafter, at any time during the neonatal period. Other features of infection in a newborn include poor feeding, vomiting, lethargy, irritability, poor skin perfusion, and low blood pressure. Risk factors for infection include maternal fever, prolonged rupture of membranes, preterm labor, group B streptococcus colonization on the mother's screening test, maternal chorioamnionitis, and frequent urinary tract infections during pregnancy. Sepsis is an important consideration in any newborn with respiratory distress because early diagnostic work-up (Escobar et al., 2000) and empirical therapy with antibiotics can prevent morbidity and mortality related to this common problem in newborns.

Metabolic Errors

Common derangement in metabolism that may cause respiratory distress is hypoglycemia (low blood glucose level), which is often noted among the infants of diabetic mothers. Rarely, inborn errors of metabolism caused by organic acidemias or amino acid disorders, urea cycle disorders, and others can present as respiratory distress. State of the art newborn screening programs have helped to identify some of these infants, and those not screened should be considered once other common causes of respiratory distress are ruled out. Usually there is a short period of time after birth, often 1–2 days, when the baby appears to be doing well and feeding, but soon afterward starts to breathe faster and heavier as a result of an accumulation of acids or toxic metabolites. Common blood tests done during the initial evaluation may point toward increased acid or ammonia accumulation and form a clue for more specific testing and diagnosis (Enns & Packman, 2001).

Management of Acute Respiratory Distress

The main goal of management of acute respiratory distress is the maintenance of adequate blood oxygen and concurrent control of blood carbon dioxide levels to prevent acidosis. Carbon dioxide diffuses more readily from blood into alveoli; therefore, higher carbon dioxide content in blood signifies a more severe lung disease. Meanwhile, the underlying and contributory causes of respiratory distress (e.g., sepsis, anemia, patent ductus arteriosus) are investigated and treated accordingly. Exogenous surfactant replacement is considered for RDS.

Supplemental oxygen is given to increase the oxygen uptake from the lungs into the blood to keep the partial pressure of oxygen in the blood from 50 to 80 millimeters of mercury. If adequate oxygen level cannot be maintained by increasing oxygen concentration to greater than 60% in the inspired air, or the carbon dioxide level in the blood rises to greater than 60 millimeters mercury, assisted ventilation should be considered. The first step is to start CPAP by placing prongs in the nose, and forcing the baby to breathe against an adjustable low pressure. If this treatment fails to achieve the targeted oxygenation and elimination of carbon dioxide, mechanical ventilation is initiated with placement of a plastic tube (i.e., endotracheal tube) that is connected to a ventilator.

Two types of ventilators are commonly used today in neonatal intensive care units. One is the traditional ventilator that gives mechanical breaths over a range of normal breathing rates (20–60 breaths per minute) and is referred to as a conventional ventilator. Another type delivers very small tidal volume breaths at a very high rate (i.e., high frequency ventilators that deliver 360–900 breaths per minute by oscillating diaphragm as in a high frequency oscillator or 420 breaths per minute by jet stream as in a high frequency jet ventilator). Blood gases and chest x-rays are monitored during mechanical ventilation, and as targeted lung volume and blood gases are achieved, the settings are weaned accordingly. Other supportive measures include providing adequate body warmth and temperature control, fluid, and electrolyte and nutrition support, which is described in detail in Chapter 10 of this book.

There are ongoing efforts for improving the management of acute respiratory distress in newborns. Newer generation surfactants, including synthetic ones, are being developed for RDS. Nitric oxide as a pulmonary vasodilator used for term and near-term infants with pulmonary hypertension is now being tested for anti-inflammatory benefits and for its lung growth promoter (Lindwall et al., 2005) effect in preterm infants with RDS. In addition to the improved versions of conventional and high frequency ventilators, other modes of ventilation-like liquid ventilation (Wakabayashi, Tamura, & Nakamura, 2006) are being tested for newborns with respiratory distress.

Chronic Lung Disease

As neonatal intensive care has advanced, the survival rates of very low birth weight, premature babies have improved remarkably. However, this improvement comes with the cost of an increased number of survivors who have neurodevelopmental and chronic respiratory issues. Infants with mild or moderate severity of respiratory distress with only short periods of mechanical ventilation recover well and seldom have any chronic pulmonary or neurodevelopmental issues, unless complicated by other medical conditions, such as infections, surgical complications, or malformations. However, very low birth weight (< 1,500 grams) and extremely low birth weight (< 1,000 grams) premature infants with severe respiratory distress may need prolonged periods of respiratory support and hospital stay (Klinger, Sirota, Lusky, & Reichman, 2006). They are at a high risk for developing chronic lung disease and adverse neurodevelopmental outcomes. About one third of extremely low birth weight babies leave the hospital with a diagnosis of chronic lung disease or bronchopulmonary dysplasia (BPD).

The term BPD was first coined by Northway, Rosan, and Porter in 1967, who defined this condition as dependence on oxygen at 28 days of life with chest x-ray changes. Because the population of infants surviving now is more premature than before, this definition has been broadened to include infants needing oxygen at a corrected gestational age of 36 weeks with or without x-ray changes; and the term has been used interchangeably with chronic lung disease as well. Frequently, infants with BPD are discharged on home oxygen therapy and require some form of home monitoring equipment. They need extra care from their parents and physicians, as well as follow-up care by pediatric subspecialties, such as pediatric pulmonology, physical and/or occupational therapy, and early intervention services.

BPD or chronic lung disease evolves from therapeutic interventions, such as oxygen therapy and ventilatory support for acute respiratory illnesses in newborns with RDS. Pathogenesis is multifactorial with prematurity and the need for ventilatory support is the most important initiating factor (Chess, D'Angio, Pryhuber, & Maniscalco, 2006; Walsh et al., 2006). These lifesaving interventions required in the initial acute phase can induce acute inflammatory changes in the lung as a result of the mechanical effect of ventilators (i.e., barotrauma and/or volutrauma) or toxic effect of high oxygen concentration. These acute inflammatory changes later perpetuate into chronic inflammation of the lung and interfere with lung function. These conditions typically lead to prolonged ventilator support and a need for oxygen, which in turn may hamper the target of achieving independent oral feeding and interaction with the environment. Infants with BPD show signs of respiratory distress in the form of chest wall retractions and have a tendency to retain excessive fluids. Due to their increased efforts at breathing, in addition to their growth, their caloric needs are higher. However, their fluid intake should be lower because of fluid retention. They frequently are treated with diuretics to get rid of retained fluid, which may cause excessive loss of minerals, such as sodium, potassium, calcium, and chloride. These losses pose further challenges to their nutrition, and the majority of these infants are undernourished by the time they are ready to be discharged.

Other common problems associated with BPD include gastroesophageal reflux (GER), which adds another barrier to the nutritional rehabilitation of these infants. It is preferable for nutritional management to be planned with the help of a trained nutritionist. The infant's nutritional planning should provide a high density calorie formula with some fluid restriction; supplementation of minerals, iron, and vitamins; and management of GER. Adequate nutrition is the cornerstone for repair and healing of chronic lung disease.

Some infants with BPD are treated with potent, anti-inflammatory drugs, such as steroids; however, in recent years there have been serious concerns raised about the adverse, long-term neurodevelopmental issues in steroid-treated babies (Parikh et al., 2007; Short et al., 2003). These drugs are now used very cautiously in select infants after their parents have been informed about the risks and the benefits of such therapy (American Academy of Pediatrics Committee on Fetus and Newborn, 2002).

After discharge, infants with BPD are susceptible to viral and bacterial infections. For example, respiratory syncytial virus (RSV), which typically causes mild cold symptoms in children during the winter, may result in life-threatening bronchiolitis or pneumonia if acquired by an infant with BPD. Therefore, premature newborns and infants with BPD need passive immunization against RSV. One such product available commercially is a monoclonal antibody called palivizumab (Synagis), which is given by injection once every month through the RSV season from late fall to early spring (Fenton, Scott, & Plosker, 2004).

Conclusion

Infants with BPD continue to be a very vulnerable group and may require a substantially high proportion of health care resources. Severe BPD invariably is associated with some degree of adverse developmental outcome; however, it is difficult to distinguish the effects of the severity of lung disease from those issues related to the intensity of interventions and associated medical complications, such as poor nutrition, infection, and intracranial hemorrhage that can affect neuron development. Frequently this population of infants has increased mortality, morbidity, and readmission to the hospital during the first 1–2 years of life as compared to their counterparts without BPD. Follow-up of infants with BPD shows a progressive improvement in the pulmonary function and weaning of oxygen in the majority of the children, varying from a few weeks to the first few years after discharge from the hospital. In that respect, BPD is entirely different from the adult onset of the chronic lung disease and has a favorable outcome most of the time. However, the same is not true in terms of frequently seen, adverse neurodevelopmental outcomes. These concerns are discussed in greater detail in other chapters of this book.

REFERENCES

Al Kharfy, T.M. (2004). High frequency ventilation in the management of very low birth weight infants with pulmonary hemorrhage. *American Journal of Perinatology, 21*(1), 19–26.

American Academy of Pediatrics Committee on Fetus and Newborn. (2002). Postnatal corticosteroids to treat or prevent chronic lung disease in preterm infants. *Pediatrics, 109,* 330–338.

Avery, M.E., & Merrit, T.A. (1991). Surfactant replacement therapy. *New England Journal of Medicine, 324,* 865–869.

Ballard, R.A. (2004). Respiratory system. In W.H. Taeusch, R.A. Ballard, & C.A. Gleason (Eds.), *Avery's diseases of the newborn* (8th ed., pp. 601–778). New York: Elsevier.

Carey, B.E. (1999). Neonatal air leaks: Pneumothorax, pneumomediastinum, pulmonary interstitial emphysema, pneumopericardium. *Neonatal Network, 18*(8), 81–84.

Chess, P.R., D'Angio, C.T., Pryhuber, G.S., & Maniscalco, W.M. (2006). Pathogenesis of bronchopulmonary dysplasia. *Seminars in Perinatology, 30,* 171–178.

Clark, D.A. (1994). Respiratory distress. In G.L. Ensher & D.A. Clark, *Newborns at risk: Medical care and psychoeducational intervention* (2nd ed.). Gaithersburg, MD: Aspen Publishers.

Clark, D.A., Neiman, G.F., Thompson, J.E., & Bredenberg, C.E. (1987). Surfactant displacement by meconium free fatty acids: An alternative explanation for atelectasis in meconium aspiration syndrome. *Journal of Pediatrics, 110,* 765–770.

Enns, G.M., & Packman, S. (2001). Diagnosing inborn errors of metabolism in the newborn: Laboratory investigations. *Neo Reviews* (AAP publications online), *2*(8), e192–e200.

Escobar, E.J., Li, D.K., Armstrong, M.A., Gardener, M.N., Flock, B.F., Verdi, J.E., Xiong, B., & Bergen, R. (2000). Neonatal sepsis work up in infants > 2000 grams at birth: A population-based study. *Pediatrics, 106,* 256–263.

Fenton, C., Scott, L.J., & Plosker, G.L. (2004). Palivizumab: A review of its use as a prophylaxis for serious respiratory syncytial virus infection. *Paediatric Drugs, 6*(3), 177–197.

Halliday, H.L. (2006). Recent clinical trials of surfactant treatment for neonates. *Biology of Neonate, 89*(4), 323–329.

Hermes-DeSantis, E.R., & Clyman, R.I. (2006). Patent ductus arteriosus: Pathophysiology and management. *Journal of Perinatology, 26*(Suppl. 1), S14–S18.

Jain, L., & Dudell, G.G. (2006). Respiratory transition in infants delivered by cesarean section. *Seminars in Perinatology, 30,* 296–304.

Jain, L., & Eaton, D.C. (2006). Physiology of fetal lung fluid clearance and effect of labor. *Seminars in Perinatology, 30,* 34–43.

Klinger, G., Sirota, L., Lusky, A., & Reichman, B. (2006). Bronchopulmonary dysplasia in very low birth weight infants is associated with prolonged hospital stay. *Journal of Perinatology, 26*(10), 640–644.

Lindwall, R., Blennow, M., Svensson, M., Jonsson, B., Berggren-Bostrom, E., Flanby, M., et al. (2005). A pilot study of inhaled nitric oxide in preterm infants treated with nasal continuous airway pressure for respiratory distress syndrome. *Intensive Care Medicine, 31,* 959–964.

McIntosh, N. (1983). Pulmonary air leaks in newborn period. *British Journal of Hospital Medicine, 29*(6), 512–517.

Munshi, U.K., & Clark, D.A. (2002). Meconium aspiration syndrome. *Contemporary Clinical Gynecology and Obstetrics, 2,* 247–254.

Northway, W.H., Rosan, R.C., & Porter, D.Y. (1967). Pulmonary disease following respiratory therapy for hyaline membrane disease. *New England Journal of Medicine 276,* 357–368.

Parikh, N.A., Lasky, R.E., Kennedy, K.E., Moya, F.R., Hochhauser, L., Romo, S., & Tyson, J.E. (2007). Postnatal dexamethasone therapy and cerebral tissue volumes in extremely low birth weight infants. *Pediatrics, 119,* 265–272.

Pfister, R.H., & Soll, R.F. (2005). New synthetic surfactants: The next generation? *Biology of Neonate, 87,* 338–344.

Raval, M.V., Laughon, M.M., Bose, C.L., & Phillips, J.D. (2007). Patent ductus arteriosus ligation in premature infants: Who really benefits, and at what cost? *Journal of Pediatric Surgery, 42,* 69–75.

Schreiber, M.D., Gin-Mestan, K., Marks, J.D., Huo, D., Lee, G., & Srisuparp, P. (2003). Inhaled nitric oxide in premature infants with respiratory distress syndrome. *New England Journal of Medicine, 349,* 2099–2107.

Short, E.J., Klein, N.K., Lewis, B.A., Fulton, S., Eisengart, S., Kercsmar, C., et al. (2003). Cognitive and academic consequences of bronchopulmonary dysplasia and very low birth weight: 8-year-old outcomes. *Pediatrics, 112,* e359–e366.

Wakabayashi, T., Tamura, M., & Nakamura, T. (2006). Partial liquid ventilation with low dose perfluoro chemical and high frequency oscillation improves oxygenation and lung compliance in a rabbit model of surfactant depletion. *Biology of Neonate, 89*(3), 177–182.

Walsh, M.C., Stanley, S., Davis, J., Allen, M., Van Marter, L., Abman, S., Blackmon, L., & Jobe, A. (2006). Summary proceedings from the Bronchopulmonary Dysplasia Group. *Pediatrics, 117*(3), S52–S59.

CHAPTER 10

Nutrition and Feeding Problems

Linda J. Levy and David A. Clark

At the conclusion of this chapter, the reader will

* *Understand the essential nutritional components of breast milk and formula*

* *Understand the limitations and difficulties of feeding preterm and sick newborns*

It is a great challenge to nourish the preterm newborn (born at less than 37 weeks of gestation) or sick newborn adequately. There are many nutritional deficiencies in neonates that have been linked to significant long-term problems, including diminished immune function, poor growth, and delays in cognitive and motor development (American Academy of Pediatrics [AAP] Committee on Nutrition, 2004f).

Development

The ability to feed depends on the normal anatomy and function of the mouth and intestinal tract (Grand, Watkins, & Torti, 1976). The mouth is formed early in the first trimester. Malformations of the lips, the failure of the palate to fuse resulting in a cleft palate (see Figure 10.1), and a small mandible all create anatomic relationships that interfere with sucking and swallowing. The ability to swallow is present by 20 weeks' gestation; by late in the third trimester, near term, the fetus swallows up to 750 milliliters of amniotic fluid each day. This important function helps to maintain an adequate volume of amniotic fluid. An inability to swallow and a blockage of the upper intestinal tract create excess amniotic fluid that commonly causes excess uterine distension and preterm birth.

The suck is not well developed at birth in preterm infants, and it is first detected at approximately 20 weeks' gestation. At this time, the suck is poorly coordinated and generates little negative pressure. During the next 6 weeks of gestation, the sucking pattern matures so that by 34 weeks' gestation it has consistent high amplitude bursts. The sucking and swallowing reflexes are not coordinated, one to the other, until approximately 34 weeks' gestation. Thus, the vast majority of young preterm infants require feeding via gavage tubes. Infants who have suffered a prenatal or perinatal insult, even though more mature, may have delayed development of suck and swallow as they recover from their perinatal asphyxia insult.

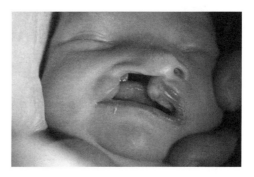

Figure 10.1. Example of cleft palate. (From Clark, D.A., private collection; reprinted by permission.)

Components of Nutrition

Nutrition prior to birth is provided by the passage of all nutrients from the mother to the fetus via the placenta (AAP Committee on Nutrition, 2004d). Waste products of protein, carbohydrate, and fat metabolism are returned to the mother for elimination via her lungs, liver, and kidneys. Once the child is born, the intestine must immediately begin the complex process of digesting breast milk or formula for the crucial nutrients that were once provided by the mother. Although there has been an exponential increase in knowledge of fetal growth and nutrition, the extrauterine growth of the preterm baby still does not match that of intrauterine growth. Newborns that are ill often are unable to tolerate the type and quality of feeding necessary for optimal growth and development. Alternately, they frequently require intravenous nutrition. Even with recent technological advances, intravenous (IV) nutritional therapy remains a poor substitute to the well-developed, properly functioning intestinal tract.

The intestinal tract will measure approximately 100–110 inches long at birth. Most of the enzymes necessary for digestion of sugars, proteins, and fats are present. Unfortunately, the more immature the infant, the more limited the digestive capability. The body composition of a full-term infant differs drastically from that of a premature baby (Moya, 1993). In a full-term baby, approximately 12%–15% of body weight is fat, and 11%–12% is protein. Premature babies have a much lower percentage of body fat—as low as 1% at 28 weeks' gestation. This difference in total body composition reflects the total calories in reserve. The full-term newborn can modulate metabolism and has sufficient stored calories to retain body heat and serum glucose concentrations.

The digestive tract has specialized functions, digestion, and absorption of nutrients (Lissauer & Fanaroff, 2006). Initially, the mature newborn's stomach has limited volume with delayed emptying and decreased acid secretion. This permits the early passage of hormones, enzymes, and protective proteins of breast milk to the lower portions of the intestinal tract, which helps control intestinal colonization. In general, protein and fat digestion is initiated in the stomach, enhanced in the first part of the small intestine (duodenum), and then completed in the remainder of the small intestine. Carbohydrate digestion is initiated in the mouth and generally is completed within the first portion of the small intestine. Water, vitamins, minerals, and other vital nutrients are absorbed throughout the small and large intestines.

In premature infants, digestion (especially of fats and carbohydrates) tends to be inefficient (AAP Committee on Nutrition, 2004e). Consequently, the number of calories available is less than the total number of calories ingested. Adequate digestion and absorption of nutrients within the intestine requires continued movement in the digestive tract from mouth to anus. This process is termed intestinal motility. Many of the hormones secreted in the intestinal tract modify digestive capabilities, which promotes more efficient digestion. Dietary components themselves can influence intestinal motility. High fat meals, increased caloric density, and casein (the curd protein in milk) slow stomach emptying and intestinal motility. Although the slow intestinal motility permits more time for thorough digestion and absorption of fats and complex proteins, this inefficient process may allow these nutrients access to the large intestine where intestinal bacteria may use them for their own growth. A diminished function of the liver or kidneys may decrease utilization of protein, carbohydrates, and fats necessary for ultimate growth. In addition, the premature infant no longer has the temperature support of his or her mother and utilizes calories to help maintain body temperature. This condition results in fewer calories available for growth.

The average 28-week gestation infant (40 weeks is full term) weighs approximately 1,000 grams. During the last 12 weeks of gestation, there will be approximately a three-fold increase of body weight and a disproportionate increase of many nutrient stores, especially glycogen (a storage form of glucose) and calcium. These nutrient stores cannot be replaced, which leaves the preterm infant at higher risk for poor growth that may have long-term ramifications. Overall growth of the infant after birth is a marker for adequate organ growth, especially of the lungs and brain. Rapid bone growth with an insufficient intake of calcium, phosphorus, vitamin E, and protein may lead to poor bone mineralization, which leaves infants vulnerable to fractures or rickets. Essential fatty acids and the long-chain, polyunsaturated fatty acids (LCPUFA) are essential components of many membranes, including the developing brain and retina. Each of these major components is discussed separately later in this chapter.

Dehydration is a common problem in preterm and low birth weight infants because of the high skin permeability and water loss through the skin. A 1,000 gram, 28-week gestation, premature baby has a water loss nearly three times that of a full-term infant. Given the limited ability of the kidney to concentrate urine, dehydration that results in a high blood sodium level may be life threatening. The immature kidneys also have a limited ability to excrete a water load in excess of fluid administration, which may result in edema and congestive heart failure. Therefore, the range of fluid that may be administered in a premature or sick newborn is much restricted compared to that which is tolerated by a full-term baby. Babies who are receiving phototherapy or being cared for under radiant warmers may have additional, unmeasured fluid losses. Poorly functioning kidneys due to perinatal asphyxia or the presence of patent ductus arteriosus (when the vessel that connects the fetal pulmonary artery to the fetal aorta fails to constrict) with excess lung fluid are two conditions that may require some fluid restriction.

Carbohydrates

Carbohydrates are the primary energy source for tissue metabolism (Lifshitz, 1988). Because carbohydrates can be derived from fat, there is no essential carbohydrate. Tissue metabolism can adjust to a carbohydrate-free diet. This is not true of protein or fat because there are essential amino acids and essential fatty acids that cannot be synthesized. However, carbohydrates are the precursors of many metabolic pathways, such as those for the formation of nucleic acids (DNA

and RNA) and for bilirubin conjugation and excretion. Dextrose, the d-isomer (dextrorotatory) of glucose, is a 6-carbon monosaccharide and is the primary carbohydrate for energy metabolism. The primary sugar of breast milk or infant formula is the disaccharide lactose, which is composed of equal portions of glucose and galactose. The outermost layer of the cell directly exposed to the intestinal contents is the intestinal brush-border; the brush-border enzyme, lactase, which splits lactose into its two components, glucose and galactose, is minimally active prior to 34 weeks' gestation. Therefore, lactose digestion in preterm infants is limited, and preterm formulas have been modified to account for this deficit.

Any undigested carbohydrate may reach and modify the growth of bacteria in the large intestine. The bacteria will ferment the carbohydrate-producing gases (carbon dioxide and hydrogen) and organic acids. These organic acids may be absorbed and metabolized and provide some recovery mechanism for calories; however, some may accumulate in the small intestine and act as an irritant and, therefore, initiate an inflammatory process.

Protein

Protein and potassium are the two critical nutrients for normal growth and development of all newborns (Clark & Miller, 1993). Dietary protein from breast milk or infant formula is broken down in the intestinal tract to amino acids, which are absorbed and transported to the liver (Raiha, 1989). The liver removes many of these amino acids and synthesizes them into the serum-circulating proteins, including serum albumin, transport proteins for metals (e.g., ferritin that transports iron), and the majority of the coagulation factors. The amino acids that bypass the liver are directly incorporated into actively growing tissue and are a major component of cell membranes, enzymes within the cell, hormones, and neurotransmitters. The majority of protein digestion occurs in the stomach and the small intestine and is detectible by 20 weeks' gestation. A preterm infant has developed gastric, intestinal, and pancreatic function for protein digestion and absorption of the proteins that were present in the amniotic fluid. Many of the amniotic fluid proteins are similar to the whey proteins that are naturally present in breast milk.

Total protein intake in preterm infants is limited to some degree by immature hepatic function and a limited capacity of the preterm kidneys to excrete the breakdown products of protein metabolism. The immature kidney cannot remove the waste products of metabolism as efficiently as the placenta, which is backed up by the maternal kidneys. Premature infants fed an excess of protein have higher blood urea nitrogen levels than full-term babies, and this may be a marker of postnatal growth retardation.

The digestion of milk proteins is a complex process (Clark & Miller, 1993). The two major groups of proteins in all milks are caseins, the proteins that curd, and whey proteins, which are the soluble proteins. The casein proteins are less readily digested. This is specifically true of the bovine casein as compared to human casein protein. Undigested bovine casein, a major component of standard infant formula, has been associated with delayed gastric emptying and lactobezoars, which are firm masses in the stomach that may require surgical removal. The undigested casein fraction may also bind crucial minerals, such as calcium, magnesium, zinc, and chromium. The whey proteins are much more easily digested with a greater than 95% utilization. This compares with the approximately 80% utilization of the casein protein fraction that is digested. The excess, unused amino acids are excreted in the urine.

Alternative Proteins   Sources for formula protein rather than cow's milk protein are the soy hydrolysates and elemental formulas derived from a variety of protein sources, including casein and beef. Taurine is an important amino acid that is derived from cysteine and is abundant in breast milk. It is important for growth and development of the central nervous system and the retina. All standard commercial formulas in the United States now contain supplemental taurine comparable to that found in breast milk.

Fats

Lipids are vital for growth and development (Hamosh, 1988), and fats are the primary energy source of newborns, accounting for more than 50% of the calories in breast milk or formula. Fats are essential for brain development (Food and Agriculture Organization [FAO]/World Health Organization [WHO], 1994). In the full-term infant, the body of fat is increased to nearly 15-fold over that of a 28-week, 1 kg infant who will triple his or her birth weight from 28 weeks to full-term gestation (40 weeks). Approximately 10% of the fat of a term baby is brown fat, which can rapidly release energy due to its high density of cellular mitochrondia. This tissue is responsive to the adrenal hormones, especially norepinephrine, which allows the energy to be rapidly mobilized. Fat digestion requires that pancreatic enzymes cleave fatty acids from the glycerol molecule, which is a 3-carbon compound and half the size of a glucose (sugar) molecule (Hamosh, Bitman, & Wood, 1985). The fat absorbed is repackaged within the intestinal mucosa to triglycerides by reattaching the fatty acids to the glycerol. These packages subsequently are transported throughout the body. If the fat is not utilized, it is placed in storage (commonly in the liver and fatty tissue throughout the body). The breakdown of glycerol and fats results in the production of energy, water, and carbon dioxide identical to the breakdown products of glucose metabolism. At the cellular level, this process is dependent on carnitine, which is considered a conditionally essential nutrient because under certain conditions its requirements may exceed the individual's capacity to synthesize it. Carnitine facilitates the transport of medium and long-train, fatty acids across mitochondrial membranes, allowing their oxidation and the subsequent production of energy. In turn, it also facilitates the transport of intermediate toxic products out of the mitochondria, which prevents their accumulation. Because of these key functions, carnitine is present primarily in tissues that utilize fatty acids as their primary fuel. These include skeletal and cardiac muscle. Any excess carnitine in the diet is excreted by the kidneys.

Because long-chain, fatty acids may be poorly digested by premature infants, approximately 50% of the fat content of preterm formula is present as medium-chain triglycerides. These are glycerol molecules that have attached fatty acids of 14 carbons less.

There are two essential fatty acids, linoleic and alpha-linolenic acid (Innis, 1991). These cannot be synthesized in the body as they are 18 carbon fats. Insufficient intake of these by any child or adult would result in an essential fatty acid deficiency. In healthy older children and adults, these fats would be used as the base to make much more complex fats, including arachidonic acid (ARA) and docosahexanoic acid (DHA). DHA and ARA are in low concentration in breast milk, comprising no more than 2% of all the fat (Jensen, 1999). However, these fatty acids have very important functions in the brain. There is rapid accumulation of DHA in the fetal brain in the last trimester. This process continues in the developing brain for the first 2 years of life. Until the 1990s, commercial formulas available in the United States and in much of the world did not include DHA and ARA. With the lack of these fats in the formula, developmental differences could be demonstrated between breast-fed and formula-fed children, especially in visual acuity and early cognitive development (Rogan & Gladen, 1993). Since then, the Food and Drug Administration has approved the use and addition of DHA and ARA to infant formula. Multiple studies since the 1990s have shown that infants fed formula containing appropriate amounts of DHA and ARA perform similarly to breast-fed babies on tests of visual acuity and cognitive development (Innis, Akrabawi, Diersen-Schade, Dobson, & Guy, 1997; Ryan et al., 1999).

Minerals

Deficiency of many minerals has been documented to delay growth and development. These include calcium, magnesium, sodium, potassium, and iron. In addition, small levels of zinc, copper, manganese, chromium, molybdenum, and selenium are important trace elements. Potassium is the most crucial mineral because it is the major intracellular metal, whereas sodium is found primarily in extracellular fluid.

The differential concentrations of these minerals, within and outside of a cell, are crucial in maintaining the polarization of the cell (electrical activity) that allows for the movement of nutrients into and waste products from cells. This po-larity also is critical for transmitting electrical impulses throughout the central nervous system, regulating muscular activity, and driving the beat of the heart.

Calcium and phosphorus are primarily responsible for bone growth. The majority of calcium is deposited in the last trimester (28–40 weeks' gestation). Infants that are born prematurely are more prone to delayed bone growth, which is known as osteopenia of prematurity. The regulation of calcium and phosphorus absorption, its metabolism, and its deposition is controlled by the parathyroid glands, the kidneys, and the liver. In addition to its crucial role in the growth of cells, phosphorus also is the base of many high energy compounds within the body, including adenosine triphosphate (ATP) and adenosine diphosphate (ADP). The metabolism of magnesium is closely linked to that of calcium. It is the second most common intracellular electrolyte in the body, and it is known to be important to many transport mechanisms that have enzyme function. In excess, it may suppress muscular activity. Mothers with preeclampsia (including high blood pressure) or premature labor may receive magnesium sulfate to quiet the uterus. If a mother has been receiving magnesium therapy and her child is born with a high level of blood magnesium, the newborn may present with lethargy, poor respiratory effort, and decreased intestinal motility.

Iron is essential in the formation of the hemoglobin of red blood cells. It is absorbed primarily in the first portion of the small intestine. Approximately 50% of the iron in breast milk is absorbed, which is much greater than the amount typically absorbed from formulas. Breast milk contains an iron-binding protein, lactoferrin, which enhances the transfer of iron across the intestinal mucosa. Lactoferrin, binding the iron, precludes its use by iron-dependent bacteria, which may be harmful to the newborn intestine. Virtually all newborns, including preterm babies, have sufficient iron stores at birth to supply their usual needs until the birth weight is nearly doubled. Preterm infants receiving transfusions may develop an iron excess as a result of receiving more iron in blood transfusions than is being lost from frequent blood sampling. Infant formulas for babies are iron fortified, and infants being breast fed receive supplemental iron well before doubling their birth weight because it is now recognized that even mild subclinical deficiency of iron may impair neurological development. Symptoms of iron deficiency include irritability, listlessness, inadequate growth, feeding difficulties, and anemia. Although beyond the scope of this text, the need for supplemental trace minerals for premature infants has been well recognized (Mertz, 1985). There have been many reports of zinc deficiency that causes delayed growth, diarrhea, hair loss, and perianal skin lesions. Copper deficiency may result in infants with poor weight gain, edema, anemia, and decreased muscle tone. A relative deficiency of chromium may lead to a poor ability to metabolize glucose. Standard parenteral (IV) nutrition, breast milk, and routine formulas provide sufficient amounts of all known trace elements.

Vitamins

Vitamins can be classified as fat soluble or water soluble (Greene & Smidt, 1993). Few deficiencies can be demonstrated in the water soluble vitamins, such as vitamin C and the B-complex vitamins (niacin, biotin, and pantothenic acid). In contrast, deficiency of fat soluble vitamins may be due to poor absorption of fat. Deficiencies of vitamins A, D, and E have been linked to specific clinical findings in newborns, especially preterm newborns. Although controversial, vitamin A supplementation may be helpful for mitigating the severity of bronchopulmonary dysplasia. Supplemental vitamin D is useful for limiting the osteopenia of prematurity. Vitamin E is an antioxidant that improves the survival of red blood cells once they have been released from the bone marrow.

Vitamin K has long been recognized as critical for preventing hemorrhagic disease in the newborn (Fomon & Suttie, 1993). Newborns are born relatively deficient in vitamin K because it is synthesized by intestinal bacteria, and the newborn intestine is sterile. During the first week, the intestine is colonized with organisms that are capable of producing vitamin K. Approximately 1% of babies who do not receive vitamin K will

hemorrhage. The bleeding may be severe and involve the central nervous system, lung, or adrenal glands.

Means of Receiving Nutrition

Infants receive nutrition through either breast milk or formula, as detailed in the following sections.

Breast Milk

Breast milk is the gold standard for nutrition (AAP Committee on Nutrition, 2004a; Anderson, Johnstone, & Remley, 1999). It is a complex biological product. The composition of breast milk varies from woman to woman, based on her nutritional status. Women who suffer poor nutrition and poor fat stores produce a poorer quantity and quality of breast milk (Heinig & Dewey, 1997). This is typical of women living in countries such as Ethiopia, whose breast milk contains insufficient fat and protein to sustain appropriate growth of the baby (Dewey, Heinig, & Nommsen-Rivers, 1995).

The composition of breast milk changes during the course of a single feeding (Picciano, 2001a; 2001b). Early mature breast milk has higher lactose (sugar) concentration that decreases during the course of a 15- to 20-minute feeding. In the same time frame, the fat content of the milk initially is low, but it increases during the course of the individual feeding. In a full sample of mature milk, 50% of the calories are derived from fat. The caloric density of the milk changes during the course of a feeding; that is, initially it is approximately 16–17 calories per 30 cc in the foremilk, which increases up to 24–25 calories per 30 cc in the hind milk. Not uncommonly, women have a dominant breast based on their handedness. As there is much better muscular and blood flow to the right arm of the right-handed mother, similarly, the right breast commonly has a better blood supply and therefore produces a higher quantity and quality of breast milk.

The primary carbohydrate of breast milk is lactose, which is readily digested by the enzyme lactase in the intestinal brush border. The proteins of breast milk are caseins, which account for 30% of the total protein, and whey proteins, which account for approximately 70% of the total protein. The primary whey protein is alpha lactalbumin, which is similar to circulating blood albumin and proteins that are found in amniotic fluid. Even the smallest preterm babies at birth have been exposed to amniotic fluid, and, therefore, the enzymes that digest lactalbumin are well developed. The fat content of human milk is complex fat, including the essential fatty acids of linoleic acid, alpha-linolenic acid, DHA, and ARA.

In addition, there are many unique substances in breast milk that are not yet present in formula (Hamosh, 2001). These include immunoglobulins, which are protein antibodies that help to coat the intestine and defend against bacteria (Goldman, Chheda, Keeney, Schmalsteig, & Schanler, 1994). Breast milk also contains cells, lymphocytes, and neutrophils, which help to protect the mouth and the first portion of the intestine against bacterial infection. There are many other compounds that help to facilitate the colonization of the newborn intestine with healthy bacteria, such as *Lactobacillus species* and *Bifidobacterium* (Heinig, 2001).

For more premature infants (less than 32 weeks' gestation or 1,500 gram birth weight), nutritional enhancement of breast milk by additional calories, calcium, potassium, and other essential nutrients is necessary for appropriate growth (Clark, 1993).

Infant Formulas

Formulas attempt to mimic the caloric composition of breast milk (AAP Committee on Nutrition, 2004b). They effectively mimic the vitamin and mineral composition. The fat blend in most infant formulas will include DHA and ARA and is very similar to breast milk. The cow's milk, protein-based formulas contain lactose, which is present in human milk. However, the soy formulas have primarily sucrose or glucose polymers as the carbohydrate source. This is of some significance in that sucrose is 100 times sweeter than lactose, and if infants are given a soy formula for even brief periods of time, they may prefer those formulas to the more standard formulas or even

to breast milk. The most significant difference in formula, as compared to breast milk, is the protein type. The quantity of protein is similar to that of breast milk or slightly greater to allow for some decreased digestibility. The proteins are from two major groups: 1) the cow's milk proteins (caseins and whey) that have been modified to some degree to make them more digestible, and 2) the soy proteins. Each of the major formula companies has a soy protein-based product. This is not whole soy protein, but soy protein that has been hydrolyzed to smaller, more digestible subgroups of proteins. These derivations of soy protein vary from one company to another.

Preterm infant formulas have been modified to adjust for the decreased ability of a newborn intestine to handle certain nutrients (Romero & Kleinman, 1993). As the enzyme lactase is only fully functional by about 34 weeks' gestation, all premature formulas have decreased amounts of lactose, usually only 40%–50% of the carbohydrate source. Lactose is not removed completely from formula in that lactose is important for calcium absorption, and these infants have a significant calcium deficit. Because preterm newborns also may have some difficulty digesting fat, the type of fat that comprises nearly 50% of the fat in preterm formulas is a medium-chain triglyceride, which is a glycerol (3-carbon molecule) to which are attached shorter chained fatty acids that are directly absorbed and metabolized without the need for pancreatic lipase or bile salts to emulsify the more complex larger fats.

Special Formulas

There are many special formulas that are designed to address particular needs. For babies that are having problems with sugar, fat, or protein absorption, there are elemental formulas where the preparations are designed to eliminate much of the digestive process. Sugars are in their simplest form; proteins have been hydrolyzed down to one, two, and three amino acids. Fats are given as medium-chain triglycerides. In general, these formulas are not as palatable because, as proteins are hydrolyzed, they become more bitter and may not be as well tolerated by the baby. For babies with specific genetic defects in metabolism (primarily disorders of protein metabolism), rarely used specialty formulas are available. A prime example of this would be children with phenylketonuria, which is a newborn metabolic disease in which excess amounts of phenylalanine accumulate in the brain and result in brain damage. Formulas have been developed that give just enough phenylalanine for appropriate growth, without providing excess that would cause the baby to have atypical development. This is true for many of the metabolic defects that are amenable to dietary therapy.

Common Neonatal Diseases Affecting the Ability to Feed

Although the intestine of preterm infants may be capable of digesting key nutrients, various disease states may make it difficult to feed the newborn. Although babies born before 34 weeks' gestation commonly do not have a fully integrated suck–swallow reflex, enteral nutrition can be accomplished by the use of a gavage or gastric feeding tube.

Intestinal motility and digestion within the intestinal tract are compromised by systemic illnesses that may affect the preterm newborn. Chief among these is respiratory distress that results from morphological immaturity of the lung and biochemical immaturity due to lack of surfactant (see Chapter 9 for more information). These infants have a high respiratory rate and do not tolerate food, even when placed in the stomach. They have an increased caloric need because of the work of breathing and require parenteral nutrition to maintain appropriate blood glucose and other key nutrients. Infants who require prolonged ventilation may develop chronic lung disease with a long-term increase in caloric need and a poor growth pattern. Infants who have been intubated for a long period of time may have aversions to oral feeding, a tonic bite reflex, abnormal tongue thrust, and/or a hyperactive gag. They may also develop grooves in their palates that interfere with the ability to form a proper seal around the nipple. A poorly coordinated suck reflux, resulting in apnea while feeding, is also common.

Acquired intestinal disease may interrupt digestion or absorption (Clark & Mitchell, 2004). The second and most common cause of death of premature infants is necrotizing enterocolitis (NEC), an inflammatory bowel disease seen more commonly in infants weighing less than 1 kg (Clark & Miller, 1996). The incidence of NEC is as high as 5%–15% of babies with less than a 1,500 gram birth weight. Mortality rates can be as high as 20%–30%. This illness of the intestine may result in necrosis and require that a portion of the intestine be removed surgically (Clark & Miller, 1990). This often results in malabsorption, a limited ability to tolerate feedings, and a need for long-term IV nutrition.

The smallest preterm infants are also at risk for intraventricular hemorrhage, which is discussed earlier in this book (see Chapter 5). One complication of intraventricular hemorrhage is the blockage of the flow of the spinal fluid, which results in hydrocephalus. In the more severe forms, the infants may have significant problems, such as cerebral palsy and intellectual disability. These babies commonly do not feed or grow well. Any infant with severe brain injury may require a permanent feeding tube for adequate nutrition. This is inserted through the abdominal wall into the stomach so that the tube does not interfere with the upper airway and respiratory function.

Newborns with congenital heart disease are at risk for malnutrition. Many have symptoms such as poor feeding, abdominal distension, and delayed gastric emptying. Some of these conditions are associated with a high metabolic rate due to strain on the maldeveloped heart. Some infants have congestive heart failure with associated mild protein malabsorption and commonly significant fat malabsorption. In one study, prior to corrective surgery, infants were found to take in, on average, only 82% of the estimated energy needs.

Conclusion

In summary, the development and function of the intestinal tract is second in complexity only to the function of the central nervous system. There are many anatomic defects of acquired illnesses that interfere with adequate nutrition. Breast milk remains the gold standard for feeding healthy, full-term infants, as well as for most neonates born after 34 weeks' gestation. For the more premature infants, nutritional enhancement of breast milk by additional calories, calcium, potassium, and other essential nutrients is necessary for appropriate growth. Alternatively, there are many preterm formulas that have been developed to address the unique needs of premature infants.

REFERENCES

American Academy of Pediatrics Committee on Nutrition. (2004a). Breastfeeding. In *Pediatric nutrition handbook* (pp. 55–85). Elk Grove Village, IL: Author.

American Academy of Pediatrics Committee on Nutrition. (2004b). Formula feeding of term infants. In *Pediatric nutrition handbook* (pp. 87–97). Elk Grove Village, IL: American Academy of Pediatrics.

American Academy of Pediatrics Committee on Nutrition. (2004c). Infant nutrition and the development of gastrointestinal function. In *Pediatric nutrition handbook* (pp.3–22). Elk Grove Village, IL: American Academy of Pediatrics.

American Academy of Pediatrics Committee on Nutrition. (2004d). Nutrition during pregnancy. In *Pediatric nutrition handbook* (pp. 167–190). Elk Grove Village, IL: American Academy of Pediatrics.

American Academy of Pediatrics Committee on Nutrition. (2004e). Nutritional needs of the preterm infant. In *Pediatric nutrition handbook* (pp. 23–54). Elk Grove Village, IL: American Academy of Pediatrics.

American Academy of Pediatrics Committee on Nutrition. (2004f). *Pediatric nutrition handbook.* Elk Grove Village, IL: American Academy of Pediatrics.

Anderson, J.W., Johnstone, B.M., & Remley, D.T. (1999). Breast-feeding and cognitive development: A meta-analysis. *American Journal of Clinical Nutrition, 70,* 525–535.

Clark, D.A. (1993). Nutritional requirement of the premature and small-for-gestational-age infant. In R.M. Suskind (Ed.), *Textbook for pediatric nutrition* (2nd ed., pp. 23–32). New York: Raven.

Clark, D.A., & Miller, M.J.S. (1990). Intraluminal pathogenesis of necrotizing enterocolitis. *Journal of Pediatrics, 117*(pt. 2), S64–S67.

Clark, D.A., & Miller, M.J.S. (1993). Nutritive proteins in feeding the infant. *Excerpta Medica, 2,* 41–55.

Clark, D.A., & Miller, M.J.S. (1996). What causes necrotizing enterocolitis and how can it be prevented? In

T. Hansen (Ed.), *Current topics in neonatology* (No. 1, pp. 160–176). Philadelphia: W.B. Saunders.

Clark, D.A., & Mitchell, A.L. (2004). Development of gastrointestinal function: Risk factors for necrotizing enterocolitis. *Journal of Pediatric Pharmacology and Therapeutics, 9*(2), 96–103.

Dewey, K.G., Heinig, M.J., & Nommsen-Rivers, L.A. (1995). Differences in morbidity between breast-fed and formula-fed infants. *Journal of Pediatrics, 126,* 696–702.

Fomon, S.J., & Suttie, J.W. (1993). Vitamin K. In S.J. Fomon (Ed.), *Nutrition of normal infants* (pp. 348–358). St. Louis: Mosby.

Food and Agriculture Organization (FAO)/World Health Organization (WHO). (1994). Lipids in early development. In *Fats and oils in human nutrition: Report of a joint expert consultation* (pp. 49–55). Rome: Author.

Goldman, A.S., Chheda, S., Keeney, S.E., Schmalsteig, F.C., & Schanler, R.J. (1994). Immunologic protection of the premature newborn by human milk. *Seminars in Perinatology, 18,* 495–501.

Grand, R.J., Watkins, J.B., & Torti, F.M. (1976). Development of the human gastrointestinal tract. *Gastroenterology, 70,* 790–810.

Greene, H.L., & Smidt, L.J. (1993). Water soluble vitamins. In R.C. Tsang (Ed.), *Nutritional needs of the preterm infant* (pp. 121–134). Philadelphia: Williams & Wilkins.

Hamosh, M. (1988). Fat needs for term and preterm infants. In R.C. Tsang & B. Nichols (Eds.), *Nutrition during infancy* (pp. 133–159). Philadelphia: Hanley & Belfus.

Hamosh, M. (2001). Bioactive factors in human milk. *Pediatric Clinics of North America, 48,* 69–86.

Hamosh, M., Bitman, J., & Wood, D.L. (1985). Lipids in milk and the first steps in their digestion. *Pediatrics, 75,* 146.

Heinig, M.J. (2001). Most defense benefits of breastfeeding for the infant: Effect of breastfeeding duration and exclusivity. *Pediatric Clinics of North America, 48,* 105–123.

Heinig, M.J., & Dewey, K.G. (1997). Health effects of breastfeeding for mothers: A critical review. *Nutrition Research Review, 10,* 35–56.

Innis, S.M. (1991). Essential fatty acids in growth and development. *Progress in Lipid Research, 30,* 39–103.

Innis, S.M., Akrabawi, S.S., Diersen-Schade, D.A., Dobson, M.V., & Guy, D.G. (1997). Visual acuity and blood lipids in term infants fed human milk or formulae. *Lipids, 32,* 63–72.

Jensen, R.G. (1999). Lipids in human milk. *Lipids, 34,* 1243–1271.

Lifshitz, C.H. (1988). Carbohydrate needs in preterm and term newborn infants. In M. Dobson, D. Guy, R.C. Tsang, & B. Nichols (Eds.), *Nutrition during infancy* (pp. 122–132). Philadelphia: Hanley & Belfus.

Lissauer, T., & Fanaroff, A. (Eds.). (2006). *Growth and nutrition in neonatalogy at a glance* (pp. 76–77). Oxford, United Kingdom: Blackwell.

Mertz, W. (1985). Metabolism and metabolic effects of trace elements. In R.J. Chandra (Ed.), *Trace elements in nutrition of children* (pp. 1–13). New York: Raven.

Moya, F.R. (1993). Nutritional requirements of the term newborn. In R.M. Suskind (Ed.), *Textbook of pediatric nutrition* (2nd ed., pp. 9–22). New York: Raven.

Orzalesi, M. (1987). Vitamins and the premature. *Biology of the Neonate, 52*(1), 97–112.

Picciano, M.F. (2001a). Nutrient composition of human milk. *Pediatric Clinics of North America, 48*, 53–67.

Picciano, M.F. (2001b). Representative values for constituents of human milk. *Pediatric Clinics of North America, 48*, 263–264.

Raiha, N.C.R. (1989). Milk protein quantity and quality and protein requirements during development. *Advances in Pediatrics, 36*, 347–368.

Rogan, W.J., & Gladen, B.C. (1993). Breast-feeding and cognitive development. *Early Human Development, 31*, 181–193.

Romero, R., & Kleinman, R.E. (1993). Feeding the very low-birthweight infant. *Pediatrics in Review, 14*(4), 123–132.

Ryan, A.S., Montalto, M.B., & Groh-Wargo, S., Mionouni, F., Sentipaul-Walerius, J., & Doyle, J. (1999). Effect of DHA-containing formula on growth of preterm infants to 59 weeks postmenstrual age. *American Journal of Human Biology, 11*, 457–487.

Wright, A.L. (2001). The rise of breastfeeding in the United States. *Pediatric Clinics of North America, 48*, 1–12.

CHAPTER 11

Physical Development and Impairment

Angel Rios and David A. Clark

At the conclusion of this chapter, the reader will

- *Understand the importance of a detailed prenatal history in assisting with the management of fetal abnormalities*

- *Understand the factors involved with fetal development*

- *Understand the fetal tests available in diagnosing fetal abnormalities*

- *Understand the approaches to evaluating the newborn with congenital abnormalities*

Newborn medicine has changed dramatically since the early 1990s. Approximately 3% of newborns are born with genetic problems. These genetic anomalies range from conditions that are benign, such as a cleft lip, in which the prognosis for the newborn infant is excellent, to life-threatening disorders, such as trisomy 13. Some of the advances that have changed the face of newborn medicine include fetal blood sampling that can be performed as early as 18 weeks of gestation. Fetal blood sampling can be used to detect fetal karyotype (appearance and characteristics of chromosome size, number, and form), hematological disorders, and congenital infections. Abnormalities can be detected by cytogenetics studies, which can be performed in two ways: 1) by obtaining amniotic fluid (amniocentesis) or 2) by performing chorionic villous sampling (CVS). The major difference between the two methods is the timing of when these tests can be performed. Amniocentesis can be performed as early as 17 weeks of gestation compared to 9 weeks for CVS tests. (These tests are described in more detail later in this text.) Maternal blood testing also can

be used as a helpful screening test. It is important to note, however, that a screening test does not make a diagnosis; rather, it is used to identify the need for further testing. One such maternal blood test is the triple screen that consists of alpha-fetoprotein, estriol, and human chorionic gonadotropin (hCG). Down syndrome is highly suggestive if the alpha-fetoprotein is low, hCG is high, and estriol is low. Many birth defects are now detected by fetal imaging.

Fetal imaging can be performed in two ways. The first involves using ultrasound and the second utilizes magnetic resonance imaging (MRI). Both techniques can be used to detect a variety of fetal malformations, such as congenital heart disease, central nervous system disorders, and malformations of organs and extremities. With the advent of these medical advances in newborn medicine, parents can be counseled before delivery, and the appropriate steps in managing these problems can be initiated (e.g., referral to a tertiary care center or early termination in the case of lethal disorders). An expecting mother should give birth in a center that is prepared to evaluate and treat her newborn. With early detection of these abnormalities, parents can be directed to appropriate treatment centers, which will be instrumental in determining the route and timing of delivery. The following are some high-risk pregnancy issues that require further testing (Milunsky, 2004).

- Maternal age of 35 years and older

- Fetal abnormality in a previous pregnancy

- Family history of genetic disease

- Co-existing maternal disease liable to affect the fetus

- Women using certain medications (e.g., isotretinoin)

- Exposure to infection

- Complication during pregnancy

- Infertility problems and recurrent losses

A detailed, comprehensive family history can uncover important clues to certain genetic disorders. Prenatal, family, and birth histories should be included when reviewing for genetic disorders. Each of these is discussed in the following sections.

Prenatal History

Inquiring about the amount of amniotic fluid can assist in the diagnosis of certain fetal problems. Adequate amounts of amniotic fluid are critical to normal growth and development. Insufficient fluid is seen in disorders involving the renal system, whereas excessive fluid typically is seen with disorders of the gastrointestinal tract or neurological disorders that impair fetal swallowing.

Maternal exposure to illicit drugs or prescription drugs, such as medications for seizure disorders, can result in specific patterns of malformations (e.g., valproic acid and fetal hydantoin syndrome). Maternal alcohol abuse can result in fetal alcohol syndrome. Figure 11.1 shows a newborn infant with fetal alcohol syndrome, in which one can see the short nose, smooth philtrum, and thin upper lip characteristic of this syndrome.

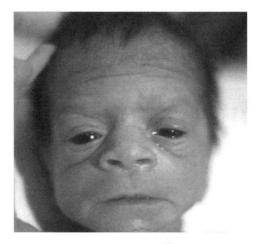

Figure 11.1. Fetal alcohol syndrome facies in premature neonate. Long, flat philtrum; thin upper lip; short palpebral fissures. (From Clark, D.A., private collection; reprinted by permission.)

Underlying medical disorders during pregnancy can result in a variety of disorders in the newborn. For example, mothers who develop HELLP (hemolysis, elevated liver enzymes, low platelets) syndrome and acute fatty liver disease during pregnancy have an increased risk of having an infant with fatty acid oxidation disorders. Another example is mothers with lupus erythmatosis who can have an infant with fetal cardiac rhythm disorders. When affected, these infants develop a slow heart rate (heart block); Figure 11.2a illustrates a normal EKG, whereas Figure 11.2b shows an EKG indicating heart block.

Previous issues with other pregnancies also may result in problems. For example, a mother who develops diabetes during pregnancy (i.e., gestational diabetes) can give birth to a very large infant (i.e., macrosomic), which can lead to a very difficult and traumatic delivery through the birth canal.

Finally, abnormalities of the placenta or uterus can compromise the fetus. Decreases in placental blood flow will decrease nutrient delivery to the fetus and thereby hamper fetal growth. Structural abnormalities of the uterus include a bicornuate uterus, which is a uterine space that is divided into two cavities and increases the incidence of preterm birth.

a

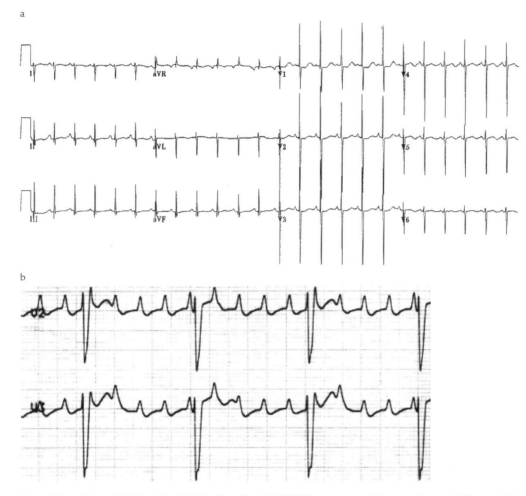

b

Figure 11.2. a) Normal EKG in a 1-day-old infant (From Tipple, M. [1999]. Interpretation of electrocardiograms in infants and children: Images. *Pediatric Cardiology, 1,* 2.) and b) an EKG of a newborn with heart block revealing a ventricular rate of 43 bpm, a wide QRS complex, and an atrial rate of 170 bpm (From Vesel, S., Zavrsnik, T., & Podnar, T. [2003]. *Ultrasound in Obstetrics and Gynecology, 21,* 190.). (*Key:* EKG = electrocardiogram; bpm = beats per minute.)

Family History

Genetic disorders can be passed along to different family members in various ways. Depending on the specific disorder, the pattern of inheritance can vary dramatically. For example, Waardenberg syndrome is an autosomal dominant disorder that carries the risk of transferring the mutant gene to 50% of offspring. In addition, there are autosomal recessive disorders, such as Hurler syndrome, in which there is a 25% risk of transferring the mutant gene to an offspring. There is a great difference in inheritance patterns, and they depend on the underlying disorder.

A prenatal history revealing repeated early miscarriages could be an important clue that one of the parents may have a balanced translocation. With a balanced translocation, chromosomal materials of one of the parents have been rearranged in such a way that important bits of one chromosome are lost and are then attached to another chromosome so that important chromosomal material is still within the cell. People who carry such a balanced rearrangement of their chromosomes usually are not affected. This condition only becomes an issue when there is a net gain or loss of chromosomal material during meiosis. This unbalanced distribution of chromosomal material can disrupt an important gene and its expression. Thus, in this situation, individuals have children who can inherit an unbalanced form of the rearrangement. For instance, if one of the parents carries a balanced translocation, it is possible for the child to inherit a rearrangement of the chromosomes where there can be an extra bit of chromosome material or a bit missing. In either case, there would be an unbalanced translocation, and, unfortunately, it can cause serious mental and physical disabilities, frequently resulting in repeated miscarriage.

Consanguinity between parents (i.e., parents descended from the same ancestors or blood origin) has been linked to various disorders. Certain cultures have a high consanguinity rate. For example, within the Saudi Arabian culture, rates of consanguinity are in excess of 50%, which results in a high incidence of autosomal recessive disorders. In this scenario, congenital disorders can be screened for early in pregnancy. One commonly discovered neurological problem found in consanguineous parents is lissencephaly (an abnormally smooth brain). When an unusual disorder is discovered, a carefully obtained family history is warranted.

Certain ethnic populations have increased frequencies of particular diseases. For example, among the Ashkenazi Jewish population, there is a high rate of Tay-Sachs and Canavan disease, which are lethal, progressive central nervous system disorders. They also exhibit high rates of familial dysautonomia, which presents with an abnormal suck, temperature insensitivity, and labile blood pressure.

Birth History

The size of the baby at birth can be very helpful in directing the health care professional in making a diagnosis. If the infant was born small for gestational age, there is a likelihood of the presence of a chromosomal abnormality, such as trisomy 13, or a possibility that the mother may have a chronic underlying disorder, such as hypertension, which can limit the blood flow through the placenta to the fetus. Commonly, maternal diabetes results in infants that are large for gestational age. Large for gestational age newborn in-

fants are also known to have genetic disorders such as Beckwith-Weidemann syndrome.

Obtaining a detailed history is critical in guiding the health care provider toward an accurate diagnosis. Ultimately, this will help in counseling and possibly determining recurrent risks. Thus, the type of delivery (i.e., vaginal or cesarean section) and the presenting reason for a cesarean section is important to know, as well as the length of gestation and reason for a premature delivery.

Structural Defects

Structural defects can be categorized as four types, including malformations, deformations, disruption, and dysplasia (Nylan, 1990).

Malformations

Malformation involves a defect in the formation of the structure of an organ. A clear example is myelomeningocele (failure of the neural tube to close during fetal development), which is shown in Figure 11.3.

Deformations

A deformation is seen when parts of the body are subjected to unusual mechanical forces. Initially, there is normal development of a fetal structure, but at some point it is subjected to unusual extrinsic forces. A baby born with club feet is a good example (see Figure 11.4).

A condition in which the mother has decreased amounts of amniotic fluid results in the uterus compressing the fetus. In Potter's se-

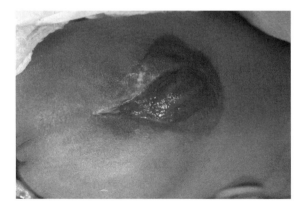

Figure 11.3.   Example of myelomeningocele. (From Clark, D.A., private collection; reprinted by permission.)

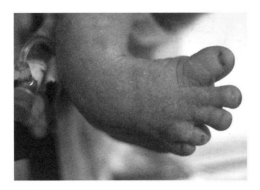

Figure 11.4. Example of club foot. (From Clark, D.A., private collection; reprinted by permission.)

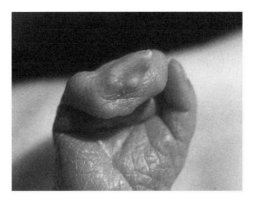

Figure 11.6. Fingers that have been amputated as a result of amnion strands disrupting the growth of fetal fingers. (From Clark, D.A., private collection; reprinted by permission.)

quence, there is an absence of kidneys (renal agenesis) resulting in a lack of amniotic fluid. This lack of amniotic fluid presents with a very characteristic facies at birth. Figure 11.5 shows a prominent skin fold below the lower eyelid, low-set ears, flattened nose, and a small recessed lower jaw. There also is an abnormal positioning of the fingers and flattening of the hands.

Disruption

Disruption, a structural anomaly that can involve an organ, part of an organ, or a larger region of the body, results from either extrinsic forces as seen with amniotic band disruption or intrinsic interferences with an originally normal developmental process. Figure 11.6 reveals fingers that have been amputated as a result of amnion strands disrupting the growth of the fetal fingers.

Dysplasia

Dysplasia involves a lack of normal cellular organization into tissue. An example of this condition is neurocutaneous melanosis and bathing trunk nevi (see Figure 11.7).

Physical Examination

The physical examination involves evaluating the infant's general appearance, as well as the head and face in particular. The following subsections provide further information guiding the health care professional's assessment.

General Appearance

General appearance should be the first assessment of the newborn infant. The health care professional observes the infant's general demeanor.

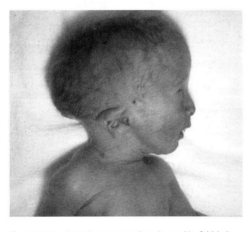

Figure 11.5. Potter's sequence: Prominent skin fold below the lower eyelid, low-set ears, flattened nose, and recessed jaw as a result of lack of amniotic fluid. (From Clark, D.A., private collection; reprinted by permission.)

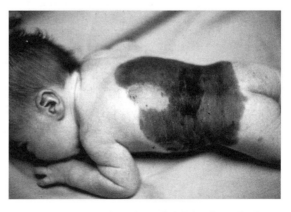

Figure 11.7. Bathing trunk nevi. (From Clark, D.A., private collection; reprinted by permission.)

Is the infant lying still with little spontaneous activity or is the infant crying inconsolably from pain? Regarding the baby's tone, are the extremities flexed or are they dangling by the infant's side? It is important to measure the baby's length, weight, and head circumference. These data are then transferred to standardized growth charts so that the physician can determine whether the infant is large, small, or appropriate for gestational age. There are the standardized growth curves for boys and girls from birth to 36 months of age. Below are growth curves for length and weight in girls (see Figure 11.8) and boys (see Figure 11.9) from birth to 36 months (Nylan, 1990).

Figure 11.10 shows two infants born at term. The newborn on the right is excessively large for

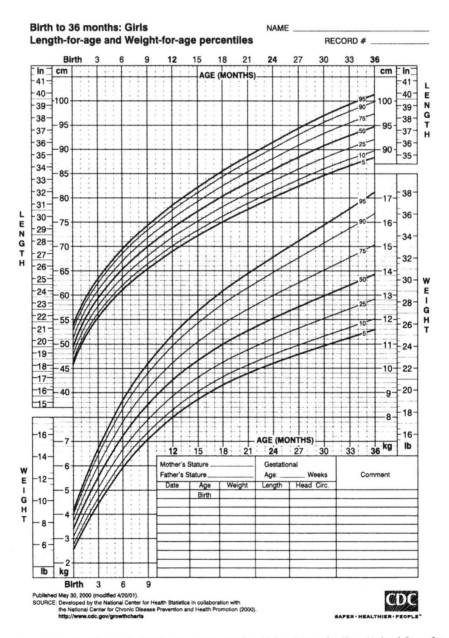

Figure 11.8.   Growth curves for length and weight in girls from birth to 36 months. (From National Center for Health Statistics. [2000]. *2000 CDC growth charts: United States*. Retrieved March 7, 2008, from http://www.cdc.gov/ growthcharts)

his gestational age, while the newborn on the left is small for gestational age as a result of maternal hypertension.

Important questions about the general appearance of the infant include: Are the body proportions normal? Are extremities shortened, and,

if so, are they uniformly shortened? If not, what parts of the extremity are shortened? There are normal neonatal standards that may be helpful in making all of these determinations. In addition, the physician needs to observe whether the baby is active or lying flaccidly in the frog-leg po-

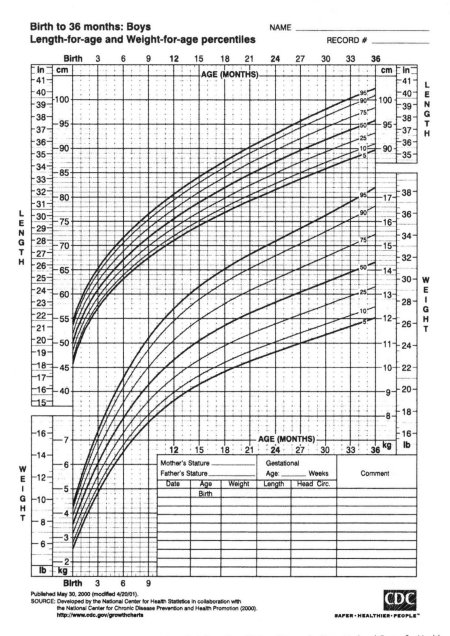

Figure 11.9.   Growth curves for length and weight in boys from birth to 36 months (From National Center for Health Statistics. [2000]. *2000 CDC growth charts: United States.* Retrieved March 7, 2008, from http://www.cdc.gov/growth charts)

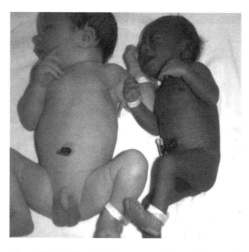

Figure 11.10. Two infants born at term. The newborn on the left is excessively large for gestational age, and the newborn on the right is small for gestational age, both as a result of maternal hypertension. (From Clark, D.A., private collection; reprinted by permission.)

sition. Also, does the child hold his mouth open with a fish mouth appearance? The physician also needs to bear in mind that neuromuscular disorders are associated with these physical findings. In Figure 11.11 there is excessive head lag when the newborn is pulled up indicating diminished muscle tone.

The Head and Face

At birth, it is important to examine the head for shape, size, defects, and malproportions. The newborn infant's skull is made up of numerous bones that have not fused; the spaces between these unfused bones are called sutures. As a re-

sult, the newborn's skull is very pliable and contributes to a considerable degree of molding. Most normal term infants have a narrowed biparietal diameter as a result of intrauterine molding during the delivery process. Figure 11.12 shows how shapes can vary depending on the external pressure applied to the skull.

Molding in the term infant is temporary and resolves over several weeks. Sutures subsequently allow for expansion to accommodate the rapid brain growth in the first year of life. There are a number of syndromes that have a characteristic head shape. These abnormalities in head shape are caused by early closure (i.e., craniosynostosis) of the sutures. Figure 11.13 demonstrates the various characteristic skull shapes as a result of craniosynostosis. The characteristic head shape results from the particular suture that has fused (see Figure 11.14). Brain growth will be constricted because of this early closure, and surgery is indicated in these cases. Some skull abnormalities occur in the absence of craniosynostosis, such as in infants with trisomy 21 who characteristically have brachycephaly and a flat occiput, as well as infants with achondroplasia.

Certain skull abnormalities are genetically associated with craniosynostosis, such as Crouzon syndrome and Apert syndrome. The craniofacial abnormalities associated with Apert syndrome include a high, large forehead, wide-spaced eyes, and flat facies. In Crouzon syndrome (see Figure 11.15), the eyes are prominent as a result of shallow orbits and, like Apert syndrome, the eyes are also widely spaced.

The face is then examined for dysmorphic features. A systematic and orderly approach

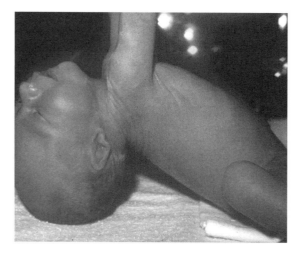

Figure 11.11. Infant with hypotonia head lag. (From Clark, D.A., private collection; reprinted by permission.)

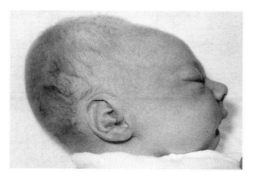

Figure 11.12. Infant with head molding. (From Clark, D.A., private collection; reprinted by permission.)

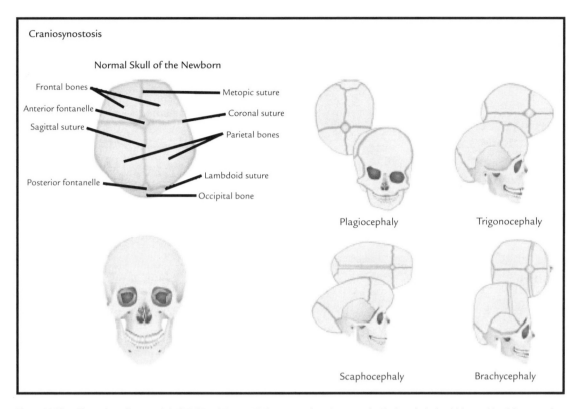

Figure 11.13. Illustration of a normal skull (left) and those with four types of craniosynostosis. Plagiocephaly, in which one side of the coronal suture closes prematurely, is the most common type. (Illustration by GGS Information Services; From Advameg. [2007]. Craniosynostosis. In *Encyclopedia of children's health: Infancy through adolescence.* Retrieved April 18, 2008, from http://www.healthofchildren.com/C/Craniosynostosis.html.)

should be developed in the evaluation of the newborn infant with dysmorphic features. In examining the face, four regions should be noted. These include the forehead, the mid-face, the malar, and the mandibular regions (see Figure 11.16).

The forehead should be examined for abnormalities, such as the sloping appearance seen with trisomy 13. The forehead can have a prominent appearance as seen in achondroplasia.

The mid-face region consists of the eyebrows to the upper vermilion border of the lip, and from the outer canthus of each eye to the commissures of the mouth. Figure 11.17 shows an infant whose mid-facial region failed to develop and resulted in shallow eye orbits and extrusion of the eyes bilaterally. The distance between an infant's eyes remains relatively constant. A very simple method of determining whether the eyes are closely spaced (hypotelorism) or widely spaced (hypertelorism) is to apply the rule of 1-1-1. The width of one eye should be

the distance between the two eyes. Hypotelorism can be observed in an infant with trisomy 13. Figure 11.18 shows an infant with hypertelorism. Cleft lip sequence and DiGeorge syndrome are disorders associated with hypertelorism. Normally one should be able to draw a straight line from one inner corner of the eye through the next inner corner of the eye. This line should intersect with the outer corner of the eye. Trisomy 21 is a genetic disorder associated with upward slanting of the eye. Treacher-Collins and Apert syndromes are examples of disorders with downward slanting eyes.

The malar region extends bilaterally from the ear to the mid-face. The normal ear should extend above a line drawn from the outer canthus of the eye. Figure 11.19 presents an infant with low-set ears that are posteriorly rotated. Examples of disorders associated with low-set ears include trisomy 18 and Treacher-Collins syndrome.

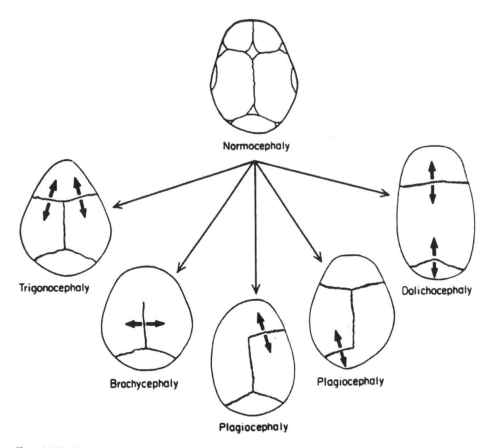

Figure 11.14.   Fused sutures and the resulting characteristic head shape. (From McMillan, J.A., DeAngelis, C.D., Feigin, R.D., & Warshaw, J.B. [1999]. *Oski's pediatrics* [3rd ed., p. 395]. Philadelphia: Lippincott William & Wilkins; Copyright © Wolters Kluwer Health; reprinted by permission.)

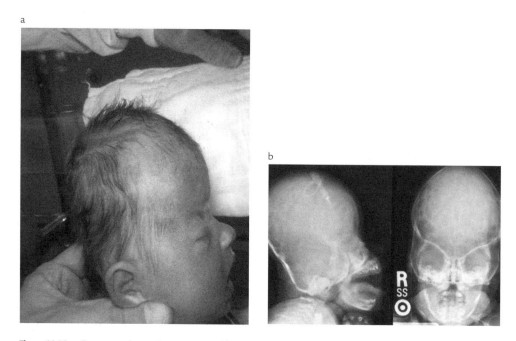

Figure 11.15.   Crouzon syndrome: a) appearance and b) x-ray. (From Clark, D.A., private collection; reprinted by permission.)

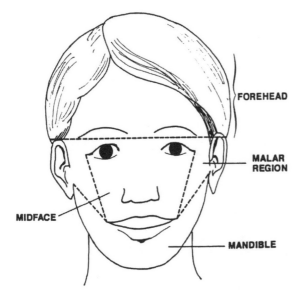

Figure 11.16. Four regions of the face. (From Marion, R.W., & Fleischman, A.R. [1991]. *The assessment and management of neonates with congenital anomalies: Reproductive births and prenatal diagnosis* [p. 346]. Stamford, CT: Appleton and Lang.)

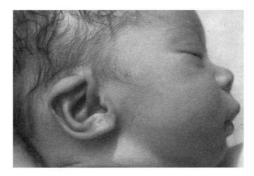

Figure 11.19. Infant with low-set ears. (From Clark, D.A., private collection; reprinted by permission.)

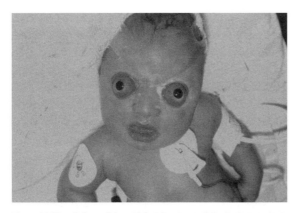

Figure 11.17. Failure of the mid-facial region to fully develop results in shallow orbits and extrusion of the eyes bilaterally. (From Clark, D.A., private collection; reprinted by permission.)

The mandibular region is comprised of the area that extends below from the lower parts of the ears and the commissures of the mouth. Normally, the jaw of the newborn is slightly retruded when viewed in profile.

The classic example of retrognathia (i.e., posteriorly displaced jaw) is the Pierre Robin syndrome, as seen in Figure 11.20. This disorder may present with significant airway obstruction because the tongue is displaced backward as a result of the retruded jaw.

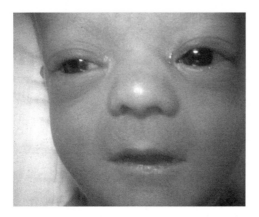

Figure 11.18. Infant with hypertelorism. (From Clark, D.A., private collection; reprinted by permission.)

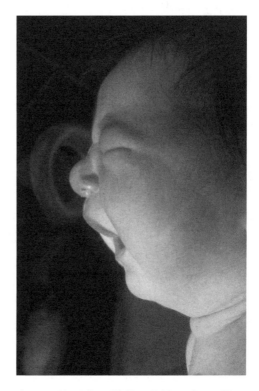

Figure 11.20. Infant with Pierre Robin syndrome. (From Clark, D.A., private collection; reprinted by permission.)

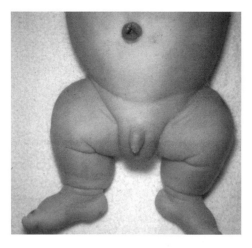

Figure 11.21.   Infant with shortened limbs (achondroplasia). (From Clark, D.A., private collection; reprinted by permission.)

The Extremities

The extremities of a newborn should also be examined for any deformities. The spectrum of deformities in the extremities can vary widely from absence of an extremity to shortened extremities to contractures. Absence of an extremity can be seen in Holt-Oram syndrome, TAR syndrome, and amniotic band sequence.

Syndromes, such as achondroplasia and osteogenesis imperfecta, are associated with shortened limbs as shown in Figure 11.21. Finally, contractures can be seen in different clinical scenarios. Infants born to mothers who have inadequate amniotic fluid can have contractures as a result of external deforming forces acting on the extremities (i.e., from the mechanical pressure from the uterus and the lack of cushioning effects because of decreased amniotic fluid). They can also be seen in newborn infants born with severe neuromuscular disorders as a result of decreased movement.

Testing for Genetic Diseases

The following subsections describe the various tests available to help guide the health care professional in detecting genetic diseases.

Newborn Screening

The newborn screen that is obtained from the blood of newborn infants and transferred onto filter paper at nursery discharge or by the 3rd day of life has been an extremely valuable tool in detecting many different disorders. The first metabolic disorder detected by newborn screening was phenylketonuria (PKU), which is a biochemical disorder detected in infants after birth. PKU is the most common amino acid disorder. Immediate detection of this disorder is critical because it can be treated simply by making some dietary changes (instituting a low-phenylalanine diet), and can, therefore, prevent intellectual disabilities. Since the inception of screening for PKU, the number of disorders that have been added to the newborn screen has expanded tremendously over the years. Table 11.1 lists the disorders that can be identified with the newborn screen in New York state. It is important to keep in mind that the disorders that are tested in newborn screening do vary from state to state. New York state, for example, tests for more than 40 disorders (New York State Department of Health, Wadsworth Center, n.d.).

Another important disorder that can be identified by routine newborn screening is congenital hypothyroidism. The incidence is ap-

Table 11.1.   Some of the disorders identified by the New York State newborn screening program

Arginemia
Biotinidase deficiency
Branch-chain ketonuria
Carnitine uptake defect
Citrullinemia
Congenital adrenal hyperplasia
Congenital hypothyroidism
Cystic fibrosis
Galactosemia
Glutaric academia type 1
Homocysteinuria
Human immunodeficiency virus (HIV) infection
Isolvalaric academia
Krabbe disease
Malonic academia
Phenylketonuria
Propionic academia
Sickle cell disease

Source: New York State Department of Health, Wadsworth Center. (n.d.).

proximately 1:3,000–1:4,000 infants. The major complication from untreated congenital hypothyroidism is growth retardation and delays in cognitive development, which ultimately result in mental deficiency. Early treatment with thyroid hormone will result in normal growth and mental development.

Molecular Cytogenetics

The tests described in this subsection are related in that the specimens obtained are sent to the laboratory for chromosomal testing. Amniocentesis is a medical procedure that doctors use to make prenatal diagnoses. An amniocentesis is performed by obtaining a small amount of amniotic fluid, which surrounds the developing fetus. The amniotic fluid is removed by inserting a needle, usually using ultrasound guidance, through the mother's uterus. The basic idea of the procedure is to isolate the fetal cells from the amniotic fluid. The next step is to culture the cells and then examine the chromosomes and/or DNA from these cells to rule out genetic abnormalities that could lead to birth defects. Amniocentesis usually is offered when there may be an increased risk for genetic abnormalities in the pregnancy, such as in mothers who are delivering a baby after the age of 35 years or when certain abnormalities are discovered during a routine ultrasound (e.g., duodenal atresia—a certain type of intestinal obstruction—is seen in an infant with trisomy 21). Amniocentesis is usually performed between 15 and 20 weeks' gestation.

Chorionic villous sampling (CVS) is another type of procedure doctors use in making a prenatal diagnosis to determine genetic abnormalities in the fetus. Unlike amniocentesis where fluid is removed, CVS involves obtaining a sample of the chorionic villous (placental tissue) by inserting a needle through the mother's abdomen, aspirating the tissue, and testing it. It is generally carried out only on pregnant women over the age of 35 years and those mothers who carry a high risk of genetic abnormalities. The advantage of CVS is that it can be carried out 10–12 weeks after the last menstrual period, earlier than amniocentesis (which is carried out at 15–20 weeks). However, this procedure is more risky than amniocentesis,

with a 1 in 100–200 risk that it will cause a miscarriage.

Percutaneous umbilical blood sampling (PUBS) is a diagnostic test that examines blood from the developing fetus to detect chromosomal abnormalities. PUBS is performed by inserting a thin needle, using ultrasound guidance, through the abdomen and uterine walls to the umbilical cord. The needle is inserted into the umbilical cord and a small sample of fetal blood is obtained. The sample is sent to the laboratory for analysis, and results are usually available within 72 hours. PUBS is done at 18 weeks or shortly thereafter. Usually it is performed when definitive diagnostic information cannot be obtained through amniocentesis, CVS, or ultrasound, or the results of these tests were inconclusive.

Fluorescent in situ hybridization (FISH) is a cytogenetic test that can be used to detect and localize the presence or absence of specific DNA sequence on individual chromosomes. The procedure uses fluorescent markers that will bind only to those parts of the chromosome, which will result in the diagnosis of the underlying disorder that is being considered (see Figure 11.22).

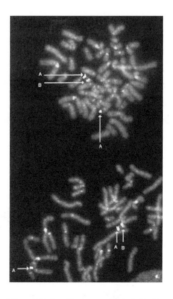

Figure 11.22.   Fluorescent in situ hybridization (FISH). (From Arn, P. [2000, March]. Genetics and the child with developmental delay. *Jacksonville Medicine.* Retrieved May 2, 2008, from http://www.dcmsonline.org/jax-medicine/2000journals/march2000/genetics.htm; reprinted by permission.)

The various probes that hybridize to a particular chromosome result in a unique colored banding pattern for each chromosome. Fluorescent microscopy can be used to determine where the fluorescent probe is bound to the chromosome. FISH is used to detect or confirm gene or chromosome abnormalities that are generally beyond the resolution of routine cytogenetics. Some disorders in which FISH is especially useful include Williams, Prader-Willi, DiGeorge, and velocardiofacial syndromes. DNA probes specific to regions of particular chromosomes are attached to fluorescent markers and hybridized with a chromosome spread. The picture shows a computer-generated false color image in which small variations in fluorescence wavelength among probes are enhanced as distinct primary colors. The combination of probes that hybridize to a particular chromosome produce a unique pattern for each chromosome.

Imaging Tests

Ultrasound (US) has several very important functions. First, it can be useful in estimating the gestational age of the fetus. Second, it can monitor the growth of the fetus. Finally, it can be used to diagnose fetal anomalies. Anomalies that can be detected by ultrasound include neurological problems, such as hydrocephalus (excess build-up of fluid in the brain), defects of the fetal abdominal wall (gastroschisis and omphalocele), cardiac defects (hypoplastic left heart and transposition of the great vessels), and neural tube de-

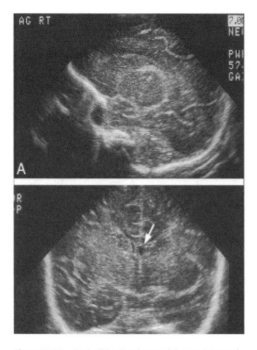

Figure 11.23. Sagittal (top) and coronal (bottom) views of a typical preterm brain. The corpus callosum is identified by the arrow. (Reproduced with permission from: William D. Rhine and Francis G. Blankenberg [Jan. 2001]. Cranial ultrasonography. *NeoReviews, 2*[1], 3–11, Copyright © 2001 by the AAP.)

fects (meningomyelocele). For example, Figure 11.23 reveals a normal ultrasound in a preterm newborn brain. Figure 11.24 shows that the ventricles of a preterm newborn brain are markedly enlarged as a result of a Grade 3 intraventricular hemorrhage.

Fetal magnetic resonance imaging (MRI) is a diagnostic imaging technique that provides high

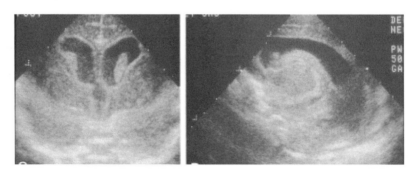

Figure 11.24. A posthemorrhagic hydrocephalus on the coronal (bottom) and sagittal (top) view. (Reproduced with permission from: William D. Rhine and Francis G. Blankenberg [Jan. 2001]. Cranial ultrasonography. *NeoReviews, 2*[1], 3–11, Copyright © 2001 by the AAP.)

quality, cross-sectional images of organs and structures within the body without x-rays or radiation. It is important to remember that ultrasound remains the imaging modality of choice for screening for fetal anomalies. US and MRI are complementary imaging techniques; for example, if a CNS anomaly is detected by ultrasound, the MRI can demonstrate additional information that cannot be obtained by US. The additional information that can be obtained from MRI image includes the chemical makeup of tissues and vascular malformations, as well as obtaining a very detailed picture of malformation as shown in Figure 11.25.

Unlike US and MRI, computer tomography (CT) uses x-rays to obtain its images. The image is constructed by a computer from a large number of pictures shot at different viewing angles, thus allowing for more precise location of abnormalities. CT is especially useful in evaluating newborn infants who experience a sudden acute

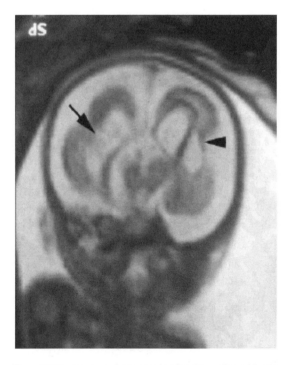

Figure 11.25. Fetal magnetic resonance imaging performed in the early second trimester showing encephalomalacia following twin demise. (Reproduced with permission from: Patrick D. Barnes [Jan. 2001]. Magnetic resonance imaging of the fetal and neonatal central nervous system. *NeoReviews, 2*[1], 12–21, Copyright © 2001 by the AAP.)

deterioration in their neurological status. This includes abnormalities such as intracranial hemorrhage, infarction, tumors, and vascular malformations.

Biochemical Testing

The principal maternal markers used for screening chromosomal abnormalities include maternal serum human gonadotropin (hCG), α-fetoprotein (AFP), and unconjugated estriol (uE_3). These markers are commonly referred to as the triple screen. An example of its benefit becomes evident when it is used for screening for Down syndrome. Typically the AFP and uE_3 is reduced while the hCG is elevated in Down syndrome. The triple screen can be used in combination with fetal ultrasound to increase the detection rate of chromosomal abnormalities.

Future Treatment

Tremendous medical advancements have been made since the 1990s, and there are many more on the horizon. For example, it may be possible in the future to replace a defective gene and totally eliminate the disease caused by that defective gene.

Gene Replacement

Due to the results of the human genome project in which the genetic origins of diseases were being deciphered, it has now become possible to identify individuals at risk for various diseases by analyzing their genetic makeup and incorporating advances in genetic technology. Along with the realization that human disease has its fundamental origins with abnormalities within each individual's genetic makeup has come the possibility of correcting many of these diseases by replacing the defective genes responsible for them. This development has been the center of a very hot and controversial topic.

Interventions

Once a fetal abnormality is diagnosed, the single most important intervention strategy is the provision of timely genetic counseling. The goal of genetic counseling is to educate the parents about the disorder and prepare them with the potential options that are available to them. Genetic counseling can only begin if and when a definitive diagnosis has been established. For example, the fetus may have a constellation of structural abnormalities that are all surgically correctable, such as umbilical hernia, polydactyly (extra digits), cleft lip and cleft palate, which are all very treatable structural abnormalities that should lead to a normal outcome. However, when these structural abnormalities are found in a fetus with trisomy 13, for example, the underlying chromosomal disorder makes this condition lethal, and surgical intervention is not warranted. Topics to be discussed with the parents are details about the fetal disorder, patterns of inheritance, appropriate referrals, and courses of action that will assist in family planning.

Three options can be offered to parents when a fetal abnormality is detected. They can continue with the pregnancy, attempt prenatal treatment if available, or, if dealing with a lethal disorder, terminate the pregnancy. At this point, it becomes exceedingly important to refer such parents to a tertiary care center. The tertiary care center then can organize the various specialists who can counsel the parents. These specialists can include perinatologists, neonatologists, surgeons, geneticists, radiologists, and cardiologists. These various specialists can inform the parents about a plan of management for the remainder of the pregnancy and for an appropriate mode of delivery, if applicable. The key is to communicate sympathetically with the parents and to offer the most comprehensive overview possible.

Conclusion

Medicine has evolved at an extremely rapid rate. Diseases that were in the past very difficult to diagnose prenatally are now identified before the delivery of the infant. In addition, there is now a better understanding of the pathophysiology involving environmental factors, drugs, and maternal diseases and their ultimate effect on the fetus.

As our knowledge of the human genome continues to expand, scientists are now developing tests and potential therapies for genetic disorders. Technological advances that include fetal imaging, molecular cytogenetic analysis, and maternal biochemical testing have revolutionized medicine by assisting health care providers in optimizing management of the fetus with a congenital abnormality. Inevitably, parents are overwhelmed with the news of a baby with a congenital abnormality; however, as result of new medical advancements, families are now informed well in advance about disease occurrence and long-term prognoses. It is now possible to intervene and develop a treatment plan before the newborn infant is born, and appropriate management can be undertaken before delivery of the baby.

REFERENCES

Advameg. (2007). Craniosynostosis. In *Encyclopedia of children's health: Infancy through adolescence.* Retrieved April 18, 2008, from http://www.healthofchildren.com/C/Craniosynostosis.html

Arn, P. (2000, March). Genetics and the child with developmental delay. *Jacksonville Medicine.* Retrieved May 2, 2008, from http://www.dcmsonline.org/jax-medicine/2000journals/march2000/genetics.htm

Barnes, P. (2001). Magnetic resonance imaging of the fetal and neonatal central nervous system. *NeoReviews, 2*(1), 12–21.

Carr, S.M. (2005). *All text material.* Hylton Park, Wessington, Sunderland, UK: Image © Applied Imaging.

Marion, R.W., & Fleischman, A.R. (1991). *The assessment and management of neonates with congenital anomalies: Reproductive births and prenatal diagnosis* (pp. 341–357). Stamford, CT: Appleton and Lang.

McMillan, J.A., DeAngelis, C.D., Feigin, R.D., & Warshaw, J.B. (1999). *Oski's Pediatrics* (3rd ed.). Philadelphia: Lippincott Williams & Wilkins.

Milunsky, A. (2004). *Genetic disorders and the fetus: Diagnosis, prevention, and treatment* (5th ed., pp. 22–33). Baltimore: The Johns Hopkins University Press.

National Center for Health Statistics. (2000). *2000 CDC growth charts: United States.* Retrieved March 7, 2008, from http://www.cdc.gov/growthcharts

New York State Department of Health, Wadsworth Center. (n.d.). Newborn screening program. Retrieved April 21, 2008, from http://www.wadsworth.org/newborn

Nylan, W.L. (1990). Structural abnormalities: A systematic approach to diagnosis. *Clinical Symposia Ciba-Geigy, 42*(2), 1–32.

Rhine, W.D., & Blankenberg, F.G. (2001). Cranial ultrasonography. *NeoReviews, 2*(1), 3–11.

Tipple, M. (1999). Interpretation of electrocardiograms in infants and children: Images. *Paediatric Cardiology, 1*, 3–13.

Vesel, S., Zavrsnik, T., & Podnar, T. (2003). *Ultrasound in Obstetrics and Gynecology, 21*, 189–191.

CHAPTER 12

Infection and Immunity

Michelle L. Eastman and David A. Clark

At the conclusion of this chapter, the reader will

- *Identify and describe the routes of infection transmission from mother to baby*

- *Understand the specific qualities of the newborn immune system*

- *Understand alterations in the maternal immune system during pregnancy*

- *Understand how specific infectious agents affect the newborn*

- *Understand antenatal initiatives and neonatal immunizations*

Infections may affect newborn development during pregnancy and after birth by disrupting the formation of tissues and organs (Remington & Klein, 2001). Bacteria, viruses, or protozoa may cause the infection. Newborns may acquire infection by three different routes: intrauterine, intrapartum, and postpartum (Romero, Athayde, Maymon, Pacora, & Bahado-Singh, 1999). A congenital infection may be acquired by an intrauterine (before the baby is born) or intrapartum (during the birth process) route (Sweet & Gibbs, 2002).

Any infection that is transmitted to the neonate after birth is acquired by a postpartum route of transmission. The route of acquisition as well as the timing of infection will affect fetal and perinatal outcomes (Newell & McIntyre, 2000).

Neonatal infection (sepsis) is delineated as early versus late onset. An early onset sepsis occurs within the first 6 days of life and most often is transmitted via an intrauterine or intrapartum route of transmission. Early onset infection of the neonate will present 85% of the time within the first 24 hours of life (Anderson-Berry, Bellig, & Ohning, 2006). Late onset neonatal infection occurs within 7–90 days of life and most often is

transmitted via a postpartum route of transmission. The incidence of sepsis is higher in premature infants versus full-term infants. Several risk factors for sepsis are identified in Table 12.1.

In this chapter, we consider alterations in the maternal immune system during pregnancy and qualities of the newborn immune system that allow sepsis to occur, as well as how specific infectious agents affect the newborn.

Diagnostic Features

The symptoms and signs of infection are diverse, and many can resemble or be disguised by other illnesses of the newborn. Although respiratory distress may be caused by infection, it more frequently results from retained lung fluid or a deficiency of surfactant in premature infants. In newborns, irritability may arise from an inflammation of the membranes surrounding the brain (meningitis), but this condition is seen more often as a result of birth asphyxia, drug withdrawal, or hemorrhage into the central nervous system. Jaundice may result from the accelerated breakdown of red blood cells with infection; it also can be due to bruising during delivery and

Table 12.1.   Perinatal infections (sepsis): Modes of transmission

Infectious agent	Transplacental	Intrapartum	Postpartum	Breast milk
Viruses				
Rubella	+	+	+	+
Cytomegalovirus	+	+	+	+
Herpes I and II	rare	+	+	–
Varicella	+	+	+	+
Enterovirus	+	+	+	+
Hepatitis B and C	+	+	–	+
Spirochete				
Syphilis (*Treponema*)	+	+	–	–
Parasites				
Toxoplasmosis	+	–	–	–
Malaria	+	–	–	–
Bacteria				
Gonorrhea	–	+	–	–
Group B *Streptococccus*	–	+	+	–

prematurity. Hypoglycemia, although evident with infection, more often is manifested in babies born preterm, with growth retardation, or large for gestational age as a result of maternal diabetes. These symptoms and signs may indicate possible sepsis within the differential diagnosis for the infant. The mortality rate for *untreated*

Table 12.2.   Symptoms and signs of neonatal infections (sepsis)

General and/or metabolic
    Temperature instability
    Hypothermia, fever (unusual)
    Jaundice
    Acidosis
    Hypoglycemia

Central nervous system
    Apnea
    Hypotonia
    Lethargy
    Poor suck
    Seizures

Cardiopulmonary
    Respiratory distress (tachypnea)
    Hypotension
    Tachycardia and/or bradycardia

Laboratory
    Abnormal blood cell counts
    Anemia—red blood cell destruction
    Leukopenia or leucocytosis—white blood cell destruction
    Thrombocytopenia

Skin
    Petechiae
    Rash
    Pustules

neonatal sepsis may be as high as 50% (Anderson-Berry et al., 2006).

If such complex and confusing patterns seem to predominate, what characteristics do serve as indicators? A few symptoms and signs are relatively useful in indicating the presence of neonatal infection (Siegel & McCracken, 1981) (see Table 12.2). These factors include poor temperature control and the early onset of apnea. Older children and adults generally respond to infection with a fever, and fever is very common among newborns. Premature infants, however, usually require intensive temperature support. Thus, if the effects of overheating and maternal medication can be ruled out as a cause of apnea in the first several days of life, the cause commonly is associated with infection (Mustafa & McCracken, 1992).

Immunity and Decreased Resistance to Infection

Prior to birth, the fetus has a limited capacity to ward off infection. For most babies, the intrauterine environment is sterile. Once delivered, however, newborns are exposed to numerous viruses and bacteria with which they must cope. Moreover, the functions of the white blood cells and circulating blood proteins are critical to the ability of the newborn to respond successfully to infection (Regelman, Hill, Cates, & Quie, 1992).

Basically, the white blood cells are divided into two subgroups: agranulocytes (without granules) and granulocytes (granules are located outside the cell nucleus). Agranulocytes include lymphocytes (i.e., small white blood cells that produce antibodies or proteins directed against infectious agents). Another primary agranulocyte is the monocyte, which enhances antibody production and is the prominent white blood cell involved in clearing the debris of infection. Granulocytes (i.e., neutrophils) contain powerful enzymes that primarily fight bacterial infection (Miller & Stiehm, 1979). For bacterial infection to be managed effectively, the neutrophil must be attracted to the site of the infection, must be capable of ingesting the bacteria, and then must be able to destroy the bacteria. In the newborn, while the process of killing bacteria is similar to that in older children and adults, the mobilization of neutrophils to the site of an infection and subsequent ingestion of bacteria is somewhat restricted (Remington & Klein, 2001).

Circulating blood proteins, primarily the antibodies (immunoglobulins), are a passive form of immunity that help in the process of neutralizing and eliminating bacteria and viruses. Immunoglobulin G (IgG) is a protein that is transferred from the mother across the placenta to the fetus, mostly during the last 10 weeks of gestation (Newell & McIntyre, 2000). If the mother has been exposed to an infection and has responded appropriately, some protection can be conveyed to the baby via the transfer of IgG. This protection helps to explain the rarity of chickenpox, mumps, measles, and rheumatic fever in newborns. However, if after birth the baby is exposed to an organism that the mother has never coped with effectively, the infant is more likely to contract that disease (Remington & Klein, 2001). The few infants who become infected with agents their mothers have acquired usually have much milder illnesses. However, the more premature an infant is, the higher the risk for infection or the more severe the illness as a result of lower levels of IgG (Anderson-Berry et al., 2006).

A second immunoglobulin, IgM, is a protein much larger than IgG and is the first antibody produced by the body in response to infection. IgM does not cross the placenta in either direction; thus, maternal IgM is distinct from the baby's IgM (Newell & McIntyre, 2000). Therefore, an elevated IgM level in the blood of a newborn suggests that the baby has been exposed to an infectious agent and is responding (Bellanti & Boner, 1981). IgM levels rise rapidly in the first month of age despite initial gestational age (Remington & Klein, 2001).

A supplementary complex of proteins found in the blood, the complement system, aids the function of white blood cells in recognizing infection and of the immunoglobulins in fighting it. Unfortunately, this mechanism also is deficient, especially in the premature infant (Remington & Klein, 2001).

In addition to these complications, babies are more prone to infection after birth because of major differences in their anatomy compared with that of adults. In particular, their skin is thinner and, therefore, cutaneous infections are more common. Preterm infants frequently are unable to feed, and when a tube is placed into the stomach to provide adequate nutrition, the limited antibacterial and antiviral capabilities of the tonsils and adenoids are bypassed. Many invasive procedures, such as placement of a tube down the trachea for respiratory support and insertion of a catheter into a blood vessel, increase the risk of infection. One of the more common sites of infection, even in healthy full-term babies, is the navel, after the dried umbilical cord is shed.

Intrauterine (Transplacental) Infections

An intrauterine infection may be acquired by the baby prior to birth if the mother has a systemic infection that infects the placenta (chorioamnionitis) or travels via the placenta (transplacental) to the baby (American Academy of Pediatrics [AAP] and the American College of Obstetricians and Gynecologists [ACOG], 2000; Newell & McIntyre, 2000). In addition, infected maternal cervical secretions may transmit an infection to the baby prior to birth by infecting the amniotic fluid (ascending infection) (Newell & McIntyre,

2000). As the baby passes through the vagina during birth, infected maternal cervical secretions, blood, and feces may cause the baby to acquire an intrapartum infection. Any breaks in skin integrity of the infant due to birth trauma or invasive procedures (e.g., a scalp electrode) will increase the chance of infection transmission to the baby (Newell & McIntyre, 2000).

The most common diseases transmitted from mother to baby transplacentally have been designated as TORCH infections (Nahmias, 1974). This acronym represents the diseases toxoplasmosis (TO), rubella (R), cytomegalovirus (C), and herpes (H). Frequently, an "S" for syphilis is added at the beginning to produce STORCH. These organisms do not produce a homogeneous group of illnesses; they include agents with very different characteristics: three viruses (rubella, cytomegalovirus, and herpes); a parasitic infection (toxoplasmosis); and a parabacterial infection (syphilis) (Cowles & Gonik, 1992; Overall, 1992).

The list of organisms proven to cause congenital infections has grown rapidly so that the acronym TORCH is no longer inclusive. Two of the more pertinent, transplacental viral infections are human immunodeficiency virus (HIV) and hepatitis B virus (HBV).

Rubella

Rubella (also known as German measles) is the prototype of viral infections. Much of the information on this disease was obtained in the 1960s (Centers for Disease Control and Prevention [CDC], 2001). The illness may be mild in the mother, and only maternal rubella with intrauterine infection in the first 4 months of gestation is likely to produce any abnormal physical finding or developmental disability. In the most severe situation, it is important to realize that infection prior to 4 months of gestation is well established before the baby's own body may be involved. Some of these effects may be transient; others may be long lasting (Overall, 1992).

Historically, the four most common and persistent problems of newborns with rubella have been 1) hearing loss (in approximately 87%) (Miller, Rabinowitz, Frost, & Seager, 1969); 2) vi-

sual problems, primarily cataracts and glaucoma (in approximately 34%); 3) heart disease (in approximately 46%) (Cooper, 1985; Preblud & Alford, 1990); and 4) intellectual disabilities (in approximately 40%). Four decades ago, the national cost of the care of these infants was excessively high as a result of the combination of physical and developmental problems (Hardy, 1973). A concerted effort in the late 1960s culminated in a rubella vaccine that was licensed in 1970. Within several years of that accomplishment, the number of identifiable cases of both rubella and congenital rubella decreased by 80%.

The classic signs of a child with congenital rubella included low birth weight, bruising, a large liver and spleen, abnormalities of bone development, meningitis, hearing loss, cataracts, abnormal retinal development, various forms of cardiac disease, intellectual disabilities, behavioral and language disorders, undescended testes, hernias, and microcephaly. Less commonly seen were jaundice, glaucoma, myopia, hepatitis, generalized enlargement of the lymph nodes, pneumonia, diabetes, thyroid dysfunction, seizures, and degenerative brain disease. Infected infants could excrete the virus for prolonged periods of time, with as many as 10% still actively shedding the organism in urine up to 1 year of age. These newborns used to be a potential source of infection to women of childbearing age (Cherry, 1990). The immunization of children against rubella has virtually eradicated fetal rubella infection (Hinman, 1985).

Cytomegalovirus

Cytomegalovirus (CMV) infection is the most common intrauterine infection in the United States and United Kingdom (Lissauer & Fanaroff, 2006). The infection rate is 0.5–1 per 1,000 live births, and it is even higher for developing countries (Lissauer & Fanaroff, 2006). CMV is a herpes virus and, like all other members of the group, the infection, once acquired, remains throughout life (see Figure 12.1). The individual may have no obvious symptoms, but in periods of decreased resistance, the organisms may be reactivated. CMV may be transmitted to the baby from the mother by an intrauterine, intrapartum, or postpartum

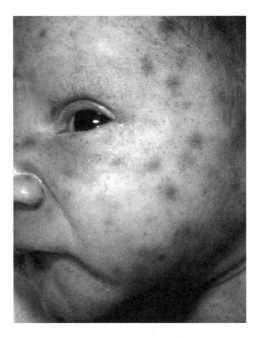

Figure 12.1. Infant with cytomegalovirus. (From Clark, D.A., private collection; reprinted by permission.)

route. The mother to infant transmission rate is 40% (Lissauer & Fanaroff, 2006). Postpartum route of transmission includes infected breast milk and blood transfusions (Lissauer & Fanaroff, 2006). Manifestations of the virus in the newborn are similar to those of rubella. Infection of the mother, however, is much more difficult to recognize clinically because she may evidence little more than flu-like symptoms. As few as 10% of infants manifest signs of congenital CMV at birth (American Academy of Pediatrics [AAP], 2006). Hearing loss and learning disability are manifestations of congenital CMV noted later on in infancy and childhood when the infant appears otherwise normal at birth (AAP, 2006). Those at greatest risk include individuals with a primary maternal infection and a fetus who acquires the infection during the first half of the pregnancy.

A specific treatment for CMV is not available; however, for those newborns with severe CMV infection, the antiviral drug ganciclovir will improve acute organ disease of the eye, liver, bone marrow, and lungs (Lissauer & Fanaroff, 2006). The long-term central nervous system benefit of ganciclovir treatment remains controversial (Lissauer & Fanaroff, 2006).

Toxoplasmosis

Toxoplasmosis differs from most of the other infections in that the *Toxoplasma* protozoan causing the disease is one of the few parasites that can be transmitted directly from the mother to the fetus (CDC, 2004). The mother usually is asymptomatic with this infection. Humans are aberrant hosts for this parasite, which primarily infects cats, but also may infect dogs. The small eggs produced by the parasite may be inhaled by the pregnant mother as she changes cat litter. Once in the human, the developing embryos complete their development within the intestinal tract and then seed to various organs throughout the body by means of the blood. Wherever a cyst forms, tissue disruption occurs (Feldman, 1968).

Mothers with infection in the first trimester of pregnancy tend to produce infants with severe congenital disease. Third trimester infections may be subclinical. Manifestations of the more severe conditions include microcephaly, deafness, retinitis, blindness, jaundice, seizures, large lymph nodes, pneumonia, and enlarged liver and spleen (Lee, 1988). Of greatest concern is the tendency of the parasite to travel to the baby's brain, with subsequent tissue disruption. The cysts may be seen by a simple x-ray of the skull because they commonly calcify. Subtle cerebral cysts may be found by computerized axial tomography (CAT) scanning. Antibiotics are available to help limit the extent of the disease, but areas of the brain or other tissue that have been affected usually do not recover adequately. The neurodevelopmental outcome of babies who have toxoplasmosis is variable depending on the distribution and number of parasites that infest the brain or other vital organs (Cowles & Gonik, 1992).

Syphilis

Neonatal syphilis is much less common than it was 30 years ago as a consequence of the aggressive screening of mothers during pregnancy. The infectious agent, *Treponema,* is a worm-like microorganism that can invade and infect any organ of the body. The severity of the disease manifestation depends on tissue disruption and the host's response to the invasion of the organism (Taber & Huber, 1975). The typical presentations of congenital syphilis are a dry skin rash, bruising, large liver and spleen, hypotonia, jaundice, anemia, and a profuse rhinorrhea (Nabarro, 1954). The illnesses may show only subtle symptoms and thus go unrecognized. One of the more common characteristics of the disease is seen in babies of several months of age who have joint swelling or limited movement of the extremities. Child abuse frequently is suspected in these cases; however, x-rays do not reveal fractures. Rather, an elevation of the outermost layer (periosteum) of the long bones that results from infection by the organism is seen. Even with this relatively late presentation, if the disease is recognized and treated, long-term developmental disability may be minimal (Wendel, 1988).

Therapy for syphilis is comparatively simple. The disease is readily treated with penicillin or one of several other antibiotics. These medications must be given for a minimum of 10 days to ensure minimal risk of recurrence. If there is involvement of the central nervous system, however, the treatment must be more aggressive and prolonged. Once infection is recognized in the child, the mother also should be examined and treated, and her sexual partners should be serologically tested and treated.

Human Immunodeficiency Virus

HIV-1 is a member of the human retrovirus family and is the most common type of HIV seen in infants. It is an RNA virus that can attach to a receptor on the surface of a helper T cell lymphocyte. Once inside the helper lymphocyte, the virus can multiply rapidly and eliminate the lymphocyte's role in the immune system. T cells promote the manufacture of antibodies by other lymphocytes (Fauci, 1988). In their absence, the child becomes vulnerable to many different opportunistic infections.

Pregnancy does not appear to aggravate the severity of HIV infection in previously asymptomatic women, but HIV transmission from mother to infant can occur across the placenta at the time of delivery, via breast feeding, or from intimate contact with body secretions (Cowan, Hellman, & Chudwin, 1984; Gonik & Hammill, 1990). The incidence of HIV infection in women

in the childbearing age group is estimated at approximately 0.15%; however, this figure may be as high as 2% in some inner city populations (AAP & ACOG, 1999a). The typical profile of an infected pregnant mother is a low income, young woman in the inner city who abuses drugs intravenously or who has an intravenous drug abuser as a sexual partner. With the benefits of medication, the rate of transmission from mother to child in the United States is approximately 1%.

In neonates, the most common clinical features of HIV infection that have progressed to AIDS are failure to thrive, hepatomegaly, and disseminated pneumonia. Without treatment, the average onset of severe immunodeficiency occurs at 5–10 months of age. The incubation period seems to be much shorter in children than in adults, and the disease course is much more aggressive, probably because of the immature immune function in combination with a larger infective initial dose of virus (Rubinstein, 1986).

At birth, most affected infants appear healthy (Hanson & Shearer, 1992). A few investigators have reported hypertelorism, a flat nasal bridge, long palpebral fissures, and other facial features as suggestive of intrauterine HIV infection. Unfortunately, many of these characteristics overlap with clinical features of babies born to mothers who abuse drugs, especially alcohol.

Historically, the long-term prognosis for infants and young children without treatment has been very poor (Mok, Giaquinto, & DeRossi, 1987). In the past, it was estimated that approximately 75% of children infected died within 1 year of the presentation of AIDS symptoms following HIV infection. As of 2008, mothers and children still need comprehensive social, medical, and supportive care. Any infant exposed to the HIV virus should have follow-up for 3 years to ascertain whether or not infection has occurred. All secondary infections, even minor ones such as a diaper rash, should be treated promptly. Recent evidence seems to suggest that the viral load may be predictive of the disease progression in young children (Bell, 2007).

Since the mid 1990s, there have been important developments in preventing the vertical transmission of HIV from mothers to their newborns in the United States. As of 2008, HIV/AIDS in the youngest populations has become a chronic disease, rather than a fatal condition, with a reduction in transmission rate from mother to infant now approximating 1% (a dramatic decline from the former estimates of 25%–30% rates of vertical transmission). At this writing, Bell summarized some of the most recent medical treatments as follows:

> Since the early 1990s, guidelines addressing the complex issues of treatment of pediatric HIV disease have been developed. In general, antiretroviral agents should be used in combination in the treatment of all children with HIV. Single drug therapy has been shown to be inferior, presumably because HIV can develop mutations that render the virus resistant to individual agents. The availability of different drugs with different actions has led to combination therapy referred to as highly active antiretroviral therapy (HAART). These regimens routinely involve the use of three or more drugs, including a protease inhibitor. Another principle that has been adopted for care of HIV infected children is the measurement of viral load. This can assess the adequacy of medical therapies with the goal being suppression of viral numbers below limits of detection of the assay. Adjustments of dosages of medications for weight are an ongoing part of good clinical care because underdosing of medications can lead to development of viral resistance. For newly diagnosed cases in infants, therapy should be started as soon as a confirmed diagnosis is established. (2007, p. 79)

In sum, as a result of much research, the prognosis in treating infants and young children is much more optimistic as of 2004, and there continues to be hope that eventually a vaccine might be developed in the near future, although there remain many questions yet to be answered.

Hepatitis B Virus

HBV is a large, double-stranded DNA virus. This virus can produce severe systemic illness that includes jaundice, fever, and rash that can progress to chronic liver failure. The virus is common in Africa and Southeast Asia. Of these Third World populations, 35%–40% are infected without overt symptoms (carriers). The great influx of immigrants from underdeveloped countries has resulted in a greater risk of hepatitis B virus (HBV) infection in the United States.

If a pregnant woman is infected with HBV, there is a 50% risk of the neonate acquiring the infection (Arevalo, 1989). The current recommendation from the CDC is that all newborns be vaccinated with the recombinant (synthetic) form of hepatitis B vaccine. Babies whose mothers are positive for hepatitis B surface antigen should also receive protective immunoglobulins. Because the HBV has a long incubation period (50–180 days), aggressive protection of the newborn can prevent a serious debilitating disease (Zeldis & Crumpacker, 1990).

Other Infections

Numerous other infections, primarily viral, can cross the placenta and infect the newborn (Amstey, 1984). Many of these illnesses have similar signs and symptoms that result in confusion about the diagnosis. The viruses that cause mononucleosis (Epstein-Barr virus), chickenpox (varicella), poliomyelitis, mumps, enterovirus, and influenza can infect the newborn after infecting the mother (Overall, 1992). In each case, an aggressive approach to the diagnosis is important, largely in order to counsel the parents and to prevent the spread of the infectious agent to other children and staff in the facility caring for the child. Although many of the presenting symptoms of infections are similar, subsequent developmental disabilities differ with the types of viruses and their predilection for certain portions of the central nervous system.

Intrapartum Infections

Intrapartum infections are those that are acquired in the birth process, with vaginal deliveries affording a greater exposure.

Herpes

One of the most serious and virulent illnesses in the newborn, most often acquired as an ascending infection, is herpes (Whitley, 1990). There are several strains of the virus. Type 1 is predominantly an oral organism that is responsible for cold sores and fever blisters. Type 2 herpes is primarily a genital organism. The sexual liberation beginning in the 1970s has led to an increase in type 1 oral infections and type 2 herpes genital infections (AAP & ACOG, 1999b).

The fetus or newborn may be affected by either form of the disease. The most frequent presenting symptom, found in approximately 80% of the cases, is lethargy (Overall, 1994). Respiratory distress is evidenced in approximately 60%. The typical rash of herpes is seen in less than 50% of affected newborns. Other signs of the disease are those usually evident with generalized infections of the newborn, including temperature instability, enlarged liver and spleen, poor coagulation of blood, and jaundice (Corey & Spear, 1986a, 1986b). Herpes, however, is an aggressive virus and what commonly appears to be a localized infection may progress rapidly to systematic disease, especially targeted toward the central nervous system. The generalized form of the disease is devastating. Although survival is better with the localized form of the disease, as many as 40% of the survivors have serious sequelae, including seizures, intellectual disabilities, and other forms of severe developmental disability (Nahmias, Keyserling, & Kerrick, 1983).

Although new antiviral agents are available, they are not a panacea for neonatal herpes. They are most beneficial when used in children who have localized disease, with the hope of preventing generalized disease and central nervous system disease. Furthermore, while the treatment of newborns with generalized illness has resulted in an increase in survival, many of the survivors still have serious sequelae (Brunell, 1980). It is difficult to prevent transmission of herpes from a mother to the newborn. Even though a mother who has had herpes may be asymptomatic at the time of delivery, the infant may become infected. If there are active herpes lesions in the mother, cesarean delivery may help limit the exposure of the baby and subsequent illness.

Gonorrhea

Gonorrhea is a sexually transmitted disease. Adult males usually have a penile discharge, whereas females may be asymptomatic. Babies born to mothers with active gonorrhea are at greatest risk for eye infection (Cowles & Gonik, 1992). Early in the 1900s in New York State, visual impairment resulting from neonatal eye in-

fection was the most common single cause of loss of vision in children enrolled in schools for the blind. As a result, nearly all states now mandate eye prophylaxis against this infection.

Generally, the baby is exposed to the bacteria at the time of descent through the birth canal. Less commonly, after rupture of the membranes, the bacteria may ascend into the amniotic fluid surrounding the infant. In either case, the organism penetrates the anterior cell layer of the eye, and within 5 days a purulent infection results. If untreated, disease in the eye may progress to meningitis or other systemic infection. The disease may be treated with antibiotics. Unfortunately, although treatment may eradicate the organism, the damage has been done once the infection in the eye becomes purulent. Therefore, eye prophylaxis is very important. As was discussed in Chapter 3 on the evaluation and care of the neonate, the most commonly used therapeutic agent is erythromycin.

Postpartum Infections

Postpartum infections can be acquired from breast milk, blood transfusions, hands, or instruments. In addition, infections may be transmitted by infected family members or hospital personnel during care (Newell & McIntyre, 2000).

Systemic Infections

Any organism in the mother's vagina or in the baby's environment after birth may infect the newborn (Klein, 2001). The symptoms usually are those of systemic disease—temperature instability, respiratory difficulty, and other evidence of specific organ involvement. One common bacterial organism acquired, in some cases at birth and in other instances from family or hospital staff, is *Streptococcus*. There are many varieties of these bacteria. Group A *Streptococcus* is predominant with strep throat and also has been associated with rheumatic fever and severe kidney disease. It is rare for the newborn to be infected with these bacteria because protective antibodies (proteins) from the mother that have crossed the placenta usually limit the bacterial proliferation. Group B *Streptococcus* infection, however, is a serious threat to the newborn (Baker

& Edwards, 1990; Gibbs, Schrag, & Schuchat, 2004). Basically, it has two forms of presentation. The early type is marked by severe respiratory distress, simulating surfactant deficiency in the newborn (Ablow et al., 1976). Despite aggressive respiratory support and the use of antibiotics, the mortality rate remains high (i.e., up to 50% in many intensive care nurseries) (Baltimore et al., 2001). A second, more subtle form of this infection is meningitis, which is generally caused by a different serotype of group B *Streptococcus.*

Typically, the illness is manifested 2 or 3 weeks after birth, but it may present as late as several months after birth. Early symptoms include poor feeding and lethargy. Fortunately, once identified, this form of infection generally is more amenable to therapy. Another bacteria with a similar pattern of neonatal disease is *Listeria monocytogenes.* There is an early respiratory form of infection and a late meningitic presentation. It can be treated with the same antibiotics (Mustafa & McCracken, 1992) used to treat streptococcal infections.

The most common, environmentally acquired infection in the newborn is produced by *Staphylococcus* (Shinefield, 1990). Its mildest form is manifested as skin pustules that can be treated topically without the use of systemic antibiotics. The bacteria can infect any portion of the body, including the breast (abscess), umbilical cord (omphalitis), circumcision site, and lungs (pneumonia). One of the more severe manifestations of staphylococcal infection is the scalded skin syndrome, which results from a toxin produced by a local colonization of the bacteria. In this disease, large patches of skin are shed and there are major problems with fluid losses, much like those in burn patients. With aggressive supportive therapy, these infants generally survive. In sum, there are many potentially harmful bacterial and viral infections. The most premature infants and those newborns requiring the greatest therapeutic intervention generally have the more serious manifestations.

Conclusion

Prevention of neonatal infection resides largely with a high index of suspicion and concern among the health care team responsible for car-

ing for the pregnant mother (CDC, 2006). She should be encouraged to avoid sexual contact with anyone with lesions or a discharge. Any meat she consumes, which is a potential source of parasitic infections, should be cooked thoroughly. To prevent toxoplasmosis, the mother should avoid contact with the feces of animals, especially cats (she should avoid contact with cat litter). She should be given no live vaccines, such as those for rubella, poliomyelitis, or mumps, during pregnancy. During visits to her health care team, the vaginal examination should include a surveillance culture for gonorrhea (CDC, 2006). Serologic testing for syphilis during the pregnancy is mandatory. If an infection is identified, it should be treated promptly to minimize the potential risk to the fetus.

Treatment of the neonate with infection is relatively straightforward. If the illness is bacterial, antibiotics for the specific organism should be used. If the child has signs and symptoms of the infection but no etiology is identified, the choice of antibiotic then is based on determination of the organism most likely to be infecting the baby (deLouvois & Harvey, 1988). Apart from general supportive therapy, transfusion with fresh frozen adult plasma or immunoglobulins may be useful (Baker & the IVIG Collaborative Study Group, 1989). These therapies may offer essential elements that the baby has in short supply but needs to cope with infection.

The viral and protozoal infections are much more difficult to remedy. The antibiotics available for treatment are generally toxic and have limited application. For viral infections such as cytomegalovirus, no therapy is available.

The prognosis for any newborn with an infection is dependent on the responsible organism and its predilection for certain body organs. Overall, viral infections, especially herpes, cytomegalovirus, and rubella, tend to cause damage to the central nervous system and, therefore, are apt to produce more devastating developmental problems. Unfortunately, with many of the perinatal infections, much of the damage is irreversible, even if therapy is instituted immediately. Understandably, every child who has had an infection as a baby should be monitored closely for developmental delay.

REFERENCES

Ablow, R.C., Driscoll, S.G., Effmann, E.L., Gross, I., Jolles, C.J., Uauy, R., et al. (1976). A comparison of early-onset Group B streptococcal neonatal infection and the respiratory distress syndrome of the newborn. *New England Journal of Medicine, 294,* 65–70.

American Academy of Pediatrics and the American College of Obstetricians and Gynecologists. (1999a). *Joint statement on human immunodeficiency virus screening. ACOG Statement of Policy.* Elk Grove Village, IL: AAP; Washington, DC: American College of Obstetricians and Gynecologists.

American Academy of Pediatrics and the American College of Obstetricians and Gynecologists. (1999b). Management of herpes in pregnancy. *ACOG Practice Bulletin 8.* Washington, DC: American College of Obstetricians and Gynecologists.

American Academy of Pediatrics and the American College of Obstetricians and Gynecologists (2000). Perinatal viral and parasitic infections. *ACOG Practice Bulletin 20.* Washington, DC: American College of Obstetricians and Gynecologists.

American Academy of Pediatrics Committee on Infectious Diseases. (2006). *Red book: 2006 report of the committee on infectious diseases* (27th ed.). Elk Grove Village, IL: Author.

Amstey, M.S. (1984). *Virus infection in pregnancy.* Orlando, FL: Grune & Stratton.

Anderson-Berry, A.L., Bellig, L.L., & Ohning, B.L. (2006). Neonatal sepsis. Retrieved July 25, 2007, from http://www.emedicine.com/ped/topic2630 .htm

Arevalo, J.A. (1989). Hepatitis B in pregnancy. *Western Journal of Medicine, 150,* 669–674.

Baker, C.J., & Edwards, M.S. (1990). Group B streptococcal infections. In J.S. Remington & J.O. Klein (Eds.), *Infectious diseases of the fetus and newborn infant* (3rd ed., pp. 742–811). Philadelphia: W.B. Saunders.

Baker, C.J., & the IVIG Collaborative Study Group. (1989). Multicenter trial of intraveneous immuno-globulin (IVIG) to prevent late-onset infection in preterm infants: Preliminary results. *Pediatric Research, 25,* 275A.

Baltimore, R.S., Huie, S.M., Meek, J.I., Schuhat, A., & O'Brien, K. (2001). Early-onset neonatal sepsis in the era of group B streptococcal prevention. *Pediatrics, 108,* 1094–1098.

Bell, M.J. (2007). Infections and the fetus. In M.L. Batshaw, L. Pellegrino, & N.J. Roizen (Eds.), *Children with disabilities* (6th ed., pp. 71–82). Baltimore: Paul H. Brookes Publishing Co.

Bellanti, J.A., & Boner, A.L. (1981). Immunology of the fetus and newborn. In G.B. Avery (Ed.), *Neonatology: Pathophysiology and management of the newborn* (2nd ed., pp. 701–722). Philadelphia: Lippincott Williams & Wilkins.

Brunell, P.A. (1980). Prevention and treatment of neonatal herpes. *Pediatrics, 66,* 806–808.

Centers for Disease Control and Prevention. (2001). Control and prevention of rubella: Evaluation and management of suspected outbreaks, rubella in pregnant women, and surveillance for congenital rubella syndrome. *MMWR Morbid Mortal Wkly Rep 50*(RR-12), 1–23.

Centers for Disease Control and Prevention. (2004). *Parasitic disease information: Toxoplasmosis.* Retrieved January 3, 2007, from http://ww.cdc.gov/ncidod/dpd/parasites/toxoplasmosis

Centers for Disease Control and Prevention. (2006). Sexually transmitted diseases treatment guidelines. *MMWR Recommendations, Rep. 55*(RR11), 1–94; published erratum in *MMWR Recommendations, Rep. 55*(997).

Cherry, J.D. (1990). Enteroviruses. In J.S. Remington & J.O. Klein (Ed.), *Infectious diseases of the fetus and newborn infant* (3rd ed., pp. 325–366). Philadelphia: W.B. Saunders.

Cooper, L.Z. (1985). The history and medical consequences of rubella. *Review in Infectious Diseases, 7*(Supplement 1), S64–S67.

Corey, L., & Spear, P.G. (1986a). Infections of herpes simplex viruses (Part 1). *New England Journal of Medicine, 314*(11), 686–691.

Corey, L., & Spear, P.G. (1986b). Infection of herpes simplex viruses (Part 2). *New England Journal of Medicine, 314*(12), 749–757.

Cowan, M.J., Hellman, D., & Chudwin, D. (1984). Maternal transmission of acquired immune deficiency syndrome. *Pediatrics, 73,* 382–386.

Cowles, T.A., & Gonik, B. (1992). Perinatal infections. In A.A. Fanaroff & R.J. Martin (Eds.), *Neonatal-perinatal medicine: Diseases of the fetus and infant* (5th ed., Vol. 1, pp. 251–271). St. Louis: Mosby.

deLouvois, J., & Harvey, D. (1988). Antibiotic therapy of the newborn. *Clinics in Perinatology, 15,* 365–388.

Fauci, A.S. (1988). The human immunodeficiency virus: Infectivity and mechanisms of pathogenesis. *Science, 239,* 617–622.

Feldman, H.A. (1968). Toxoplasmosis. *New England Journal of Medicine, 279,* 1370–1375, 1431–1437.

Gibbs, R.S., Schrag, S., & Schuchat, A. (2004). Perinatal infections due to group B streptococci. *Obstetrics and Gynecology, 104,* 1062–1076.

Gonik, B., & Hammill, H.A. (1990). AIDS in pregnancy. *Seminars in Pediatric Infectious Disease, 1,* 82–88.

Hanson, C.G., & Shearer, W.T. (1992). Pediatric HIV infections and AIDS. In R.D. Feigin & J.D. Cherry (Eds.), *Textbook of pediatric infectious diseases* (3rd ed., pp. 990–1011). Philadelphia: W.B. Saunders.

Hardy, J.B. (1973). Clinical and developmental aspects of congenital rubella. *Archives of Otolaryngology, 98,* 230–236.

Hinman, A.R. (1985). Prevention of congenital rubella: Symposium summary. *Pediatrics, 75,* 1162–1165.

Klein, J.O. (2001). Bacterial sepsis and meningitis In J.S. Remington & J.O. Klein (Eds.), *Infectious diseases of the fetus and newborn infant* (5th ed., pp. 943–998). Philadelphia: W.B. Saunders.

Lee, R.V. (1988). Parasites and pregnancy: The problems of malaria and toxoplasmosis. *Clinics in Perinatology, 15,* 351–364.

Lissauer, T., & Fanaroff, A.A. (Eds.). (2006). *Neonatology at a glance.* Malden, MA: Blackwell.

Miller, M.E., & Stiehm, E.R. (1979). Host defenses in the fetus and neonate. *Pediatrics, 64,* 705–833.

Miller, M.H., Rabinowitz, M.A., Frost, J.O., & Seager, G.M. (1969). Audiological problems associated with maternal rubella. *Laryngoscope, 79,* 417–426.

Mok, J.Q., Giaquinto, C., & DeRossi, A. (1987). Infants born to mothers seropositive for human immunodeficiency virus: Preliminary findings from a multicenter European study. *Lancet, 1,* 1164–1168.

Mustafa, M.M., & McCracken, G.H., Jr. (1992). Perinatal bacterial diseases. In R.D. Feigin & J.D. Cherry (Eds.), *Textbook of pediatric infectious diseases* (3rd ed., pp. 891–923). Philadelphia: W.B. Saunders.

Nabarro, D. (1954). *Congenital syphilis.* London: E. Arnold.

Nahmias, A.J. (1974). The TORCH complex. *Hospital Practice, 9,* 65–72.

Nahmias, A.J., Keyserling, H.I., & Kerrick, G.M. (1983). Herpes simplex. In J.S. Remington & J.O. Klein (Eds.), *Infectious diseases of the fetus and newborn infant* (3rd ed., pp. 636–678). Philadelphia: W.B. Saunders.

Newell, M.L., & McIntyre, J. (Eds.). (2000). *Congenital and perinatal infections.* New York: Cambridge University Press.

Overall, J.C., Jr. (1992). Viral infections of the fetus and neonate. In R.D. Feign & J.D. Cherry (Eds.), *Textbook of pediatric infectious diseases* (3rd ed., pp. 924–959). Philadelphia: W.B. Saunders.

Overall, J.C., Jr. (1994). Herpes simplex virus infection of the fetus and newborn. *Pediatric Annals, 23,* 131–136.

Preblud, S.R., & Alford, C.A., Jr. (1990). Rubella. In J.S. Remington & J.O. Klein (Eds.), *Infectious diseases of the fetus and newborn infant* (3rd ed., pp. 196–240). Philadelphia: W.B. Saunders.

Regelman, W.E., Hill, H.R., Cates, K.L., & Quie, P.G. (1992). Immunology of the newborn. In R.D. Feigin & J.D. Cherry (Eds.), *Textbook of pediatric infectious diseases* (3rd ed., pp. 876–890). Philadelphia: W.B. Saunders.

Remington, J.S., & Klein, J.O. (Eds.). (2001). *Infectious diseases of the fetus and newborn infant* (5th ed.). Philadelphia: W.B. Saunders.

Romero, R., Athayde, N., Maymon, E., Pacora, P., & Bahado-Singh, R. (1999). Premature rupture of the membranes. In A. Reece & J. Hobbins (Eds.), *Medicine of the fetus and mother* (pp. 1581–1625). Philadelphia: Lippincott Williams & Wilkins.

Rubinstein, A. (1986). Pediatric AIDS. *Current Problems in Pediatrics, 16,* 361–409.

Sauerbrei, A., & Wutzler, P. (2000). The congenital varicella syndrome. *Journal of Perinatology, 20,* 548–554.

Schrag, S., Gorwitz, R., Fultz-Butts, K., & Schuchat, A. (2002). Prevention of perinatal group B streptococcal disease. *Revised guidelines from CDC. MMWR Recommendations, Rep. 51,* (RR-11):1–22.

Shinefield, H.R. (1990). Staphylococcal infections. In J.S. Remington & J.O. Klein (Eds.), *Infectious diseases of the fetus and newborn infant* (3rd ed., pp. 866–900). Philadelphia: W.B. Saunders.

Siegel, J.D., & McCracken, G.H., Jr. (1981). Sepsis neonatorum. *New England Journal of Medicine, 304,* 642–646.

Sweet, R.L., & Gibbs, R.S. (2002). *Infectious diseases of the female genital tract* (4th ed.). Philadelphia: Lippincott Williams & Wilkins.

Taber, L.H., & Huber, T.W. (1975). Congenital syphilis. In S. Krugman & A.A. Gershon (Eds.), *Infections of the fetus and newborn infant* (pp. 183–190). Philadelphia: W.B. Saunders.

Wendel, G.D. (1988). Gestational and congenital syphilis. *Clinics in Perinatology, 15,* 287–304.

Whitley, R.J. (1990). Herpes simplex viruses. In B.N. Fields & D.M. Knipe (Eds.), *Virology* (2nd ed., pp. 1843–1887). New York: Raven.

Zeldis, J.B., & Crumpacker, C.S. (1990). Hepatitis. In J.S. Remington & J.O. Klein (Eds.), *Infectious diseases of the fetus and newborn infant* (3rd ed., pp. 574–600). Philadelphia: W.B. Saunders.

CHAPTER 13

The Interface of Physiology and Medical Environments

Gail L. Ensher and David A. Clark

At the conclusion of this chapter, the reader will

- *Understand the ways in which neonatal intensive care unit (NICU) environments have affected the development of newborns with medical problems*

- *Understand recent changes in how the physical environment of light, sound, touch, and smell have been modified within NICU hospital settings to address issues of adverse outcomes for newborns*

- *Understand the meaning of developmentally supportive and relationship-based care in NICU nurseries*

- *Understand ways in which families can participate meaningfully in the care of their newborns in NICU nurseries*

Concerns for high-risk newborns are not only centered on medical treatments. With new abilities to save infants born at as early as 23–24 weeks of gestation, improved survival rates have required the use of aggressive, highly technological therapies. As a result, professionals across both medical and educational fields since the mid- to late 1980s have become keenly interested in the developmental environments of neonates hospitalized for extended periods of time. Among those infants born prematurely in the United States annually, the smallest and most acutely ill babies continue to be especially vulnerable to the stressful influences of neonatal intensive care as a result of their neurological immaturity and physiological instability. As we consider the care that is now available for the earliest and most premature infants, it is apparent that medical technology can provide intervention for conditions affecting almost every organ system. However, these amazing contributions for the preservation of life have also presented us with new challenges in terms of developmental care before and after hospital discharge.

Impact of the Neonatal Intensive Care Unit Environment on Development of the Brain and the Senses

The following subsections cover developmental issues encountered in prematurity and addressed in the NICU.

Intervention in the Neonatal Intensive Care Unit

When we refer to the high-risk infant, we need to remember that the concept of risk applies to more than the neonate's chance of survival. As a result of life-threatening medical events, the infant admitted to the NICU has experienced major physiological and environmental conditions that often interfere with and/or compromise typical development. Thus, as the infant's medical needs are addressed, so too should the developmental, psychosocial, and family concerns be addressed. Accordingly, there are at least two primary goals for infants during their hospital stays in neonatal intensive care: 1) reduce adverse and potentially detrimental stimuli to the lowest possible level, and 2) create supportive and developmentally appropriate environments for both babies and their families. Significant changes have been implemented in Level 3 and Level 4 regional hospitals since the late 1990s to address both of these issues. (Level 1 hospitals are equipped to care for typical newborns, and Level 2 hospitals are equipped to care for those infants with less acute medical needs for brief stays.) Commenting on these new NICU developments, Rais-Bahrami and Short wrote,

> As survival rates of preterm infants have improved, the focus of care is now including a consideration of the optimal environment within the NICU for the premature infant to develop. Traditional NICU care has focused on medical protocols and procedures. A newer approach uses a more relationship-based, individualized, developmentally supportive model. This approach recognizes that the usual NICU setting is not optimal for the premature infant's developmental progress. Typical NICU care has involved the infant experiencing prolonged diffuse sleep states, unattended crying, a high ambient noise level, a lack of opportunity for sucking, and poorly timed social and caregiving interactions. (2007, p. 117)

In an effort to achieve more developmentally appropriate environments and practices within the NICU, at least three components are essential. The first involves education of nursery staff who provide daily medical and/or interactive care to infants, as well as education of the families who will assume caregiving when the baby is discharged. Increasingly, educators, child development specialists, and medical personnel are acknowledging the strong interaction among physiological, environmental, and developmental processes that determine the well-being and ultimate outcomes of preterm infants (Als, 1997). In short, NICU staff need to have an awareness

and knowledge of the types of stimulation and protection that are most beneficial to the newborns whom they care for, as well as approaches to optimize interactions with these infants.

Likewise, parents and caregivers need to learn about their premature babies who are vulnerable and at risk. Most importantly, they need to understand the many behavioral cues that newborns demonstrate and the ways in which they can most appropriately respond. In addition, they need to be prepared for frequent, common problems that they may encounter with at risk or early delivery babies, such as excessive irritability, mixed wake and sleep cycles, difficulties with feeding, and slow attention and response patterns. In working with families, nursery staff can encourage mothers and fathers to touch, hold, and care for their infants in ways that can develop attachment, decrease anxiety, minimize stress, and ease the transition to home.

The second component of the process for developing more appropriate nursery environments is the monitoring and assessment of infant states, including attention to muscle tone, reflexes, regulation of behavioral states, neurobehavioral responses, and feeding issues. It is important to keep in mind that newborns are differentially sensitive and responsive to various types of stimulation depending on their gestational ages, illness, neurophysiology, and temperament (Lester & Tronick, 1990). With ongoing daily observations and assessment, hospital staff can apply various types of intervention and strategies for needed environmental protection.

The third aspect of intervention for high-risk infants and families is providing smooth transitions to home and services if deemed appropriate following discharge. Ideally, this planning process is not limited to family education only when a baby is in intensive care, but will continue in developmental follow-up and with early intervention, as needed. In particular, both discharge and postdischarge programs need to include basic education and preparation for home care by families, information about equipment, and referrals for community-based services that need to be in place before an infant leaves the NICU. An essential dimension of this process is developing a means for maintaining contact with families after discharge to facilitate the transition from hospital to home and to address parent concerns in a timely manner. Research findings support the need for further development of hospital-to-home approaches for low birth weight newborns because they demonstrate improved outcomes. Indeed, with relatively short hospital stays now common practice, support for parents of high-risk infants that begins in the NICU has emerged as one of the most promising strategies for educating families as well as enhancing the growth and development of young children (Broedsgaard & Wagner, 2005).

Risks of Prematurity to Brain Development

Basic to any discussion of specific developmental intervention with hospitalized newborns is a fundamental understanding of the changes that take place when an infant is born several weeks or months early. These are described in depth in the chapter on neonatal neurology (see Chapter 5). In review, however, the brain develops through a continuous process, which begins in utero and proceeds beyond birth until approximately 2 years of age. Preterm infants are delivered before in utero stages of brain development are complete, which places them at considerable risk for potential abnormal brain growth and development. Brain development can be classified into the following four categories (Barb & Lemons, 1989, p. 8):

1. Neuronal proliferation is a process that involves the rapid and repeated production of neurons, which are made up of the axon, cell body, and the dendrite. Neuronal production initially occurs between 2 and 4 months gestation and is followed by development of glial cells (supportive tissue of the central nervous system) at approximately 5 months gestation.
2. Migration refers to the movement of nerve cells from their site of origin to the area they eventually occupy within the mature central nervous system. Migration occurs primarily between 3 and 5 months gestation.
3. Organization involves several changes including: (a) the alignment and layering of the cortex, (b) further development and expansion of the axons and dendrites, (c) establishment of synaptic contacts, (d) selective elimination via cell death of neuronal processes, and (e) additional differentiation and proliferation of the glial cells. Organization takes place primarily in the third trimester and establishes the elaborate network of the central nervous system.
4. Myelinization is the development of the myelin sheath covering the axon, which enhances conduction of impulses in the nervous system. This process begins at 20 weeks gestation and continues into adult life.

As described here and in the chapter on neonatal neurology (see Chapter 5), much of the brain growth and maturation in the preterm infant that would have occurred in utero takes place in an extrauterine environment that is characterized by a variety of medical insults during the perinatal period. Conditions such as hypoxia, acidosis, infection, and inadequate nutrition may lead to intraventricular hemorrhage or other cerebral insults that may have serious consequences for immediate and later brain development. As discussed in the chapter on pain management in infants and young children (see Chapter 14), researchers increasingly are focusing on the physiological changes, responses of the premature newborn to pain, and the long-term consequences of exposure to pain. Given the fact that the human brain has powerful, plastic or adaptable capabilities that allow the central nervous system to cope with a variety of conditions, including damage, two questions inevitably rise to the forefront of this discussion and to future research efforts on NICU intervention. First, what can be done in terms of prevention when infants are in hospital environments? Second, when damage does occur, how can predictable delays be attenuated? Speaking directly to this issue, Als wrote,

It appears that development in the extrauterine environment leads to different and potentially maladaptive developmental trajectories. Understanding the neurodevelopmental expectations of the fetal infant is increasingly providing a basis for modification of traditionally delivered newborn intensive care, which appears to inadvertently increase the stress and challenge to the vulnerable preterm nervous system. Furthermore, understanding the neurodevelopmental expectation of the fetal infant is increasingly leading to the abandonment of first-generation skill teaching and task-oriented intervention approaches in the NICU for the sake of a process-oriented, relationship-based, individualized, developmentally focused frame-work of care delivery. (1997, p. 48)

Infant Behavior: Keys to Intervention in Neonatal Intensive Care Unit Environments

Infants communicate through the windows of their behavior. They offer clues as to "what they need, how much they need, and when they need it" (Cole, 1985, p. 24). Preterm infants differ from their full-term counterparts, as well as from each other, in their capacities to respond to their environments—variables that are largely determined by their gestational ages and the status of their health, illness, and any residual disability. Als, a pioneer in research on newborns in intensive care, offered a meaningful framework for studying and understanding individual differences via her description of five subsystems and their respective behavioral manifestations related to premature infants:

The detailed behavioral observations document the language of the infant's behavior along three channels of communication: the autonomic system, motor system, and state system (Als & Duffy, 1982). The autonomic nervous system's functioning can be observed in the infant's breathing patterns, color fluctuation, visceral stability or instability, and autonomic behaviors such as tremors and startles (Als, in press-b). . . .
   Simultaneously, motor system functioning can be observed in the infant's body tone, postural repertoire, and movement patterns. . . .

The infant's state organization can be observed in terms of the infant's range of states, the robustness and modulation of the available states, and the patterns of transition from state to state.

- Is this an infant who shows the full continuum of states, moving from deep sleep to light sleep, to a drowsy state, to quiet alertness, to an active aroused state, to upset and crying; or does the infant typically move from sleep to aroused states and immediately back down to sleep again, skipping the alert state?
- When the infant is sleeping, is the sleep robust, or does the infant never quite settle, showing facial movements, vocal discharges, and general restlessness?

- What is the quality of the infant's alert state? Is the infant's expression animated, with shiny-eyed alertness and gently forward-shaped mouth, available for engagement and interaction? Does the infant quickly move to panicked wide-eyedness, or barely seem to muster the energy to interact through a lidded, glassy-eyed strained appearance? . . .

All observations are seen in the context of the infant's efforts at taking the next step and regulating efforts through approach and avoidance behavior (Als, 1982, in press-b). This framework assumes that the infant has strategies available to move toward and take in stimuli, if the input is appropriate in timing, complexity, and intensity in relation to the infant's thresholds of functioning; and, conversely, that the infant has strategies to move away from or avoid inputs that are too complex or intense or are inappropriately timed. (1997, pp. 58–59)

Initial responses of a preterm newborn who is ill to environmental stress are very different from those of healthy infants. These responses often have been manifested in observable physiological changes, such as crying, gaze aversion, color change, and even vomiting (Catlett & Holditch-Davis, 1990). These initial behavioral changes frequently are followed by rapid physiological deterioration and state disorganization, evidenced by multiple sudden swings in state during which the infant may withdraw into lower levels of consciousness or "shut down" (appear to be asleep) or stare fearfully or worriedly at his or her surroundings. Given the compelling data, changes in best practice NICU intervention have been indicated for more than a decade (White, 2004). No longer are professionals and families asking whether changes are necessary. The issue before medical staff, clinicians, and educators is the nature of NICU intervention.

Research focused on various types of environments and stimulation is not new. Data gathered since the mid 1980s on intervention with premature, high-risk, and developmentally delayed newborns in NICUs have been extensive. Reviews on the effectiveness of programming, however, leave many questions unanswered and consistently raise the need for refinement of methodology and design of such studies, not to mention the ethical concerns involved.

To move beyond this point of controversy, research in the future will have to address multiple issues about the appropriateness and timing of intervention with varying degrees of prematurity. These questions include the nature of specific programming for purposes of protection as well as stimulation, sensitive measures of developmental change, the diversity of high-risk populations, and the guidance that needs to be offered to families in relation to earlier versus later stimulation and interaction. As is evident in prior research, in most instances it is not possible to involve in a study adequate numbers of infants within given risk categories, define such groups accurately, or impose control conditions in which babies are denied programming that is considered beneficial. Thus, future studies will need to be developed and carried out around all of these constraints. In addition, contemporary researchers and practitioners are advocating intervention for preterm infants that is individualized and adapted to the apparent abilities of the child to respond to various stimuli.

Developmentally Appropriate Practices with Newborns and Their Families

Along with all of the previously noted infant-related considerations, focus also must be directed toward the family—the ultimate and continuing caregiver for the newborn.

Caring for Infants

In a very real sense, interaction with newborns in neonatal intensive care settings has come full circle. Historically, prior to the 1960s, preterm infants were considered too fragile to tolerate stimulation. The prevailing philosophy was one of minimal handling (Als, 1997; Lester & Tronick, 1990). This thinking began to change with heightened concerns that the NICU environment might be, in reality, depriving the most vulnerable newborns of sensory stimulation. These concerns ushered in a new period of research and intervention carried out with a variety of strategies

focused on tactile-kinesthetic (Hasselmeyer, 1964; Korner, Kraemer, Haffner, & Cosper, 1975; Neal, 1968; Solkoff & Matuszak, 1975); auditory (Katz, 1971; Segal, 1972); and multimodal (Kramer & Pierpont, 1976; LaRossa & Brown, 1982; Leib, Benfield, & Guidubaldi, 1980) stimulation protocols. Since those earliest efforts and studies, work in neonatal intensive care nurseries has evolved toward establishing more sensitive, family-centered, protective environments for infants and families alike. Als detailed these changes as follows:

> Since the mid-1980s, newborn intensive care units have been involved in a transformation of care that has been described as the most profound change that has occurred in neonatal care practice since its beginning (Gilkerson & Als, 1995). Nurseries are moving from task- and teaching-oriented models toward a new model of family-centered, developmentally supportive care—a professional and family alliance that supports the parents' cherishing of their child and the child's neurobiologically based expectations for nurturance. (1997 p. 55)

The Senses: Protection from Visual Stimulation in the Neonatal Intensive Care Unit
For years, it has been recognized that light and other "competing stimuli (sensory interference) such as intense noise, pain, unusual movement" can have many adverse effects on humans (Graven, 2004, p. 211). Light affects biological rhythm, endocrine glands (pituitary and pineal), gonadal function, and vitamin D synthesis. Consequently, there have been ongoing concerns about the possible detrimental effects for infants exposed to high intensity light. Miller and Menacker (2007) noted that the most common cause of retinal damage in infants is retinopathy of prematurity (ROP), and that recently the incidence of babies affected by ROP has increased as a result of the survival of early-for-dates, very low birth weight newborns Moreover, studies from the early 1990s documented evidence of higher percentages (a greater than 30% incidence among babies weighing less than 1,000 grams) of ROP among preterm neonates exposed to standard bright NICU environments (Glass et al., 1985). Such findings are not surprising in view of the differences that very low birth weight infants ex-

perience when they are thrust into a world of bright light versus the protected, muted environment of the mother's uterus where they are exposed only to filtered cycles of night and day (i.e., red spectrum only).

Addressing the need for visual protection, NICU environments are now being modified to accommodate the vulnerabilities of the newborns with medical complications, especially those of very low birth weight infants. Accordingly, increasing numbers of NICU and pediatric units are being designed with individual, overhead reduced lighting, as well as capacities for simulating day and night cycles to offer time-out periods and protection from light exposure. They are also implementing circadian rhythms, which include the sleep-wake cycle and daily rhythms in hormone production (Rivkees, 2004). Although circadian rhythms in preterm infants constitute a new area of research, Rivkees pointed out the importance of this area of inquiry in future studies of infant development. He wrote,

> Increasing evidence indicates that the circadian timing system is a fundamental homeostatic system that potently influences human behavior and physiology throughout development. After birth, there is progressive maturation of the circadian system with day–night rhythms in activity and hormone secretion developing between 1 and 3 months. Recent evidence shows that the circadian system of primate infants is responsive to light at very premature states and that low intensity lighting can regulate the developing clock. With continued elucidation of circadian system development and influences on human physiology and illness, it is anticipated that consideration of circadian biology will become an increasingly important component of neonatal care. (2004, pp. 225–226)

The Senses: Protection from Noise and Auditory Stimulation in the Neonatal Intensive Care Unit

Not unlike the visual surroundings of the NICU, random and unpredictable sounds in the NICU have been a major source of environmental stress for the preterm infant (Gray & Philbin, 2004). High-risk newborns have a much higher incidence of moderate to profound hearing loss than do infants in the general population. For example, Rais-Bahrami and Short noted that

> ELBW [extremely low birth weight] infants are at increased risk for hearing loss because of multisystem illness and the frequent use of medications, such as aminoglycoside antibiotics and diuretics, that can be toxic to the auditory [cochlea] system. The overall prevalence of sensorineural hearing impairment is about 4 per 10,000 in full-term infants. This increases to 13 per 10,000 in LBW [low birth weight] infants and to 51 per 10,000 among VLBW [very low birth weight] infants. (2007, pp. 113–114)

In addition, Gray and Philbin (2004) discussed in depth concerns about increased distractibility and inattention as a result of unpredictable noise environments, such as the NICU.

Again, sensitivity to excessive and/or unexpected noise of human voices, radios, alarms, charts being placed on top of incubators, and other extraneous sounds is not new to hospitals, and in particular to NICUs. In utero, infants are exposed primarily to the mother's heartbeat, her voice, bowel sounds, and muted sounds from the outside world. In keeping with our knowledge of the risks of noxious environmental stimuli, a higher incidence of hearing impairment among children born at very early gestational ages, and the need for more protected environments in NICUs, medical staff are becoming increasingly aware of noise levels and ways to implement more developmentally appropriate practices, such as eliminating radios, talking in areas away from infants in incubators, muffling sounds of objects placed on top of incubators, clustering medical procedures with infants, and talking softly to infants when in quiet, alert states. Furthermore, if signs of stress, such as crying, grimacing, changes in skin color, or hiccupping appear, medical staff should advise families to discontinue their efforts until such a time that their infants have reached a more stable state. Lastly, given the risks of hearing impairment among premature infants, the majority of hospitals (now law in New York State) screen all babies meeting a certain criteria of birth weight, gestational age, and nature of illness who were admitted to NICUs before hospital discharge, as well as recommending semiannual follow-up of audiological evaluations throughout the first 3 years of life (Herer, Knightly, & Steinberg, 2007).

***The Senses: Protection from Adverse Tactile,
Kinesthetic, and Vestibular Stimulation***   As
discussed previously, NICUs used to be characterized by too much and inappropriate visual
and auditory stimulation, with the amount of
soothing tactile, kinesthetic, and vestibular intervention being extremely limited. In utero, infants
are floating in amniotic fluid, are in a flexed position, and have opportunities for firm, but protected resistance against the walls of the mother's
womb. Historically, in the NICU, however, stark
exposure to the NICU environment included numerous experiences with touch and interaction,
but they were often associated with pain and dis-
comfort. As Furdon (see Chapter 14) points out,
the prevailing view used to be that pain is a
learned response and that infants (especially
preterm babies) do not experience such sensations. Recent research has offered strong evidence
to the contrary, revealing a decline in oxygenation
and increased heart rate in the presence of
painful, aversive touch procedures. In fact, infants exposed to excessively painful procedures,
such as circumcision, have been known to "shut
down" completely because of the noxious overload. Although medical research is far from
understanding completely the management of
pain with preterm infants (especially low birth
weight neonates), we now know that within the
neonatal unit environment, there are interventions that can be implemented to lessen the stress.
Addressing the issue of painful stressors for
acutely ill newborns, Catlett and Holditch-Davis
recommended the following, which now has become common practice in many NICUs:

> The effects of procedural touch can be lessened by
> grouping care in short intervals and watching oxy-
> gen monitors so that procedures can be stopped
> whenever possible before hypoxemia occurs. For
> the sickest and smallest premature infants, long
> rest periods must be provided before and after pe-
> riods of procedural touch to optimize oxygen lev-
> els and minimize prolonged stress. . . .
>
> Because acutely ill prematures are so sensitive
> to stimulation, interactional touch must be ap-
> proached with great care and a good deal of expert-
> ise. If not, infants will respond as negatively to in-
> teractional touch as to procedural touch. Several
> studies have shown that gentle, interactional touch
> during the neonatal period can decrease crying, in-

> crease weight gain, increase bowel motility, and
> improve developmental status at one year of age.
> (1990, p. 24)

Several other researchers have noted the
association between continuous handling of critically ill infants in neonatal settings and the potential for periventricular-intraventricular hemorrhage (Bada et al., 1990; Evans, 1991).

Given that precautions and specifications
are now receiving endorsement from medical
and developmental fields, NICU intervention
programs focusing on tactile, kinesthetic, and
vestibular stimulation is constituting an active
area of research and inquiry (Westrup, Kleberg,
von Eichwald, Stjernqvist, & Lagercrantz, 2000)
in the United States and in other countries. Studies from the late 1980s and early 1990s reported
findings that newborns given tactile-kinesthetic
stimulation with massage, stroking, and passive
movement of the limbs for very brief periods of
time (Field et al., 1986; Scafidi et al., 1990) gained
weight more quickly; were more active and alert
during behavioral observations; and showed
more mature habituation, orientation, motor,
and range of state behavior, as well as briefer
hospital stays. More recently, the method of kangaroo care, which involves parent–infant, skin–
skin contact with the newborn nestled in the parent's or caregiver's chest, is now being used in
various forms in NICUs across the United States
(Feldman, Eidelman, Sirota, & Weller, 2002). This
type of tactile stimulation originated in Bogata,
Columbia in 1979 for larger infants and has been
associated with decreased hospital stays, shorter
periods on ventilators, and increased alert states
(Browne, 2004). Equally important, such non-
technological strategies have also yielded changes
in parent interactions with their infants. For example, Feldman and colleagues reported the following results with a small sample of 73 preterm
infants who received kangaroo care in a NICU in
Israel compared with a similar group of babies
who served as a control group:

> After KC [kangaroo care], interactions were more
> positive at 37 weeks GA [gestational age]: mothers
> showed more positive affect, touch, and adaptation
> to infant cues, and infants showed more alertness
> and less gaze aversion. Mothers reported less de-

pression and perceived infants as less abnormal. At 3 months, mothers and fathers of KC infants were more sensitive and provided a better home environment. At 6 months, KC mothers were more sensitive and infants scored higher on the Bayley Mental Developmental Index . . . and the Psychomotor Developmental Index. (2002, p. 16)

Other studies (Ferber & Makhoul, 2004) found similar results with full-term newborns, indicating that kangaroo care seems to "influence state organization and motor system modulation of the newborn shortly after delivery" (p. 858). Given the potential benefits in terms of both infants and their families, albeit short-term findings at this point, strategies such as kangaroo care may have some long-term benefits for families in terms of attachment issues and possible prevention of child abuse and neglect with often difficult to care for populations of young children. In conclusion, Browne summarized the favorable outcomes as follows:

> Skin-to-skin practices for premature infants in the NICUs provide significant support for physiologic stability, behavioral organization, and positive attachment relationships. With care, even the smallest intubated infants can benefit from this practice. Additionally, there are benefits to the mother that include stress reduction, better breast-feeding outcomes, and more positive attachment behavior. STS care benefits the infant by providing both a buffer from the physical environment of the NICU as well as assistance with regulation after environmental disruption. Thus, the parent's bodies may be conceptualized as the most optimal environment for the fragile infant. (2004, pp. 294–295)

Calming Techniques

Calming techniques have been used in NICU nurseries to address some of the adverse environmental influences to which preterm infants are exposed daily. In particular, three strategies continue to be widely used to pacify newborns and to facilitate more typical sleeping patterns. The topics of positioning, swaddling, and nonnutritive sucking are discussed in the following sections.

Positioning   The full-term infant comes into the world with well-developed flexor tone (phys-

iological flexion) of all extremities. In contrast with these more mature patterns of development, the preterm baby usually presents with generalized low muscle tone and may assume more extended positions of the limbs. Thus, positioning of the premature neonate should be focused on promoting the development of flexor tone. Developmental specialists often suggest that, among the options, prone positions in incubators can be very beneficial as compared to the recommended placement of typically developing newborns in supine position (as newborns with medical problems demonstrate increasing wellness, the transition can be made to supine position). In addition, placing a roll along the baby's abdominal surfaces can be helpful in facilitating the development of flexion of the trunk and extremities (Pergolizzi, 2007) and can provide the child with boundaries that simulate the uterine environment, as well as keeping the infant in a more self-regulated state (Als et al., 2004).

Swaddling   Historically, swaddling is a technique that has been found to be effective for promoting sleep and calming and pacifying infants who are fussy, crying, and/or colicky (especially infants withdrawing from maternal opioid abuse). Specific to the preterm neonate, specialists have reported that swaddling increases oxygenization and decreases heart rate.

Observations in contemporary NICUs continue to reinforce the importance of this simple, but beneficial technique. For instance, Als and her colleagues (2004) advocate an individualized developmental care and assessment program in which observation plays a major role for reading infant cues and determining appropriate intervention strategies. Part of that protocol with many newborns will involve swaddling them with soft blankets or "bedding" infants in "comfortable bunting" to assist with a "return to restful sleep" (Als et al., 2004, p. 848).

Nonnutritive Sucking   The third simple technique for calming both the full-term and preterm infant is nonnutritive sucking. For years, mothers and fathers have confirmed the fact that babies who use their fingers, hands, or pacifiers early tend to soothe themselves more easily and quickly. With our growing knowledge and increased awareness of the impact of pain on premature infants, nonnutritive sucking has been adopted more frequently in NICUs. Kimble and Dempsey summarized the several positive effects of nonnutritive sucking that have been suggested in various research and observational studies.

> Nonnutritive sucking has been found to affect movement, sleep, state regulation and arousal, oxygenation, and nutrition and growth. Its quality is used as an indicator of central nervous system well-being. Speculations have been suggested about improved outcomes from respiratory distress syndrome, patent ductus arteriosus. . . . The possible effect of sucking movement on attachment between mother and infant has also been described. (1992, p. 32)

As the reader can discern from this discussion of intervention strategies for the high-risk and vulnerable newborn in the NICU environment, there are no clear answers about the optimal approach to offering developmental care. Unquestionably, problems of small sample size, short-term follow-up, insufficient descriptions of programming, and other methodological issues have limited the extent of our understanding of very complex issues with respect to the preterm and acutely ill infant, as well as our ability to generalize from findings of such studies. The challenge now lies in taking what we know to be most helpful and harmful and moving forward with further research to address questions, to protect children as individuals starting from their earliest days in intensive care, and to enhance opportunities for a better start in the first year of life. Some of the current work conducted by Als and her colleagues (2004) with preterm infants offers research-based evidence that represents best practices in hospital settings for both infants and their families and that simultaneously marries the study of both physiology and environment.

Shepley (2004) offered promise for significant future changes in the design and development of NICUs for critically ill newborns and their families. Shepley wrote,

> These developments lead one to believe that the future for evidence-based design for infants and staff in the NICU is hopeful. The stage has been set to enable the design disciplines, the medical establishment, and academicians to work together to significantly improve the quality of life for infants, families, and staff in neonatal intensive care units. (2004, p. 309)

Conclusion

Caring for newborns in neonatal intensive care cannot proceed successfully without assisting and working with families. Chapter 21 emphasizes this point, as have Als and her colleagues:

> The developmental care model tested views the infant as an active participant who seeks ongoing caregiver support for self-regulation during the initial stabilization phase and in the course of continuing developmental progression. Individualized developmental care provided by the preterm infants' parents in collaboration with their nursery teams, and supported by a developmental specialist, may provide an extrauterine environment that supports cortical development by providing more stable autoregulation to the immature autonomic system in a challenging sensory environment by focus and consistent assurance of calm behavioral function in the course of all medical and daily care procedures. (2004, pp. 854–855)

These findings also have been supported by research in multicenter, randomized trials of individualized developmental care for very low birth weight preterm infants (Als et al., 2003).

In conclusion, parents need to join with medical staff as full partners (Johnson, Abraham, & Parrish, 2004) in the numerous daily routines of feeding, holding, dressing, carrying out simple medical procedures, reading infant cues, offering developmentally appropriate stimulation with growth and change, among others. Most important, however, they must provide the affection and love so critical to the well-being of their babies. They need to do so despite the frequent, lingering anxieties and concerns about the future of their children that never seem to leave their side. They will learn to appreciate, perhaps like no other families, those moments of success and next steps that often are taken for granted with the delivery and developmental progression of "typical children." Therefore, it is vitally important for all of us who work with young children and their families to be mindful of the need to offer guidance and support for these families who may feel and, in fact, be just as vulnerable as the tiny babies entrusted to their care. Finally, as some researchers and authors are recommending, families justifiably should be involved with others in the design and development of future intensive care nurseries based on their own personal experiences and perspectives.

REFERENCES

Als, H. (1986). A synactive model of neonatal behavioral organization: Framework for the assessment of neurobehavioral development in the preterm infant and for support of infants and parents in the neonatal intensive care environment. *Physical and Occupational Therapy in Pediatrics, 6*, 3–53.

Als, H. (1997). Earliest intervention for preterm infants in the newborn intensive care unit. In M.J. Guralnick (Ed.), *The effectiveness of early intervention* (pp. 47–76). Baltimore: Paul H. Brookes Publishing Co.

Als, H., Duffy, F. H., McAnulty, G.B., Rivkin, M.J., Vajapeyam, S., Mulkern, R.V., et al. (2004). Early experience alters brain function and structure. *Pediatrics, 113*(4), 846–858.

Als, H., Gilkerson, L., Duffy, F.H., McAnulty, G.B., Buehler, D.M., Vandenberg, K., et al. (2003). A three-center, controlled trial of individualized developmental care for very low birth weight preterm infants: Medical, neurodevelopmental, parenting, and caregiving effects. *Journal of Developmental & Behavioral Pediatrics, 24*(6), 399–409.

Bada, H.S., Korones, S.B., Perry, E.H., Arheart, K.L., Pourcyrous, M., Runyan, J.W., et al. (1990). Frequent handling in the neonatal intensive care unit and intraventricular hemorrhage. *Journal of Pediatrics, 117*(1, pt. 1), 126–131.

Barb, S.A., & Lemons, P.K. (1989). The premature infant: Toward improving neurodevelopmental outcome. *Neonatal Network, 7*(6), 7–15.

Broedsgaard, A., & Wagner, L. (2005). How to facilitate parents and their premature infant for the transition to home. *International Nursing Review, 52*, 196–203.

Browne, J.V. (2004). Early relationship environments: Physiology of skin-to-skin contact for parents and their preterm infants. In R.D. White (Ed.), *The sensory environment of the NICU: Scientific and design-related aspects. Clinics in Perinatology, 31*(2), 287–298.

Catlett, A.T., & Holditch-Davis, D. (1990). Environmental stimulation of the acutely ill premature infant: Physiological effects and nursing implications. *Neonatal Network, 8*(6), 19–26.

Cole, J.G. (1985). Infant stimulation reexamined: An environmental- and behavioral-based approach. *Neonatal Network, 3*(5), 24–31.

Evans, J.C. (1991). Incidence of hypoxemia associated with caregiving in premature infants. *Neonatal Network, 6*(5), 23–28.

Feldman, R., Eidelman, A.I., Sirota, L., & Weller, A. (2002). Comparison of skin-to skin (kangaroo) and traditional care: Parenting outcomes and preterm infant development. *Pediatrics, 110*(1), 16–26.

Ferber, S.G., & Makhoul, I.R. (2004). The effect of skin-to-skin (kangaroo care) shortly after birth on the neurobehavioral responses of the term newborn: A randomized, controlled trial. *Pediatrics, 113*(4), 858–865.

Field, T.M., Schanberg, S.M., Scafidi, F., Bauer, C.R., Vega-Lahr, N., Garcia, R., et al. (1986). Tactile/kinesthetic stimulation effects on preterm neonates. *Pediatrics, 77*(5), 654–658.

Glass, P., Avery, G.B., Subramanian, K.N.S., Keys, M.P., Sostek, A.M., & Friendly, D.S. (1985). Effect of bright light in the hospital on incidence of retinopathy of prematurity. *New England Journal of Medicine, 313*, 401–404.

Graven, S.N. (2004). Early neurosensory visual development of the fetus and newborn. In R.D. White (Ed.), The sensory environment of the NICU: Scientific and design-related aspects. *Clinics in Perinatology, 31*(2), 199–216.

Gray, L., & Philbin, M.K. (2004). Effects of the neonatal intensive care unit on auditory attention and distraction. In R.D. White (Ed.), The sensory environment of the NICU: Scientific and design-related aspects. *Clinics in Perinatology, 31*(2), 243–260.

Hasselmeyer, E.C. (1964). The premature neonate's response to handling. *American Nursing Association, 1*, 15–24.

Herer, G.R., Knightly, C.A., & Steinberg, A.G. (2007). Hearing: Sounds and silences. In M.L. Batshaw, L. Pellegrino, & N.J. Roizen (Eds.), *Children with disabilities* (6th ed., pp. 157–183). Baltimore: Paul H. Brookes Publishing Co.

Johnson, B.H., Abraham, M.R., & Parrish, R.N. (2004). Designing the neonatal intensive care unit for optimal family involvement. In R.D. White (Ed.), The sensory environment of the NICU: Scientific and design-related aspects. *Clinics in Perinatology, 31*(2), 353–382.

Katz, V. (1971). Auditory stimulation and developmental behavior of the preterm infant. *Nursing Research, 20*, 196–201.

Kimble, C., & Dempsey, J. (1992). Nonnutritive sucking: Adaptation and health for the neonate. *Neonatal Network, 11*(2), 29–33.

Korner, A.F., Kraemer, H.C., Haffner, M.E., & Cosper, L.M. (1975). Effects of waterbed flotation on premature infants: A pilot study. *Pediatrics, 56*, 361–367.

Kramer, L.I., & Pierpont, M.D. (1976) Rocking waterbeds and auditory stimuli to enhance growth of preterm infants. *Journal of Pediatrics, 88*, 297–299.

LaRossa, M.M., & Brown, J.V. (1982). Foster grandmothers in the premature nursery. *American Journal of Nursing, 82*, 1834–1835.

Leib, S.A., Benfield, D.G., & Guidubaldi, J. (1980). Effect of early intervention and stimulation of the preterm infant. *Pediatrics, 66*, 63–90.

Lester, B.M., & Tronick, E. (Eds.). (1990). Introduction: Guidelines for stimulation with preterm infants. *Clinics in Perinatology: Stimulation and the Preterm Infant, 17*(1), xiii–xvii.

Miller, M.M., & Menacker, S.J. (2007). Vision: Our window to the world. In M.L. Batshaw, L. Pellegrino, & N.J. Roizen (Eds.), *Children with disabilities* (6th ed., pp. 137–155). Baltimore: Paul H. Brookes Publishing Co.

Neal, M. (1968). Vestibular stimulation and the development behavior of the small premature infant. *Nursing Research Reports, 3*, 2–5.

Pergolizzi, J. (2007, September 26). *Care of newborns in the neonatal intensive care unit.* Unpublished lecture delivered at Syracuse University, School of Education, Syracuse, NY.

Rais-Bahrami, K., & Short, B.L. (2007). Premature and small-for-dates infants. In M.L. Batshaw, L. Pellegrino, & N.J. Roizen (Eds.), *Children with disabilities* (6th ed., pp. 107–122). Baltimore: Paul H. Brookes Publishing Co.

Rivkees, S.A. (2004). Emergence and influences of circadian rhythmicity in infants. In R.D. White (Ed.), The sensory environment of the NICU: Scientific and design-related aspects. *Clinics in Perinatology, 31*(2), 217–228.

Scafidi, F.A., Field, T.M., Schanberg, S.M., Bauer, C.R., Tucci, K., Roberts, J., et al. (1990). *Infant Behavior and Development, 10*, 199–212.

Segal, M.V. (1972). Cardiac responsivity to auditory stimulation in preterm infants. *Nursing Research, 21*, 15–19.

Shepley, M.M. (2004). Evidence-based design for infants and staff in the neonatal intensive care unit. In R.D. White (Ed.), The sensory environment of the NICU: Scientific and design-related aspects. *Clinics in Perinatology, 31*(2), 299–311.

Solkoff, N., & Matuszak, D. (1975). Tactile stimulation and behavioral development among low birthweight infants. *Child Psychiatry and Human Development, 6*, 33–39.

Westrup, B., Kleberg, A., von Eichwald, K., Stjernqvist, K., & Lagercrantz, H. (2000). A randomized, controlled trial to evaluate the effects of the newborn individual developmental care and assessment program in a Swedish setting. *Pediatrics, 105*(1), 66–72.

White, R.D. (Ed.). (2004). The sensory environment of the NICU: Scientific and design-related aspects. *Clinics in Perinatology, 31*(2), 199–393.

CHAPTER 14

The Management of Pain in Infants and Young Children

Susan Arana Furdon

At the conclusion of this chapter, the reader will

- *Understand the history of pain management for newborns in neonatal intensive care units (NICUs) in the United States*

- *Understand some of the myths surrounding pain management for newborns*

- *Be knowledgeable about some of the research-based evidence for pain management for newborns*

- *Understand some of the challenges and contemporary approaches to pain management for critically ill newborns*

- *Understand some of the developmental consequences of newborn exposure to pain*

Newborn pain is a complex clinical problem. The impact of the high-risk environment of the neonatal intensive care unit (NICU) on the newborn is just beginning to be defined in research. Exposure to painful procedures and therapy in the newborn period and the effect on the developing brain influences a child's response to future painful events. The challenge of adequate pain assessment and management in the NICU has significant implications for infants leaving the NICU for an outpatient setting.

Pain is an unpleasant sensory or emotional experience associated with actual or potential tissue damage. Pain is whatever the person experiencing pain says it is, and it exists whenever that person says it does (Bonica, 1979; Merskey, 1980). This definition of pain, described by the International Association for the Study of Pain (Bonica, 1979), was formulated within an adult model. Traditionally, pain is defined in the con-

text of the adult framework. It is subjective, and it is based on emotions, beliefs, verbal communication, and previous experiences with pain.

Neonatal care developed its roots in the 1960s. The birth, transport to Boston, and death of President Kennedy's son at the gestational age of 34 weeks spotlighted the issue of prematurity in the United States. In the subsequent decades, technology advanced, and the survival of premature infants increased. The physiological instability of the newborn in the intensive care unit necessitated various painful, invasive procedures. Research related to pain assessment and management of pain during these procedures lagged behind advances in technology. The vulnerability of this premature or critically ill newborn population was identified. An initial understanding of the anatomy and physiology of the brain related to pain came via laboratory research conducted in the 1980s. Research has since focused on identifying a standardized approach to the assessment of neonatal pain as a basis for determining the effectiveness of preventative and treatment strategies of pain in the clinical setting. The impact of the extrauterine environment (the NICU) and the long-term sequelae of repetitive pain on this vulnerable population continue to be investigated.

This chapter provides an overview of the evidence relating to the assessment of neonatal pain and the contemporary clinical approach to pain management in the neonatal intensive care setting. Effective strategies and barriers toward management of neonatal pain are identified. Short-term and long-term effects of pain in infants who had been in the NICU are also described.

Dispelling Myths About Pain

Traditional beliefs about pain affect our recognition of pain and approach to pain management in newborns. Certainly, adults and verbal children have the ability to verbalize their pain and rate the intensity of the experience. Children are reliable reporters of their own pain by age 5 (Bieri, Reeve, Champion, Addicoat, & Ziegler, 1990; Varni, Walco, & Katz, 1989). Instead of verbal expression of pain, preverbal children exhibit their pain through expressive behavior and subjective, complex physiological responses (Craig, Whitfield, Grunau, Linton, & Hadjistavropoulos, 1993; Grunau & Craig, 1987; Stevens & Johnston, 1994). The health care worker must recognize physiological indicators and provide a systematic observation of behaviors. Preverbal children rely on the recognition of pain responses by the caregiver.

Although painful procedures often can be reduced in a coordinated health care environment, complete elimination of these procedures is not possible. Newborns are regularly exposed to painful procedures in order to evaluate their responses to treatment (e.g., blood draws for blood gas determination after ventilator changes); to determine a diagnosis (e.g., lumbar puncture to culture cerebrospinal fluid); or to treat an illness (e.g., chest tube for a pneumothorax) (see Table 14.1).

The beliefs, experience, and techniques used by nurses and medical staff have an effect on the pain assessment and management practices utilized in their daily practice. Appropriate pharmacological measures and nonpharmacological measures to minimize pain during these procedures often are underutilized and inconsistent, despite the understanding that the procedures are painful (Franck, 1991, 1992; Porter, Wolf, Gold, Lotsoff, & Miller, 1997; Simons, van Dijk, Anand, et al., 2003).

Explanations for undertreatment of neonatal pain include incorrect assumptions (myths) by the health care provider. Scientific evidence is essential in undermining the myths that lead to attitude formation (Porter, 1989; Schechter, 1989; Schuster & Lenard, 1990). Since the 1980s, clinical and laboratory research has focused on dispelling three major myths related to neonatal pain:

1. Infants do not feel pain.

2. Infants cannot respond to pain.

3. Infants cannot remember pain.

Notable in the initial advances to our understanding of neonatal pain was anesthesiologist Dr. Sunni Anand. His research provided the foundation for fetal and neonatal pain research that followed. His research specifically dispelled the myth that infants have a nervous system that is too immature to experience pain so therefore they do not feel pain. Neurophysiological pathways from the peripheral receptors to the cerebral cortex for feeling pain are developed even in premature newborns (Anand & Carr, 1989; Anand & Hickey, 1987; Anand, Sippell, & Aynsley-Green, 1987). Important neurodevelopmental milestones occur in the second trimester between the gestational ages of 20 and 25 weeks; yet, extremely low birth weight infants are born and survive during this vulnerable period. These milestones include development of nociceptive receptors, which allow the ability to feel through the skin. Nociceptive receptors are one of the first fibers to grow in the spinal cord. A fetus is capable of feeling pain by the gestational age of 20 weeks (Anand & Hickey, 1987). Electroencephalograms (EEG) and ultrasounds can differentiate

Table 14.1.   Painful procedures that newborns may experience during the course of medical care

Procedure	Description	Purpose
Heel lance	Puncture of the lateral aspect of the newborn's heel	Laboratory testing of blood is necessary to guide the clinical management of the newborn
Vascular Access	Insertion of a catheter into a vein or an artery; some catheters are sutured in place	Provides mechanism for intravenous fluid management and/or withdrawing blood for testing
Chest tube	Flexible tube inserted into the chest between the ribs and pleural cavity, a space that enfolds the lungs; tube is secured with sutures for several days before being removed	Drains blood, fluid, or air and allows the lungs to fully expand
Lumbar puncture	Needle temporarily placed between third and fourth lumbar vertebrae into cerebral spinal column	Withdraws cerebral spinal fluid for the purpose of diagnostic testing for infection
Bladder aspiration	Needle inserted into the skin and then the bladder	Withdraws urine for the purpose of diagnostic testing for infection
Intubation	Insertion of an endotracheal tube into the trachea; tube can be required for a short period or for months	Provides mechanism for providing for mechanical ventilation when lungs are immature or have disease
Suctioning	Temporary insertion of a catheter into the endotracheal tube	Provides means to withdraw secretions from the endotracheal tube/prevents occlusion of the endotracheal tube
Insertion of gastric tube	Tube inserted through the mouth or nose, down the esophagus, and into the stomach; generally left in place for a day or a week	Feeds a premature infant who is unable to coordinate suck and swallow coordination; coordination generally occurs around 32–34 weeks of gestation
Removal of tape	Reinsertion of tubes results in replacement of tape; premature skin is very fragile and removal of tape easily removes several layers of skin, resulting in excoriation	Resecures devices (tubes and drains) that provide necessary, life-saving services
Circumcision	Removal of penile foreskin	Surgically excises foreskin due to religious, cosmetic, or sanitary considerations
Immunization	Injection subcutaneously or into the muscle	Creates immunity again a specific disease

sleep–wake cycles and responses to touch and sound at this gestational age (Bhutta & Anand, 2002). By 28 weeks of gestation, the density of the nociceptive nerve endings in the skin is similar to that of the adult (Humphrey, 1964). After that time, the density of the nerve endings becomes greater than the adult's until 2 years of age. Pain fibers are unmyelinated (without a fatty sheath) until the gestational age of 30 weeks. Myelination was originally believed to have an impact on the conduction of the pain impulse, but it is now known that impulses travel well along unmyelinated nerve tracks (Coskun & Anand, 2000). Myelination of the brain stem and along the nerve tracks in the spinal cord is complete by 37 weeks of gestation. This increases the speed of the sensory input to the brain (Gilles, Shankle, & Dooling, 1983).

During this critical period, the anatomic foundation (prerequisites) for functional maturity develops (Schuster & Lenard, 1990). Neuronal migration, a step in brain development, is essential in moving the appropriate types of cells to the appropriate section of the brain. This process is the cornerstone of our ability to think and respond as humans (Anand & Hickey, 1987).

During the same period, in Boston, another pioneer in neonatal behavioral care, Heidelise Als provided evidence that the developing central nervous system was vulnerable to the environmental influences of care, which are pain, noise, lighting, and sensory overload (Als et al., 1994). The process of being born at an early gestational age does alter the infant's brain physiology so that it cannot be compared to the brain that develops in utero in a protected environment. Adverse environmental experiences including repetitive or prolonged pain can result in neuronal injury at a vulnerable time in development (Bhutta & Anand, 2002).

Subsequent clinical research attempted to describe neonatal responses to pain. These studies provide the framework for the development of standardized assessment tools to be used in the clinical arena (Craig et al., 1993; Grunau & Craig, 1987; Johnston & Stevens, 1990; Johnston & Strada, 1986). Infants do respond to pain with a physiological response (i.e., an increase in heart rate, an increase in blood pressure, a decrease in oxygen saturation); a hormonal response (i.e., an increase in catecholamine, cortisol); a metabolic response (e.g., an increase in glucose, a breakdown in protein); and a behavioral response (e.g., crying, change in tone and facial features) (Anand & Hickey, 1987).

Pain is subjective and complex and has an impact on the health care worker's belief in the patient's claim to pain. Standardized neonatal assessment tools were developed based on observed pain responses to reduce that subjectivity. This framework defines pain in ways that the health care worker can understand by translating physiological responses and behaviors into an adult scoring tool that rates pain on a scale from 0 to 10. Initial research was done to establish the validity and reliability of various assessment tools. Clinical utility for use in the intensive care units also was determined. The research provides straightforward evidence that the gestational age of the infant has an impact on his or her ability to respond. Not all assessment tools include this variable within the scoring tool, which limits the reliability of tools that do not include gestational age as a variable (Puchalski & Hummel, 2002; Stevens, Johnston, & Horton, 1993). Another major concern in the clinical arena is the infant who is too clinically ill to respond at all. Currently, there is no single tool utilized that provides a gold standard for pain assessment in the NICU (Duhn & Medves, 2004).

Most tools were validated in acute pain models. Tools related to chronic disease states in the neonatal period have yet to be developed. Despite these limitations, it is important for each institution to adopt a standardized assessment tool in order to provide a uniform approach when discussing infant pain (Furdon, Pfeil, & Snow, 1998).

Approaches to Infant Pain Management

In the early decades of neonatology, limiting or avoiding narcotics was the only safe and practical way for surgery. The belief in the underdeveloped cortex was compounded by limited pharmokinetic data related to the use of opioids in premature infants (Koren et al., 1985; Schuster & Lenard, 1990). Minimal analgesics and the use of muscle relaxants or neuromuscular blocking agents (i.e., paralyzing agents) were the mechanisms in accomplishing surgery in the premature infant during the 1960s and 1970s.

Research defined the physiological and philosophical rationale for safety in narcotic analgesia in infants. Higher hormonal and metabolic stress responses and higher rates of complications and mortality were noted in infants with analgesia as compared to those not given analgesia (Fisher, Robinson, & Gregory, 1982; Robinson & Gregory, 1981). Morphine was often used for its analgesic potency and sedative effect. Maintenance of blood pressure stability was possible. Adverse effects (e.g., apnea and decreased blood pressure) could be reversed or minimized with dose reduction, slower administration, and adequate monitoring. It was further shown that a steady plasma concentration with a constant infusion provided the best relief in the presence of pain and resulted in the fewest side effects (Hester & Foster, 1993; Lynn, Nespeca, Bratton, & Shen, 2000). There were no data that indicated that children were more susceptible to adverse effects of respiratory depression than adults. This research led to the current pain management approach in the care of acute ongoing pain, usually in the postoperative period.

Acetaminophen (Tylenol) is an appropriate drug for dull, continuous pain that results from inflammatory conditions (e.g., circumcision or immunizations). Concerns regarding potential toxicity in preterm and term infants are not supported in the literature (Bhatt-Mehta & Rosen, 1991; Jacqz-Aigrain & Anderson, 2006). Acetaminophen evidence supports the positives because if given 2 hours prior to a circumcision, it decreases crying time during skin excision and improves postprocedure comfort scores. Around the clock administration of acetaminophen for 24 hours after the procedure improved feeding behavior and sleep–wake cycles (Howard, Howard, & Weitzman, 1994; Taddio, 2001).

Analgesics for painful procedures include the application of eutectic mixtures of local anesthetics (EMLA) and buffered lidocaine (i.e., lidocaine attenuated with sodium bicarbonate to remove the stinging sensation). Approved in the mid-1990s, EMLA is a topical anesthetic for superficial cutaneous and medical procedures (Taddio, Stevens et al., 1997). Buffered lidocaine can provide an effective local anesthetic for chest tube insertion and lumbar puncture and does not have an adverse impact on the success rate of the procedure (Pinheiro, Furdon, & Ochoa, 1993).

A consensus statement published in 2001 provided an evidenced-based guideline for prevention or treatment of pain and adverse consequences related to specific procedures (Anand,

2001). Strategies that support implementation of these research-based guidelines in the NICU are outlined in Table 14.2.

On average, each newborn in the NICU has 14 painful procedures per day (Simons et al., 2003). Included in these procedures were intubation, endotracheal suctioning, nasal-gastric tube insertion, intravenous insertion, venipuncture, and chest tube insertion. A 23-week gestational age infant is likely to have, on average, 488 procedures during his or her initial hospitalization (Johnston, Collinge, Henderson, & Anand, 1997; Simons et al., 2003).

A main source of procedural pain in the newborn period is the process of intubation, which is placing a tube into the trachea for the purpose of ventilating the infant. Adults and children are routinely medicated for this procedure. In the past, premedication for newborns was relatively uncommon. The manual for physicians in training, *The Harriet Lane Handbook*, states that "medications should be used for sedation prior to

Table 14.2.   Evidence-based strategies for improved amelioration of pain in the neonatal intensive care unit

Strategy	Purpose
Multidisciplinary staff education	Provide information on relevant topics: Neurophysiology of pain Assessment in the preverbal patient Nonpharmacological treatment Analgesics Adjunctive treatment
Parent/family education	Address fears and lack of knowledge Encourage parents to be advocates and fully participate in care
Development of written population-specific protocol	Standardize pain assessment: Define minimum frequency of assessment Define uniformity of approach (tool) Standardize approach to pain management procedures and postoperative procedures Use preemptive analgesia (when pain is expected, provided appropriate pretreatment) Recognize that procedures hurt, organize care, and coordinate required testing to minimize their frequency Standardize approach to pain management in the postoperative period Standardize documentation standards Standardize reportable conditions related to pain response (i.e., nursing communication to medical team for predetermined pain score)
Discussion of pain daily on interdisciplinary rounds	Cultivate a climate for collegial discussion Utilize resources as consults—pharmacist, clinical nurse specialist, anesthesiologist, and intensivist
Quality improvement initiatives	Define and discuss strategies to improve compliance with the standards within the multidisciplinary team Define the process of patient advocacy within the institution

Sources: Anand et al. (2006); The Joint Commission (2008); Schechter, Blankson, Pachter, Sullivan, & Costa (1997); Schmidt, Holida, Kleiber, Petersen, & Phearman (1994).

intubation except in the unconscious or the new-born" (Soileau-Burke, 2002, p. 3). Research now shows that premedication for intubation minimizes hypertension and tachycardia, decreases pain, decreases intracranial pressure, and there is less time required for the procedure and fewer attempts made (Barrington & Byrne, 1998; Marshall, Deeder, Pai, Berkowitz, & Austin, 1984; Oei, Hari, Butha, & Lui, 2002). Administration of an analgesic prior to elective intubation is now the standard (Anand, 2001).

The best approach for minimizing pain is still undetermined. The best approach, once researched well in randomized controlled studies, can result in opposing conclusions. This is true of the approach to infants who are on a ventilator for prolonged periods. It was thought that the use of morphine or a sedative (i.e., midazolam) would be better than no analgesic or sedative in the long-term management of the infant on the ventilator. Many neonatal ICUs adopted this approach prior to its scientific study. In two research controlled trials, routine use of morphine infusions as a standard of care in the management of ventilated preterm newborns was not supported (Simons et al., 2003). It is thought that the effects of surgery without anesthesia, as well as anesthesia without surgery, may be equally detrimental to the developing brain (Anand et al., 2004). Thus, more is not always better, and we have to remain cautious as we proceed with new analgesics or nonevidence-based approaches. Randomized controlled trials are necessary to provide the health care arena with an evidence-based approach.

Health Care Workers' Attitudes, Beliefs, and Practices

The health care professional's knowledge and belief about the need for pain management strategies are more congruent with the scientific evidence than their actual utilization of pain management strategies in their practice (Porter, Wolf, Gold, Lotsoff, & Miller, 1997). Adoption of standards for the management of pain in hospi-

talized patients began with the publication of the Agency for Health Care Policy and Research (AHCPR) national guidelines in 1992 (Schmidt, Holida, Kleiber, Petersen, & Phearman, 1994). Inclusive in these guidelines were the following:

- The call for multidisciplinary involvement in the management of pain

- A standardized approach to the assessment of pain

- Clear documentation of assessment at regular intervals

- Development of a written protocol or policy or unit standard

- A systematic review of effectiveness of pain relief strategies

- Education of children and their families

- Utilization of family preferences when determining methods to use

- Development of a quality improvement program

These guidelines were the precursor to the Joint Commission on Accreditation of Healthcare Organizations (JCAHO) standards. A systematic approach to the assessment and management of pain in the hospitalized patient was mandated. The age of the patient could no longer be a factor in the decision not to treat pain (The Joint Commission, 2008). The institution is required to promote family involvement in all aspects of care, including decisions regarding pain management. Pain prevention and treatment needs to be a high priority in the patient's management, and JCAHO is committed to this as an outcome measure related to patient rights, patient satisfaction, patient outcome, and health care costs (Schechter, Blankson, Pachter, Sullivan, & Costa, 1997). A patient's pain has an impact on his or her ability to progress toward expected outcomes. For example, a newborn experiencing pain will limit movement, which has an impact on the mobilization of fluids and potentially increases his or her length of time on a ventilator. This will ultimately affect the length of time in the hospital and the cost of his or her health care.

Surveys of health care workers consistently have shown problems related to both underprescription and underadministration of medications. The adoption of a written multidisciplinary standard for care in a tertiary intensive care nursery offered staff the education and management expertise to provide a standardized approach to postoperative neonatal care. The use of morphine had been associated with a poor respiratory drive; thus, continuous infusions of morphine often were limited. Through a quality improvement initiative, data related to all infants who had abdominal surgery were collected during a 2-year period 1 year prior to initiation of continuous infusion of morphine postoperatively and 1 year after adoption of the standard. Despite a continuous infusion of morphine, this center demonstrated that postoperative infants were extubated (removed) from the ventilator an average of 20 hours earlier with the use of a continuous infusion of morphine (Furdon, Eastman, Benjamin, & Horgan, 1998).

Surveys of tertiary centers continue to indicate that pain management strategies are not consistently being utilized in these vulnerable patients (Porter et al., 1997). Preemptive analgesic therapy was provided in less than 35% of infants studied (Simons et al., 2003). Systematic assessment and documentation of pain by the medical care providers was noted to be the only significant predictor of postsurgical analgesic use across 10 participating NICUs. Postoperative pain in 14 Canadian NICUs was consistently treated, usually with opioid analgesics. Opioid or nonopioid analgesics were rarely given, however, for nonsurgical invasive procedures (Johnston et al., 1997).

Despite increased knowledge related to infant pain, pain management strategies continue to be implemented based on attitudes and perceptions. There are differences in perceptions of pain related to specific procedures among health care professionals. Generally speaking, the nurse (often the observer of the procedure) perceives that the procedure is more painful than the physician (who is doing the procedure and who can prescribe analgesics) (Simons et al., 2003). Gender was not discussed as a contributing factor. If the medical health care provider had a signifi-

cant past pain experience, they were likely to rate the painfulness of the procedures higher. This association was not noted among nurses (Page & Halvorson, 1991).

Reasons for not premedicating for a procedure include a lack of time or an inconvenience in waiting for medications to take effect. Education and lack of available information about pharmacological measures continue to be cited as contributing factors (Porter et al., 1997). Obstacles to nonpharmacological strategies also can be based on insufficient knowledge but additionally include the factor of time. Certainly the perception or reality of inadequate staffing and insufficient resources play a role in dedicating time to administer comfort measures (Porter et al., 1997).

Nonpharmacological strategies for pain reduction are effective in the management of pain during painful procedures, especially when behavioral strategies are provided in a consistent approach and when pharmacological strategies are added as needed, depending on the level of invasiveness (Franck & Lawhon, 2000). Rocking, swaddling, facilitated tucking (i.e., placing infant prone with legs drawn upward), and nonnutritive sucking are all proven methods of pain reduction (Campos, 1989; Corff, Seideman, Venkataramna, Lutes, & Yates, 1995). Swaddling following a heel stick in infants 27–34 weeks of gestational age immediately quiets crying infants, decreases their heart rate, and facilitates their return to sleep state (Fearon, Kisilevsky, Hains, Muir, & Tranmer, 1997; McIntosh, van Veen, & Brameyer, 1994). The same infants who were not swaddled after a heel stick took a minimum of 10 minutes to return to baseline physiological state levels (Fearon et al., 1997). Skin–skin (kangaroo) care has been shown to release endorphins due to closeness, warmth, and rhythmic breathing of the parent. Skin-to-skin care during a heel lance procedure is effective in decreasing the infant's pain response (Johnston et al., 2003).

Pediatric patients with chronic, severe pain found acupuncture treatment pleasant and helpful (Kemper et al., 2000). In the newborn period, complementary therapies of acupuncture, Reiki, and aromatherapy have not been extensively studied. Recently published evidence concluded that the use of a 5-minute gentle leg massage of the ipsilateral leg decreases pain responses to a heel stick in preterm babies as measured by a standardized assessment tool and heart rate (Jain, Kumar, & McMillan, 2006).

Parents

Consumers' involvement in their own health care has greatly focused and redirected parents' attention to pain and pain management in the intensive care nursery. In a recent survey of parents, they reported that their NICU infants experienced more pain than they expected. More than half were educated on how to comfort their newborns, but the parents still had unmet informational needs related to their infants' pain. In addition, they wished for more involvement in their infants' care (Franck, Cox, Allen, & Winter, 2004). Certainly information about an infant's condition and treatment is empowering. Bridging communication barriers with the medical and nursing staff provides a foundation for the parents' role of advocacy that is essential for their infants' care.

Long-Term Consequences

There is a growing body of evidence to support the likely long-term effects of pain on the newborn, which includes neurodevelopmental, cognitive, and behavior disabilities that manifest later in childhood and ameliorate future pain responses (Anand et al., 2006; Puchalski & Hummel, 2002). Research supports pain control for the management of current pain but also for the protection from future pain experiences (McClain & Kain, 2005).

Initial research on long-term consequences focused on the effect of pain management for circumcision on the infant boy's response to 2 and 4 month immunizations (Taddio, Goldbach, Ipp, Stevens, & Koren, 1995). The use of a topical anesthetic for circumcision attenuates the vaccination response. The research was replicated in a comparison of boys circumcised with an analgesic, boys circumcised without an analgesic, and uncircumcised boys with their responses to

vaccinations several months later (Taddio, Katz, Ilersich, & Koren, 1997). The conclusion was that infants remember the pain they experienced.

Conditioning and hypersensitivity responses were noted in infants exposed to repeated painful stimuli. Infants of diabetic mothers, who require frequent heel sticks for glucose monitoring, displayed behavior that indicated that they anticipated pain. Their facial expressions, body movements, and crying showed more intense pain responses than newborns not exposed to repeated heel lances (Taddio, Shah, Gilhert-MacLeod, & Katz, 2002). Pain has an impact on future pain responses, even in the smallest of patients. The number of invasive procedures that the extremely low birth weight infant experiences in the preceding 24 hours significantly predicts behavioral response (grimacing) when undergoing the next procedure (Grunau, Holsti, Whitfield, & Ling, 2000).

Research links pain sensitivity ratings and child temperament to early pain experiences (Grunau, Whitfield, & Petrie, 1994). Subsequent research concluded that former extremely low birth weight infants, at the age of 8–10 years, rated pictures of medical events as more painful (Grunau, Whitfield, & Petrie, 1998). Additional research determined that the behavioral reactions to pain decreased in children born prematurely, the more pain that the infant had initially experienced. This has enormous implications for factoring the history of prematurity into the assessment of pain of a formerly premature child because that child may not have changes in behavior that would provide the health care worker with the necessary information to treat pain. The same conclusion was reached after a case control study evaluating the tenderness threshold of adolescents born prematurely compared to those born at term. The former preterm adolescents had significantly more tender points and lower tender thresholds (girls more than boys), which displayed higher somatic pain sensitivity. Despite increased tenderness, most preterm children did not report pain or other symptoms (Buskila et al., 2003).

Children born prematurely and who have had multiple surgeries need a higher dose of analgesics when they have additional surgery

(Peters et al., 2005). This study, comparing children hospitalized at birth with those who did not require previous hospitalizations, concluded that changes in behavior persist after discharge from the hospital. These children had less facial expression of pain, but a statistically higher heart rate when compared to previously nonhospitalized children. The differences were more pronounced the more ill the newborn was at birth, the longer the infant was in the NICU, the more procedures the infant experienced, and the more morphine sulfate the infant received.

The stress hormones of premature infants at age 8 and 18 months were compared with fullterm infants at the same age. Repeated invasive procedures contribute to higher levels of stress hormones, including cortisol levels (Grunau, Holsti, & Peters, 2006). Prolonged exposure to cortisol has been shown to produce changes in the brain in areas responsible for learning and memory (Anand & Scalzo, 2000; de Kloet, Sibug, Helmerhorst, & Schmidt, 2005). The full implication of pain in the neonatal period is not understood. Continued research in this area is essential in providing accurate behavioral and pain assessments in children.

Challenges for Providing Care

Research has provided an understanding of pain during fetal and neonatal development and evidenced-based standards to manage pain in the newborn period. This information is not always effectively translated into routine clinical practice. The evidence supports the need for the medical community to be more responsive and sensitive in the management of pain in children. There continue to be barriers that prevent clinicians from using known, effective means of relieving pain (i.e., cognitive, attitudinal, and institutional barriers). There often is an inconsistency between knowledge and practice. The health care provider needs to use the evidenced-based conclusions within his or her own practice. Disseminating the research can help dispel the myths. How health care providers incorporate research into their practices is up to each one of them, as

professionals, to decide. Quality improvement activities surrounding pain management strategies are expected. Those initiatives help modify behaviors toward compliance to a unit pain management protocol. Ultimately, the responsibility of health care professionals is prevention, assessment, intervention, and advocacy related to pain.

Conclusion

Assessment and treatment of pain in children is an important part of pediatric practice. Despite the evolving body of evidence related to pain assessment and management of newborns, there are still vast gaps in knowledge. Chronic pain in children is one of those areas. A reported 75 million adults currently have chronic pain issues (DeAngelis, 2003). Those numbers will expand as more premature infants survive to adulthood. We need to be attentive to the cues of newborns and young children. If they say it hurts, then it does. Prevention of pain and effective treatment of pain are determinants in the long-term effects of pain. Long-term effects of analgesics utilized in the newborn period are unknown. We need to continue to be advocates for newborns in order to minimize painful procedures and provide adequate pharmacological and nonpharmacological pain management. JCAHO standards provide institutional support for the treatment of pain in all patient populations. Providing information to parents and including them in the care of their newborns is essential.

REFERENCES

Als, H., Lawhon, G., Duffy, F.H., McAnulty, G.B., Gibes-Grossman, R., & Blickman, J.G. (1994). Individualized developmental care for the very low birthweight preterm infant: Medical and neurofunctional effects. *Journal of the American Medical Association, 272,* 853–858.

Anand, K.J.S. (International Evidence-Based Group for Neonatal Pain). (2001). Consensus statement for the prevention and management of pain in the newborn. *Archives of Pediatric & Adolescent Medicine, 155,* 173–180.

Anand, K.J.S., Aranda, J.V., Berde, C.B., Buckman, S., Capparelli, E.V., Carlo, W., et al. (2006). Summary proceedings from the neonatal pain-control group. *Pediatrics, 117,* S9–S22.

Anand, K.J.S., & Carr, D.B. (1989). The neuroanatomy, neurophysiology and neurochemistry of pain, stress and analgesia in newborns and children. *Pediatric Clinics of North America, 36,* 795–822.

Anand, K.J.S., Hall, R.W., Desai, N., Shephard, B., Bergqvist, L.L., Young, T.E., et al. (2004). Effects of morphine analgesia in ventilated preterm neonates: Primary outcomes from the NEOPAIN randomized trial. *Lancet, 363,* 1673–1682.

Anand, K.J.S., & Hickey, P.R. (1987). Pain and its effects in the human neonate and fetus. *The New England Journal of Medicine, 317,* 1321–1329.

Anand, K.J.S., & Scalzo, F.M. (2000). Can adverse neonatal experiences alter brain development and subsequent behavior? *Biology of the Neonate, 77,* 69–82.

Anand, K.J.S., Sippell, W.G., & Aynsley-Green, A. (1987). Randomized trial of fentanyl anaesthesia in preterm neonates undergoing surgery: Effects on the stress response. *Lancet, 1,* 243–248.

Barrington, K.J., & Byrne, P.J. (1998). Premedication for neonatal intubation. *American Journal of Perinatology, 15,* 213–216.

Bhatt-Mehta, V., & Rosen, D.A. (1991). Management of acute pain in children. *Clinical Pharmacy, 10,* 667–684.

Bhutta, A.T., & Anand, K.J.S. (2002). Vulnerability of the developing brain: Neuronal mechanisms. *Clinics in Perinatology, 29*(3), 357–372.

Bieri, D., Reeve, R.A., Champion, G.D., Addicoat, L., & Ziegler, J.B. (1990). The Faces Pain Scale for the self assessment of the severity of pain experienced by children: Development, initial validation and preliminary investigation for ratio scale properties. *Pain, 41,* 139–150.

Bonica, J.J. (1979). The need for a taxonomy. *Pain, 6,* 247–248.

Buskila, D., Neumann, L., Zmora, E., Feldman, M., Bolotin, A., & Press, J. (2003). Pain sensitivity in prematurely born adolescents. *Archives of Pediatric & Adolescent Medicine, 157,* 1079–1082.

Campos, R.G. (1989). Soothing pain-elicited distress in infants with swaddling and pacifiers. *Child Development, 60,* 781–792.

Corff, K.E., Seideman, R., Venkataramna, P.S., Lutes, L., & Yates, B. (1995). Facilitated tucking: A nonpharmacologic comfort measure for pain in preterm neonates. *Journal of Obstetric, Gynecologic, & Neonatal Nursing, 24,* 143–147.

Coskun, V., & Anand, K.J.S. (2000). Development of supraspinal pain processing. In K.J.S. Anand, B.J. Stevens, & P.J. McGrath (Eds.), *Pain in neonates: Pain research and clinical management* (2nd ed., pp. 23–54). New York: Elsevier.

Craig, K.D., Whitfield, M.F., Grunau, R.V.E., Linton, J., & Hadjistavropoulos, H.D. (1993). Pain in the preterm neonate: Behavioural and physiological indices. *Pain, 52,* 287–299.

de Kloet, E.R., Sibug, R.M., Helmerhorst, F.M., & Schmidt, M.V. (2005). Stress, genes and mechanism of programming the brain for later life. *Neuroscience & Biobehavior Reviews, 29,* 271–281.

DeAngelis, C.D. (2003). Pain management. *Journal of the American Medical Association, 290,* 2480–2481.

Duhn, L.J., & Medves, J.M. (2004). A systematic integrative review of infant pain assessment tools. *Advances in Neonatal Care, 4,* 126–140.

Fearon, I., Kisilevsky, B.S., Hains, S.M., Muir, D.W., & Tranmer, J. (1997). Swaddling after heel lance: Age-specific effects on behavioral recovery in preterm infants. *Journal of Developmental and Behavioral Pediatrics, 18,* 222–232.

Fisher, D.M., Robinson, S., & Gregory, G.A. (1982). Additional causes of post-operative complications in premature infants. *Anesthesiology, 57,* 428–429.

Franck, L.S. (1991). Issues regarding the use of analgesia and sedation in the critically ill neonate. *AACN Clinical Issues, 2,* 709–719.

Franck, L.S. (1992). The influence of sociopolitical, scientific and technologic forces on the study and treatment of neonatal pain. *Advances in Nursing Science, 15,* 11–20.

Franck, L.S., Cox, S., Allen, A., & Winter, I. (2004). Parental concern and distress about infant pain. *Archives of Disease in Childhood: Fetal and Neonatal Edition, 89,* F71–F75.

Franck, L.S., & Lawhon, G. (2000). Environmental and behavioral strategies to prevent and manage neonatal pain. In K.J.S. Anand, B.J. Stevens, & P.J. McGrath (Eds.), *Pain in neonates: Pain research and clinical management* (2nd ed., pp. 203–216). New York: Elsevier.

Furdon, S.A., Eastman, M., Benjamin, K., & Horgan, M. (1998). Outcome measures after standardized pain management strategies in postoperative patients in the neonatal intensive care unit. *Journal of Perinatal & Neonatal Nursing, 12,* 58–69.

Furdon, S.A., Pfeil, V., & Snow, K. (1998). Operationalizing Donna Wong's principle of atraumatic care: Pain management protocol in the NICU. *Pediatric Nursing, 24,* 336–342.

Gilles, F.J., Shankle, W., & Dooling, E.C. (1983). Myelinated tracts: Growth patterns. In F.J. Gilles, A. Leviton, & E.C. Dooling (Eds.), *The developing human brain: Growth and epidemiologic neuropathology* (pp. 117–183). Boston: John Wright.

Grunau, R.V.E., & Craig, K.D. (1987). Pain expression in neonates: Facial action and cry. *Pain, 28,* 395–410.

Grunau, R.V.E., Holsti, L., & Peters, J.W.B. (2006). Long-term consequences of pain in human neonates. *Seminars in Fetal & Neonatal Medicine, 11,* 268–275.

Grunau, R.V.E., Holsti, L., Whitfield, M.F., & Ling, E. (2000). Are twitches, startles and body movements pain indicators in extremely low birthweight infants? *Clinical Journal of Pain, 16,* 37–45.

Grunau, R.V.E., Whitfield, M.F., & Petrie, J.H. (1994). Pain, sensitivity and temperament in extremely low birthweight premature toddlers and preterm and full term controls. *Pain, 58,* 341–346.

Grunau, R.V.E., Whitfield, M.F., & Petrie, J.H. (1998). Children's judgements about pain at age 8 to 10 years: Do extremely low birthweight (< or = 1000g) children differ from full birthweight peers? *The Journal of Child Psychology & Psychiatry, 39,* 587–594.

Hester, N.O., & Foster, R.L. (1993). Integrating pediatric postoperative pain management into clinical practice. *Journal of Pharmaceutical Care in Pain and Symptom Control, 1,* 5–34.

Howard, C.R., Howard, F.M., & Weitzman, M.L. (1994). Acetaminophen analgesia in neonatal circumcision: The effect on pain. *Pediatrics, 93,* 641–646.

Humphrey, T. (1964). Some correlations between the appearance of human fetal reflexes and the development of the nervous system. *Progress in Brain Research, 4,* 93–135.

Jacqz-Aigrain, E., & Anderson, B.J. (2006). Pain control: Non-steroidal anti-inflammatory agents. *Seminars in Fetal & Neonatal Medicine, 11,* 251–259.

Jain, S., Kumar, P., & McMillan, D.D. (2006). Prior leg massage decreases pain responses to heel stick in preterm babies. *Journal of Pediatric Child Health, 42,* 505–508.

Johnston, C.C., Collinge, J.M., Henderson, S.J., & Anand, K.J.S. (1997). A cross-sectional survey of pain and pharmacological analgesia in Canadian neonatal intensive care units. *Clinical Journal of Pain, 13,* 308–312.

Johnston, C.C., & Stevens, B. (1990). Pain assessment in newborns. *Journal of Perinatal & Neonatal Nursing, 4,* 41–52.

Johnston, C.C., Stevens, B., Pinelli, J., Gibbins, S., Filion, F., Jack, A. et al. (2003). Kangaroo care is effective in diminishing pain response in preterm neonates. *Archives of Pediatric & Adolescent Medicine, 157,* 1084–1088.

Johnston, C.C. & Strada, M.E. (1986). Acute pain response in infants: A multidimensional description. *Pain, 24,* 373–382.

The Joint Commission. (2008). *Health care issues: Pain management.* Retrieved April 21, 2008, from www.jointcommission.org/NewsRoom/health_ca re_issues.htm#9

Kemper, K.J., Sarah, R., Silver-Highfield, E., Xiarhos, E., Barnes, L., & Berde, C. (2000). On pins and needles? Pediatric pain patients' experience with acupuncture. *Pediatrics, 105,* 941–947.

Koren, G., Butt, W., Chinyanga, H., Soldin, S., Tan, Y.K., & Pape, K. (1985). Postoperative morphine infusion in newborn infants: Assessment of disposition characteristics and safety. *Journal of Pediatrics, 107,* 963–967.

Lynn, A.M., Nespeca, M.K., Bratton, S.L., & Shen, D.D. (2000). Intravenous morphine in postoperative infants: Intermittent bolus dosing versus targeted continuous infusion. *Pain, 88,* 89–95.

Marshall, T.A., Deeder, R., Pai, S., Berkowitz, G.P., & Austin, T.L. (1984). Physiologic changes associated with endotracheal intubation in preterm infants. *Critical Care Medicine, 12,* 501–503.

McClain, B.D., & Kain, Z.N. (2005). Procedural pain in neonates: The new millennium. *Pediatrics, 115,* 1073–1075.

McIntosh, N., van Veen, L., & Brameyer, H. (1994). Alleviation of the pain in heel prick in preterm infants. *Archives of Disease in Childhood: Fetal & Neonatal Edition, 70,* F177–F181.

Merskey, H. (1980). Some features of the history of the idea of pain. *Pain, 9,* 3–8.

Oei, J., Hari, R., Butha, T., & Lui, K. (2002). Facilitation of neonatal nasotracheal intubation with premedication: A randomized controlled trial. *Journal of Paediatrics and Child Health, 38,* 146–150.

Page, G.G., & Halvorson, M. (1991). Pediatric nurses: The assessment and control of pain in preverbal infants. *Journal of Pediatric Nursing, 6,* 99–106.

Peters, J.W., Schouw, R., Anand, K.J.S., Van Dijk, M., Duvenvoorden, H.J., & Tibboel, D. (2005). Does neonatal surgery lead to increased pain sensitivity in later childhood? *Pain, 114,* 444–454.

Pinheiro, J.B., Furdon, S.A., & Ochoa, L. (1993). Role of local anesthesia during lumbar puncture. *Pediatrics, 91,* 379–382.

Porter, F.L. (1989). Pain in the newborn. *Clinics in Perinatology, 16,* 549–563.

Porter, F.L., Wolf, C.M., Gold, J., Lotsoff, D., & Miller, J.P. (1997). Pain and pain management in newborn infants: A survey of physicians and nurses. *Pediatrics, 100,* 626–632.

Puchalski, M., & Hummel, P. (2002). The reality of neonatal pain. *Advances in Neonatal Care, 2,* 233–244.

Robinson, S., & Gregory, G.A. (1981). Fentanyl-air-oxygen anesthesia for ligation of patent ductus arteriosus in preterm infants. *Anesthesia Analog, 60,* 331–334.

Schechter, N.L. (1989). The undertreatment of pain in children: An overview. *Pediatric Clinics of North America, 36,* 781–834.

Schechter, N.L., Blankson, V., Pachter, L.M., Sullivan, C.M., & Costa, L. (1997). The ouchless place: No pain, children's gain. *Pediatrics, 99,* 890–894.

Schmidt, K., Holida, D., Kleiber, C., Petersen, M., & Phearman, L. (1994). Implementation of the AHCPR pain guidelines for children. *Journal of Nursing Care Quality, 8,* 68–74.

Schuster, A., & Lenard, H.G. (1990). Pain in newborns and prematures: Current practice and knowledge. *Brain & Development, 12,* 459–465.

Simons, S.H., van Dijk, M., Anand, K.S., Roofthooft, D., van Lingen, R.A., & Tibboel, D. (2003). Do we still hurt newborn babies? A prospective study of procedural pain and analgesia in neonates. *Archives of Pediatric & Adolescent Medicine, 157,* 1058–1064.

Simons, S.H., van Dijk, M., van Lingen, R.A., Roofthooft, D., Daivenvoorden, H.J., Jongeneel, N., et al. (2003). Routine morphine infusion in preterm newborns who received ventilatory support: A randomized controlled trial. *Journal of the American Medical Association, 290,* 2419–2427.

Soileau-Burke, M. (2002). Emergency management. In V.L. Gunn & C. Nechyba (Eds.), *The Harriet Lane handbook* (16th ed., p. 3). St. Louis: Mosby.

Stevens, B.J., & Johnston, C.C. (1994). Physiological responses of premature infants to a painful stimulus. *Nursing Research, 43,* 226–231.

Stevens, B.J., Johnston, C.C., & Horton, L. (1993). Multidimensional pain assessment in premature infants: A pilot study. *Journal of Obstetric, Gynecologic, & Neonatal Nursing, 22,* 531–541.

Taddio, A. (2001). Pain management for neonatal circumcision. *Paediatric Drugs, 3,* 101–111.

Taddio, A., Goldbach, M., Ipp, M., Stevens, B., & Koren, G. (1995). Effect of neonatal circumcision on pain responses during vaccination in boys. *Lancet, 345,* 291–292.

Taddio, A., Katz, J., Ilersich, A.L., & Koren, G. (1997). Effect of neonatal circumcision on pain response during subsequent routine vaccination. *Lancet, 349,* 599–603.

Taddio, A., Shah, V., Gilbert-MacLeod, G., & Katz, J. (2002). Conditioning and hypersensitivy to pain in newborn infants exposed to repeated heel lances. *Journal of the American Medical Association, 288,* 857–861.

Taddio, A., Stevens, B., Craig, K., Rastogi, P., Ben-David, S., Shennan, A., et al. (1997). Efficacy and safety of lidocaine-prilocaine cream for pain during circumcision. *The New England Journal of Medicine, 336,*(17) 1197–120.

Varni, J.W., Walco, F.A., & Katz, E.R. (1989). Assessment and management of chronic and recurrent pain in children with chronic diseases. *Pediatrician, 16,* 56–63.

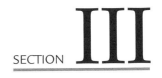

Families as the
Social Foundation
for Growing and Learning

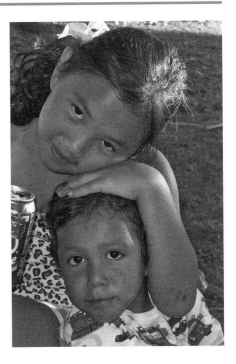

CHAPTER 15

Cultural Diversity

DIFFERENT WAYS OF LOOKING AT THE ROLES
OF FAMILIES, YOUNG CHILDREN, AND DISABILITY

Margo A. Nish and Gail L. Ensher

At the conclusion of this chapter, the reader will

- *Understand how families of varying cultures perceive issues of ability and disability in their young children*

- *Understand how diverse cultural perspectives of abilities and disabilities in young children can be addressed as best practice in early education*

- *Understand some of the challenges of working with families and young children of diverse cultures*

- *Understand how personnel working with families can be best prepared and trained to address differences across cultures*

As adults, we are undoubtedly products of our many environments. Who we are, what we believe, and how we respond to the world around us has been shaped by the influences of our life experiences. These experiences are as different and complex as we are as human beings.

The process of developing who we are is clearly rooted in how we are raised. Thus, an infant begins immediately to respond and develop in accordance with the feedback received in his or her environment. This environmental feedback generally comes from primary caregivers within the infant's family, and it varies from family to family due to the diversity of our culture. Indeed, the United States is becoming an increasingly diverse society. Based on a population clock maintained by the U.S. Census Bureau, the U.S. population as of February 24, 2008, was 303,496,765 (U.S. Census Bureau, 2006). In 2006, there were 4,265,996 births; 2,309,833 (54.15%) were to non-Hispanic whites, 617,220 (14.47%) were to non-Hispanic blacks, 47,494 (1.11%) were

to Asian Indians, 239,829 (5.62%) were to Asians, and 1,039,051 (24.36%) to Hispanics (U.S. Census Bureau, 2006). In keeping with the spirit of such diversity, Lynch and Hanson wrote,

As U.S. society has become more heterogeneous, cross-cultural effectiveness has emerged as an essential skill for all service providers who work with children and their families. The need to be cross-culturally competent is just as critical for neonatal intensive care nurses, social workers, or physicians in health care environments as it is for child care providers, educators, psychologists, physical therapists, occupational therapists, speech-language pathologists, and aides in educational environments. . . .

Because of the young age of the children, the issues on which families and professionals focus in providing services for infants, toddlers, and preschoolers are closely related to the family's values, beliefs, and traditions. The most basic issues—health care, sleeping, eating, regulating body states, building relationships, and exploring the environment—are central concerns for those who work with young children. They also are primary concerns for families and ones for which typically no "outside" interference takes place unless there has been some evidence of gross maltreatment. When a child has a disability, however, many outsiders may become involved with the child and family. The potential for conflict related to child-rearing practices thus emerges. Developing a respect for the values and beliefs of different cultures can help diminish these possible clashes. (2004, pp. 7–8)

Diversity and Family Viewpoints

The cultural construct of family is usefully defined as the intimate, interpersonal aspect of the sociocultural surroundings in which a person develops. A child is both profoundly influenced by and has a profound influence on those surroundings (Coople, 2003). For some children, this experience is a continuous, consistent one. For others, it is a discontinuous experience and may involve a complete change in the family. For most, membership changes over time.

The term family covers a large range of circumstances. How stable is it? Who decides who belongs? Are some people included by virtue of function who might not be included by designation? There are formal and informal kinship systems, any of which may provide the essential functions of the family. There are temporary caregivers who may provide many of those things expected of family or very few. Children with disabilities reside in all kinds of families and in all kinds of circumstances (Pawl & Milburn, 2006).

Family viewpoints, often rooted strongly in cultural perspectives, greatly influence how disability is acknowledged, viewed, discussed, and responded to beginning in infancy. Medical and educational professionals charged with caring for a child with a disability first must examine and understand these various family and cultural viewpoints. The development and implementation of an effective treatment plan is dependent on this understanding.

Beliefs regarding typical child development and differences in goals for children exist in large part due to societal expectations. These expectations are evidenced by the ways in which parents view and respond to characteristics and behavior across cultural groups. In Okagaki and Stern-

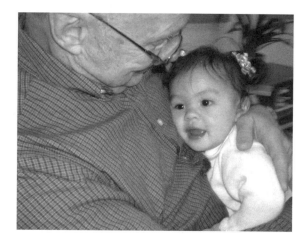

berg's 1993 study, developing obedience and conformity to external standards were rated as very important for children's development by parents from four immigrant groups—Cambodian, Filipino, Mexican, and Vietnamese. In fact, these qualities were considered by these immigrant parents to be far more important than the development of independent thinking and problem-solving skills.

Contrasting sharply, parents who were born in the United States identified the development of independent behaviors and creative thinking skills as most important in their children's development. Okagaki and Sternberg (1993) also examined parental beliefs across cultures relative to how "intelligent" behavior in children is judged. Latino parents ranked social skills as an indicator of a child's intelligence, whereas Filipino and Vietnamese parents identified motivation as a

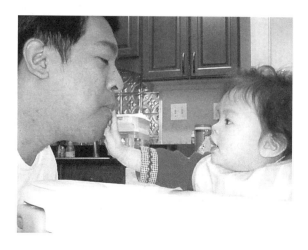

very important characteristic in determining intellectual abilities. The beliefs held by both of these groups contrast sharply with the Western psychological model of intelligence that embraces the identification and measurement of innate cognitive capabilities.

The contrast in these beliefs and expectations becomes even greater when we apply them to at-risk infants and children identified as having disabilities. The stresses faced by the parents of a child with a disability are incalculable. Depending on the severity of the disability and the time of diagnosis (i.e., in utero, at birth, in infancy, or in early childhood), many complex factors have an impact on the family who is ultimately responsible for the daily care of the child. Some parents fall victim to the "whose fault is it" pattern of coping and blame their behaviors for the child's disability. These may include the use of both legal and illegal substances (past or present); overconsumption of alcohol (past or present); work schedules and professional responsibilities; exercise regimes; prenatal nutrition; marital difficulties; or not arriving at the hospital early enough for adequate medical observation prior to delivery.

In some cultures, the presence of a child with a disability signals the influence of some higher power. The book *The Spirit Catches You and You Fall Down* (Fadiman, 1997) depicts such a scenario. A Hmong family of a young girl with a severe seizure disorder is in conflict with medical professionals caring for her. The doctors had prescribed medication that the family refused to give because they believed that the girl had embodied a powerful spirit. To the family, good fortune had been bestowed upon them through this child.

Given the fact that medical and educational professionals will encounter and play significant roles in the lives of young children and families who represent a myriad of diverse cultures, clearly the knowledge of and sensitivity to differing cultures is critical (Foley & Hochman, 2006). This is not to suggest the use of a "one size fits all" approach when working with young children and families from specific cultural groups, but rather to bring to the forefront the notion that cultural sensitivity has as its cornerstone the qualities of respect and appreciation.

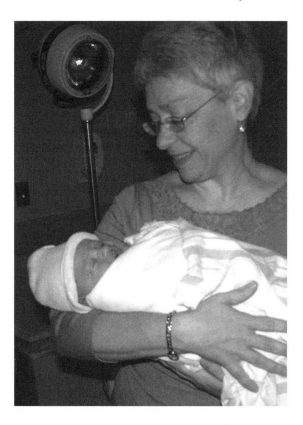

As discussed by Anderson and Fenichel (1989, as cited in Lynch and Hanson, 2004),

> Cultural sensitivity cannot mean knowing everything there is to know about every culture that is represented in a population to be served. At its most basic level, cultural sensitivity implies, rather, knowledge that cultural differences as well as similarities exist. . . . For those involved in early intervention, cultural sensitivity further means being aware of the cultures represented in one's state or region, learning about some of the general parameters of those cultures, and realizing that cultural diversity will affect families' participation in intervention programs. Cultural knowledge helps a professional to be aware of possibilities and to be ready to respond appropriately. (p. 5)

Places Where We Live, Learn, and Receive Services

The birth or adoption of a new baby always is a very emotional time for everyone involved. It forever changes an existing family structure and places many individuals in new relationships.

Parents become grandparents, new sets of couples or individuals become parents, and children gain siblings while their place within the family structure changes. Within many cultures, these changes resonate deeper and influence the relationships within large, multigenerational extended families. A new baby has some impact on each and every member of the family.

The addition of a child with a disability to a family brings a multitude of additional, significant issues that influence the family, as well as all professionals involved. Although knowledge of a child's disability prior to birth or adoption often allows a family to be connected with medical and early intervention and education services sooner, it also increases the number and variety of people who will have a significant impact on the family dynamics. In many situations, the delivery of these services begins in the hospital setting. Professionals must be attuned to and respectful of the many cultural factors that influence the ways in which families make medical choices. Many medical procedures, surgeries, and the use of particular drugs that are considered appropriate protocols may, in fact, be objectionable and forbidden by some families.

Early intervention and education services that are provided to an infant or young child with a disability and his or her family often take place in the home. Within every home is found the patterns, relationships, and unwritten rules that are unique to the particular family. These encompass beliefs about childrearing to include sleeping patterns, eating, toilet training, developmental milestones, and discipline. Each family and home setting also is unique in terms of leisure time activities, mealtimes, physical characteristics of the home, and interpersonal relationships. These patterns and characteristics, although very familiar and comfortable for the particular family, may seem unusual or feel uncomfortable to the early childhood provider. Differences of this type even exist between families and early intervention providers who share the same culture. These concerns are magnified many times over when cultural differences are added to the equation.

As young children with or without disabilities enter school environments for the first time,

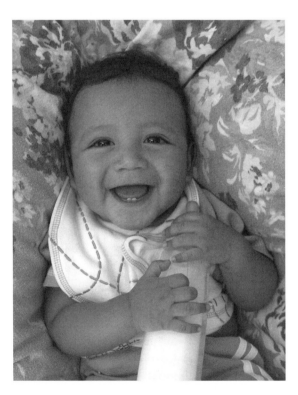

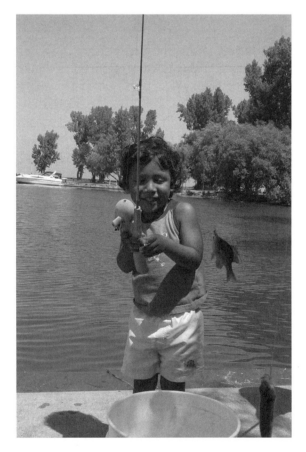

there are many factors that influence the success of this experience for children, families, and educators (Hanson & Lynch, 2003). Children interact with others and respond to the world around them according to what they have learned in their homes from their families. Parents arrive with expectations for their children, as well as conceptions about education that are based on all of their own prior school and life experiences.

Some parents view the relationship between themselves and educational professionals as a partnership. Other parents view the educational process as one that is conducted within the confines of the school and does not involve the home. It is incumbent upon educational professionals to assess family viewpoints regarding the educational setting and process in a sensitive manner. The method that is used to gain cultural, linguistic, family, and developmental information is extremely critical because this process forms the foundation of the relationship between the family and the educational professionals.

Undoubtedly, one of the first questions on a preschool educator's mind at the beginning of the school year is "Who are these children in my class?" Answering this question is complicated enough when there is a match between the cultural and linguistic backgrounds of the teacher and the children (Howard, 1999). When this is not the situation, the task of gaining information about the children may be even more complicated. A further case in point is the fact that there yet remains within the United States such a great divide or gap between largely Caucasian communities of early educators and populations of inner city multiracial groups of young children who reside with less than affluent families (Fadiman, 1997; Johnson, Gallagher, LaMontagne, Jordan, Gallagher, Hutinger, et al., 1994; Kuykendall, 1991; Ladson-Billings, 1994). Almost inevitably, there is much room for miscommunication and misunderstanding (McKracken, 1993; Payne, 1996; Yatvin, 2004).

Tabors (2008) detailed the following information-gathering framework that is useful for educators working with young children. It includes some guidelines for early childhood educators to use as benchmarks when initiating the process of

gathering information about children in an early childhood preschool education classroom.

Rule #1: Do not make any assumptions about a child's cultural or linguistic background without getting further information. This is clearly the starting point for any data-gathering activity and should apply equally to all of the children in a classroom. In the process of collecting information from the families, interesting and helpful characteristics may be discovered, such as other languages spoken or countries visited, that would otherwise never be known. . . .

Rule #2: Decide what information is important to know. If the primary interest is in collecting cultural and linguistic information, then there are certain categories of information that will be important as children move into the early childhood education situation. These include 1) basic demographic information, 2) linguistic practices in and outside of the home, and 3) relevant cultural practices. . . .

Rule #3: Plan how to get this information. This type of information can be collected via formal questionnaires, trips to the library, or searches on the Internet and/or informal chats with parents or other cultural representatives. In many situations, there is an intake interview when a family applies for admission to a preschool education program or a home visit is within the first few weeks of the school year. In either of these situations, basic demographic and linguistic information could be developed from questions asked at that time. If sitting down with the family to answer questions is not an option, sending home a questionnaire with demographic and linguistic questions is a possibility, but one that does not always yield results. If a questionnaire is sent home without response, it may be necessary to have someone with the appropriate linguistic skills visit or call the family to get the answers.

Information on cultural practices may be more difficult to acquire. One good starting point for the preschool educator is the library, where books on individual countries, religions, or linguistic groups might provide some insights and relevant background information. Books or magazine articles also provide historical information that might be important in understanding why a particular family has recently arrived in the community. . . .

Again, however, it is certainly helpful for a preschool educator to have the option of asking parents about their cultural practices. As one Head Start teacher remarked,

On the home visit paperwork, we have a form that the office wants anyway. What country are you from? What foods do you eat? Do you celebrate any holidays? But those, they don't get down to the behaviors and the traditions, the taking off the shoes things. For me, it depends on the parent a lot; if they seem like they're the willing kind, I'll come out and ask them.

The early childhood educator may also consider asking the parents to include him or her in a communitywide celebration, which could provide important cultural information as well as let the parents know that the educator values their cultural traditions and is interested in knowing more.

Rule #4: Think about using a variety of ways to get this information. Getting information from second-language families can be a challenge. One of the most basic hurdles is, of course, finding an effective way to communicate. Here are some suggestions.

First, face-to-face communication in the second language may be the most difficult for the parents. Face-to-face communication requires quick processing and formulation of a response in real time. This takes a relatively high level of proficiency in a language. It is important to remember that if face-to-face communication is used in a language that is a second language for the parents, the questions may be difficult for them to understand, and they may have difficulty putting together their answers. Therefore, if face-to-face communication is used, the same question should be asked more than once, using slightly different wording to confirm that consistent responses are being given.

Second, written communication in the parents' second language may give them a chance to read and respond in a way that is less pressured than face-to-face communication. Reading ability in a second language may be stronger than speaking ability. Furthermore, written communications can be shared with other members of the same first-language community who can read and write the second language. Parents with low levels of proficiency may seek out a translator to help complete a questionnaire. For this reason, it is important to remember that a completed questionnaire may not represent the actual language abilities of the parents but may represent their ability to recruit translation help when needed.

Third, communications that can be arranged in the parents' home language (either oral or written) likely will be the most comfortable for the parents. Many programs have parent liaisons that are bilingual in English and in one of the languages spoken by parents in the program. In this case, both written and oral communications can be translated into the home language, and responses can then be translated for the benefit of staff members who do not speak that home language. If a program does not have access to parent liaisons, it will be necessary to develop relationships with community members who can act as translators. Public schools, churches, community agencies, community newspapers, and even local grocery stores are good places to ask about translation services. . . . (pp. 86–89)

Addressing Diverse Cultural Perspectives in Early Education

As discussed in the introduction to this chapter, infants, young children, and, ultimately, adults are all products of our life experiences that begin with our family construct. Child-rearing practices within individual families invariably reflect the underpinnings of the cultural group with whom they identify. In addition, these child-rearing practices are heavily influenced by factors such as socioeconomic status and level of education. Second-language acquisition and the length of time a family has resided in the United States also greatly influence child-rearing practices (Handel, 1999).

The parenting of a child with special needs joins typical child-rearing issues with the added complexity of individual family and cultural views related to religion, medicine, and causes of disability. Providing medical and educational services to a child with a disability and his or her family requires an understanding of and sensitivity to the many ways in which the lives of each and every member of the family have been and will be affected.

Within our current educational system, parental or family involvement is mentioned with the same frequency as many core content areas. Parents are viewed as playing critical roles in the educational process. At the core of the philosophy for many programs is a commitment to parents, whose involvement is sought and encouraged. Within the arena of early intervention programs for infants and toddlers with disabilities, parental or family involvement is not simply encouraged, it is a legally mandated component. This goes beyond the parent acting as an advocate for particular services and requires that the parent has a role as a member of the intervention team. Specific language regarding this role is detailed in the Individuals with Disabilities Education Improvement Act (IDEA) of 2004 (PL 108-446).

The involvement of the parent or family in early intervention programs, for example, is facilitated through the development of an individualized family service plan (IFSP). The IFSP provides a vehicle through which all intervention and program goals, activities, and outcomes are constructed in a collaborative process, which involves the evaluation team members, service providers, the parent(s), and the child's case coordinator. The IFSP is a working document that is reviewed at regular intervals and revised to meet the changing needs of both the child and his or her family. It is the platform from which a child's early intervention program is launched and at all times requires parent and family involvement and agreement. Similar requirements are mandated in the development and implementation of individualized education programs (IEP) for young children.

Given that family involvement is essential to the early intervention process, an emphasis should be placed on the development of professional skills related to how family systems function across cultures. Beckman and colleagues (1984) outlined the following:

> It is clear that truly family-centered programs must consider the ways in which the entire family will be influenced by the decisions that are made. Second, intervention strategies must be flexible enough to accommodate diversity in family beliefs, values, functioning styles, as well as in the manner and intensity of family involvement. Third, families are dynamic units that change over time in multiple ways, such as in composition, priorities, strengths, and concerns. The intervention system must be flexible enough to respond to these changes on a continual basis. (p. 23)

As medical and educational professionals strive to understand and develop flexibility in responding to diverse family styles and cultures, it is essential to recognize that just as child-rearing practices differ across families and cultures, so do the ways in which disabilities are viewed. A common occurrence within the same cultures is that of individual families with vastly differing opinions related to disability and child rearing.

The effective early interventionist needs to take careful stock of and utilize such information in the development of relationships with family members and ultimately in the development and delivery of intervention and service plans. In all of these situations, it is important that the service provider (medical or educational) be familiar with different intervention options, but it is most important for the provider to be receptive to and as objective as possible about values and beliefs that may be in contrast to his or her own. The one caveat, of course, is related to life-saving medical procedures that may conflict with religious beliefs of the family (e.g., blood transfusions for a newborn) but without which the child would not survive. Despite this exception, Lynch and Hanson (2004) succinctly stated,

> A cardinal rule in working with all families is to make no assumptions about their concerns, priorities, and resources. This is even more critical when the family's cultural and socioeconomic background and identification are different from that of the service provider. However, becoming familiar with information about other cultures and life experiences and determining their relevance to individual families and family members can reduce the potential for tension between service providers and families from different cultural backgrounds. (p. 58)

It is through the understanding of and respect for each and every family's uniqueness that strong and effective programs for young children are built.

Language Difference or Disability?

This chapter would be remiss without a clear reference to those issues separating language differences from language disabilities in young children. Decisions, based on inaccurate and inappropriate assessment, for example, can have serious consequences without sensitive consideration of cultural contexts. In particular, Slentz and colleagues suggested the following potentially devastating results for young children in the assessment process (1997, p. 13; also cited in Ensher et al., 2007):

- Without knowledge of the demands and standards of the home environment, the young child's behaviors may be negatively misinterpreted.
- Typical developmental competence in other languages and cultures may be mistakenly identified as delay or disability.
- Preschoolers may receive special education services instead of more appropriate bilingual or culturally relevant interventions.
- Children may be wrongly identified as having developmental delays or disabilities if the expectations of the primary culture are different from the mainstream developmental standards reflected in evaluation instruments.
- Self-esteem can suffer if children perceive that their languages and cultures are devalued, considered inferior, or a disadvantage to development.
- Children may lose contact with immediate family if parents interpret results of evaluation and assessment as an indictment of their efforts to socialize their children in their own life-ways.
- In the long-term, educational, social, and vocational opportunities may be curtailed if children are labeled as having less potential for learning.
- Beneficial services may be overlooked if genuine disabilities/delays are masked or obscured by cultural differences.

Training for Best Practice

To gain an understanding of an individual family's unique beliefs and values about childrearing and disability, professional training must include sensitive and competent methods through which to gather needed, culturally sensitive in-

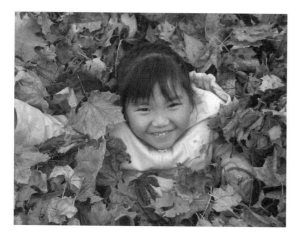

formation. Because infants and young children are dependent upon their families for survival, it is logical to begin the information-gathering process of an intervention program within the family setting. Barrera and Kramer (1997) commented on the complexity of learning about diverse cultures as follows:

> Promoting the development of the competencies needed to become culturally competent is not an easy task. Acquisition of these competencies often challenges all that lies at the core of how we define ourselves (e.g., worldviews, values). It also challenges the objective, mechanistic paradigm that generates our certainty that knowledge is something to be transmitted from teacher to learner rather than coconstructed between expert and novice (or, as is often the case with cultural competence, between novice and novice). (pp. 229–230)

Accordingly, these authors identified 12 essential competencies for nurturing and developing cultural sensitivities when working with diverse families and their young children. They suggested the need for the following (Barrera and Kramer, 1997, p. 232):

Knowledge and understanding

a. Of culture and cultural dynamics on a general level and as applied to self and others
b. Of cross-cultural research on diverse patterns of child rearing, developmental support, and teaching/learning in various cultural contexts
c. Of knowledge construction, paradigms, and diverse worldviews (e.g., "objective scientific," "social constructivist")
d. Of cultural diversity (i.e., definitions, components, impact on children's learning and development)
e. Of power and social positioning dynamics that affect behavior and performance across cultural boundaries
f. Of elements of effective teaching of children who are culturally and linguistically diverse
g. Of mediation as a tool for culturally responsive intervention

Abilities/skills

a. Reconsider one's role and understandings in light of different paradigms and cultural parameters
b. Locate early intervention within professional culture and community

c. Understand and respect children and family's understandings, especially when they differ significantly from my own

d. Creatively and collaboratively problem-solve with colleagues, families, and children to find best ways for bridging or mediating between understandings

e. Use these ways to mediate interactions and learning situations for children and communications and interactions with families.

Training students and practicing professionals to work with culturally diverse populations of families and their young children involves a multifaceted process. In the least, this will require

- Reading and learning about new value systems and how these might translate into behavior within U.S. cultures

- Knowledge of how families view receiving and accepting help and services from others

- Knowledge of how families perceive their own present needs and priorities in relationship to those of their child who may have special needs

- Knowledge of how families feel about unfamiliar people entering their homes

- Knowledge of ways in which families and professionals who may speak different languages might best communicate and dialogue with one another

- Understanding the significant people within families who may speak for others

Equally important, students and professionals always need to be reflective about their practices and maintain dialogue with their mentors and colleagues. Learning about other cultures is a lifelong process. One should not assume a philosophy that all people are alike, because within specific cultures and ethnic groups, families need to be viewed as individuals with their own sets of challenges and strengths.

Finally, throughout the course of interactions with families and growing to know individual family members, service providers must be mindful that they are working with the child's primary caregivers and teachers through whom services and early intervention take place. With-

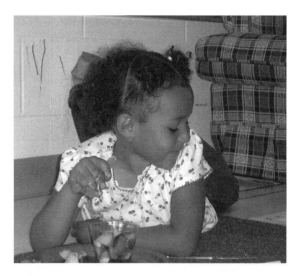

out their partnership and understanding, whatever professionals might offer will be less effective for the child. In the end, families hold the primary knowledge about their children and are in the most central position to carry out recommendations and suggestions made by others. Students and professionals must understand that the term family centered must be "lived" and practiced, no matter how differently approaches must be configured to accommodate difference across diverse cultural and ethnic groups.

Conclusion

Most professionals—physicians, teachers, social workers, and others—readily acknowledge the realities of the changing and increasingly diverse populations with whom they are called to interact and offer services. In so doing, there will be unique issues and situations to problem solve; for example, different ways of raising children, different values and priorities in terms of lifestyles, different perceptions of a child's abilities and disabilities, and different languages and interpretations.

Learning about difference is a challenging task because we inevitably turn back to our own ways of doing things and view particular situations from our own backgrounds that are more familiar and comfortable. In the long term, building relationships with families will be the key to successful intervention efforts, and these endeavors will require much more than knowing

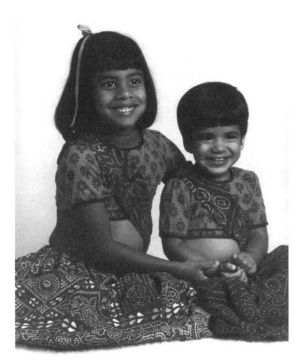

special holidays, foods, music, or other information that is interesting but not relevant to the task. This process will demand that both families and professionals meet in the middle when opening themselves to acceptance, respect, communication, and being willing to agree that there are different ways for accomplishing goals on behalf of a child. Genuine dialogue in which ownership is shared and participants admit to not knowing all of the answers is essential. Those qualities ultimately will sustain relationships across all cultures, regardless of the respective ethnic group or professional discipline.

REFERENCES

Anderson, P., & Fenichel, E. (1989). *Serving culturally diverse families of infants and toddlers with disabilities.* Washington, DC: National Center for Clinical Infant Programs.

Barrera, I., & Kramer, L. (1997). From monologues to skilled dialogues: Teaching the process of crafting culturally competent early childhood environments. In P.J. Winton, J.A. McCollum, & C. Catlett (Eds.), *Reforming personnel preparation in early intervention: Issues, models, and practical strategies* (pp. 217–251). Baltimore: Paul H. Brookes Publishing Co.

Beckman, P., et al. (1984). A transactional view of stress in families of handicapped children. In M. Lewis

(Ed.), *Social connections: Beyond the dyad.* New York: Plenum.

Copple, C. (Ed.) (2003). *A world of difference: Readings on teaching young children in a diverse society.* Washington, DC: National Association for the Education of Young Children.

Ensher, G.L., Bobish, T.P., Gardner, E.F., Reinson, C.L., Bryden, D.A., & Foertsch, D.J. (2007). *Partners in play: Assessing infants and toddlers in natural contexts.* Clifton Park, NY: Thomson Delmar Learning.

Fadiman, A. (1997). *The spirit catches you and you fall down.* New York: Farrar Straus Giroux.

Foley, G.M., & Hochman, J.D. (2006). *Mental health in early intervention: Achieving unity in principles and practice.* Baltimore: Paul H. Brookes Publishing Co.

Handel, R. (1999). *Building family literacy in an urban community.* New York: Teachers College Press.

Hanson, M.J., & Lynch, E.W. (2003). *Understanding families: Approaches to diversity, disability, and risk.* Baltimore: Paul H. Brookes Publishing Co.

Howard, G. (1999). *We can't teach what we don't know: White teachers, multiracial schools.* New York: Teachers College Press.

Individuals with Disabilities Education Improvement Act (IDEA) of 2004, PL 108-446, 20 U.S.C. §§ 1400 *et seq.*

Johnson, L.J., Gallagher, R.J., LaMontagne, M.J., Jordan, J.B., Gallagher, J.J., Hutinger, P.L., et al. (Eds.). (1994). *Meeting early intervention challenges: Issues from birth to three.* Baltimore: Paul H. Brookes Publishing Co.

Kuykendall, C. (1991). *From rage to hope: Strategies for reclaiming Black & Hispanic students.* Bloomington, IN: National Educational Service.

Ladson-Billings, G. (1994). *The dreamkeepers: Successful teachers of African American children.* San Francisco: Jossey-Bass.

Lynch, E.W., & Hanson, M.J. (Eds.). (2004). *Developing cross-cultural competence: A guide for working with children and their families* (3rd ed.). Baltimore: Paul H. Brookes Publishing Co.

McKracken, J. (1993). *Valuing diversity: The primary years.* Washington, DC: National Association for the Education of Young Children.

Okagaki, L., & Sternberg, R. (1993). Parental beliefs and children's school performance. *Child Development, 64,* 36–59.

Pawl, J.H., & Milburn, L.A. (2006). Family- and relationship-centered principles and practices. In G.M. Foley & J.D. Hochman (Eds.), *Mental health in early intervention: Achieving unity in principles and practice* (pp. 191–226). Baltimore: Paul H. Brookes Publishing Co.

Payne, R. (1996). *A framework for understanding poverty.* Highlands, TX: aha! Process.

Slentz, K., Lewis, G., Fromme, C., Williams-Appleton, D., Milatchkov, L., & Shureen, A. (1997). Evaluation and assessment in early childhood special education: Children who are culturally and linguistically diverse. In T. Bergeson, B.J. Wise, D.H. Gill, & A. Shureen (Eds.), *Special education . . . a service, not a place* (pp. 1–69). Olympia: Washington Office of State Superintendent of Public Instruction.

Tabors, P.O. (2008). *One child, two languages: A guide for early childhood educators of children learning English as a second language* (2nd ed.). Baltimore: Paul H. Brookes Publishing Co.

U.S. Census Bureau. (2006). *2006 American Community Survey data profile highlights.* Retrieved April 21, 2008, from http://factfinder.census.gov/servlet/ACSSAFFFacts?_submenuld=factsheet_0&_sse=on

Yatvin, J. (2004). *A room with a differentiated view: How to serve all children as individual learners.* Portsmouth, NH: Heinmann.

CHAPTER 16

The Cycle of Substance Abuse

Heidi Baldwin, Nancy S. Songer, and Gail L. Ensher

At the conclusion of this chapter, the reader will

- *Be knowledgeable about drug and alcohol abuse during pregnancy*

- *Understand some of the influences and factors that lead to addiction*

- *Become familiar with the various in utero and neonatal problems associated with exposure to drugs and alcohol*

- *Have an understanding of the challenges faced by children living in substance abusing homes*

- *Be knowledgeable about a variety of approaches to working with young children who have had in utero exposure to damaging, illegal, and toxic substances*

The prevalence of substance abuse (including alcohol, drugs, and tobacco) among women in America continues to be an alarming concern, especially in light of the fact that a percentage of these women are pregnant. Exposure to various substances in utero has been shown to cause irreparable damage to the developing fetus, which results in a variety of compromising situations for the newborn, ranging from low birth weight to severe birth defects. As these children grow, they may present with a range of learning disabilities and developmental delays that could have been prevented. In addition, the use and/or abuse of alcohol, drugs, and tobacco in the home (either by the maternal or paternal figure in the household) throughout the child's developing years creates additional adverse situations that may affect development.

Prevalence of Alcohol and Drug Use During Pregnancy

Alcohol use and abuse during pregnancy leads to an array of problems for the developing fetus, ranging from minor developmental delays to fetal alcohol syndrome (FAS). According to a report from the National Conference of State Legislatures (NCSL) at the January 2000 conference, "alcohol is the most commonly used addictive substance in the United States, and of the approximately 4 million women who give birth each year in the United States, 2.6 million use some amount of alcohol during their pregnancy." The report also cited that an estimated 22,000 children per year "experience mild, moderate, or severe adverse effects as a result of their mothers' alcohol ingestion" (Steinberg & Gehshan, 2000, p. 3). Educating people about the dangers of any alcohol consumption during pregnancy needs to be at the front of the campaign to improve this statistic.

With the overall number of Americans using cocaine increasing from 1.5 million in 1997 to 2 million in 2002, there is a significant increase in the number of potential childbearing women who are using this drug (Schiller & Allen, 2005). A 2002 report by the National Survey on Drug Use and Health (NSDUH) found that 3.3% of pregnant women ages 15–44 reported using illicit substances and 0.9% reported current use of cocaine (Schiller & Allen, 2005). Cocaine continues to be one of the most widely used illicit substances among pregnant women, second only to marijuana (Schiller & Allen, 2005).

The rates of illegal drug use among pregnant women have been more prevalent among those who are unmarried, have less than 16 years of formal education, are unemployed, and are on some form of public assistance. The same data indicated that although abuse of illegal substances has been more prevalent among African Americans in general, the rate of drug use among pregnant women has been much greater among white women than other ethnic groups. The use of legal drugs (specifically alcohol and cigarettes in this study) was highest among white women as compared to African American women and Hispanic women. The National Institute on Drug Abuse (NIDA; 2005b) also indicated that marijuana use is highest among pregnant women younger than 25 years of age, and the rate of cocaine use is higher among those who are 25 years of age or older.

Although findings suggest that this trend in overall drug use among different ethnic groups is shifting, marijuana continues to be the most widely used illicit drug among pregnant women of all ethnicities. The National Survey on Drug Use and Health study conducted by the Office of Applied Studies, Substance Abuse and Mental Health Services Administration (2005) indicated that greater numbers of pregnant African American women reportedly used illicit drugs more than their white or Hispanic peers. Cigarette use among pregnant white women continues to be

most prevalent. Figures 16.1, 16.2, 16.3, and 16.4 represent the most recently documented data on the trends of substance use among pregnant women. The term "past month" on these figures indicates the month prior to the survey, as reported by those in the survey. The survey also outlines the number of women who began using substances after delivering their children, as indicated by the "nonpregnant, recent mother" statistics in Figure 16.4.

There has not been as much research on the effects of prescription drug use and abuse among pregnant women as there has been on the prevalence of illegal drugs. Research findings by NIDA indicate that prescription drug abuse is on the rise in the United States, particularly among older adolescents and women. Citing the 2003 National Survey on Drug Use and Health (NSDUH), NIDA (2006c) reported that an estimated 4.7 million Americans used prescription drugs (including, in order of prevalence, pain relievers, tranquilizers, stimulants, and sedatives) nonmedically for the first time in 2002. They also stated that "in 2002, more than half (55 percent) of the new users were females, and more than half (56 percent) were ages 18 or older" (p. 1). Because the majority of these new users were of childbearing age, the possibil-

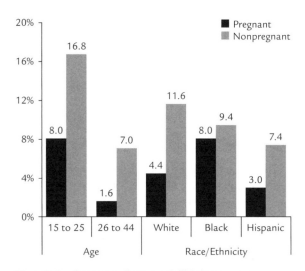

Figure 16.1.   Percentages of past month illicit drug use among women age 15–44, by pregnancy status, age, and race and/or ethnicity: 2002 and 2003. (From Office of Applied Studies, Substance Abuse and Mental Health Services Administration. [2005]. *The NSDUH report: Substance use during pregnancy: 2002 and 2003 update.* Retrieved June 25, 2007, from http://www.oas.samhsa.gov/2k5/pregnancy/pregnancy.htm)

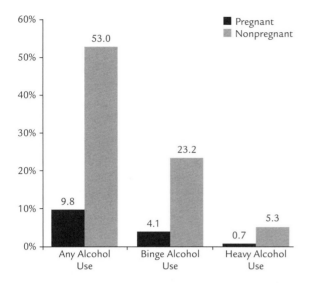

Figure 16.2. Percentage of past month alcohol use among women age 15–44, by pregnancy status: 2002 and 2003. (From Office of Applied Studies, Substance Abuse and Mental Health Services Administration. [2005]. *The NSDUH report: Substance use during pregnancy: 2002 and 2003 update.* Retrieved June 25, 2007, from http://www.oas.samhsa.gov/2k5/pregnancy/pregnancy.htm)

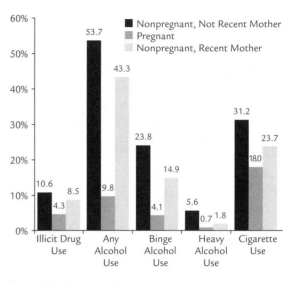

Figure 16.4. Percentage of women age 15–44 who reported past month substance use, by pregnancy and recent motherhood status: 2002 and 2003. (From Office of Applied Studies, Substance Abuse and Mental Health Services Administration. [2005]. *The NSDUH report: Substance use during pregnancy: 2002 and 2003 update.* Retrieved June 25, 2007, from http://www.oas.samhsa.gov/2k5/pregnancy/pregnancy.htm)

ity of pregnant women being among these previously cited statistics undoubtedly have increased (NIDA, 2008b).

Also included in this report were findings of the Drug Abuse Warning Network (DAWN), which monitors medications and illicit drug use reported in emergency departments across the

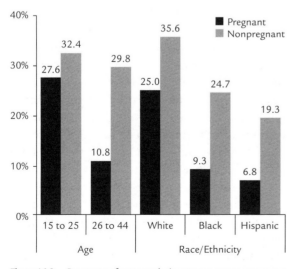

Figure 16.3. Percentage of past month cigarette use among women age 15–44, by pregnancy status, age, and race and/or ethnicity: 2002 and 2003. (From Office of Applied Studies, Substance Abuse and Mental Health Services Administration. [2005]. *The NSDUH report: Substance use during pregnancy: 2002 and 2003 update.* Retrieved June 25, 2007, from http://www.oas.samhsa.gov/2k5/pregnancy/pregnancy.htm)

country. In 2002, two of the most frequently reported prescription medications in drug abuse related cases were benzodiazepines (e.g., diazepam, alprazolam, clonazepam, lorazepam) and opioid pain relievers (e.g., oxycodone, hydrocodone, morphine, methadone, combinations of these drugs) (NIDA, 2006b). More research needs to be conducted on the effects of these drugs on the developing fetus in order to educate people about their danger. Moreover, Ensher and Clark wrote about the effects of prescription drugs when a mother is nursing:

In general, drugs should be avoided during lactation. Medications are frequently prescribed for the nursing mother, with only marginal indications. If a maternal drug is necessary and there is a known hazard for the newborn, a more innocuous therapy can often be prescribed. Ultimately, the physician must consider every time a drug is recommended whether benefits to the mother outweigh dangers to the infant. Regrettably, problems arise inadvertently when mothers do not realize that they are pregnant. (1994, p. 186)

The effects of cigarette smoke, both in utero and during the childhood years, have serious health implications and quite often lead to conditions that interfere with a child's learning. According to research conducted by Pressinger (1998), the decline of smoking in the general population is slowest among those of childbearing age. Citing documentation from the National Household Survey on Drug Abuse, Pressinger noted that approximately one third of women of reproductive age smoke cigarettes on a regular basis. Another concern is that estimates by the Office of Smoking and Health indicate that "one-third to one-half of nonsmoking pregnant women are exposed to significant levels of involuntary or second hand smoke" (Pressinger, 1998, p. 1). NIDA noted that an estimated 18% of women in the United States smoke during their pregnancy, which results in an estimated 910 infant deaths annually (from 1997 to 2001) and more than $350 million per year in neonatal care costs related to smoking (NIDA, 2006c).

The majority of incidents of substance abuse are not stand-alone situations. Research indicates a strong link between cigarette, alcohol, and drug use, with polydrug use among those who are abusing drugs during pregnancy. The effects these substances can have on the developing fetus escalate and intensify as more and more substances are used in conjunction with one another (Schiller & Allen, 2005).

Contributing Factors Leading to Addiction

Researchers have identified several risk factors that typically are associated with those who develop drug abuse problems, including lack of stable family environments, peer influences, and drug availability. These risk factors are not necessarily a prediction for a particular individual; however, they are useful in defining levels of risk for initial drug use. Likewise, researchers have examined protective or resilience factors (e.g., parental involvement in the life of a child) that often reduce the chances of children with potential risk factors from advancing to substance abuse. Understanding research on biological, psychological, and environmental factors and their interactions has been helpful toward comprehending the influences involved in a person's first use of drugs and the risks for subsequent progression to addiction. Some studies are now focusing on how specific risk factors, such as unstable family environments, can be offset by increasing the impact of protective factors, such as surrogate parenting or mentoring programs (NIDA, 2004).

Nature versus Nurture

The issue of nature versus nurture in the development of addictions has been debated for years. There are those who believe that individuals who abuse drugs and alcohol choose to continue the behavior of using substances of their choice. The presumption is that they can stop any time they wish. There are others who believe that addiction is a biological or physical condition over which people have little to no power. They are unable to stop using the substance once they have started. Although there are multiple factors that may precede an individual's decision to begin to use drugs or alcohol, one must consider why some people who begin using drugs and alcohol become addicted and why others do not.

Research has suggested that personality and behavioral traits and styles that are evident in early childhood may have important implications for later substance use behaviors. These traits may include aggressiveness (e.g., children with histories of physical abuse or violence); early onset of behavior problems; difficulties with peer relations; and difficulties with learning. Early initiation of drug use in young people likewise has been identified as a strong predictor of later abuse. More recent evidence (Biederman, Faraone, Monuteaux, & Feighner, 2000; U.S. Department of Health and Human Services, Administration for Children and Families, Office of Planning, Research and Evaluation, 2006) shows a strong association between low levels of competency in multiple areas (as reported by both children and teachers) and tobacco and alcohol use among elementary school children. Although initial use of alcohol may be driven more by social influences, such as peers, later stages of problem drinking appear to be linked developmentally to intrapersonal problems. Over time, high school students who were more susceptible to social influences and who displayed lower levels of competency were more likely to exhibit increased drinking behavior. One group of investigators speculated that cognitive deficits may precede and predispose some individuals to drug use initiation. Therefore, weaknesses in cognitive skills and learning disabilities may be undetected risk factors that underlie other identified risk factors, such as low self-esteem and academic failure. *Preventing Drug Abuse Among Children and Adolescents,* a recent report by the National Institute on Drug Abuse (2008), likewise addresses issues of the critical importance of early life experiences and the exposure of young children to substance abusing parents. The report states,

> Studies such as the National Survey on Drug Use and Health, formally called the National Household Survey on Drug Abuse, reported by the Substance Abuse and Mental Health Services Administration, indicate that some children are already abusing drugs at age 12 and 13, which likely means that some begin even earlier. Early abuse often includes such substances as tobacco, alcohol, inhalants, marijuana, and prescription drugs such as sleeping pills and anti-anxiety medicines. If drug abuse persists into adolescence, abusers typically become more heavily involved with marijuana and then advance to other drugs, while continuing their abuse of tobacco and alcohol. Studies have also shown that abuse of drugs in later childhood and early adolescence is associated with greater drug involvement. (p. 3)

In a publication from Brigham and Women's Hospital in Massachusetts, Gottleib (2007) stated that according to a 2001 survey conducted by the Substance Abuse and Mental Health Services Administration (SAMHSA), there were 16 million drug users, 13 million heavy drinkers, and 66 million smokers in the United States in 2001. Neuroscientists consider addiction a brain disease that is chronic and relapsing. It is considered such because it alters the brain in fundamental, lasting, and life-changing ways. Neuroimaging techniques (e.g., magnetic resonance imaging [MRI]) have documented actual changes in the size and shape of nerve cells in the brains of those who abuse drugs and alcohol. According to Dr. Stephen Hyman, former Director of the NIMH, networks of nerve cells determine our feelings and behavior, and drugs influence behavior by transforming the way these networks function. Dopamine, the brain chemical that is released

during pleasurable activities, is the biological link among all addictions. When drinking and using drugs result in a large spike of dopamine, the chances are significant that people will repeat the behavior that caused this chemical spike, thus beginning the cycle of addiction. Crack cocaine is a powerful drug that elevates the dopamine levels much faster than normal activities associated with pleasure, which makes it much more addictive (Gottleib, 2007).

Alan Leshner (1997) of NIDA hypothesized that once a person crosses the line from user to addiction, he or she can no longer control his or her behavior. Addiction is not a voluntary behavior, but actually a different state of compulsive, uncontrollable drug use. Leshner (1997) further hypothesized that this transformation helps to explain why it is so difficult to break an addiction because drug cravings are the most powerful motivator to continue using. Cravings are more significant than physical withdrawal in keeping addicts "hooked," and drugs such as cocaine and methamphetamine (unlike heroin or alcohol) do not produce intense physical withdrawal symptoms, but they do produce overpowering cravings.

Drugs such as methadone, naltrexone, and more recently buprenorphine (a partial opioid agonist) are commonly used to ease the withdrawal from alcohol and narcotics addiction. Aerobic exercise has also been found to be a safer alternative to using a prescription drug to counteract drug addiction. During exercise, dopamine levels are increased in the areas of the brain involved with addiction, and there is a decrease in feelings of depression and anxiety (Gottleib, 2007).

Legrand, Iacono, and McGue (2005) focused on the importance of prevention as the best line of defense against fighting addiction because failure to overcome an addiction is common even when there is strong family support. Typically, less than one third of alcoholics are recovered 1–2 years after treatment. These authors concurred with other reports and studies that those who are addiction vulnerable tend to be more impulsive and easily bored. These individuals are generally outgoing, sociable, expressive, rebellious, and enjoy taking risks. Moreover, they are more likely to question authority and challenge tradition.

Having these traits does not doom one to addiction; however, it does place individuals at an elevated risk. Having a parent with a substance abuse problem is an established predictor of a child's future addiction. Studies have shown that the more a parent drinks within a 24-hour period, the greater the risk factor for his or her offspring.

Although DNA is never an ultimate determining factor, parents with addiction problems tend to share a genetic vulnerability with their children, which is coupled with a home where alcohol and drugs are available and where abuse is common. These findings indicate that there are many factors that influence an individual to use alcohol or drugs; however, genetics and home environment both have a major influence on whether or not someone begins that cycle (Legrand et al., 2005).

Familial Factors

Children in substance abusing homes generally are exposed to drugs and alcohol at much earlier ages than those whose parents are not users. Parental substance use has been implicated as a risk factor for child substance use. For example, among children in the primary grades early onset of smoking was associated with exposure to parental smoking. Among adolescents, substance use by an important adult was a potential risk for substance use experimentation. Adolescents who reported exposure to adult use of alcohol, tobacco, or marijuana were likely to be further advanced in the onset process than other students in grades 7 through 9 (NIDA, 2004). Children in substance abusing homes see adults engaged in using substances on a fairly regular basis, and thus are more likely to accept these behaviors as typical and acceptable.

According to Kevin Conway (Associate Director of the Division of Clinical Neuroscience and Behavioral Research at NIDA) and colleagues (Compton, Thomas, Conway, & Colliver, 2005; Swendsen, Conway, Rounsaville, & Merikangas, 2002), familial alcoholism has long been known to increase the risk of alcoholism in offspring, but the risk is not 100%. Family history is just one of many variables that may contribute to develop-

ing alcoholism. Exposure to heavy drinking or antisocial behavior in parents or offspring may increase the incidence of their children developing alcoholism. However, warm parent–child relationships often decrease this risk, despite a parent's alcoholism, suggesting that an individual's personality influences how he or she responds to familial problems.

Thrill seeking also may play a role in children being affected by familial alcoholism. The more thrill seeking a child is, the greater his or her risk for developing alcoholism; whereas children with low thrill seeking tendencies may have a significantly lower chance of developing alcoholism. As noted in the previously cited research, Conway commented that the notion of an addictive personality has been largely rejected, but there are personality traits that may enhance the probabilities of addiction to substances. Richard A. Grucza, an epidemiologist at Washington University School of Medicine, suggested that rethinking the relationship between personality and addiction may be an important step in determining the risk of developing an addiction (Grucza et al., 2006). Rather than thinking about an addictive personality, it is important to think about how personality might influence a person's response to other genetic and environmental risk factors. He also noted that thrill seeking may be a family trait and seems to be a significant risk factor for alcoholism, which creates more complicated familial patterns to study. Studying patterns of substance abuse in families is important, but one must look at a variety of influences and conditions, such as attention-deficit/hyperactivity disorder (ADHD; NIDA, 2006d), to gain more insight into how and why some people become addicted to various substances and others do not.

Mental Health Issues Leading to Substance Abuse

The onset of drug abuse seems to occur later for females, and the paths toward abuse are more complex than for males. Typically, there is a pattern of breakdown of individual, familial, and environmental protective factors and an increase in childhood fears, anxieties, phobias, and failed relationships that lead to abuse in females. The etiology of female drug use often lies in predisposing psychiatric disorders prior to using drugs. For instance, childhood sexual abuse has been associated with drug use in females in several studies. Research indicates that higher numbers of women in drug use treatment report histories of physical and sexual abuse, with victimization beginning in the early primary years and occurring repeatedly. These findings are not surprising in light of the consistent close correlation between substance abuse and child abuse and neglect (see Chapter 17).

Studies of drug use among young women who became pregnant before reaching 18 years of age reported that 32% had a history of early forced sexual intercourse (rape or incest). These adolescents, compared with nonvictims, used more crack, cocaine, and other drugs (Hillis et al., 2004); had lower self-esteem; and had long-term psychosocial consequences. Data from studies of women with substance use problems and schizophrenia often have associated noteworthy histories of traumatic life events and posttraumatic stress experiences in their younger years (Gearon, Kaltman, Brown, & Bellack, 2003).

Prenatal Impact of Substance Abuse

The use of alcohol, drugs, and tobacco has several adverse effects on the developing fetus, many of which prevail throughout childhood and into adulthood. In addition to the physical impact that these substances have on development in utero, there are numerous developmental delays whose implications are seen throughout the stages of a child's life. Physical implications, such as low birth weight, premature births (with accompanying issues), physical abnormalities and malformations, developmental delays, and a variety of other complications, are commonly associated with maternal substance use and abuse during pregnancy (see Chapter 5). Understanding the effects of these substances is an important factor in educating women on the importance of avoiding such substances during and after pregnancy.

Developmental Issues Related to Alcohol Use

With alcohol being the most commonly used addictive substance in the United States, approximately 22,000 children each year experience mild to severe adverse effects as a result of their mothers' alcohol consumption (Steinberg & Gehshan, 2000). Fetal growth retardation, malformations, developmental disabilities, and spontaneous abortions are some of the many problems that can occur (Cogswell, Weisberg, & Spong, 2003). In addition, alcohol consumption can result in fetal alcohol syndrome (FAS), which slows growth, damages the nervous system, and produces facial abnormalities and intellectual disabilities. It can also result in fetal alcohol effects (FAE), which produce a milder group of intellectual and behavioral difficulties, including short attention spans, memory problems, and disorganization (Steinberg & Gehshan, 2000).

Beyond FAS and FAE, there are other related effects of in utero alcohol consumption. *Fetal alcohol spectrum disorder (FASD)* is the current terminology used to encompass this variety of complications. If there are signs of alcohol-related neurodevelopmental problems in the absence of other criteria of FAS, the term *alcohol-related neurodevelopmental disorder (ARND)* is used (Batshaw, Pellegrino, & Roizen, 2007).

It is important to note that *FAS* describes the "simultaneous occurrence of several birth defects associated with alcohol consumption during pregnancy and consists of fetal growth restriction, central nervous system impairment and facial deformities. This diagnosis requires the presence of all three defects" (Cogswell et al., 2003, p. 1726S). Fetal growth restriction involves growth deficiency in both the prenatal and postnatal periods. Central nervous system impairment includes intellectual disabilities and behavior problems. Certain abnormalities in facial and skull structure are present, such as small eye openings (i.e., short palpebral fissures); alterations in nose and forehead structure; an absent or elongated groove between the upper lip and nose (i.e., philtram); a thin upper lip; a flattened mid-face; and underdevelopment of the upper or lower jaw (Larkby & Day, 1997).

Traditionally, alcohol use and abuse during pregnancy has been seen as taboo in our society, and often the mother who drinks continuously throughout her pregnancy is perceived as causing the most damage to her unborn child. Studies, however, suggest that frequent binge drinking is more dangerous to fetal development than one or two drinks on a daily basis (Abel, 1998). This is due to alcohol concentrations, levels of toxicity, and the duration of such in the womb. According to Abel in *Fetal Alcohol Abuse Syndrome*, "bingeing, especially chronic bingeing, is more dangerous for the unborn child than consumption of the same amount of alcohol over an extended period of time" (1998, p. 160). Binge drinking is much more common in the United States than in other countries, and a typical episode includes at least five drinks. This is a likely explanation for the fact that the United States has a greater rate of FAS than other countries. Abel goes on to explain that the more chronic the binge drinking, the greater the damage because this extends the time period of alcohol toxicity over a longer duration of the pregnancy. The greater the level of toxicity, the greater the risks are for the unborn child.

In addition to binge drinking, women who abuse alcohol consistently pose a great risk to their unborn children, depending on the severity of their alcoholism. The beginning stages of alcoholism pose less risk to the developing fetus than the later stages, especially if severe enough to cause cirrhosis of the liver. Abel emphasized that a mother's health status with respect to her alcoholism is a key factor in determining "ultimate embryonic toxicity" and that the length of a woman's alcoholism is "less important than the severity of her alcohol-related pathology (e.g., alcoholic liver disease, DTs)" (p. 161).

Cirrhosis is the most common condition among this population. It is associated with increased rates of spontaneous abortion and preterm birth. In addition, many of the effects directly attributed to alcohol exposure in utero may instead be due to the combined effects of maternal cirrhosis and alcohol consumption (Abel, 1998). These health factors, as well as the fact that alcoholic women are often malnourished, have a negative impact on fetal development in a number of ways, regardless of the stage of alcoholism.

Abel (1998) also discussed the fact that metabolism plays a significant role on the effects of the alcohol, including a reduction of fetal growth and the development of malformations. He continued to explain that metabolite acetaldehyde of alcohol is exceedingly more toxic to the embryo than ethanol and may affect fetuses directly or augment ethanol's fetal toxicity. Findings indicate that women who are alcoholics are also at a higher risk for giving birth to a child with FAS because they produce a higher than normal amount of acetaldehyde when they drink. Abel further noted that women in advanced stages of alcoholism produce a greater amount of this substance than other drinkers, despite equal amounts of alcohol intake.

Finally, Abel suggested that although FAS clearly occurs in all races, individuals living in poverty are more likely to become known to authorities as having children with FAS than are people from more affluent circumstances. He noted that environmental and social correlates of poverty that are directly related to FAS further enhance adverse consequences for infants and young children; these factors include diet or poor nutrition, violence, psychological stress, excessively large families, smoking, and abuse of other drugs. Because maternal diet and nutrition directly influence the developing fetus, maternal diet is the most critical factor affecting growth and development in utero. Unfortunately, nutrition is compromised in women who abuse alcohol because alcohol can reduce nutrition absorption. Women who are alcoholics also have decreased water and food intake and decreased weight gain during pregnancy, which can cause additional adverse outcomes on their children (Abel, 1998). It must again be emphasized, however, that FAS crosses all types of families, from all economic and educational backgrounds and settings.

Cogswell and her colleagues (2003) have also considered the effects of alcohol on nutrition absorption. Because energy from alcohol often replaces energy from food, it leads to an overall decline in nutrient intake. Alcohol intake can disturb gastrointestinal function, which leads to reduced or enhanced absorption of vitamins and minerals. Zinc absorption is a cofactor for alcohol dehydrogenase (the ethanol-metabolizing enzyme) and may be impaired. Excessive alcohol intake can mobilize vitamin A from the liver and cause vitamin A toxicity, which can result in birth defects and tends to increase the incidence of malformations. The full effects of alcohol on the metabolism of B vitamins are not yet clear; however, in vitro studies suggest that short-term exposure to alcohol inhibits the transport of vitamin B_6, but not thiamin or biotin. The metabolism of iron also may be affected, but more research needs to be conducted to support preliminary data findings. In addition, alcohol consumption increases metabolic demands, increases DNA and RNA needed for synthesis and regeneration of liver cells, and impairs utilization of nutrients (Cogswell et al., 2003).

Based on all of these findings, it is conclusive that alcohol ingestion during pregnancy can cause irreparable damage to the developing fetus. Whether a pregnant mother is binge drinking or suffers from alcoholism, the toxicity created in her system when drinking will cause an unhealthy environment for her child. Nutrition as well is compromised in situations where the mother is drinking alcohol during her pregnancy, which further complicates the situation for the unborn child. Because all of these dangers can be avoided with the absence of alcohol, educating women before, during, and after pregnancy is crucial.

Developmental Issues Related to Drug Use

A variety of complications can be attributed to maternal drug use during pregnancy, including shortened gestational periods, low birth weight, smaller than normal head (and brain) size, miscarriages, genital and urinary tract malformations, and nervous system damage. Moreover, research has suggested that perhaps fewer negative outcomes affect children, depending on environmental factors and genetic vulnerability to exposure, the type of drug of exposure, the frequency and magnitude of drug use, and the quality of prenatal and postnatal care (Steinberg & Gehshan, 2000).

Marijuana is one of the many drugs that can have an impact on fetal development. Research has indicated that marijuana use during pregnancy may slow fetal growth, slightly decrease the length of pregnancy, and possibly increase the risk of premature delivery. These factors also can increase the chance of delivering a low birth weight infant. These effects are seen most often in women who use marijuana on a regular basis (at least 4–6 times per week) (Hulse, Milne, Holman, & Bower, 1997). Hulse et al. (1997) also noted that cigarette smoking, which is a known cause of low birth weight, often is associated with the use of cannabis.

Cocaine is another illegal drug whose effects in utero have been studied and debated at length. There are those who believe that the initial reports about the effects of cocaine are inaccurate and that cocaine is not as devastating as once originally believed. One should consider this notion with caution, as there are numerous studies indicating serious risks with in utero cocaine exposure. In particular, it is well documented that exposure to cocaine in the early months of pregnancy can increase the risk of miscarriage, whereas exposure in the later months can trigger preterm labor or cause a baby to grow poorly (i.e., intrauterine growth restriction [IUGR]). Cocaine-exposed babies are more likely to be born with low birth weight, face an increased risk of intellectual disabilities, have cerebral palsy, and have smaller heads. Studies also suggest that cocaine places the fetus at an increased risk of stroke or heart attack and may cause placental abruption (Vidaeff & Mastrobattista, 2003).

Schiller and Allen (2005) highlight the significant obstetric complications with cocaine use that pose a risk to both the mother and the fetus. Women using cocaine have a higher incidence of poor weight gain and cardiac complications, such as hypertension, arrhythmia, cardiac ischemia, and hemorrhagic stroke. Cocaine normally stresses the cardiovascular system; however, in pregnant women the toxicity of cocaine increases, which elevates the risk for cardiovascular events, such as stroke and seizures. Uterine rupture, hepatic rupture, placental abruption, and maternal death occur more frequently in women using cocaine.

The physiological effects of cocaine, such as vasoconstriction, hypertension, and tachycardia, can have devastating consequences in terms of the placenta and the developing fetus. Cocaine causes vasoconstriction of the maternal uterine blood vessels during pregnancy. Specifically, oxygen and nutrients normally transferred to the fetus via these vessels are unable to reach the placenta and fetus, which results in uteroplacental insufficiency and fetal hypoxemia. Spontaneous abortion, premature labor and delivery, abruptio placentae (premature detachment of the placenta), and fetal intracranial hemorrhage are complications that may occur as a primary result of this vasoconstriction.

The physical properties of cocaine (low molecular weight, hydrophilic, and lipophilic) allow it to cross the placenta and pass through the blood–brain barrier. Not only is cocaine transferred to the fetus via diffusion into the umbilical cord and within the placental vessels, but it also is found in the amniotic fluid and is swallowed by the fetus. Metabolism of cocaine in the fetus is known to be considerably slower than in adults; thus, fetal exposure to cocaine is prolonged. This condition often results in IUGR, including low birth weight, low birth length, and deficits in head circumference (Schiller & Allen, 2005). NIDA has stated that the full extent of prenatal cocaine exposure is yet unknown; however, they concur that babies born to mothers who abused cocaine during their pregnancies frequently are born prematurely, have low birth weights, have smaller head circumferences (which may or may not be affected), and are often shorter in length (NIDA, 2006a).

Heroin, one of the most addictive opiates, is another illicit drug that can create complications when used during pregnancy. The reported use of heroin among the general population continues to rise, which correlates with an increased risk of pregnant women using this drug (Coles & Black, 2006; NIDA, 2005a). Common pregnancy complications associated with heroin use include miscarriage, placental abruption, poor fetal growth, premature rupture of the membranes, premature delivery, and stillbirth. As many as half of these babies are born with low birth weight, and most of them experience serious prematurity-related

health issues during the newborn period, such as breathing problems and brain bleeds that can result in lifelong disabilities.

There are cautions that pregnant women using heroin should not attempt to stop taking the drug suddenly, as immediate withdrawal may place mothers and babies at increased risk of miscarriage or premature birth. The suggested course of treatment to withdraw from the drug is to use methadone under the supervision of a doctor or a drug treatment center. There are some concerns about the effects of methadone as well, and babies often show signs of dependence on the drug, but these can be treated quite effectively in the nursery. Babies who are exposed to methadone generally do far better than those babies born to mothers who continue to use heroin throughout the pregnancy (Briggs, Freedman, & Yaffe, 2005).

A study conducted by the National Institute on Drug Abuse (2007b) indicated that the use of crystal methamphetamine in young adults is higher than previously reported. Specifically, the study published in the journal *Addiction* (NIDA, 2007b) cited that 2.8% of young adults in the United States between the ages of 18 and 26 years acknowledged use of this drug versus a previously reported prevalence rate of 1.4% (Hulse et al., 1997). It would stand to reason that this trend would reflect an increase among women of childbearing age abusing this substance as well. An article published in the *Journal of Drug Issues* (Derauf, Katz, Frank, Grandinetti, & Easa, 2003) indicated that the rise in methamphetamine abuse is most prevalent in the Western regions of the United States, with the highest rates (considered an epidemic by many) in Hawaii. As a result of drug prevalence in Hawaii, a study was conducted to determine the rate of methamphetamine use among pregnant women in that state; however, this research was inconclusive.

There have been very few studies on the risks of the use of amphetamines, such as ecstasy, during pregnancy. However, recent results of a 2005 national survey on drug use and health (Substance Abuse and Mental Health Administration, 2006) indicated that use of ecstasy has increased dramatically in recent years and that in utero it may lead to the same risks and problems associated with other types of amphetamines. Another commonly abused amphetamine is methylamphetamine, which is more commonly known as speed, ice, crank, and crystal meth. Some studies suggest that this drug also has increased risks of birth defects associated with use during pregnancy, such as cleft palate and heart and limb malformations (Smith et al., 2006). Amphetamines also can contribute to maternal high blood pressure, which can slow fetal growth and cause other complications for both the mother and the baby, such as premature delivery and excessive bleeding in the mother following delivery (Smith et al., 2006).

In addition to illegal drug use, NIDA (2006b) has reported an increase in the abuse of prescription and over-the-counter medications in recent years; however, similar to methamphetamine use, little if any research has been conducted to determine the in utero effects of these drugs during pregnancy. This report by NIDA noted a statistic provided by the Drug Abuse Warning Network (DAWN) that indicated that the two most frequently reported prescription drugs in abuse-related cases are benzodiazepines (e.g., diazepam, alprazolam, clonazepam, lorazepam) and opioid pain relievers (e.g., oxycodone, hydrocodone, morphine, methadone). As rates of abuse of these drugs continue to rise, there is an increasing need for studies to be done on the rates of exposure and the effects on fetal development when they are used by pregnant women.

Developmental Issues Related to Smoking

With an estimated 18% of pregnant women smoking tobacco products during their pregnancies, the numbers of children who are affected by this problem are immense (NIDA, 2006c). Smoking during pregnancy can introduce toxic substances, such as nicotine, hydrogen cyanide, and carbon monoxide into the fetal blood supply (Steinberg & Gehshan, 2000) and can create many adverse effects, such as IUGR decreased birth weights, as well as spontaneous abortions. One report by the NIDA (2006c) noted that the decreased birth weights seen in infants of mothers who smoke reflect a dose-dependent relationship,

which means that the more a woman smokes during pregnancy, the greater the reduction of infant birth weight. Moreover, by-products such as carbon monoxide and nicotine from tobacco smoke may interfere with the oxygen supply to the fetus. Nicotine also readily crosses the placenta, with concentrations in the fetus reaching as much as 15% higher than maternal levels. Nicotine concentrates in fetal blood, amniotic fluid, and breast milk, which can have severe consequences for the fetus. The same NIDA report (2006c) stated that there were 910 infant deaths annually from 1997 through 2001 as a result of smoking, and neonatal care costs related to smoking are estimated to be more than $350 million per year.

According to an article by Cogswell and colleagues (2003), cigarette smoking during pregnancy can cause spontaneous abortions in the first trimester, premature placenta abruption, preterm delivery, decreased birth weight, and sudden infant death syndrome (SIDS). The risk of being small for gestational age among those born to women who smoke during pregnancy is at least 2 times as high, and these infants weigh, on average, 150–300 grams less. Cogswell and colleagues (2003) also noted that cigarette smoking is a source of oxidant stress and that carbon monoxide and nicotine are both components of cigarettes that may affect birth weight and cause preterm delivery. More specifically, carbon monoxide binds to hemoglobin to form carboxyhemoglobin, which causes fetal hypoxia and is related to sudden infant death syndrome. Nicotine and carbon monoxide may lead to vasoconstriction and reduced blood flow, and nicotine specifically can increase maternal blood pressure and heart rate, which reduces uterine blood flow. There are other components of cigarette smoke, such as lead, thiocyanate, and cadmium, that may also damage the fetus.

The effects that smoking has on micronutrients and how those affect pregnant women and their fetuses quite often lead to adverse pregnancy outcomes (Cogswell et al., 2003). Cigarette smoking is known to decrease appetite and may consequently decrease the amount of nutrients consumed by a pregnant woman. Cigarette smokers are also less likely to consume micronutrient supplements and are more likely to consume alcohol or other substances that interfere with nutrient metabolism. Cigarette smoking may also decrease the absorption of micronutrients in the intestine and increase the utilization of nutrients, a condition that indicates that nutrient requirement values should be increased for cigarette smokers. More specifically, studies suggest that smokers have lower blood and tissue levels of vitamin B_6, folate, and vitamin B_{12} than do nonsmokers. The amount of zinc available to the fetus is lower as well because the cadmium from cigarette smoke accumulates and binds to zinc in the placenta, which causes higher placental zinc levels in smokers. Cadmium also has been found to cause severe anemia in the fetus, but only mild anemia in the mothers, which suggests that cadmium might interfere with transplacental availability of iron. Anemia may be associated with an increased risk of SIDS, and that risk almost doubles when the mother not only smokes, but is anemic herself. Finally, smoking increases hemoglobin concentration related to carbon monoxide exposure, as well as perhaps hemoglobin levels in the cord blood and in neonates (Cogswell et al., 2003)

Neonatal and Childhood Problems Related to Maternal Substance Abuse

Infants who are exposed to alcohol, drugs, and tobacco in utero have a significant chance of some type of physical disability as a result of this exposure. Furthermore, exposure leads to addiction, withdrawal, and a range of physical and developmental difficulties after birth.

Addiction and Withdrawal

Many substances that a child might be exposed to in utero can create a physical dependence that may result in withdrawal soon after birth. The onset of the withdrawal symptoms depends on the type of narcotic the infant has been exposed to in utero. Heroin and methadone are both known to be addictive to the fetus. Heroin has a short half-life (4 hours), and as a result, withdrawal symptoms are apparent on the first day. Methadone (an opiate used to help withdraw from drugs such as heroin), however, has a very long half-life (32 hours in newborns) and remains in the infant's system for days. Withdrawal symptoms for this drug occur 24–48 hours after birth, and are evident as late as 7–10 days after birth. Methadone is excreted in the infant's urine for 10–14 days after birth, which may account for the prolonged withdrawal period for methadone-exposed infants (Zuckerman, Frank, & Brown, 1995).

Heroin appears to create the most intense withdrawal symptoms for babies, such as increased metabolic activity, trembling, irritability, diarrhea, vomiting, continual crying, and sometimes seizure-like activity (The American College of Obstetricians and Gynecologists [ACOG], 2005). Respiratory symptoms of heroin withdrawal include tachypnea, hyperpnea, respiratory alkalosis, cyanosis, and apnea. Autonomic nervous system signs of withdrawal include sneezing, yawning, tearing, sweating, and hyperpyrexia (Randall, 1995). Methadone withdrawal is characterized by restlessness, agitation, tremors, and sleep disturbance. These symptoms may last 3–6 months after birth, and they may be a reflection of the prolonged metabolism and excretion of methadone (Zuckerman et al., 1995).

Onset of withdrawal symptoms, especially in infants with methadone exposure, may be delayed as late as 4 weeks. Infants born to mothers who have used multiple drugs are reported to have more frequent and more severe neonatal withdrawal symptoms than those exposed to a single drug in utero (Bada et al., 2002). In addition to heroin and methadone, numerous other substances that are used and abused during pregnancy create a physical dependency and can result in withdrawal-like symptoms in babies after they are born and no longer exposed to the substance. Babies who are regularly exposed to marijuana in utero appear to display symptoms after birth that include excessive crying and trembling. Babies who are exposed to amphetamines in utero also appear to have withdrawal-like symptoms after birth, such as jitteriness, drowsiness, and breathing problems.

Infants who are exposed to barbiturates (e.g., phenobarbital) in utero up to 12 weeks prior to delivery also exhibit symptoms of withdrawal after delivery. The symptoms are similar to infants exposed to opiates (e.g., hyperactivity, tremors, crying, vomiting, diarrhea). These symptoms usually appear 4–8 days after birth (Randall, 1995).

Although most people do not associate cigarette smoking during pregnancy with addiction, newborns who have been exposed to tobacco byproducts in utero display signs of stress and drug withdrawal that are consistent with symptoms reported in infants exposed to other drugs (NIDA, 2006c).

Physical Difficulties

In utero exposure to alcohol, as well as a variety of drugs, can result in lasting physical difficulties that can have an impact on a child's development and well-being. Infants born to mothers who drank heavily during pregnancy have been described as being fitful sleepers, and their electroencephalogram (EEG) patterns during sleep cycles reveal consistent hypersynchrony and delayed maturation of sleep-related EEG. EEG sleep synchronies in these children were often as much as 200% higher than normal during active REM sleep (Abel, 1998).

In addition to sleep disturbances, feeding patterns often are disrupted in children who have FAS or FAE. Hypotonia can reflect a general muscle weakness that may contribute to this problem, but it is more common to see fine motor dysfunction that results in underlying feeding difficulties for some infants with FAS or FAE (e.g., an abnormal, weak, or easily tired suck). Attempts to overcome these early feeding difficulties may create a conditioned emotional response that is associated with physical contact. This may explain why some children with FAS prefer not to be touched. Gross motor function impairment is also common in these children, who often are described as being developmentally delayed in their motor skills, as well as manifesting evidence of balance and coordination difficulties. These developmental delays are much more prevalent if the mothers continued drinking through-

out the pregnancy rather than drinking during the first and second trimesters only (Abel, 1998).

Drug exposure in utero also can lead to a variety of serious physical problems for newborns. According to NIDA (2005c), research has shown that some babies born to women who used marijuana during their pregnancies display altered responses to visual stimuli, increased tremulousness, and a high-pitched cry, which may indicate problems with neurological development. Cocaine exposure also creates a variety of physical symptoms that are apparent after birth. These babies often have feeding difficulties and experience sleep disturbances. Many of these newborns appear jittery and irritable, and they may startle easily and cry at the gentlest touch or sound. As a result, these babies frequently are difficult to comfort and are described as withdrawn or unresponsive. Many cocaine-exposed babies "turn off" surrounding stimuli and go into a deep sleep for most of the day. These behavioral disturbances are sometimes temporary and tend to resolve themselves during the first few months of life. Cocaine-exposed babies also have a greater chance of dying from SIDS. Amphetamine exposure can cause many long-lasting physical problems in newborns. Physical impairments, such as heart defects, cleft palate, limb and skeletal defects (club foot), are most commonly seen as a result of this type of drug exposure.

Exposure to heroin often results in a number of health-related problems, including prematurity, breathing difficulties, and brain bleeds in newborns, which can lead to lifelong disabilities. Exposure to heroin before birth, similar to cocaine, significantly increases a child's risk of SIDS. Another study (Bada et al., 2002) that was highlighted in the *Archives of Disease in Childhood* focused on the risk for central nervous system (CNS) and autonomic nervous system (ANS) symptoms following in utero exposure to cocaine and/or opiates. There were signs of abnormal posture, sweating, hiccupping, bradycardia, hyperthermia, and hypothermia. More common symptoms include the prevalence of hypotonia, weak cry, lethargy, mottling, tachycardia, and nasal flaring. Hypertonia and a high-pitched cry were even more common, and the symptoms most frequently noted were jitteriness, tremors, and irritability. Infants who were exposed to cocaine and/or opiates were 2–3 times more likely to exhibit jitteriness and/or tremors, irritability, hypertonia, high-pitched cry, and difficulty in consoling. They were 1½ times more likely to show poor suck and nasal stuffiness, and 4 times more likely to have an excessive suck. Difficulties with arousal were often observed in infants exposed to cocaine (Bada et al., 2002).

With methamphetamine use on the rise and fetal exposure to this drug a growing problem in the United States, more studies are being conducted on the effects of this drug on neonatal development and the subsequent physical problems associated with exposure. The most current research indicates that methamphetamine abuse during pregnancy may result in prenatal complications, increased rates of premature delivery, and altered neonatal behavioral patterns, such as abnormal reflexes and extreme irritability. Methamphetamine abuse during pregnancy also may be linked to congenital deformities (NIDA, 2005d).

Inhalant abuse is increasing across the United States. Although no formal studies have been carried out in terms of the effects of inhalant use during pregnancy, there are a number of case reports noting abnormalities in infants born to mothers who chronically abuse solvents. Further animal studies conducted suggest that prenatal exposure to toluene or trichlorethylene (TCE) can result in reduced birth weights, occasional skeletal abnormalities, and delayed neurobehavioral development. Case reports (although limited) note abnormalities in these newborns, and there is evidence of subsequent developmental impairment among some of these children (NIDA, 2006a).

Phenobarbital, although the logical choice to treat neonatal dependence on barbiturates, has some potential disadvantages. It can produce depression of neonatal respiration and sucking, especially when used at higher dosages (Randall, 1995). There always are possibilities of complications from drugs that are used to ease withdrawal from illicit drugs; however, these complications are generally much less significant than those that would result if the mother continued using the illicit substance.

Mothers who smoke cigarettes during pregnancy expose their babies to nicotine and carbon monoxide in utero, which can have many adverse effects on the health of their children. As noted previously, smoking during pregnancy can cause fetal growth delays and decreased birth weights. Smoking during pregnancy also may be associated with spontaneous abortions and SIDS (NIDA, 2006c).

Developmental Challenges and School-Related or Learning Issues

Developmental problems resulting from alcohol and drug exposure can be far reaching and continue throughout a child's lifetime. By the time children with FAS reach preschool age, not only are sleep problems and poor coordination still an issue, but new problems begin to emerge. The most commonly mentioned behavioral characteristics of these children are highlighted in Table 16.1.

At this early age, speech and communication difficulties are most commonly found in African American and Native American children with FAS (Abel, 1998). FAS-related communication difficulties may be due to articulation prob-

Table 16.1. Frequently mentioned behavioral characteristics of preschool children with fetal alcohol syndrome

Hypersensitivity to touch

Attention Deficit Disorder (ADD)

Hyperactivity ("always on the go," "never sits still," "never seems to listen")

Impulsiveness

Accident prone (Possibly a combination of hyperactivity and poor coordination)

Extreme mood changes (laughs or cries too readily)

Heightened anxiety

Constantly demands attention

Low threshold for frustration

Unusual aggressiveness

Frequent temper tantrums over trivial problems

Disobedient in response to requests from parents

Unable to adapt easily to changes in routine activities

Requires more direct supervision than other children

Difficulty forming friendships with other children

Overly friendly and social towards adults

Does not distinguish friends from strangers; has no fear of strangers

Overly talkative; little meaningful content to speech

Talks at inappropriate times

From Abel, E.L. (1998). *Fetal alcohol abuse syndrome* (p. 121). New York: Plenum; Copyright © 1998 Plenum; reprinted with kind permission from Springer Science and Business Media.

lems that arise from anomalies in the physical structure of the jaw, teeth, palate, and gums (Committee on Substance Abuse and Committee on Children with Disabilities, American Academy of Pediatrics, 2000). Fine motor dysfunction involving coordination of muscles in the tongue or larynx may be responsible for the inability to articulate vowels and consonants. Articulation problems also may be related to the effects of alcohol on the auditory system. In addition, when compared to children of the same age, gender, and socioeconomic background, children with FAS were less advanced in their use of complex grammatical structures, and their short-term memories were not as developed as their peers. These communication disorders and related problems in children with FAS likewise appear to be a result of difficulties in cognitive processing rather than receptive abilities. It is believed that these disturbances in information processing also may be responsible for behavioral problems later seen in the classroom. Teachers often believe that these children understand what they have been told, even though they probably do not, and, therefore, their behavior is interpreted as disrespectful (Abel, 1998).

Once children enter school, FAS- and FAE-related cognitive difficulties and behavioral problems become recognized more readily. These children are quickly labeled as having ADHD or being hyperactive because of their restlessness, distractibility, and their inability to focus on their work and adhere to the rules. (It is important to note that although FAS and ADHD have many common behavioral characteristics, they are clinically distinct disorders with different underlying pathologies [Abel, 1998].) Academically, these children often begin to lag behind their peers in arithmetic and reading skills. The same impaired information-processing skills that influence their communication problems likewise may contribute to their delayed reading comprehension. It has been noted, too, that the writing and drawing skills of these populations of children are delayed, perhaps due to fine motor dysfunction.

Outside of the classroom, children with FAS and/or FAE frequently are described as having poor social skills. They are observed to be playing alongside of, but not with, their peers, and if they engage in play at all, it is with children younger than themselves. As a result, these children are teased or bullied, and they often withdraw and/or isolate themselves.

Students with FAS and/or FAE are unable to generalize from one situation to another and, therefore, do not appear to learn from their mistakes as quickly as others, which interferes with success both in school and at home. Short-term memory difficulties and inabilities to retrieve information may lead to frustration and temper tantrums, as well as the need to be taught the same material repeatedly. It has been suggested that these children perform much better in structured learning environments because of fewer cognitive demands for processing and responding to new information (Abel, 1998).

One of the most serious consequences of FAS and/or FAE is intellectual disability, which has a prevalence rate of approximately 50% (Committee on Substance Abuse and Committee on Children with Disabilities, American Academy of Pediatrics, 2000). At this writing, the potential for improved intellectual abilities among children with FAS and/or FAE is yet unknown. Stimulating home environments certainly can provide a foundation for change and, conversely, being raised in a neglectful or cognitively disadvantaged environment is a deterrent to enhancing intellectual growth (Abel, 1998). Creating the most conducive environments for learning and improving cognition should be a priority for those raising and educating children with FAS and/or FAE.

Studies indicate that there often are significant neuropsychological problems among children who are exposed to alcohol in utero but do not have FAS. Slower information processing, difficulty with complex decision making, and difficulty with particular mathematical tasks are all challenges for these children. Researchers also have found that children who were exposed to alcohol throughout the gestational period (as opposed to those who were only exposed during the first and/or second trimester) had deficits in short-term memory, encoding, and overall mental processing. These children frequently are less attentive, more active, and require a longer time to respond to their environment. Not unlike children with FAS, in school these individuals often are noted as having poor attention, social difficulties, anxiety, depression, and behavior problems, as well as lower performance in reading, spelling, and mathematics (Larkby & Day, 1997).

NIDA (2006a) reported that researchers are now finding evidence that cocaine exposure during fetal development may lead to "subtle, yet significant, later deficits in some children, including deficits in some aspects of cognitive performance, information-processing, and attention to tasks–abilities that are important for success in school." In *The Sixth Triennial Report to Congress,* NIDA (2003) indicated that children with histories of prenatal polydrug exposure that included cocaine scored significantly lower on standardized measures of language development than did nonexposed children and should be considered at risk for language delay. Other studies also have found significant language delays among infants prenatally exposed to cocaine, including difficulties in auditory comprehension (Beeghly, Martin, Rose-Jacobs, Cabral, Heeren, Augustyn, et al., 2006; Cone-Wesson, 2005; Potter, Zelazo, Stack, & Papageorgiou, 2000). Schiller and Allen (2005) noted a trend toward lower IQ scores among this group. Finally, although the research findings are somewhat controversial, some studies have shown that exposure to cocaine during fetal development may lead to subtle but significant deficits later on, especially with behaviors that are crucial to success in the classroom, such as blocking out distractions and concentrating for long periods, as well as continuing cognitive and learning problems well into middle school and beyond.

The outlook for heroin-exposed children depends greatly on a variety of factors, including whether or not newborns present serious complications from prematurity. In particular, children exposed to heroin in utero may have an increased risk of lower cognitive functioning and serious behavior problems (Briggs et al., 2005).

Although some studies (Smith et al., 2006) have suggested that babies exposed to ecstasy and other amphetamines in utero have altered levels of a specific brain chemical and may suffer lifelong difficulties in memory and learning,

more research needs to be conducted on the effects of amphetamines to gain deeper insight into the outlook for the children who have been exposed to these drugs before birth.

Although some researchers attempt to minimize the dangers of smoking during pregnancy, evidence is clear that exposure to tobacco byproducts in utero can lead to learning and behavioral problems in children. Perhaps the most significant issue associated with maternal smoking during pregnancy that affects learning is the link to behavioral difficulties and ADHD. Several clinical studies have found a significant association between maternal smoking during pregnancy and ADHD symptoms in their offspring, even when other potential confounding factors were taken into account for these symptoms (Thapar et al., 2003). In addition to the more immediate effects, smoking more than a pack of cigarettes a day during pregnancy nearly doubles the risk that the affected child will become addicted to tobacco if that child starts smoking later in life (NIDA, 2006c).

Often children of parents who continue to smoke experiment with smoking at earlier ages than their peers and are more likely to become addicted to nicotine before they are of legal age to purchase cigarettes. Smoking at a young age has a number of ramifications in the school setting, from an increase in discipline issues to a decrease in physical activities, such as participation in sports. There are also increased health concerns when young people start smoking while their bodies are still developing. Smoking at any age has known health risks associated with it; however, children who smoke or those who are in homes with parents who smoke seem to have an increase in health complications, ranging from more frequent colds and ailments, such as bronchitis, to increased episodes of asthma.

In 2006, NIDA reported that nearly 4 million American adolescents had used a tobacco product within a given month and that nearly 90% of smokers started smoking by age 18. Of those smokers under 18 years of age, more than 6 million would die prematurely from a smoking-related disease (NIDA, 2006c).

Implications of Children Living in Substance Abusing Homes

It is clear that the risks for children living in homes where substance abuse is present include both emotional and physical dangers. The rate of abuse and neglect in these situations is alarming, and the immediate dangers of firsthand exposure to these substances create a new set of problems above and beyond the dangers of in utero drug exposure.

Exposure to Alcohol

Parents or caregivers who abuse alcohol have a significant impact on their children, their safety, and the behaviors that are considered acceptable in such households. Clearly, safety is an issue to be considered while children are living in these circumstances. Issues such as driving while intoxicated with children in the vehicle, not supervising children as a result of intoxication, and children having access to substances that can cause them great harm or injury are all of concern. Alcoholic parents frequently neglect their children as a result of their drinking. Physical safety and emotional well-being often is compromised in these situations as well. In addition, neglect may come in the form of nutritional deprivation when an alcoholic purchases alcohol with money that should be used for nutritional food for the family.

As discussed in Chapter 17 in this text, alcoholics may become violent and abusive when under the influence, which poses an enormous safety risk for children (and spouses) in the home. Enduring abuse can result in issues of low self-esteem and can lead to a variety of mental health issues, which eventually revisit substance abuse among those who grew up in alcoholic homes. Thus, another vicious cycle begins.

The stability of growing up in a loving, nurturing environment is virtually nonexistent in homes where families abuse alcohol. There may be very little, if any, day-to-day stability for anyone living in the household. The only consistent factor may be the knowledge that life in that home is anything but predictable, and that one should be ready for almost anything to happen. Each day can be one filled with uncertainty and hesitation in which the members of the household try to be on their best behavior to avoid setting off a drinking binge that will result in unpredictable behavior and upturned emotions.

Children of alcoholics often blame themselves for a parent's behavior and believe that if they try harder, get better grades, or behave better, then perhaps the alcoholic parent might not drink as much. Obviously, the child has little or no control over these kinds of parent behaviors. Yet, the child may feel this is the only possibility for control and change; thus, they attempt to manipulate situations in the home to make things better. When they are unsuccessful in their efforts, these children often blame themselves, which creates more stress and uncertainty in their lives.

The influence of the parent who abuses alcohol typically is far reaching. In the *Sixth Triennial Report to Congress*, NIDA (2003) noted a recent study suggesting that the "sensitive period" for the influence of a father's substance use on a son's behavioral problems starts when the son is about 6 years of age. These findings suggest the importance of early intervention to reduce paternal substance abuse to prevent intergenerational transmission of behavioral problems and substance abuse. Externalizing behavioral problems in male children and adolescents are among the best predictors of subsequent substance use in early and late adolescence. Educating parents as to the dangers of their behaviors, as well as educating children so that they are aware of common behaviors of alcoholics (in an attempt to help them realize they are not to blame in the situation) is a first step in confronting the devastating effects that alcoholism has on families.

Exposure to Drugs

In similar ways, there are significant safety and stability issues for those growing up in homes where drugs are used or abused as in homes where alcohol is abused. In the *Sixth Triennial Report to Congress*, NIDA (2003) noted that drug use can have a significant negative impact on the health of children who are exposed to nicotine or illegal drugs by growing up in a household where drugs and tobacco are abused. Exposure often leads to the use of drugs during childhood and adolescence, which can be especially damaging to the child's developing body and emotional well-being. Similarly, neglect is a serious concern for these children. Substance abuse and addiction greatly impair the caretaking abilities of these parents. Life at home often is chaotic and uncertain, and the needs of the child are left unmet. When a caregiver responds appropriately to their needs for comfort, stimulation, and food, infants develop a sense of security. Once they have a sense of security, infants can explore their environment and develop other relationships. Addiction prevents a mother from responding to her infant's needs, as her primary focus is on the drug of her choice, not her child. The addicted mother's life is organized around attaining the drug or drugs of choice, not caring for her children (Zuckerman et al., 1995), despite her affection for them.

Children who grow up in homes where methamphetamine is produced are perhaps in the greatest danger of being exposed to toxic substances that can cause severe damage to their developing bodies. According to the NIDA (2005d), the number of children who were found at seized methamphetamine laboratory sites in the United States more than doubled from 1999 to 2001. These children typically lack proper immunizations, medical care, dental care, and necessities, such as food, water, and shelter.

In addition to the high rate of abuse and neglect (which creates emotional and behavioral problems) that are a result of the preoccupation with this drug by those running "meth labs," these children are being exposed to the toxic chemicals produced at these sites. They often inhale dangerous chemical fumes or gases or ingest toxic chemicals or illicit drugs. This exposure can cause serious short- and long-term health problems that include damage to the brain, liver, kidneys, lungs, eyes, and skin. Inhaling or ingesting these toxic substances may cause cancer or even death in these children. The risk of exposure to toxic chemicals at these sites is greater in children than in adults as a result of the nature of childhood behavior (e.g., touching nearly everything

in their environment and then putting their hands, as well as exposed objects, in their mouths). The states reporting the highest number of children found in these labs in 2001 were California, Washington, Oregon, and Missouri, in that order. Table 16.2 illustrates the increasing problem of exposure to methamphetamine. Table 16.3 illustrates the wide variety of chemicals that children are exposed to in these labs.

Children at methamphetamine laboratories may absorb these chemicals into their bodies via ingestion, inhalation, skin contact, or accidental injection. Ingestion poses the greatest risk to a child's health; however, exposure is most frequent through inhalation and contact with the skin. Immediate physical problems from ingesting toxic chemicals and/or methamphetamine may result in potentially fatal poisoning, internal chemical burns, damage to organ function and development, and harm and inhibition to neurological and immunologic development and functioning (NIDA, 2005d). Inhaling the chemical vapors that are created during methamphetamine production causes shortness of breath, cough, and chest pain. These vapors may cause intoxication, dizziness, nausea, disorientation, poor coordination, pulmonary edema, chemical pneumonitis, and other serious respiratory problems when absorbed into the body through the lungs. Serious burns can result when the chemicals used to produce methamphetamine come into contact with the skin, either through direct spills or by contact with surfaces that are contaminated with chemical spills.

There are many long-term risks with exposure as well because a child's developing brain and other organs are more susceptible to damage throughout these periods of maturation. In addition, children may be less able than adults to pro-

Table 16.2.   Children and methamphetamine laboratories

Year	Number of children present at seized laboratories	Number of children tested positive for toxic levels of chemicals
1999	950	150
2000	1,748	340
2001	2,028	700

From National Drug Intelligence Center. (2002). *Information bulletin: Children at risk* (Document ID: 2002-L0424-001). Retrieved June 27, 2007, from http://www.usdoj.gov/ndic/pubs1/1466/1466p.pdf

Table 16.3. Hazardous chemicals used in methamphetamine production

Chemical	Hazards
Pseudoephedrine	Ingestion of doses greater than 240 mg. causes hypertension, arrhythmia, anxiety, dizziness, and vomiting. Ingestion of doses greater than 600 mg. can lead to renal failure and seizures.
Acetone/ ethyl alcohol	Extremely flammable, posing a fire risk in and around the laboratory. Inhalation or ingestion of these solvents causes severe gastric irritation, narcosis, or coma.
Freon	Inhalation can cause sudden cardiac death or severe lung damage. It is corrosive if ingested.
Anhydrous ammonia	A colorless gas with a pungent, suffocating odor. Inhalation causes edema of the respiratory tract and asphyxia. Contact with vapors damages eyes and mucous membranes.
Red phosphorous	May explode on contact or friction. Ignites if heated above 260°F. Vapor from ignited phosphorous severely irritates the nose, throat, lungs, and eyes.
Hydrophosphorus acid	Extremely dangerous substitute for red phosphorous. If overheated, deadly phosphine gas is released. Poses a serious fire and explosion hazard.
Lithium metal	Extremely caustic to all body tissues. Reacts violently with water and poses a fire or explosion hazard.
Hydriodic acid	A corrosive acid with vapors that are irritating to the respiratory system, eyes, and skin. If ingested, causes severe internal irritation and damage that may cause death.
Iodine crystals	Gives off vapor that is irritating to respiratory system and eyes. Solid form irritates the eyes and may burn skin. If ingested, it will cause severe internal damage.
Phenylpropanolamine	Ingestion of doses greater than 75 mg. causes hypertension, arrhythmia, anxiety, and dizziness. Quantities greater than 300 mg. can lead to renal failure, seizures, stroke, and death.

From National Drug Intelligence Center. (2002). *Information bulletin: Children at risk* (Document ID: 2002-L0424-001). Retrieved June 27, 2007, from http://www.usdoj.gov/ndic/pubs1/1466/1466p.pdf

Key: mg = milligrams; °F = degrees Fahrenheit.

cess and eliminate chemicals. Thus, acute or chronic diseases, such as neurodevelopmental problems in babies, cancer, and internal organ damage (Science Daily, 2005), may develop when children are exposed to these toxic chemicals. Furthermore, children who have lived in homes where methamphetamine was produced often exhibit emotional and behavioral problems that may persist indefinitely. With the increasing methamphetamine epidemic, officials predict that the number of children exposed to the toxins of these meth labs is likely to continue to increase at alarming rates without major efforts toward education and intervention (NIDA, 2007b).

Secondhand Smoke and Children

The relationship between secondhand smoke and children has become the target of an intense commercial campaign on major television networks as recently as 2006. Unfortunately, children do not have a choice when their parents or other caregivers are smoking around them. The negative health effects from smoking that can affect the adults who are choosing to smoke are the same health issues that can have an impact on children who take in secondhand smoke. It is, therefore, not surprising in schools to see large numbers of children suffering from asthma- and other respiratory-related conditions that may be a result of exposure to secondhand smoke.

School-Related and Learning Issues

In addition to the physical effects of exposure to drugs and alcohol that have already been discussed, numerous issues surface for children who live in homes where substance abuse is present. Aside from the physical difficulties that arise from in utero exposure to drugs and alcohol, there are obstacles that are present for children living in these environments, whether they were exposed in utero or not. Children of alcoholics and drug abusers are commonly living in unforgivable chaos and uncertainty. The amount of energy spent on worrying about their situations, fearing for their well-being, and fulfilling basic survival needs can take a physical as well as an emotional toll on these children. Physical complaints such as headaches and stomachaches are common, especially in school. General feelings of malaise may be common; however, children may not be able to pinpoint "what hurts."

Moreover, trying to maintain a balance between school and the chaos at home can be an emotional drain on children that interferes with their abilities to concentrate and learn. Frequently, children in such situations go to great lengths to protect their families. Unfortunately, these children are generally not willing to share their experiences with anyone at school. Consequently, no one knows the cause of their behaviors, and they may be labeled as lazy and unwilling to complete their work. Educators always need to remember that "behavior is communication" and that there are reasons behind the ways that children present themselves in school.

Breaking the Cycle

Prevention of drug abuse is the best course of action for reducing the number of children who are adversely affected by the damaging effects of drugs and alcohol. According to NIDA (2004), communitywide coalitions working on comprehensive prevention programs that involve the family, schools, communities, and the media in delivering consistent and persistent antidrug messages can be effective in reducing drug abuse. Other approaches to breaking the cycle are discussed next.

Laws Protecting the Unborn

According to a January 2000 report by the National Conference of State Legislatures (Steinberg & Gehshan, 2000), 16 states consider alcohol and drug ingestion during the perinatal period to be child abuse or neglect, including Florida, Illinois, Massachusetts, Minnesota, New York, South Carolina, South Dakota, and Virginia. Such legislation, at a minimum, should trigger an investigation of parental fitness and confirmation of drug use during pregnancy that is made through testing for cocaine, opiates, and alcohol of the newborn at birth. If drug use is revealed, the infant (as well as other children under the mother's care) may be placed in foster care while the mother is referred to a treatment program. In some instances, the child (or children) may be permanently removed from the home if the family fails to participate in a treatment program. However, fear of losing their children may be the main reason that women hesitate to seek treatment and counseling for addiction during pregnancy. Furthermore, women often fear criminal penalties, even though this system is in place to protect children rather than to punish the substance abusing mother. Removing children from their homes generally is a last resort, and when this happens, reunification after treatment is seen

as a goal and one of the measures of success of the program (Steinberg & Gehshan, 2000). Unfortunately, however, appropriate rehabilitation services are yet to be established and/or maintained in many communities throughout the United States, and child protective workers are greatly overworked and increasingly being held accountable for monitoring far too many families.

Early Intervention and Support Systems for Families

In a statement on October 29, 1997, before the U.S. House of Representatives Subcommittee on Labor, Health and Human Services, and Education Committee on Appropriations, Alan I. Leshner, the Director of NIDA and NIH, highlighted the importance of the family environment and the parent–child relationship in deterring young people from engaging in drug use (Leshner, 1997). He noted that one aspect of drug abuse and addiction that may affect the overall health of a child is the environment in which he or she is brought up. This is related to how families play a crucial role in human development throughout the lifespan. Furthermore, a number of NIDA-supported studies accordingly have focused on understanding the role of early family environments in determining later drug use and determining the kinds of family-based interventions, such as strengthening parenting skills, that can be used to offset these early effects (NIDA, 2007a). Because drug use often is a cyclical problem that continues from generation to generation, it is imperative to focus on prevention, education of parents, and formal and informal support systems for families.

Implications for Practice

With information that is now available about the effects of substance abuse on child development, we are now able to focus on improving the learning capacities of young children. To realize the full potential of such efforts, however, appropriate training for educators is imperative (Miller, 2006). Educators must know more about the nature of learning styles and patterns of young children that result from prenatal exposure to both drugs and alcohol so that they and other professionals can offer learning environments and curricula suitable to the needs of their students. It is important for educators to be aware of the behaviors that reflect executive function and self-regulation problems that can affect abilities to attend, remain on task, control impulses and motor function, recall and retrieve information, and plan.

Children of substance abusers are often described as having little concept of time or direction and having difficulty with planning and engaging in unstructured or creative activities. They also may display resistance to change, experience problems with transitions, and forget information or directions. Frequently they are unable to understand the relationships between behavior and consequences and have trouble monitoring their emotions. Cognitive delays and difficulties with processing information may be problematic as well. Without the appropriate training, such behaviors may cause educators themselves to act inappropriately, which often confuses these children and creates more issues that are disruptive to the learning environment. Accordingly, educators need to be prepared to address a range of learning and behavioral challenges of varying degrees of severity (Watson & Westby, 2003).

There are a number of approaches and strategies that educators can use to assist children who are struggling with family addiction. Some children, for instance, may need individual instructions after general instructions have been given to the whole class. Extra time or a reduced workload can sometimes make a significant difference. If a child is unable to focus for a period of time, activities may need to be shortened. Children who are overly active or who may not be aware of their behaviors may need to be allowed to stand for part of their work time and may need reminders about their behaviors. Verbal reminders and physical proximity often are successful in assisting children with maintaining attention. Small-group instruction, games, short and specific directions, and repetition in academic tasks are approaches that can be successfully implemented by general and special education early childhood teachers and other clinical personnel in a variety of settings.

Conclusion

Writing on this same topic, Ensher and Clark (1994) summarized the issues around substance abuse. In many ways, we have moved forward in our efforts to develop new partnerships to address many of these problems that continue to plague infants, young children, and their families in the United States. They wrote the following:

The youngest casualties of the current drug epidemic in the United States are the thousands of infants born each year who are exposed prenatally to drugs, alcohol, and cigarette smoking. Although the media have focused primarily on "crack" cocaine use by pregnant women, that attention ignores the immense number of expectant mothers who use and abuse one or more other legal and illegal substances. Unfortunately, the fact that substance abuse often involves more than one agent makes it exceptionally difficult to determine the effects of any particular agent in subsequent child development. Furthermore, the complexity of situations in which drug-using mothers live certainly contributes to the commonly observed developmental lags of children born into such circumstances [Miller & Hyatt, 1992]. In many situations, prenatally drug-exposed children look much like other children who reside in similarly chaotic homes and neighborhoods and who exhibit behaviors that appear to be excessively negative. Unless prenatally drug-exposed children are referred by neonatal, perinatal, pediatric, or other medical professionals, their problems—subtle or overt—may go undetected for months and sometimes years. (p. 170)

In an effort to address the incidence of prenatal drug and alcohol exposure, education must be at the forefront of preventative measures. It is imperative that schools and health care facilities alike warn people of the dangers of substance abuse on prenatal, neonatal, and childhood development. Unlike many environmental and genetic factors that can have an impact on development, exposure from substance use and/or abuse is one area that is completely avoidable. Most certainly, not every child who is exposed to drugs, alcohol, and tobacco products in utero will have adverse reactions and develop disabilities as a result of this exposure. However, the risks are high and the incidence of adverse outcomes is widespread.

Once the child enters school, there may be educational difficulties that arise from exposure to the various substances discussed in this chapter. It is paramount for educators to gain an awareness not only of the impact that substance use may have had on a child's development, but also of the measures that must be taken in school to help that child meet his or her goals with success. If a child's home life remains chaotic, the roles of the educator, physician, and other professionals become even more significant; and school may be the only stable environment to which the child is exposed.

Regardless of the severity of the disabilities and struggles that might arise in children who are affected by substance use and/or abuse, there is potential for learning and improvement in a child's abilities. Patience, caring, nurturing, and focusing on the individual needs of the child becomes critically important. Perhaps the most inspiring and noteworthy dimensions of children who are affected by drug, alcohol, and tobacco exposure is the resiliency that they demonstrate and their determination to move forward. The literature is filled with stories about the importance of role models and supportive adults. One or two significant people in their lives can make the critical difference between living up to higher expectations and realizing their potentials in the future. Isolation versus supportive community, whether dealing with single parenthood, substance abuse, child abuse and neglect, or many of the other ills that affect young children and their families, very often is the determining factor in the courses that young lives and their families take in eventually breaking the cycle of substance abuse and all that goes with it.

REFERENCES

Abel, E.L. (1998). *Fetal alcohol abuse syndrome.* New York: Plenum.

American College of Obstetricians and Gynecologists. (2005). *Your pregnancy and birth* (4th ed.). Washington, DC: Author.

Bada, H.S., Bauer, C.R., Shankaran, S., Lester, B., Wright, L.L., Das, A., et al. (2002). Central and autonomic signs with in utero drug exposure. *Archives of Disease in Childhood: Fetal and Neonatal Edition, 87*(2), F102–F116.

Batshaw, M.L., Pellegrino, L., & Roizen, N.J. (Eds.). (2007). *Children with disabilities* (6th ed.). Baltimore: Paul H. Brookes Publishing Co.

Beeghly, M., Martin, B., Rose-Jacobs, R., Cabral, T., Heeren, T., Augustyn, M., et al. (2006). Prenatal cocaine exposure and children's language functioning at 6 and 9.5 years: Moderating effects of child age, birthweight, and gender. *Journal of Pediatric Psychology, 31,* 98–115.

Biederman, J., Faraone, S.V., Monuteaux, M.C., & Feighner, J.A. (2000). Patterns of alcohol and drug use in adolescents can be predicted by parental substance use disorders. *Pediatrics, 106*(4), 792–797.

Briggs, G.G., Freedman, R.K., & Yaffe, S.J. (2005). *Drugs in pregnancy and lactation: A reference guide to fetal and neonatal risk* (7th ed.). Philadelphia: Lippincott Williams & Wilkins.

Cogswell, M.E., Weisberg, P., & Spong, C. (2003). Cigarette smoking, alcohol use, and adverse pregnancy outcomes: Implications for micronutrient supplementation. *The Journal of Nutrition, 133*(5), 1722S–1731S.

Coles, C.D., & Black, M.M. (2006). Introduction to the special issue: Impact of prenatal substance exposure on children's health, development, school performance, and risk behavior. *Journal of Pediatric Psychology, 31*(1), 1–4.

Committee on Substance Abuse and Committee on Children with Disabilities, American Academy of Pediatrics. (2000). Fetal alcohol syndrome and alcohol-related neurodevelopmental disorders. *Pediatrics 106*(2), 358–361.

Compton, W.M., Thomas, Y.F., Conway, K.P., & Colliver, J.D. (2005). Developments in the epidemiology of drug use and drug use disorders. *American Journal of Psychiatry, 162,* 1494–1502.

Cone-Wesson, B. (2005). Prenatal alcohol and cocaine exposure: Influences on cognition, speech, language, and hearing. In D. Kendel (Ed.), ASHA 2004 research symposium. *Journal of Communication Disorders, 38,* 279–302.

Derauf, C., Katz, A.R., Frank, D.A., Grandinetti, A., & Easa, D. (2003). The prevalence of methamphetamine and other drug use during pregnancy in Hawaii. *Journal of Drug Issues, 33*(4), 1001–1016.

Ensher, G.L., & Clark, D.A. (1994). *Newborns at risk: Medical care and psychoeducational intervention* (2nd ed.). Gaithersburg, MD: Aspen.

Gearon, J.S., Kaltman, S.I., Brown, C., & Bellack, A.S. (2003). Traumatic life events and PTSD among women with substance use disorders and schizophrenia. *Psychiatric Services, 54,* 523–528.

Gottleib, E. (2007). *The science of addiction.* EBSCO Publishing. Retrieved March 24, 2008, from search.ebscohost.com

Grucza, R.A., Cloninger, C.R., Bucholz, K.K., Constantino, J.N., Schuckit, M.A., Dick, D.M., et al. (2006).

Novelty seeking as a moderator of familial risk for alcohol dependence. *Alcoholism: Clinical & Experimental Research, 30*(7), 1176–1183.

Hillis, S.D., Anda, R.F., Dube, S.R., Felitti, V.J., Marchbanks, P.A., & Mark, J.S. (2004). The association between adverse childhood experiences and adolescent pregnancy, long-term psychosocial consequences, and fetal death. *Pediatrics, 113*(2), 320–327.

Hulse, G.K., Milne, E., Holman, C.D.J., & Bower, C.I. (1997). Maternal cannabis use and birth weight: A meta-analysis. *Addiction, 92*(11), 1553–1560.

Larkby, C., & Day, N. (1997). The effect of prenatal alcohol exposure (morphologic and neurologic manifestations). *Alcohol Health & Research World, 21,* 192–198. Retrieved March 24, 2008, from http://pubs.niaaa.nih.gov/publications/arh21-3/192.pdf

Legrand, L.N., Iacono, W.G., & McGue, M. (2005). Predicting addiction. *American Scientist, 93,* 140–147.

Leshner, A.I. (1997). Statement on children's health issues appearing before the Subcommittee on Labor, Health, and Human Services, and Education Committee on Appropriations, United States House of Representatives. National Institute on Drug Abuse.

Miller, D. (2006). Students with fetal alcohol syndrome: Updating our knowledge, improving their programs. *Teaching Exceptional Children, 38*(4), 12–18.

National Drug Intelligence Center. (2002). *Information bulletin: Children at risk* (Document ID: 2002-L0424-001). Retrieved June 27, 2007, from http://www.usdoj.gov/ndic/pubs1/1466/1466p.pdf

National Institute on Drug Abuse. (1999). *The sixth triennial report to Congress from the Secretary of Health and Human Services: Drug abuse and addiction research: 25 years of discovery to advance the health of the public.* National Institute on Drug Abuse (NIDA) and National Institutes of Health (NIH), a component of the U.S. Department of Health and Human Services. Retrieved June 25, 2007, from http://www.drugabuse.gov/STRC/STRCindex.html

National Institute on Drug Abuse. (2003). NIDA research priorities and highlights: Role of research: Women's Health and Gender Differences. In *Drug abuse and addiction research: The sixth triennial report to Congress.* Bethesda, MD: National Institute on Drug Abuse (NIDA) and National Institutes of Health (NIH), U.S. Department of Health and Human Services. Retrieved August 17, 2007, from http://www.drugabuse.gov/STRC/Role6.html

National Institute on Drug Abuse. (2004). *NIDA research priorities and highlights: Role of research: Prevention of drug use and addiction.* Bethesda, MD: National Institute on Drug Abuse (NIDA) and National Institutes of Health (NIH), U. S. Department of Health and Human Services. Retrieved June 25, 2007, from http://www.drugabuse.gov/STRC/Role5.html

National Institute on Drug Abuse. (2005a). *Research report series: Heroin abuse and addiction.* Bethesda, MD: National Institute on Drug Abuse (NIDA) and National Institutes of Health (NIH), U.S. Department of Health and Human Services. Retrieved March 25, 2008, from http://www.nida.nih.gov/PDF/RRHeroin.pdf

National Institute on Drug Abuse. (2005b). *Research report series: Marijuana abuse: How does marijuana use affect school, work, and social life?* Bethesda, MD: National Institute on Drug Abuse (NIDA) and National Institutes of Health (NIH), U.S. Department of Health and Human Services. Retrieved June 26, 2007, from http://www.drugabuse.gov/researchReports/Marijuana/Marjuana4.html

National Institute on Drug Abuse. (2005c). *Research report series: Marijuana abuse: What are the acute effects of marijuana use?* Bethesda, MD: National Institute on Drug Abuse (NIDA) and National Institutes of Health (NIH), U.S. Department of Health and Human Services. Retrieved June 25, 2007, from http://www.nida.nih.gov/ResearchReports/Marijuana/Marijuana3.html

National Institute on Drug Abuse. (2005d). *Research report series: Methamphetamine abuse and addiction: How is methamphetamine different from other stimulants, such as cocaine?* Bethesda, MD: National Institute on Drug Abuse (NIDA) and National Institutes of Health (NIH), U.S. Department of Health and Human Services. Retrieved June 26, 2007, from http://www/drugabuse.gov/ResearchReports/Methamph/methamph4.html#medical

National Institute on Drug Abuse. (2006a). *Research report series: Inhalant abuse: What are the medical consequences of inhalant abuse?* Bethesda, MD: National Institute on Drug Abuse (NIDA) and National Institutes of Health (NIH), U.S. Department of Health and Human Services. Retrieved June 25, 2007, from http://www.drugabuse.gov/ResearchReports/Inhalants/Inhalants4.html

National Institute on Drug Abuse. (2006b). *Research report series: Prescription drugs: Abuse and addiction: Trends in prescription drug abuse.* Bethesda, MD: National Institute on Drug Abuse (NIDA) and National Institutes of Health (NIH), U.S. Department of Health and Human Services. Retrieved June 22, 2007, from http://www.drugabuse.gov/ResearchReports/Prescription/prescription5.html

National Institute on Drug Abuse. (2006c). *Research report series: Tobacco addiction: Are there other chemicals that may contribute to tobacco addiction?* Bethesda, MD: National Institute on Drug Abuse (NIDA) and National Institutes of Health (NIH), U.S. Department of Health and Human Services. Retrieved June 25, 2007, from http://www.nida.nih.gov/researchreports/nicotine/Nicotine3.html

National Institute on Drug Abuse. (2006d). *Substance-abusing adolescents show ethnic and gender differences in psychiatric disorders.* Retrieved March 25, 2008, from http://137.187.56.161/NIDA_notes/NNVol 18N1/Substance.html

National Institute on Drug Abuse. (2007a). *Congressional and legislative activities: NIDA legislative resources.* Retrieved June 28, 2007, from http://www .drugabuse.gov/about/legislation/legislation.html

National Institute on Drug Abuse. (2007b). *NIDA study suggests crystal methamphetamine use in young adults higher than previously reported.* Retrieved June 22, 2007, from http://www.nida.nih.gov/news room/07/NR6-15.html

National Institute on Drug Abuse. (2008a). *Preventing drug abuse among children and adolescents: Risk factors and protective factors.* Retrieved March 24, 2008, from http://www.nida.nih.gov/prevention/risk .html

National Institute on Drug Abuse. (2008b, March 12). *Scientific research on prescription drug abuse, before the Subcommittee on Crime and Drugs Committee on the Judiciary and the Caucus on International Narcotics Control United States Senate.* Retrieved March 24, 2008, from http://www.nida.nih.gov/Testimony/ 3/12/08Testimony.html

Office of Applied Studies, Substance Abuse and Mental Health Services Administration. (2005). *The NSDUH report: Substance use during pregnancy: 2002 and 2003 update.* Retrieved June 25, 2007, from http://www .oas.samhsa.gov/2k5/pregnancy/pregnancy.htm

Potter, S.M., Zelazo, P.R., Stack, D.M., & Papageorgiou, A.N. (2000). Adverse effects of fetal cocaine exposure on neonatal auditory information processing. *Pediatrics, 105,* e40.

Pressinger, R.W. (1998). *Cigarette smoking during pregnancy: Links to learning disabilities, attention deficit disorder—A.D.D.—hyperactivity and behavior disorders.* Retrieved June 25, 2005, from http://www .chem-tox.com/pregnancy/smoking.htm

Randall, S.R. (1995). Treatment options for drug-exposed infants. In C.N. Chiang & L.P. Finnegan (Eds.), *Medications development for the treatment of pregnant addicts and their infants: NIDA Research Monograph 149* (pp. 78–99). Rockville, MD: National Institute on Drug Abuse and U.S. Department of Health and Human Services.

Schiller, C., & Allen, P.J. (2005). Follow-up of infants prenatally exposed to cocaine. *Pediatric Nursing, 31*(5), 427–436.

Science Daily. (2005, July 27). One hit of crystal meth causes birth defects, affects fetuses at all stages of development. *Science News.* Retrieved March 26, 2008, from http://www.science daily.com/releases/ 2005/07/050727063759.htm

Smith, L.M., LaGasse, L.L., Derauf, C., Grant, P., Shah, R., Arria, A., et al. (2006). The infant development,

environment, and lifestyle study: Effects of prenatal methamphetamine exposure, polydrug exposure, and poverty on intrauterine growth. *Pediatrics, 118*(3), 1149–1156.

Steinberg, D., & Gehshan, S. (2000). *State responses to maternal drug and alcohol use: An update.* Retrieved June 22, 2007, from http://www.ncsl.org/ programs/health/forum/maternalabuse.htm

Substance Abuse and Mental Health Administration. (2006). *Results from the 2005 national survey on drug use and health: National findings.* Office of Applied Studies, NSDUH Series H-30, DHHS, Publication No. SMA 06-4194, Rockville, MD.

Swendsen, J.D., Conway, K.P., Rounsaville, B.J., & Merikangas, K.R. (2002). Are personality traits familial risk factors for substance use disorders? Results of a controlled family study. *American Journal of Psychiatry, 159,* 1760–1766.

Thapar, A., Fowler, F., Rice, F., Scourfield, J., van den Bree, M., Thomas, H., et al. (2003). Maternal smoking during pregnancy and attention deficit hyperactivity disorder symptoms in offspring. *The American Journal of Psychiatry, 160,* 1985–1989.

U.S. Department of Health and Human Services, Administration for Children and Families, Office of Planning, Research and Evaluation. (Updated September 16, 2006). *Revised Final FY 2001 Performance Plan, and FY 2000 Annual Performance Report for the Government Performance and Results Act of 1993: Youth programs.* Retrieved March 24, 2008, from http://www.acf.hhs.gov/programs/opre/ acf_perfplan/ann_per/apr2002/apr02_yth_prog .html

U.S. Department of Justice, National Drug Intelligence Center. (2002). *Information bulletin: Children at risk* (Document Product No. 2002-L0424-001). Retrieved June 27, 2007, from http://www.usdoj .gov/ndic/pubs1/1466/1466p.pdf

Vidaeff, A.C., & Mastrobattista, J.M. (2003). In utero cocaine exposure: A thorny mix of science and mythology. *American Journal of Perinatology, 20*(4), 165–172.

Watson, S.M.R., & Westby, C.E. (2003). Prenatal drug exposure: Implications for personnel preparation. *Remedial & Special Education, 24*(4), 204–214.

Zuckerman, B., Frank, D., & Brown, E. (1995). Overview of the effects of abuse and drugs on pregnancy and offspring. In C.N. Chiang & L.P. Finnegan (Eds.), *Medications development for the treatment of pregnant addicts and their infants: NIDA Research Monograph 149* (pp. 16–38). Rockville, MD: National Institute on Drug Abuse and U.S. Department of Health and Human Services.

CHAPTER 17

The Web of Family Abuse, Neglect, and Violence

Gail L. Ensher and David A. Clark

At the conclusion of this chapter, the reader will

- *Understand some of the intersecting factors and environments that contribute to the web of family abuse and neglect of young children*

- *Understand the short- and long-term effects of child abuse and neglect*

- *Understand some of the newest challenges confronting American schools with growing incidences of bullying and violence*

- *Understand some of the research and educational interventions that have been helpful in ameliorating conditions of maltreatment of young children*

- *Be knowledgeable about some of the preventative strategies that have been effective in defusing violence in American families, communities, and schools*

In their 2004 article, Wu et al. wrote conclusions to their study of infant maltreatment as follows:

> Of the approximately 900,000 children who were determined to be victims of abuse or neglect by US child protective services in 2002, the birth-to-3 age group had the highest rate of victimization (1.6%) and children younger than 1 accounted for the largest percentage of victims (9.6%). (p. 1253)

Poverty, substance abuse, adolescent pregnancy, poor parent mental health and depression, poor health care, minority race and/or ethnicity, single parenthood, social isolation, lack of resources, lower levels of education, parental histories of violence and neglect, special populations of children (e.g., preterm infants or children with disabilities), and communities of violence all have been linked to abuse and neglect of young children within families. With an eye on prevention, many researchers have sought to tease out those factors that seem to contribute most to maltreatment and neglect (Dong et al., 2004; Kelley, 2003; Kerr, Black, & Krishnakumar, 2000; Stevens-Simon, Nelligan, & Kelly, 2001; Windham et al., 2004; Zelenko, Lock, Kramer, & Steiner, 2000). Other researchers have attempted to examine those protective factors that contribute to resilience or appear to buffer children in high-risk situations (Heller, Larrieu, D'Imperio, & Boris, 1999; Osofsky, 1999; Rutter, 2000).

Magnitude of the Problem in the United States

Some researchers have characterized violence in the United States as a growing "public health epidemic" (Osofsky, 1999, p. 33). Although sources of data continue to be controversial, statistics (considered to be an underestimation in the best of circumstances) tell part of the story of the ever-increasing problems of neglect, abuse, and violence against children in this country:

- Some children, especially those living in low-income areas, experience chronic violence in their communities, with frequent, continued exposure to guns, knives, drugs, and random violence (Osofsky, 1999).

- Estimates have revealed that 3.3 million children witness physical and verbal spousal abuse each year, including insults, hitting, and fatal assaults with guns and knives (Osofsky, 1999).

- Estimates have revealed that as many as 3 million children are physically abused by their parents (Osofsky, 1999).

- "Violence in the media . . . touches virtually every child. . . . The typical American child watches 28 hours of television a week, and by the age of 18 will have seen 16,000 simulated murders and 200,000 acts of violence" (Osofsky, 1999, p. 34).

- "Commercial television for children is 50 to 60 times more violent than prime-time programs for adults, and some cartoons average more than 80 violence acts per hour" (Osofsky, 1999, p. 34).

- "With the advent of videocassette sales and rentals of movies, pay-per-view TV, cable TV, video games, and online interactive computer games, many more children and adolescents are exposed to media with violent content than ever before" (Osofsky, 1999, p. 34).

- Statistics from 2003 showed that approximately 80% of perpetrators of child maltreatment were parents; other relatives accounted for 6% and unmarried partners of parents and "others" accounted for 4% of the perpetrators (National Association of Counsel for Children, 2007).

- Many adults cite past incidences of verbal abuse by teachers as the most overwhelming, negative experiences in their lives (Brendgen, Wanner, & Vitaro, 2006). Indeed, some would say that such abuse is "epidemic" in our schools.

- Children with special health care needs (Giardino, Hudson, & Marsh, 2003) and children with disabilities (Orelove, Hollahan, & Myles, 2000) are known to be at increased risk in terms of all forms of child maltreatment when compared to children without such needs.

- Although the retrospective reporting of these experiences cannot establish a causal association with certainty, exposure to parental alcohol abuse is highly associated with experiencing adverse childhood experiences (Dube et al., 2001).

- Although most everyone agrees that "it shouldn't hurt to be a child," how to prevent this hurt and at what cost is unclear, often resulting in benign neglect (Daro & Donnelly, 2002).

- Thousands of U.S. children experience abuse and neglect every day. Although state child protective service (CPS) agencies identify and help many of these children and their families, many cases of abuse or neglect go unreported. In addition, not all states provide detailed case-level data to the National Child Abuse and Neglect Data System (American Humane, 2007).

- Even when prevention programs use a strength-based service delivery approach, most families "will leave before reaching their service goals or achieving the service levels articulated in the program's model"; this tendency "and the absence of solid outcomes among many of the families served suggest that the full promise of prevention has yet to be realized" (Daro & Donnelly, 2002, p. 737).

Meanings and Definitions

Throughout the years, numerous issues have complicated our ability to comprehend this epidemic that plagues so many children and families in this country. When a child has been violated, it is so clear that wrongdoing has taken place. Those professionals in the educational, medical, and social work fields invariably are dismayed and enraged. However, where lines are drawn across different ethnic groups, cultures, and child-rearing practices often is unclear. In addition, documenting instances of neglect and emotional abuse continues to be a daunting challenge for all involved in protecting children, especially those within our youngest populations. Azar (2002), for example, wrote,

> The legally identified categories of abuse and neglect are umbrellas for a heterogeneous set of events occurring to children. For example, Zuranvin (1991) defined 13 types of behaviors included in neglect: supervisory neglect, refusal or delay in providing health or mental health care, custody refusal or related neglect, abandonment/desertion, failure to provide a home, personal hygiene neglect, housing hazards or sanitation problems, nutritional neglect, and educational neglect. Some definitions include emotional neglect (a marked indifference to children's needs for affection, attention, and emotional support), as well as exposure to chronic or extreme abuse. Emotional abuse has been seen as both central to all maltreatment and as a distinct entity. It includes acts that are psychologically damaging to children's behavioral, cognitive, affective, or physical functioning . . . Clearly, this heterogeneity has been difficult to encompass in a single psychological theory of parenting. (p. 367)

Inevitably, a central issue is the determining line between where child maltreatment begins and ends. Developmental stages of children must be considered. Moreover, other factors include the presence of a disability, the timeframe of abuse and/or neglect, and special family circumstances or stressors. Azar (2002) noted,

> Although the earliest decades of the field of child maltreatment suffered from a lack of sophisticated theory (Azar, Fantuzzo, & Twentyman, 1994; Crittenden, 1998), the last two have seen a growth of more sophisticated attempts to explain the origins of physical abuse. Etiological theories specific to neglect, however, continue to lag behind, perhaps because of the heterogeneity of the behaviors under this label and sociopolitical issues that surround behaviors so closely linked to poverty in the United States. This lack of progress is striking, given the high prevalence of neglect. (p. 368)

Having acknowledged the realities of these statements, one should not be lulled into a belief or assumption that maltreatment of children occurs only within families below the poverty line. Such families, especially those from various ethnic backgrounds or from underrepresented groups, undoubtedly come to the attention of the authorities more frequently and more readily. However, abuse and neglect of those within our care indeed cuts across all financial and educational sectors of our country, despite the fact that researchers have repeatedly attempted to connect abuse and/or neglect to specific ethnic groups and cultures (Ferrari, 2002; Korbin, 2002). Over the years, perhaps the most promising development in attempting to understand the various dimensions and etiologies of child abuse and neglect is that we have come full circle to the realization that a multiple perspective, ecological view rather than a single explanation of causation comes closest to the truth of what happens in most families where maltreatment occurs.

To date, despite the troubling incidence of child abuse and neglect of children, there is no one commonly accepted definition of *child abuse and neglect* (National Association of Counsel for Children, 2007; Straus & Kantor, 2005). Every state has established its own definition of child abuse and neglect, thus adding to the complexities of reaching any consensus. Key federal legislation that addresses child abuse and neglect is the Child Abuse Prevention and Treatment Act (CAPTA) that was originally enacted in 1974 as PL 93-247. This legislation most recently was amended and reauthorized on June 25, 2003, as the Keeping Children and Families Safe Act of 2003 (PL 108-36) (Title I–Child Abuse Prevention and Treatment Act–117 Stat. 801). Accordingly, in its broadest terms, the federal government defines *child abuse and neglect* as

> The physical and mental injury, sexual abuse, negligent treatment, or maltreatment of a child under the age of 18 by a person who is responsible for the child's welfare under circumstances which indicate that the child's health or welfare is harmed or threatened. (Child Abuse Prevention and Treatment Act, 1974; Keeping Children and Families Safe Act, 2003)

Pieces of the Puzzle ————

Given the ambiguities of definition, the realities persist every year, with child protective services receiving approximately 2.9 million referrals alleging child maltreatment and, after investigation, confirmation that more than 900,000 children annually have been the victims of maltreatment (National Association of Counsel for Children, 2007). With the recognition that this figure undoubtedly is an underestimation of actual events, the statistics are staggering and growing again (American Humane, 2007). The next questions to be asked inevitably are: Why in this country of affluence and technology are we faced with such social tragedies? What can be done to address these problems? Clearly, answers need to focus on both sides of the issues, including policies and strategies for prevention before such acts are committed, and then, in the face of perpetration, policies and strategies that establish pathways toward remediation. Depending on the causes or origins of any given family's problems, solutions will vary.

At best, the pieces of the puzzle are complex and always evolving over time. To date, what seems evident from research are the following scenarios:

- Child abuse and neglect reportedly are more prevalent in families of very young (adolescent) parents (Dukewich, Borkowski, & Whitman, 1999; Landy & Menna, 2006; Stevens-Simon, Nelligan, & Kelly, 2001). Such elements of risk undoubtedly stem from several problems, including the immaturities of adolescence, lack of understanding of appropriate developmental milestones of infants and young children, choice of partners, and/or lack of skill in caregiving and guiding challenging behavior as young children enter their toddler years.

- Child abuse, neglect, and violence are more likely to be evident in families where parents and caregivers are engaging in substance abuse (Dube et al., 2001; Dube et al., 2003; Kelley, 2003; Landy & Menna, 2006; Nair, Schuler, Black, Kettinger, & Harrington, 2003; Osofsky & Thompson, 2000; Smith & Testa, 2002).

Overall, such families tend to be multirisk, dysfunctional, isolated, and difficult to reach, despite the advantages of long-term intervention programs. Adverse effects may begin early with prenatal exposure to drugs and alcohol, continuing with later environmental influences that exert a cumulative negative impact on psychosocial and cognitive development throughout the primary years.

- Although the mechanisms of transmission remain controversial (Newcomb & Locke, 2001), in the absence of a significant caregiver, ally, or person of influence, children who have been the victims of child abuse and neglect or who have witnessed noteworthy violence in their families (directed toward a sibling or between caregivers) are more likely to grow up to abuse and/or neglect their own children (Pears & Capaldi, 2001). Such intergenerational patterns, once again, are often resistant to change, even though they may have been the preventative and remediation recipients of many therapeutic intervention programs (Schuler, Nair, & Black, 2002).

- Moreover, within families with histories of chronic child abuse, neglect, and violence, it is common to find mothers and fathers who suffer from a lack of resources and resilience (Kerr, Black, & Krishnakumar, 2000; Zelenko, Lock, Kraemer, & Steiner, 2000) and who also may struggle with issues of depression or other social-emotional issues (Berger, 2005; Mammen, Kolko, & Pilkonis, 2002) These circumstances place their children at further risk for abuse and neglect. Indeed, much of the research carried out to date has emphasized the complexity in trying to understand child maltreatment because of the multiple and interacting dimensions of the problems within families. In other words, etiologies are anything but simple or singular.

- Finally, research on child abuse and neglect has focused on issues and considerations other than family factors. For example, a number of studies have dealt specifically with child-related concerns, such as the presence of learning challenges and the dynamics of child attachment that may have been affected by prematurity and extended stays in neonatal intensive care nurseries.

The Youngest Victims of Abuse and Neglect: Lifelong Effects

One concern that has been well documented over the years is that for the youngest victims of abuse and neglect, the effects typically are lifelong and leave a permanent handprint. This is reflected in the following poem.

The Secret's Shadow

A secret came into my life
And made my soul to cry
No matter what I do
Its shadow will never die
Memories planted too deeply
Pain I can never erase
Guilt and shame engulf me
They follow me place to place
I couldn't face reality
So slowly I withdrew
I only wanted love
But no one ever knew
I never told in words
My actions told the truth
A shadow left by a secret
Stole my very youth
The judge asked me questions
As tears welled in my heart
He never believed my story
And my world crumbled apart
The silent shadows deepened
The lines you can trace
For every hurt of life
Is written on my face
Now a counselor I must see
More questions she will ask
God please grant me more faith
If I am to finish this task
No Band-Aid for this wound
No medicine for the pain
The secret never goes away
It's embedded in my name.
—Virginia Anonymous (1997)

Pediatric Markers for Child Neglect and Abuse

Although there are typical variations in the scheme of normal development in terms of growth in height and weight, as well as the progression of intellectual, emotional, social, and sexual changes in young children, there are at the same time pediatric markers for child neglect and abuse. Physicians attending to children are in a prime position to be the first to identify these risks in families. Prevention and referral for outside services always should be the goal, rather than waiting until after the fact. Thus, if parents or caregivers fail to keep routine appointments for well-child care and checkups, or if children do not go to community and/or medical facilities for pediatric care, physicians should be alert to such failures to keep or make appointments and attempt to make contact with families to see the child. Well-child examinations typically take place at 2–4 weeks of age, and subsequently at 2, 4, 6, 9, 12, 18, and 24 months of age, followed by routine, annual well-child checkups after the age of 2 years. Moreover, a child's failure to gain weight (e.g., decreased weight for length and height [less than the 5th percentile], actual weight loss that is possibly accompanied by psychosocial problems) likewise should raise concerns on the part of a competent physician, who should be able to rule out issues of child neglect and abuse with good family history, physical examination, and minimal laboratory tests.

When there is evidence of a developmental delay or potential developmental disability (it is estimated that 16% of children have some form of developmental delay and/or disability), physicians have the training and responsibility to discuss such issues with families and make referrals to appropriate early intervention or pre-K services as early as possible. Such services are free-of-charge to families. In the event that families refuse to explore or access therapeutic and educational programs that might allow their children access to long-term benefits of improved health and later school outcomes, pediatricians need to be concerned and raise alarms about the well-being and health of the children involved.

Among the most revealing markers for ongoing child abuse and neglect are the behaviors of children, symptoms that may be evident even in the earliest years. For example, Table 17.1 presents some of the behavioral indicators that should serve as "red flags" to medical, educational, and social service personnel. Table 17.2 lists some of the risk factors associated with child abuse and

Table 17.1. Variations in childhood sexuality and possible indicators of sexual abuse

Natural behavior	Behavior of concern	Behavior requiring immediate help
Interest in urination and defecation	Plays with feces, urinates purposely outside toilet bowl	Plays or smears feces repeatedly, purposely urinates on furniture
Plays house	Simulates sexual intercourse with other children with clothes on, imitates sexual behavior with dolls	Simulates sexual intercourse while naked
Wants privacy in the bathroom	Becomes upset when observed	Aggressive or fearful in demand for privacy
Looks at nude pictures	Continuous fascination with nude pictures	Masturbates to nude pictures
Masturbates	Masturbates in public after being told not to	Masturbates in public to exclusion of other childhood activities

Table 17.2. Risk factors for abuse and neglect

Factors related to the family	Factors related to the child
Alcohol and/or drug abuse	Chronic illness
Domestic violence	Difficult temperament
Lower levels of parental education	Multiple births (e.g., several children in a given family, multiple gestations)
Parental depression	
Stress factors within the family (financial, food, and/or housing)	Prematurity
	Young age
Unstable family situations	
Young and/or single parents	

neglect. In addition, as noted earlier in this chapter, certain populations of children and families historically have been at higher risk than others for child abuse and neglect. These include families of teen and/or single parents, infants and young children who are difficult to care for (e.g., preterm babies and children with developmental disabilities and/or chronic illness), families experiencing financial stress, families with evidence of substance abuse and violence, and families struggling with depression. When these factors are known to physicians, they should continue to be vigilant to family situations and crises. Should the pediatrician have concerns, he or she should contact other adults who see the child in different settings, such as teachers or school counselors, early intervention and pre-K providers, psychologists, and possibly CPS case workers. Moreover, anticipatory guidance always needs to be offered to families, especially to young and/or inexperienced parents in terms of safety at home and in the car, strategies for the prevention of injury, smoking, supervision around water and family pools, helmets when riding bikes, and the importance of smoke detectors.

It is a well-documented fact that the majority of young children in the United States who are the victims of child abuse and neglect are younger the age of 5 years, with a significant number of those children being between 1 and 2 years (Clark, 2007). Within the first 12 months of life, infants are especially vulnerable to an extremely dangerous form of child abuse called shaken baby syndrome (SBS), which is violently shaking the infant with or without impact. It is estimated that between 600 and 1,400 children annually (Clark, 2007) are the silent victims of SBS, often occurring as a result of a caregiver or parent being unable to calm a child from inconsolable crying. The consequences for the child are usually devastating and can result in one or more of the following injuries:

- Subdural hemorrhages (bleeding in the brain under the skull)

- Retinal hemorrhages (bleeding in the back of the eye)

- Damage to the spinal cord and neck

- Fractures of the ribs and bones and skin bruising

Moreover, many infants have a history of having been abused or shaken in the past. Approximately 60% of the cases are children who have a history of having been shaken or maltreated, and approximately 22% of the families have had prior involvement with child welfare authorities (Clark, 2007). In addition, there are discernible patterns in terms of the perpetrators of these injuries, most of which are committed by individuals known to families:

- Male perpetrators outnumber females 2.2 to 1.

- More than 60% of the crimes are committed by fathers, 37% by stepfathers, and 20% by mothers' boyfriends.

- 17.3% are committed by female baby sitters.

- 12.6% are committed by mothers.

Unfortunately, unless the perpetrators of these crimes are familiar to law or child protection agencies, there have not been any truly effective ways to prevent such heinous crimes. Death is the outcome in 20% of the cases, neurological injury in 55%, and visual impairment in 65%.

Developmental Consequences

When child maltreatment happens, inevitably there are serious, short- and long-term effects for young children. Depending on the severity, frequency, age of the child, availability of other significant people to buffer situations, and the type of abuse (i.e., sexual, social-emotional, or physical) or neglect (i.e., social-emotional or physical), the developmental and social-emotional consequences will vary, which points to diverse needs in intervention and/or remediation and treatment programs. For example, a number of studies have focused on short- and long-term developmental and/or cognitive functioning difficulties as a result of cumulative child maltreatment factors (Mackner, Starr, & Black, 1997; Osofsky, 1999). Hilyard and Wolfe wrote,

> Past as well as very recent findings converge on the conclusion that child neglect can have severe, deleterious short- and long-term effects on children's cognitive, socio-emotional, and behavioral development. Consistent with attachment and related theories, neglect occurring early in life is particularly detrimental to subsequent development. Moreover, neglect is associated with effects that are, in many areas, unique from physical abuse, especially throughout childhood and early adolescence. Relative to physically abused children, neglected children have more severe cognitive and academic deficits, social withdrawal and limited peer interactions, and internalizing (as opposed to externalizing) problems. (2002, p. 679)

Similarly, findings from a study of 6-year-old children and their families that was conducted by Kerr, Black, and Krishnakumar (2000) indicated that "children who simultaneously have a history of both FTT [failure to thrive] and maltreatment demonstrate more behavior problems and worse school functioning and cognitive performance than children who have neither of these risk factors" (p. 593).

Likewise, of particular interest to physicians, educators, and other professionals working with families has been the social-emotional and behavioral effects of various types of maltreatment on children at different ages. Some research, for example, has examined the impact of child abuse on play and peer interactions (Darwish, Esquival, Houtz, & Alfonso, 2001) and found that "the experience of maltreatment has a negative impact on children's developing interpersonal skills above and beyond the influence of factors associated with low socioeconomic status and other environmental stressors" (p. 31). The American Academy of Pediatrics (2000) stressed the especially devastating effects of child abuse, neglect, violence, and possibly placement of children in foster care on brain development during the earliest years of life. In particular, the Committee on Early Childhood, Adoption and Dependent Care cited the paramount importance of continuity with primary attachment figures during the critical, developing years of young children. By extension, Osofsky (1999) has cited a number of developmental differences in infants and young children who witness violence in their homes, including excessive irritability, immature behavior, sleep disturbances, emotional distress, fears of being alone, and regression in toileting and language. Among school-age children, such differences may be manifested as sleep disturbances, reluctance to play and explore their environments, distractibility, and even symptoms associated with posttraumatic stress disorder (PTSD).

Later Manifestations of Exposure to Violence

Finally, as noted previously, a number of authors have pointed to the fact that although not all individuals who suffer from maltreatment as young children become adults who abuse and neglect their own children, this population of parents is found to be overrepresented among families who are considered dysfunctional and/or violent (Shonkoff & Phillips, 2000). In essence, there is a cycle of neglect, abuse, and violence that carries from one generation of families to another. This transmission of child maltreatment and household dysfunction is especially troubling because it emphasizes the chronicity of problems of multirisk families and the historical resistance to addressing such difficulties across the life span (Newcomb & Locke, 2001; Pears & Capaldi, 2001).

Bullying and Violence in American Schools ____

Violence is, unfortunately, a common phenomenon in the United States. At very young ages, children are exposed to extremely concerning situations via the media, printed materials, and in their neighborhood communities. Furthermore, since the late 1990s, there has been a dramatic increase in violent events that have involved children and adolescents in our American schools that are either self-inflicted or perpetrated by grievous adults. They include verbal abuse and "put downs" by teachers and bullying by peers. Depending on the longevity of the abuse and the age of exploitation, both can have extremely devastating effects. Sadly, both types of events have become common occurrences in contemporary American schools, where parents send their children with the assumption that they are "safe" places that are protected from verbal and physical harm.

Relating to child treatment and experiences in the early grades and to possible verbal maltreatment by teachers, Entwisle and Alexander (1999) wrote,

> A major source of social inequity is that elementary schools are exceedingly homogeneous in terms of their students' socioeconomic background. The boundaries of U.S. neighborhoods faithfully mirror the fault lines in the larger society, and elementary schools function along lines dictated by the socioeconomic characteristics of the neighborhoods in which they are located rather than along lines determined by the school's own educational goals. Children who live in good neighborhoods effectively land on a fast academic track because their

parents and teachers perceive them and treat them as "high-ability" children, whereas children who live in poor neighborhoods land on a slow academic track because they are perceived and treated as "low-ability" children. The myth that elementary schools share the same curriculum is false. Even when all schools use the same lesson plans and textbooks, as in Baltimore City, the SES [socioeconomic status] of the neighborhood determines the way instruction proceeds and the quality of life children experience in their classrooms. (p. 19)

Paralleling this statement, Brendgen, Wanner, and Vitaro (2006) wrote,

> Many adults mention past incidences of verbal abuse by the teacher as the most overwhelming negative experience in their lives. The present study examined the course and stability of verbal abuse by the teacher from kindergarten through grade 4 ... Verbal abuse by the teacher seems to be a highly stable phenomenon for at-risk children. Children who are relatively well adjusted are at low risk of becoming the target of verbal abuse by the teacher. If they do, however, these children are the most vulnerable to subsequent developmental difficulties. (p. 1585)

Extrapolating from the statements of these researchers, it appears that not infrequently those children who might be considered the most vulnerable in their early school years continue to be so throughout their elementary educational experiences and further into adolescence. Not surprisingly, a cycle of maltreatment—or at least neglect—is perpetuated and may have long-lasting social-emotional, behavioral, and academic consequences for children that are very difficult to redirect and remediate. Therefore, for these children, teacher abuse is highly likely to become a self-fulfilling prophecy that is relived repeatedly in negative scenarios. As a result, children who are already disadvantaged may find themselves even more isolated, threatened, and spiraling into environments of hostility with no apparent end in sight.

Similarly, debilitating patterns of maltreatment for young children may emerge when they find themselves the target of bullying at the hands of their peers in school settings. Interestingly, studies about bullying often have appeared in medically related publications; however, the issues are a concern for physicians and educators alike and are not insignificant in terms of the magnitude of the problem. Lyznicki, Mc-Caffree, and Robinowitz indicated that

> In 1999, the U.S. Departments of Education and Justice estimated that almost 1 million students 12 to 18 years of age (4 percent) reported being afraid during the previous six months that they would be attacked or harmed in the school vicinity; about 5 percent reported avoiding one or more places in school, and 13 percent reported being targets of hate-related language. (2004, p. 1723)

Bullying may take any of three forms, that is, verbal, physical, or threatening behavior (Lyznicki, McCaffree, & Robinowitz, 2004). Most researchers writing about this issue have indicated that the prevalence of bullying among American youth is substantial (The Center for Health and Health Care in Schools, 2004) and deserves serious attention. Similar to child maltreatment in family homes, the magnitude of the problem undoubtedly is much more widespread than is presently known, with long-term consequences for children and adolescents. Finally, not surprisingly, and supportive of the research on transmission of child maltreatment, those engaging in bullying behavior have often been the victims of bullying or interparental violence themselves (Baldry, 2003).

Resilience in Children and Families

In the end, some children from a very early age succumb more easily to the risks and disadvantages of their environment, whereas others seem to escape less scathed or protected from the ravages of violence and maltreatment in their families, schools, and neighborhoods. Within this latter group that represents a smaller percentage, these children are being referred to as "resilient" (Landy & Menna, 2006; Rutter, 2000). Such differences are seen both within families and across populations of children subjected to abuse and/or neglect. Inevitably, in the face of such variation, we are left with the haunting question as to why some children are so vulnerable, whereas others appear not to be in response to a

continuum of adversity. Moreover, given the benefit of intervention, how can we tip the balance more heavily toward a venue of protection? How can some children look so good, given their known family situations?

There is much to consider in attempting to answer these questions and in developing intervention programs that bring about change in both children and their families. Some of the differences reside in the severity of exposure to violence, the presence of a significant other who can serve to "protect" the child, the age of exposure to maltreatment, the length of time during which the child was subjected to abuse and/or neglect, the relief or removal from the violence, and child-specific characteristics. Most likely, resilience or an ability to adapt beyond adversity for more favorable outcomes ultimately will reside with the benefit of a combination of factors influencing any given child within the context of his or her family. Also, how we determine and who identifies positive outcomes and when in the lives of children these questions are examined may vary across agencies, teachers, or those making such judgment calls. Children change. They may "look" well adjusted at one point in their lives; yet, given a different set of circumstances, they may need support and intervention at another time. Thus, on the continuum of living from day to day, these are indeed difficult determinations to make. However, there are children who, in reality, do better than others, and it is imperative to examine why and how that can be and then to translate that evidence into practice whenever possible.

In his insightful chapter, *Resilience Reconsidered*, Michael Rutter (2000) pointed out just how complex it is to attempt to define processes of resilience over time. Drawing from the research of another author (Garmezy, 1985), Rutter cited three sets of protective factors that may be considerations in defusing or mitigating against childhood adversity. They are as follows (Rutter, 2000, p. 658):

1. Personality features such as autonomy, self-esteem, and a socially positive orientation
2. Family cohesion, warmth, and an absence of discord
3. The availability of external support systems

Clearly, duration, intensity, and consistency of exposure to such factors, as well as what might be considered physiological and/or psychological susceptibility to events of risk, weigh heavily in terms of the impact of adversity. In addition, Rutter (2000) indicated that there will be no single solution that fits or addresses the variety of conditions and situations faced by children coping with adversity. Most likely, implications for developing preventative or remediation programs will include strategies such as

- A reduction of stress, adversity, and negative chain reactions

- An increase in positive chain reactions

- Exposure to new opportunities that can break a cycle of maltreatment or adversity

- Participation in "compensatory experiences"

- The "cognitive processing of experiences" (Rutter, 2000, p. 674).

In conclusion, Rutter wrote,

> The realization that resilience is not a fixed characteristic of individuals but rather represents several somewhat different types of dynamic processes operating over time has considerably opened up the opportunities for considering how the findings may be used to develop more effective preventive policies. Because the risk and protective factors involved in different kinds of maladaptive outcome are not the same, and because the processes leading to resilience are greatly influenced by context, it is not likely that the results will translate into a single coherent program. In the past, there has sometimes been a wish to search for the hallmarks of resilience, as if once one knew what it "looked like," it should be a relatively straightforward matter to design interventions to bring it about. That no longer appears to be a sensible aim. . . . Nevertheless, although a lot has still to be learned, there is now a much better understanding of the different sorts of processes that are likely to be implicated. (2000, p. 675)

Programs of Promise: Using the Best of What We Know _____

As many family and community factors seem to contribute to events of child maltreatment, likewise multiple processes and practices are critical

for successful prevention and/or the remediation of child abuse and neglect. Moreover, numerous researchers have argued that those programs or interventions that carry the most promise are those that have been designed with ecological and empowerment perspectives and have been tied in partnerships to existing community and neighborhood resources (Chaffin & Friedrich, 2004) that are readily available to families (Fantuzzo, Manz, Atkins, & Meyers, 2005; MacLeod & Nelson, 2000). The timing of intervention and the age of the child at the onset of the program also are critical factors, as well as important considerations of whether programs are preventative or reactive in the cycle of abuse or neglect.

Models

Both preventative and remediation models of intervention have focused on a variety of strategies with families and children, including the following:

- Home visitation by professionally trained nurses, social workers, and others (Alexander et al., 2003; Daro & Harding, 1999; Leventhal, 1997) or lay paraprofessional personnel with various components of parent education, skill development, and guidance (Anisfeld, Sandy, & Guterman, 2004)

- Parent–child interaction therapy (Timmer, Urquiza, Zebell, & McGrath, 2005)

- Peer-mediated interactions among preschool children during play sessions (Fantuzzo, Manz, Atkins, & Meyers, 2005)

- Family preservation (McCroskey & Meezan, 1998) with intensive follow-up, crisis management, and a focus on family strengths

- Out-of-home foster care placement of children

To date, findings on outcomes for children and families have been promising but are inconclusive. Such results are not surprising, given the complexity in terms of the severity and forms of child maltreatment, problems of evaluation, issues concerning sustainability of positive changes, variations in vulnerability and risk across the life spans of families, as well as numerous other factors that are not well controlled or predictable.

Most certainly, the collective prevention efforts of the home visiting model of Healthy Families America (HFA), first initiated in Hawaii and now extending to more than 270 programs in 38 states and the District of Columbia, stands as one example of a network that has produced very positive, short-term changes in parent–child interactions among high-risk families and community systems of support (Daro & Harding, 1999). Daro and Harding wrote about the program,

> As such, the current pool of evaluative findings provides only partial evidence of the initiative's overall impact and the utility of developing programs that embrace HFA's 12 critical elements. Within this context, however, these initial findings suggest that continued program development along the lines of the HFA model offers significant hope for reducing child maltreatment rates and enhancing parental capacity. (1999, p. 168)

Indicators of Success

The field of research on issues and models of child maltreatment is replete with numerous iterations of what constitutes a successful intervention program. Among those cited, researchers have indicated changes in

- Parent–child interactions
- Play-related behaviors of children with peers
- Skills of parents or caregivers in managing the behavior of their children
- Substance use and abuse
- Numbers of subsequent pregnancies
- Sustained engagement with intervention programs over time
- Subsequent reported incidents of child maltreatment and family crises and violence
- Incidence of depression among mothers and fathers
- Regular participation in community support groups

Clearly, not all of these indicators apply to every family involved in proactive and/or preventative or reactive and/or remediation programs. Moreover, there are inevitable, standing questions to be answered relative to the duration of positive effects. For example, how do we consider relapses of family and child behavior in the face of success? For what periods of time do families need to sustain positive change in order for interventions to be considered effective? What percentages of families need to reflect positive change for us to consider model programs to be successful? What are the signature indicators that programs are working? Such issues continue to surface as we think about how to address the enormous concerns of child abuse, neglect, and violence on a large-scale basis. Finally, how should and can the field of research about child maltreatment move from smaller projects to the broad-scale adoption of training and implementation across diverse disciplines? It is well known within the medical, educational, and clinical professions that those families most in need of services often are the most difficult to engage and retain. In response to prevention and remediation programs, trends of parents leaving programs before targeted goals are met were seen frequently. Therefore, the most severe cycles of abuse and neglect likely continued.

Conclusion

We do not pretend to have any simple solutions to remedy problems of such magnitude; however, programs of promise do seem to point to some important considerations for future endeavors. The following is clear from our perspective:

1. Services need to be accessible and connected to real neighborhoods and communities in which families reside (e.g., universal pre-K programs, kindergartens, community health centers, physicians). Family practice doctors and pediatricians will be especially crucial to such efforts because they are at the frontline and very likely to see both parents and children in the events of trouble and violence.

2. To the extent possible, services need to adopt a proactive and positive stance that attempts to build on family strengths rather than deficits and failure. There will be times that such attitudes and perspectives cannot be pursued because of the imminent danger for children; however, thus far, much of what

we have done has been developed by taking away privileges without replacing skills and abilities. When programs are no longer involved with families, parents must be able to sustain the gains that they have made, even in the face of adversity.

3. Services need to be tied to the real, everyday tasks and responsibilities of raising children, rather than adding new and unfamiliar components to family lives. Furthermore, such services must be ethnically and culturally sensitive, as long as they do not violate the protection and safety of young children.

4. Services must demand that professionals develop new partnerships and collaborations that possibly share funding sources, but most definitely share training efforts, information, and expertise. The old adage that "each tub sits on its own bottom" has proven to be unsuccessful. Preventing families from becoming isolated is a high priority because it is a well-documented observation that parents who find themselves alone, without community and neighborhood resources, are much more likely to face difficulties of crisis magnitude.

5. Better ways to translate and integrate the positive findings from research more immediately into practice on the frontlines needs to be developed, and these will need to be adaptable to the differences across communities and neighborhoods in which families reside.

6. Early signs of family trouble must alert physicians, educators, and other clinical personnel to be proactive rather than wait. Adequate documentation has been a stumbling block in the past and too often has prevented professionals from moving ahead to put services and supports in place until after an incident. In the long run, in terms of both human and financial cost, the end result for everyone would be far greater if we are able to reach families and children much earlier, especially given that most abuse and neglect takes place within the first 5 years of a child's life.

7. To change the increasing and cyclical trajectories of child maltreatment, efforts will need to be multifaceted and will need to offer families grassroots information about a number of danger points that are likely to lead to abuse and neglect. In this regard, families need to utilize their own strengths toward empowerment and change in their own lives. As professionals, it is unlikely that we can prevent families from making their own mistakes, but we always should strive to help them learn from their past so that they can move forward toward more conflict- and violence-free lives.

In conclusion, we draw upon the words of Chaffin and Friedrich:

Ultimately, moving the child welfare and child abuse service systems toward EBP [evidence-based practice] will require a combination of organization, leadership, policy changes, and marketing. More fundamentally, however, it will require a fundamental change in the estranged practitioners taking up models handed down from clinical scientists. It also means that practice must become more like research and research must become more like practice. The path toward cumulative progress and refined interventions lies in partnerships, and in synergistic efforts of clinical scientists and frontline practitioners to innovate and refine models, systematically test the results, and then feed this information back into the service system. This iterative approach has proven fruitful in other fields. For example, the treatment of childhood leukemia has been one of the success stories of medicine, moving in a few decades from no long-term survival to longer-term survival by a large majority of children. Rather, it came by treatment centers and researchers organizing into research practice collaboratives, and conducting large-scale randomized field trials of progressively more refined and effective treatment protocols. Thus, progress was evolutionary, rather than revolutionary. To the extent that we can form similar partnerships in child abuse, we can see our own evolutionary development. (2004, p. 1111)

REFERENCES

Alexander, R., Baca, L., Fox, J.A., Frantz, M., Glanz, S., Huffman, L.D., et al. (2003). New hope for preventing child abuse and neglect: Proven solutions to save lives and prevent future crime. Retrieved August 5, 2007, from http://www.fightcrime.org

American Academy of Pediatrics, Committee on Early Childhood, Adoption and Dependent Care. (2000). Developmental issues for young children in foster care. *Pediatrics, 106*, 1145–1150.

American Humane. (2007). *Child fact sheet: Child abuse and neglect: How are we really doing?* Retrieved April 1, 2008, from http://www.americanhumane.org/site/Pageserver?pagename=nr_fact_sheets_childabuse data

Anisfeld, E., Sandy, J., & Guterman, N.B. (2004). *Best beginnings: A randomized controlled trial of a paraprofessional home visiting program. Final Report submitted to the Smith Richardson Foundation and New York State Office of Children and Family Services.* Sponsored by Columbia University College of Physicians and Surgeons, Department of Pediatrics, Alianza Dominicana, Inc. and Columbia University School of Social Work.

Azar, S.T. (2002). Parenting and child maltreatment. In M.H. Bornstein (Ed.), *Handbook of parenting: Vol. 4* (2nd ed., pp. 361–388). Mahwah, NJ: Lawrence Erlbaum Associates.

Baldry, A.C. (2003). Bullying in schools and exposure to domestic violence. *Child Abuse & Neglect, 27,* 713–732.

Berger, L.M. (2005). Income, family characteristics, and physical violence toward children. *Child Abuse & Neglect, 25,* 107–133.

Brendgen, M., Wanner, B., & Vitaro, F. (2006). Verbal abuse by the teacher and child adjustment from kindergarten through grade 6. *Pediatrics, 117*(5), 1585–1599.

The Center for Health and Health Care in Schools. (2004, December 15). *Bullying: Is it part of growing up, or part of school violence?* Retrieved August 5, 2007, http://www.healthinschools.org/News-Room/In Focus/2004/Issue-2.aspx

Chaffin, M., & Friedrich, B. (2004). Evidence-based treatments in child abuse and neglect. *Children and Youth Services Review, 26,* 1097–1113.

Child Abuse Prevention and Treatment Act (CAPTA) of 1974, PL 93-247, 42 U.S.C.5101.

Clark, D.A. (2007, February 15). Presentation entitled *Child abuse and neglect in infants and young children* (Lecture to graduate students in Early Childhood Special Education), Syracuse University, Syracuse, NY.

Daro, D.A., & Donnelly, A.C. (2002). Charting the waves of prevention: Two steps forward, one step back. *Child Abuse & Neglect, 26,* 731–742.

Daro, D.A., & Harding, K.A. (1999). Healthy families America: Using research to enhance practice. *The Future of Children, 9,* 152–176.

Darwish, D., Esquivel, G.B., Houtz, J.C., & Alfonso, V.C. (2001). Play and social skills in maltreated and non-maltreated preschoolers during peer interactions. *Child Abuse & Neglect, 25,* 13–31.

Dong, M., Anda, R.F., Felitti, V.J., Dube, S.R., Williamson, D.F., Thompson, R.J., et al. (2004). The interrelatedness of multiple forms of childhood abuse, neglect, and household dysfunction. *Child Abuse & Neglect, 28,* 771–784.

Dube, S.R., Anda, R.F., Felitti, V.J., Croft, J.B., Edwards, V.J., & Giles, W.H. (2001). Growing up with parental alcohol abuse: Exposure to childhood abuse, neglect, and household dysfunction. *Child Abuse & Neglect, 25,* 1627–1640.

Dube, S.R., Felitti, V.J., Dong, M., Chapman, D.P., Giles, W.H., & Anda, R.F. (2003). Childhood abuse, neglect, and household dysfunction and the risk of drug use: The adverse child experiences study. *Pediatrics, 111,* 564–572.

Dukewich, T.L., Borkowski, J.G., & Whitman, T.L. (1999). A longitudinal analysis of maternal abuse: Potential and developmental delays in children of adolescent mothers. *Child Abuse & Neglect, 23,* 405–420.

Entwisle, D.R., & Alexander, K.L. (1999). Early schooling and social stratification. In R.C. Pianta & M.J. Cox (Eds.), *The transition to kindergarten* (pp. 13–38). Baltimore: Paul H. Brookes Publishing Co.

Fantuzzo, J., Manz, P., Atkins, M., & Meyers, R. (2005). Peer-mediated treatment of socially withdrawn maltreated preschool children: Cultivating natural community resources. *Journal of Clinical Child and Adolescent Psychology, 34,* 320–325.

Ferrari, A.M. (2002). The impact of culture upon child rearing practices and definitions of maltreatment. *Child Abuse & Neglect, 26,* 793–813.

Garmezy, N. (1985). Stress-resistant children: The search for protective factors. In J.E. Stevenson (Ed.), *Recent research in developmental psychopathology* (pp. 213–33). Oxford, United Kingdom: Pergamon Press.

Giardino, A.P., Hudson, K.M., & Marsh, J. (2003). Providing medical evaluations for possible child maltreatment to children with special health care needs. *Child Abuse & Neglect, 27,* 1179–1186.

Heller, S.S., Larrieu, J.A., D'Imperio, R., & Boris, N.W. (1999). Research on resilience to maltreatment: Empirical considerations. *Child Abuse & Neglect, 23,* 321–338.

Hilyard, K.L., & Wolfe, D.A. (2002). Child neglect: Developmental issues and outcomes. *Child Abuse & Neglect, 26,* 679–695.

Keeping Children and Families Safe Act of 2003, PL 108-36, 42 U.S.C. §§ 5106(g) *et seq.*

Kelley, S.J. (2003). Cumulative environmental risk in substance abusing women: Early intervention, parenting stress, child abuse potential and child development. *Child Abuse & Neglect, 27,* 993–995.

Kerr, M.A., Black, M.M., & Krishnakumar, A. (2000). Failure-to-thrive, maltreatment and the behavior and development of 6-year-old children from low-income, urban families: A cumulative risk model. *Child Abuse & Neglect, 24,* 587–598.

Korbin, J.E. (2002). Culture and child maltreatment: Cultural competence and beyond. *Child Abuse & Neglect, 26*, 637–644.

Landy, S., & Menna, R. (2006). *Early intervention with multi-risk families: An integrative approach.* Baltimore: Paul H. Brookes Publishing Co.

Leventhal, J. (1997). The prevention of child abuse and neglect: Pipe dreams or possibilities. *Clinical Child Psychology and Psychiatry, 2*(4), 489–500.

Lyznicki, J.M., McCaffree, M.A., & Robinowitz, C.B. (2004). Childhood bullying: Implications for physicians. *American Family Physician, 70*, 1723–1728.

Mackner, L.M., Starr, R.H., & Black, M.M. (1997). The cumulative effect of neglect and failure to thrive on cognitive functioning. *Child Abuse & Neglect, 21*, 691–700.

MacLeod, J., & Nelson, G. (2000). Programs for the promotion of family wellness and the prevention of child maltreatment: A meta-analytic review. *Child Abuse & Neglect, 24*, 1127–1149.

Mammen, O.K., Kolko, D.J., & Pilkonis, P.A. (2002). Negative affect and parental aggression in child physical abuse. *Child Abuse & Neglect, 26*, 407–424.

McCroskey, J., & Meezan, W. (1998). Family centered services: Approaches and effectiveness. *The Future of Children, 8*, 54–71.

Nair, P., Schuler, M.E., Black, M.M., Kettinger, L., & Harrington, D. (2003). Cumulative environmental risk in substance abusing women: Early intervention, parenting stress, child abuse potential and child development. *Child Abuse & Neglect, 27*, 997–1017.

National Association of Counsel for Children. (2007). Child maltreatment. Retrieved August 5, 2007, from http://www.naccchildlaw.org/childrenlaw/childmaltreatment.html

Newcomb, M.D., & Locke, T.F. (2001). Intergenerational cycle of maltreatment: A popular concept obscured by methodological limitations. *Child Abuse & Neglect, 25*, 1219–1240.

Orelove, F.P., Hollahan, D.J., & Myles, K.T. (2000). Maltreatment of children with disabilities: Training needs for a collaborative response. *Child Abuse & Neglect, 24*, 185–194.

Osofsky, J.D. (1999). The impact of violence on children. *The Future of Children, 9*, 33–49.

Osofsky, J.D., & Thompson, M.D. (2000). Adaptive and maladaptive parenting. In J.P. Shonkoff & S.J. Meisels (Eds.), *Handbook of early childhood intervention* (2nd ed., pp. 54–75). New York: Cambridge University Press.

Pears, K.C., & Capaldi, D.M. (2001). Intergenerational transmission of abuse: A two-generational prospective study of an at-risk sample. *Child Abuse & Neglect, 25*, 1439–1461.

Rutter, M. (2000). Resilience reconsidered: Conceptual considerations, empirical findings, and policy implications. In J.P. Shonkoff & S.J. Meisels (Eds.), *Handbook of early childhood intervention* (2nd ed., pp. 651–682). New York: Cambridge University Press.

Schuler, M.E., Nair, P., & Black, M.M. (2002). Ongoing maternal drug use, parenting attitudes, and a home intervention: Effects on mother-child interaction at 18 months. *Developmental and Behavioral Pediatrics, 26*, 87–94.

Shonkoff, J.P., & Phillips, D.A. (Eds.). (2000). *From neurons to neighborhoods: The science of early childhood development.* Washington, DC: National Academy Press.

Smith, B.D., & Testa, M.F. (2002). The risk of subsequent maltreatment allegations in families with substance-exposed infants. *Child Abuse & Neglect, 26*, 97–114.

Stevens-Simon, C., Nelligan, D., & Kelly, L. (2001). Adolescents at risk for mistreating their children. Part II: A home- and clinic-based prevention program. *Child Abuse & Neglect, 6*, 753–769.

Straus, M.A., & Kantor, G.K. (2005). Definition and measurement of neglectful behavior: Some principles and guidelines. *Child Abuse & Neglect, 29*, 19–29.

Timmer, S.G., Urquiza, A.J., Zebell, N.M., & McGrath, J.M. (2005). Parent–child interaction therapy: Application to maltreating parent–child dyads. *Child Abuse & Neglect, 29*, 825–842.

Windham, A.M., Rosenberg, L., Fuddy, L., McFarlane, E., Sia, C., & Duggan, A.K. (2004). Risk of mother-reported child abuse in the first 3 years of life. *Child Abuse & Neglect, 28*, 645–667.

Wu, S.S., Ma, C.-X., Carter, R.L., Ariet, M., Feaver, E.A., Resnick, M.B., et al. (2004). Risk factors for infant maltreatment: A population-based study. *Child Abuse & Neglect, 28*, 1253–1264.

Zelenko, M., Lock, J., Kraemer, H.C., & Steiner, H. (2000). Perinatal complications and child abuse in a poverty sample. *Child Abuse & Neglect, 24*, 939–950.

CHAPTER 18

Parents with Developmental Disabilities Caring for Infants and Young Children

Ava E. Kleinmann and Nancy S. Songer

At the conclusion of this chapter, the reader will

- *Understand some of the legal issues associated with families with parents with developmental disabilities*

- *Understand the risks and issues associated with parents with developmental disabilities raising young children*

- *Understand research that has been carried out in examining issues surrounding families raising young children*

- *Understand ways in which physicians, educators, and other professionals can support families and parents with developmental disabilities who are raising young children*

When a parent is identified with intellectual disabilities, this diagnosis invariably becomes a family affair. Parents of "the parent" may find themselves in the role of caregiver again, children of the mother or father (depending upon the disability of the family member) likely will require additional support, and the parent him- or herself invariably will need assistance. In the best of circumstances, such situations are complex, as reflected in the following vignette.

Rhea

Rhea is a 32-year-old woman with mild intellectual disabilities who has a 1-year-old son, Kyle. Although she was urged to give up Kyle for adoption, Rhea decided to maintain her parental rights. The outcome of a competency evaluation recommended a number of options that varied in terms of intrusiveness, and Rhea opted to receive family support. She currently

resides with her parents who provide financial and social support, and a social worker provides consultative assistance once per week. Rhea has actively sought additional assistance through participation in parent training. Although Kyle has been identified as being at risk for developmental delays because of his mother's history, recent developmental assessment revealed that Kyle was functioning within the range of average intellectual abilities. Continued monitoring of Kyle's progress toward developmental milestones is planned, and support for Kyle's eventual transition to school is being investigated.

Definitions

The Developmental Disabilities and Bill of Rights Act Amendments of 1990 (PL 101-496) define a developmental disability as a severe, chronic disability of a person 5 years of age or older, which manifests before the age of 22 and is likely to continue indefinitely. It can be attributable to intellectual or physical disability or a combination of both. A significant developmental disability also results in substantial functional limitations in three or more major life activities (e.g., self-care, communication, learning, mobility, self-direction, capacity for independent living, economic self-sufficiency). A diagnosis of developmental disability reflects a person's need for a combination and sequence of special, interdisciplinary services that are individually planned and coordinated.

Developmental disabilities can be attributed to diagnoses such as intellectual disabilities, cerebral palsy, and epilepsy. Clearly, disabilities vary; however, the hallmark features of a developmental disability include substantial impairment in intellectual and/or adaptive functioning. Impairment of intellectual functioning typically is identified by having an IQ score that is at least 2 standard deviations below average. These scores correspond to 70 or less on measures of intelligence in which the mean is 100 and the standard deviation is 15. Because some individuals with developmental disabilities are unable to complete intelligence tests under standardized conditions, licensed professionals can use other sources of data to provide evidence of impaired intellectual functioning. Adaptive behavior deficits are characterized by overall significantly below average skills in areas considered to be major life activities according to the federal definition of developmental disabilities. Adaptive skills usually are assessed by standardized interviews or rating scales that often are administered by individuals who know the person well (e.g., parent).

Individuals with developmental disabilities face a number of challenges in their daily lives, primarily centering on issues of independence. Skill delays can have an impact on abilities, which include, but are not limited to, obtaining and maintaining employment, accessing appropriate educational opportunities and services, and forming appropriate social relationships. During childhood, a number of laws and dedicated organizations protect the rights of these individuals and facilitate access of appropriate services. Funding usually is in place to support

individuals with developmental disabilities when they are children, but the system is markedly different for adults. Part of the change has to do with the laws protecting adults with disabilities. During childhood, disability legislation such as the Individuals with Disabilities Education Improvement Act (IDEA) of 2004 (PL 108-446) entitles a child to a free appropriate public education in the least restrictive environment to meet a variety of needs. Adults with disabilities are served primarily by the Americans with Disabilities Act (ADA) of 1990 (PL 101-336), which provides accommodations to level the playing field in higher education, work, and the community. The goal is to offer access to participation in those activities that would be very challenging in the absence of accommodations. For children, emphasis is placed on maximizing success. For adults, however, disability legislation prohibits discrimination on the basis of a disability so that they can access various opportunities. As adults, there often exists a tacit expectation of increased independence, even though the level of support in place to help them be successful is much more limited.

When an individual with a developmental disability becomes a parent, an additional set of responsibilities arises. The challenges are striking, given the demands of being a parent and the limitations of having a developmental disability. Caring for an infant or young child is a full-time job that requires an advanced skill set and a strong support system. Given these realities, some children whose parents have developmental disability may be at risk for a number of negative outcomes. This chapter focuses on several issues that pertain to individuals with developmental disabilities who become parents and their children.

Challenges of Parents with Developmental Disabilities

The challenges of a parent with a developmental disability sometimes begin before the child is born. Some individuals believe that adults who are unable to be fully independent because of significant cognitive and adaptive skill impairments should not have the right to be parents. At the core of the debate is the well-being of the child. If the parents' limitations put their children at risk in any way, a number of possible approaches emerge as to how to address these challenges. Some have proposed restricting parental rights. This may include removing children from the care of their biological parents, obtaining legal joint custody with a fully capable adult, and arranging for supportive services. When these determinations are being made, an independent professional conducts a thorough competency assessment with the goal of maximizing a child's developmental trajectory. Although the assessment is impartial and objective, the emotions surrounding parenting become complex. In some instances, a parent might not fully understand what is in the child's best interest, and goals for the child may differ from those held by other family members. The parent may be confronted or criticized for his or her limitations, which may have an impact on self-esteem. In instances where the parent is able to maintain primary custody of the child or is fairly independent, he or she may be challenged on competency issues throughout the course of his or her parenting, whereas typically developing parents (who may lack the same parenting skills) may never be subject to this kind of scrutiny (Aunos, Goupil, & Feldman, 2002).

Historically, attitudes toward parents with severe developmental disabilities have not been favorable (Feldman, 1986; 1994; 1998a). In the beginning of the 20th century, compulsory sterilization was mandated in many states for individuals with intellectual disabilities, severe mental illness, and certain other impairing conditions. Although many motivations existed for this practice, the eugenics movement served as a major impetus. Eugenics postulates that manipulation of the gene pool through artificial selection may, in turn, alter the probability of certain conditions in the population at large. Whereas there is some evidence of a hereditary basis for many of the conditions that fall under the developmental disability classification, many parents with developmental disabilities have healthy, viable, and typically developmentally offspring. Although discriminatory laws pertaining to marriage and children abated following World War II, public

opinions toward parents with developmental disabilities still have been associated with numerous, unfounded blanket assumptions. Fortunately, legislation governing the rights of adults with disabilities has attenuated some of the criticism that had existed for years.

Legal Issues

A number of legal issues arise when a woman with a developmental disability becomes pregnant and has a child. They typically center on matters of competency (Aunos et al., 2002). Competency is the state of being physically or intellectually qualified to make a number of legal decisions. The first related issue pertains to consent, or the parents' ability to make an informed decision. In this discussion, consent about one's body and child are of primary importance. At times, questions also may arise about a woman's consent to have sex, whether the full implications of the act were understood, and whether there was possible misconduct by the partner who may be higher functioning. If a woman is unable to care for her child, to what extent does she consent to supportive services or allow for another individual to assume guardianship or even parent status? If the issue of terminating the pregnancy is raised, to what extent does the woman play a role in making that type of decision? Furthermore, what are the legal rights of a father with a developmental disability whose competency likewise may be questioned? For many of these concerns, a competency evaluation would be appropriate because without it any legal consent might be challenged. One might also look to a woman's history of consent for other medical care or even ordinary contracts (e.g., credit card). Another related legal issue is guardianship, which dictates who will provide care and make decisions on behalf of the child. Sometimes issues of guardianship are determined before the child is born, but, given the lengthy legal process at times, this can last for months or even years. A final related legal issue is the right to privacy. Inquiries into very personal decisions about one's body or family may be a threat to one's personal privacy. In instances where an evaluation is in progress and support from professionals is required to assess, evaluate, and assist with parenting, a danger of "watching" the family too closely may arise, particularly when the goals of the parents diverge from those of the professionals. A careful balance of ensuring competency to consent and/or holding guardianship while being mindful of one's right to privacy is critical to the needs of parents with developmental disabilities and their children.

Central to the discussion on parenting is the fact that there is no agreed-upon standard about what constitutes adequate parenting. Various regional and cultural differences exist in terms of the parental role and goals for a child's well-being. Aside from clear health benchmarks, the field has been slow to operationalize standards of care. Unfortunately, parents with developmental disabilities are overrepresented in child custody cases, and sometimes decisions about their rights are made without their input or independent of appropriate data.

System Abuse

Although systems are in place to support parents with developmental disabilities, a number of possible abuses of the system exist, which create additional challenges for these parents. First, well-meaning professionals and family members sometimes treat these parents unfairly. They frequently are treated as lesser adults and can be placed in situations where their input on major life decisions is not valued. Even in instances in which they are at least partially and legally competent to make decisions, professionals may override these desires. The ethical implications of honoring an adult's decision while keeping in mind the possible risks that may be apparent to a service provider is complicated to balance.

Second, there may be an increased likelihood of discontinuity in service delivery. Parents with a developmental disability may be less likely to follow through with maintaining services, obtaining new services, and/or ensuring that they are getting the maximum services to which their family is entitled. In addition, it is important to recognize that support systems are complicated for typically functioning individuals and require persistence, clarity, and often so-

phistication. The skill set required to navigate the web of available services also can be a limiting factor to parents with developmental disabilities.

A third issue is unwanted and unsubstantiated intervention in family affairs. Similarly, parents may not be sufficiently involved in decisions affecting their children and their families. This can create a difficult dynamic at home because parent authority is undermined by other family members or professionals.

Family Issues

Urie Bronfenbrenner's (1977) ecological framework is helpful in understanding the dynamics of families with parents who have developmental disabilities. This perspective is based on the notion that a child does not develop in a vacuum, rather within specific contexts that individually and collectively have implications for the outcome of the child and possible avenues for intervention. Applying this system to families with a parent with a developmental disability can be useful. At the microsystem level is the reality that many parents with disabilities experience low self-esteem. This can be attributed to the high level of dependence and low level of assertiveness that often characterize parents with developmental disabilities. At the mesosystem level, which refers to the relationship between the parent and various systems (e.g., schools, agencies), two major challenges include limited communication and concomitant social isolation. These situations present a challenge for parents with developmental disabilities to gain access to services and form the important social networks critical to success. The macrosystem, on the other hand, involves recognition of the societal factors that play a role in the lives of people with developmental disabilities, including widespread discrimination and generalizations made about skills of parents with disabilities. The macrosystem also includes the landmark legislation that protects individuals from discrimination and provides for appropriate services.

In addition, the role of extended family is very important to consider as a protective factor. Where support within the immediate family may be attenuated by the cognitive status of a parent, extended family members may have the opportunity to provide the necessary support that can compensate for lack of parental competence. For example, sometimes a child forms a positive attachment to a member of his or her extended family, which is a very important option for the sake of the child. Finally, parents need parents as well. Just as in families in which parents are typically developing, the continued social-emotional and financial support of grandparents is a critical factor. Additional parenting for individuals with developmental disabilities may have positive effects on them and their children.

In one study, Ehlers-Flint (2002) surveyed mothers with cognitive limitations. One interesting finding was that mothers reported higher levels of support than interference in their social networks. This finding contrasts with other research that has suggested overinvolvement by well-meaning but unwanted relatives or professionals. Given the reality that social support for parents with developmental disabilities often is generally limited, if not absent, any type of social support usually is welcome, especially given the demands of parenting.

Carlson (1997) identified a number of additional issues that pertain to families in which a parent has a developmental disability. The first is the recognition that cognitive limitations have an impact on the development of problem-solving skills. There is also a higher rate of domestic violence in families with a parent who has a developmental disability. As noted previously, mothers with developmental disabilities often have lower self-esteem than typically developing adults. However, there *is* a lower prevalence of alcohol use among parents with developmental disabilities (Christian & Poling, 1997), and a relatively lower rate of substance abuse is a protective factor for children.

Child Risk Factors ⸻

Taken together, the challenges posed to parents with developmental disabilities not surprisingly also present risks for their children. If parents are unable to access services, ensure that they are not being taken advantage of, and advocate for their children, the therapeutic value of services can be limited. Research has been slow to clarify the causal factors associated with outcomes for children of parents with developmental disabilities; however, a number of qualities typically associated with these parents are considered to be risk factors for children. In addition, the characteristics of the parents themselves also may influence child behavior, particularly in instances where the disability interferes with their ability to provide the appropriate resources and consistency that a child needs to be successful. Having other support systems (e.g., extended family, family friends, formal services) can certainly provide a broad array of supports for a child.

Perhaps the first risk factor to consider is the reality that individuals with developmental disabilities also tend to have a low socioeconomic status (SES) (Feldman, 1998a). Among typically developing parents, low SES often is correlated with relatively lower academic achievement, poor nutrition, and weaker verbal skills of the children. For parents with developmental disabilities, the challenges of low SES are compounded. To the extent that SES provides support for a family to have access to a variety of community resources (e.g., health care and education), this can be an important factor in the process of intervention.

Poverty can also be viewed as one example of parental stress, which may be related to poor child outcomes. Additional stressors, such as marital problems and the normative challenges of raising a child, can be stressful as well. Parents with developmental disabilities frequently have histories of stigmatization, learned helplessness, unemployment, social isolation, and poor supports. The compounded effects of these variables can certainly put these parents at risk for engaging in behaviors that do not augur well for a child's success. Accordingly, intervening to address deficiencies in one or more of these areas may have important implications for the reduction of parenting stress and, ultimately, improve child outcomes.

Another dimension of concern with having a parent with a developmental disability is the increased risk that the child may also have a developmental disability and/or a lower IQ. In a review of research on child outcomes, Feldman

(1986) reported higher rates of intellectual disabilities (39%–61%) for children born to two parents with delayed cognitive abilities. However, IQ in and of itself was not very predictive of parenting skill and child outcomes unless it was below 50 (i.e., severe—more than 3 standard deviations below the mean on an IQ test). Also noted were qualitative and quantitative differences in parent–child interactions. Parents were described as engaging in more negative and critical parenting styles and also spoke to their children less. These differences were related to subsequent differences in child development.

Poor academic achievement is another possible outcome for children of parents with developmental disabilities. Because IQ, level of parental involvement, and even finances account for variance in academic performance, children of parents with developmental disabilities may be at increased risk for poor academic achievement. In particular, there seems to be an increased risk for boys born to parents with developmental disabilities (Feldman, 1998a). Specifically, these boys tend to have lower school achievement and higher rates of utilization of special education services. It is possible that typical gender differences associated with boys' externalizing behavior is a factor in the relatively higher identification of school difficulties, as compared to female peers.

Additional child outcomes that have been documented include psychosocial problems (Gillberg & Geijer-Karlsson, 1983) and multiple delays in young children (Feldman, 1998a). In a longitudinal study by Feldman (1998a), children born to parents with developmental disabilities were followed for a period of 20 years, and problems documented in the national register of Sweden were tracked using this database. Although 85% of the cases identified for the study demonstrated psychosocial difficulties at some point in life, little information was given as to the extent of the disability or prevalence rates in other samples. It is also difficult to attribute any apparent difficulties to the parenting style or the fact that these children were raised by parents with developmental disabilities. In Feldman's review (1998a), developmental delays were reported for young children in terms of both communication and psychomotor skills. In addition, some conduct disorders were documented among these children, but they were found to be related more to the home environment than the parent's IQ.

Another important child outcome *can* be related to parent cognitive ability. In particular, literacy skills among individuals with developmental disabilities invariably are less developed. This fact usually has an impact on their abilities to access services or in many cases utilize simple elements of services, such as reading appointment cards supplied by a provider. In some instances, parents with developmental disabilities do not disclose their diagnosis to service providers because of the stigma associated with it. In turn, the service provider may view their behavior as incompetence, rather than making simple accommodations to benefit the child and parent (Keltner, Wise, & Taylor, 1999). In short, although it is difficult to identify causal factors associated with poor child outcomes or child resilience, what is clear is that young children of parents with developmental disabilities are at increased risk for a variety of reasons.

Also important to this discussion is the child maltreatment literature, which addresses the common assumption that parents with developmental disabilities are more likely to abuse or neglect their children. Certainly there is evidence that parents with cognitive delays are overrepresented in child custody cases related to alleged maltreatment (Feldman, 1998a). Some service providers have speculated that there is a relationship between intelligence and the rates of child maltreatment, presumably for reasons such as, but not limited to, a parent's lack of skills in being able to care for the child and impaired judgment. Although this may certainly be true in some cases, many other variables contribute to a child's overall well-being and a parent's behavior. As such, making a simple assumption such as this one is not empirically supported. However, this assumption might be a factor for individuals making referrals to agencies that protect children (e.g., child protective services). What the literature does reveal is that among parents with developmental disabilities, it is the lack of support rather than absolute level of intelligence that is the better predictor of neglect. In fact, parents who abuse their children have some commonalities that do not include intellectual level (as discussed in Chapter 17); that is, social isolation, unemployment, limited interpersonal skills, and personal histories of deprivation are all correlated characteristics of parents who abuse and/or neglect their children.

Research

The empirical research on parents with developmental disabilities and their children is fairly sparse. Awareness of the research highlights, however, is useful toward understanding the challenges of parents with developmental disabilities and the outcomes for their children. This section provides a brief review of some important work in this area. This review is by no means exhaustive; it is merely representative of the types of studies currently available in the field.

Keltner and colleagues (1999) conducted a longitudinal, between group study in which children born to mothers with and without intellectual disabilities were followed for 2 years. In this investigation, the groups were matched on a number of variables, including SES. Results indicated that in this study children were at increased risk for developmental disabilities (42%) when born to mothers with developmental disabilities, as compared to children born to mothers without developmental disabilities (12%). This finding is significant in that it highlights parental developmental disability as a risk factor while minimizing the relative risk of poverty.

Llewellyn, McConnell, Honey, Mayes, and Russo (2003) conducted a randomized, controlled trial of a home-based intervention for parents with intellectual disabilities. A 10-week, in-home training program was presented to mothers and some fathers with limited, although variable, levels of intellectual and adaptive skill. This intervention focused on teaching parents health and safety skills for their children. The results demonstrated that parents were able to increase their knowledge and skills in specified areas and maintain gains over time.

Feldman and colleagues examined reported stress levels in parents with developmental disabilities who had children of various ages (Feldman, Léger & Walton-Allen, 1997). Results indi-

cated overall that mothers reported high levels of stress and parenting problems compared to a normative group. In particular, parents of school-age children reported the highest levels of stress. As such, these children were identified as being at-risk for learning and developmental delays, as well as poor academic achievement. The authors concluded that overall stress places children at risk for both behavioral and developmental problems, as well as emotional maladjustment in school.

Although the three studies briefly reviewed here represent some of the most elegantly designed studies in the field, they are limited in scope. Review of a broader literature base also revealed that a number of general methodological limitations exist in the research on parents with developmental disabilities and their children. Consequently, conclusions drawn from this work are extremely limited. One particular issue is the use of maternal education alone as an indicator of cognitive ability. Furthermore, many of these studies have small sample sizes and may not be generalizable to or representative of a broad range of parents with developmental disabilities. Moreover, typically mothers are the focus of studies; very few investigations have focused on training fathers. Interestingly, whereas parent training studies demonstrate positive outcomes for parenting skill acquisition, even less information is known about the long-term effects for the children. As such, programming for generalization and continued demonstration of maintained effects over time are critical considerations. Another important factor to recognize is that in some states where the research was conducted, services for at-risk children were not available. Thus, any delays evident among these children also could be attributed to lack of intervention in cases where it would otherwise be indicated.

Taken together, the research results suggest that the findings with respect to child outcomes must be interpreted with caution. Findings also indicate that additional work needs to be done to address the methodological limitations present in some of the studies. Hur (1997) reviewed 20 years of research in this area of study and was able to identify only 27 articles related to the topic, many of which contained significant methodological problems. Accordingly, a number of directions for future research emerge from this discussion. For example, further work to identify risk factors is important to demystify and reduce stereotyping of parents with developmental disabilities and their children and to clarify areas for intervention. In particular, intervention studies need to examine various models and strategies of skill building for parents and children, with particular emphasis on generalizing across settings and maintaining effects over time. Finally, research needs to focus on parenting needs and training outcomes for fathers, as well as developing programs within the natural context of the entire family and community, rather than exclusive concentration on the behavior of primary maternal caregivers.

How Parents and Their Young Children Can Best Be Supported

In light of the challenges faced by parents with developmental disabilities, a number of important considerations are indicated in working with this population. First, professionals must be careful about evaluating parental adequacy by using middle class standards because SES often is lower among parents with developmental disabilities. The same resources and opportunities for child enrichment do not always exist, and likely finances are a limiting factor to optimal parenting. Putting these individuals in touch with community support resources or advocates that have external funding is therefore indicated.

Second, given that isolation and lack of support is a major risk factor for children, it would follow that another major goal of supporting parents with developmental disabilities would be to increase their utilization of community resources and interdependence with social support networks. Empowering parents to access these resources and be advocates (or seek advocates) for their children and their families is critical. Assertiveness training is one strategy to increase the advocacy skills of these individuals.

Considering history with service providers likewise is very important. Parents may always have been in a position where someone was advocating for them or where their roles in making their own major life decisions have been limited. Again, meeting parents where they are (with the challenges that they may or may not have) is essential to being able to support them appropriately. Creating individualized goal plans that take into account their skill set, cognitive strengths and limitations, as well as their personal priorities for their families is a way to structure programming for these families. On a related note, it is also important to be sensitive to the parenting difficulties of families that are at risk, although not necessarily formally identified as in need of services.

As with any family, the parents and children present with a unique set of strengths and challenges. Careful consideration of the positive aspects (e.g., protective factors) present in a family is important to assess so that these strengths can be reinforced and utilized. Concomitantly, recognition of areas of particular need that exist is important for the purposes of developing ongoing intervention strategies. When perceptions about what constitutes a weakness differ, clinical judgment should be used to prioritize intervention for areas that will most benefit the family and that hopefully are also consonant with parent priorities.

In the past, a number of parent training programs have been proposed and developed to teach parents with (and without) developmental disabilities important skills related to caring for their young children. Some strategies that have been useful for these parents include real-life coaching situations and audio aids. Parents also benefit from extended support to ensure that change has taken place and that skills are mastered. Follow-up data on progress toward appointed goals is a good way to determine the extent of program effectiveness and justify the need for continued services.

As work on parent training continues to be developed, several other strategies are worthy of consideration. For instance, teaching appropriate behavior with the use of modeling and a prompting hierarchy can be helpful. In modeling, the instructor can demonstrate desired behaviors through role play or training videos. Parents then actively engage in practicing new skills at which time they receive feedback and assistance to meet mastery criteria. This assistance or prompting subsequently can be faded at a schedule that is appropriate with skill level, with the goal that the parent ultimately use these skills with the highest level of independence possible. Being mindful of the instructional match of program curricula with parent skills and cognitive level is of crucial importance. Based on existing research, Feldman (1998b) described an interactional parent training model that addressed assessment and intervention issues pertinent to competency. He utilized a behavioral and data-based approach wherein parents were trained to certain levels of accuracy on various skill tasks. This approach offered an advantage of having records to demonstrate adaptive skills that were central to competency evaluations related to custody issues.

Other proactive approaches have concentrated efforts on parent training and educating youth with developmental disabilities about safe sex and family planning, which provides training to prospective parents preventatively before children are conceived. Feldman (1998b) described a number of strategies that have demonstrated empirical support with this population. His findings have suggested the need to train parents first on matters of health and safety, subsequently educating them about parent–child relationship skills, such as nurturing and sensitivity skills. Using picture manuals for parents to practice skills independently, in addition, has been a useful strategy for individuals who have limited literacy skills.

Also examining parent training programs, Tymchuk and Andron (1988; 1992) carried out two studies. In their earlier study, a multiple baseline design was used to train a mother and her three children. Although this study provided support for the efficacy of the training model, the generalizability of the results was limited given the sample size. In their second study, training was focused on increasing the quality and quantity of verbal interactions from mother to child. Although the program initially was successful, the acquisition effects did not maintain over time. Accordingly, whereas there appears to be evidence supporting the utility of parent training

programs, these efforts must be individually tailored, as well as programmed for skill maintenance and generalization.

Finally, service assessment is critical to best practice. Walton-Allen and Feldman (1991) conducted a survey of mothers with intellectual disabilities and their service providers to assess various service needs. Results indicated that from both perspectives a number of common needs were identified. However, groups disagreed on the nature of the services that should be pursued. With respect to social service needs, mothers with developmental disabilities reported receiving too much parent training, but not enough vocational and interpersonal skills training. In contrast, the social workers indicated that parents overestimated their skills, and reported that parent training was the most important area for intervention. What is important to glean from this study is an awareness of divergent perspectives between consumers and service providers. When these two groups disagree on the goals of training or have different service priorities, resistance may emerge and can be counterproductive. Rather than making assumptions about parent training needs, skill and needs assessments are indicated to support the development of a collaborative, positive, focused skill-training effort.

Conclusion

Parents with developmental disabilities and their children face a number of challenges that exceed the typical difficulties that any parent might encounter. Fortunately, the prognosis for families with parents with developmental disabilities has improved in recent decades with the advancement of legislation to protect their rights, development of research and training programs, and increased valuing and appreciation of people with special needs.

REFERENCES

Americans with Disabilities Act (ADA) of 1990, PL 101-336, 42 U.S.C. §§ 12101 *et seq.*
Aunos, M., Goupil, G., & Feldman, M. (2002). Mothers with intellectual disabilities who do or do not have

custody of their children. *Journal of Developmental Disabilities, 2*, 65–79.

Bronfenbrenner, U. (1977). Toward an experimental ecology of human development. *American Psychologist, 32*, 513–531.

Carlson, B.E. (1997). Mental retardation and domestic violence: An ecological approach to intervention. *Social Work, 42*(1), 79–89.

Christian, L., & Poling, A. (1997). Drug abuse in persons with mental retardation: A review. *American Journal of Mental Retardation, 102*, 126–136.

Developmental Disabilities and Bill of Rights Act Amendments of 1990, PL 101-496, 42 U.S.C. §§ 6000 *et seq.*

Ehlers-Flint, M.L. (2002). Parenting perceptions and social supports of mothers with cognitive disabilities. *Sexuality and Disability, 20*, 29–51.

Feldman, M.A. (1986). Research on parenting by mentally retarded persons. *Psychiatric Clinics of North America, 9*, 777–796.

Feldman, M.A. (1994). Parents with intellectual disabilities. *Network, 4*, 41–47.

Feldman, M.A. (1998a). Parents with intellectual disabilities. In J.R. Lutzker (Ed.), *Handbook of child abuse research and treatment* (pp. 401–420). New York: Plenum.

Feldman, M.A. (1998b). Preventing child neglect: Child-care training for parents with intellectual disabilities. *Infants and Young Children, 11*, 1–11.

Feldman, M.A., Léger, M., & Walton-Allen, N. (1997). Stress in mothers with intellectual disabilities. *Journal of Child and Family Studies, 6*(4), 471–485.

Gillberg, C., & Geijer-Karlsson, M. (1983). Children born to mentally retarded women: A 1–21 year follow-up study of 41 cases. *Psychological Medicine, 13*, 891–894.

Hur, J. (1997). Review of research on parent training for parents with intellectual disability: Methodological issues. *International Journal of Disability, Development and Education, 44*, 147–162.

Individuals with Disabilities Education Improvement Act (IDEA) of 2004, PL 108-446, 20 U.S.C. §§ 1400 *et seq.*

Keltner, B.R., Wise, L.A., & Taylor, G. (1999). Mothers with intellectual limitations and their 2-year-old children's developmental outcomes. *Journal of Intellectual and Developmental Disability, 24*, 45–57.

Llewellyn, G., McConnell, D., Honey, A., Mayes, R., & Russo, D. (2003). Promoting health and home safety for children of parents with intellectual disability: A randomized controlled trial. *Research in Development Disabilities, 24*, 405–431.

Tymchuk, A.J., & Andron, L. (1988). Clinic and home parent training of a mother with mental handicap caring for three children with developmental delay. *Mental Handicap Research, 1*, 24–38.

Tymchuk, A.J., & Andron, L. (1992). Project parenting: Child interactional training with mothers who are mentally handicapped. *Mental Handicap Research, 5*, 4–32.

Walton-Allen, N.G., & Feldman, M.A. (1991). Perception of service needs by parents who are mentally retarded and their social service workers. *Comprehensive Mental Health Care, 1*, 137–147.

CHAPTER 19

Teen Parents

TRENDS IN ADOLESCENT PREGNANCY

Nancy S. Songer and Gretchen Kinnell

At the conclusion of this chapter, the reader will

- *Know the demographics of teen parents*

- *Identify the effects of having a teen for a parent*

- *Understand the effects on adolescents when they become parents*

- *Recognize the qualities of programs and interventions that have been successful in helping teen parents achieve good outcomes for themselves and their children*

The demands of parenting are challenging for adults who understand the needs of young children, who have planned for children, and who are emotionally stable and financially secure enough to provide for them. When the parents are teenagers, children themselves in many ways, the likelihood that they have those same intellectual, emotional, intentional, and financial assets is very small. In many ways, they are parents before their time. When adolescents have babies, the changes to their lives are immediate, immense, and ongoing. The lives of the teens are not the only lives that are affected; the lives of their babies also are greatly affected by being born to teenage parents.

Who Are the Teens Having the Babies?

Before presenting actual data, it is helpful to understand that researchers who study and report about teen pregnancy present their findings by age group. This is not surprising when one considers the differences in maturity and life sit-

uation of a 19-year-old woman compared with that of a 13-year-old girl. In research on teen pregnancy, the term *younger teens* refers to girls younger than age of 15. Many researchers also create a separate category for 18- and 19-year-old women.

The birth rate for adolescent girls in the United States actually has been declining steadily from its highest point in the 1950s and 1960s. During those years, abortion was not legal, and contraceptives that are currently being used were not widely available and, in some cases, not yet developed (Piccinino & Mosher, 1998). In 2004, the birth rate of 41 per 1,000 adolescent females (15–19 years) was the lowest ever recorded (Hoffman, 2006). This 15- to 19-year-old age group is one that is commonly used in measuring and reporting data on teen pregnancy. Often, however, data are presented in more distinct age groups (10–14, 15–17, and 18–19 years of age) because the issues and statistics typically vary depending on the age at which an adolescent becomes pregnant. In the case of the overall decline in the birth rates for teenagers, the rate has fallen in all age groups; and the rates have dropped more steeply for 10-

to 14-year-olds and 15- to 17-year-olds than for 18- to 19-year-olds. Table 19.1 shows that the decrease in the birth rate during a 10-year period was almost 36% for girls who were 10–14 years old, nearly 29% for girls 15–17 years old, and almost 16% for girls 18–19 years old.

This drop in the teen birth rate is seen not only in all age groups, but also in all racial groups in the United States. During the 1990s, the steepest decline in the birth rate, a decrease of almost one third, was seen among African American teenagers. Table 19.2 shows the decline in the birth rate for frequently identified racial groups in the United States (Ventura, Mathews, & Hamilton, 2001).

Although there were declines in all five identified racial groups, the birth rates vary a great deal, as shown in Table 19.3. The birth rates for Hispanic and black adolescents are still substantially higher than for other groups.

Similar to the United States, other developed countries have experienced a decline in the teen birth rate since the early 1990s. Nine countries—Denmark, Finland, France, Germany, Italy, the Netherlands, Spain, Sweden, and Switzerland—had teen birth rates under 10 per 1,000. Furthermore, as shown in Figure 19.1, comparing the birth rates of the Netherlands, Japan, Norway, Israel, Australia, Canada, the United Kingdom, the Russian Federation, and the United

Table 19.2. Decline in teenage birth rate by racial group in the United States 1991-2000

Racial group	% decline
Black	31%
Non-Hispanic white	24%
American Indian	20%
Asian or Pacific Islander	20%
Hispanic	12%

From Ventura, S.J., Mathews, T.J., & Hamilton, B.E. (2001, September 25). Births to teenagers in the United States, 1940-2000. *National Vital Statistics Reports, 49*(10). Retrieved June 7, 2007, from http://www.cdc.gov/nchs/data/nvsr/nvsr49/nvsr49_10.pdf

States, the United States still has the highest teen birth rate.

Although teen pregnancy in all age groups and in all racial and ethnic groups is falling in the United States, 4 out of 10 adolescent girls will have been pregnant at least once before they turn 20 (Federal Interagency Forum on Child and Family Statistics, 2006). At this writing, with the population of the United States at approximately 300 million, this represents approximately 900,000 teen pregnancies per year. Of these pregnancies, 51% result in live births, 35% are terminated, and 14% end in miscarriage or stillbirth, as shown in Figure 19.2.

Based on the percentages given in Figure 19.2 and the total number of adolescent girls becoming pregnant as 900,000, the number of live births is 459,000, the number of miscarriages or still births is 126,000, and the number of abortions is 315,000. In the absence of the noted number of abortions, the number of live births would be close to 774,000, and the percentage of live births could be as high as 86%.

At the same time that the birth rate for teenagers has been declining, another rate has been increasing—the proportion of teenage births to

Table 19.1. Birth rates in the United States for teenagers by age from 1991 to 2000

Year	Birth rate per 1,000 teenagers		
	10–14 years old	15–17 years old	18–19 years old
2000	0.9	27.5	79.5
1999	0.9	28.7	80.3
1998	1	30.4	82.0
1997	1.1	32.1	83.6
1996	1.2	33.8	86.0
1995	1.3	36.0	89.1
1994	1.4	37.6	91.5
1993	1.4	37.8	92.1
1992	1.4	37.8	94.5
1991	1.4	38.7	94.4
% change	−35.7	−28.9	−15.8

From Ventura, S.J., Mathews, T.J., & Hamilton, B.E. (2001, September 25). Births to teenagers in the United States, 1940-2000. *National Vital Statistics Reports, 49*(10). Retrieved June 7, 2007, from http://www.cdc.gov/nchs/data/nvsr/nvsr49/nvsr49_10.pdf

Table 19.3. Teenage birth rate by racial groups in the United States in 2000 (births per 1,000 teenage girls)

Racial group	Teen birth rate
Hispanic	94
Black	79
American Indian	67
Non-Hispanic White	33
Asian or Pacific Islander	22

From Ventura, S.J., Mathews, T.J., & Hamilton, B.E. (2001, September 25). Births to teenagers in the United States, 1940-2000. *National Vital Statistics Reports, 49*(10). Retrieved June 7, 2007, from http://www.cdc.gov/nchs/data/nvsr/nvsr49/nvsr49_10.pdf

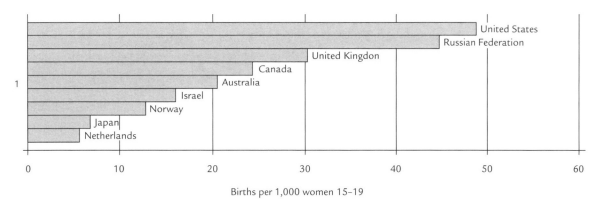

Births per 1,000 women 15–19

Figure 19.1. Teenage birth rates in selected countries. (*Source:* United Nations Department of Economic and Social Affairs, Statistical Office, 1998.)

unmarried women. In 1957, most teenagers who had babies were married; 1 infant in 7 was born to unmarried teens. In 2000, this proportion was vastly different; 4 out of 5 babies born to teenage mothers were born to unmarried teens. These proportions have risen for both younger and older teenagers (Ventura, Mathews, & Hamilton, 2001). This significant increase mirrors major changes in marriage patterns in our society. There has been an increase in the birth rate of unmarried women of all child-bearing ages, and teen parenting is following the child-bearing patterns of the larger society.

Contrary to many assumptions, far more children are born to unmarried women who are more than 20 years old than to teenagers. In 2000, 1 child in 3 was born to unmarried women. Of those unmarried mothers, 28% were teens and 72% were women older than 20. In the mid-1970s, the percentages were far different when 50% of unmarried mothers were teens and 50%

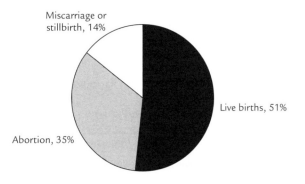

Figure 19.2. Results of teen pregnancies. (*Source:* Federal Interagency Forum on Child and Family Statistics, 2006.)

were older than 20 years (Ventura & Bachrach, 2000). This increase reflects the acceptance of single women having and raising children across all segments and age groups in the United States.

Motherhood in High School

We have seen that whereas the number of teenage girls having babies has been steadily decreasing since the 1960s, the number of children being raised by their teenage mothers is increasing because more adolescents who do give birth are choosing to keep and raise their babies rather than give them up for adoption. What accounts for or contributes to this change? One factor is the change in society's attitude toward single women of all ages having and raising children. We can see all these trends unfolding by looking at the experiences of pregnant teenagers at Thomas J. Corcoran High School in Syracuse, New York, from the late 1960s to 2006.

In the late 1960s, the Syracuse City School District worked with a social services agency to create a separate program for pregnant girls from the four high schools and six middle schools in the district. The Young Mothers Educational Development (YMED) Program provided comprehensive services, such as medical, social, education, and child care, for teens and their infants in a single, separate location. According to the principal who was at Corcoran from 1970 to 1985, pregnant girls were not required to leave their home high schools to attend the special program, but most of them did because they felt more comfortable with other girls in similar situations. In the class of 1971, an obviously pregnant graduate was the first to ask the principal for permission to participate in the graduation ceremony and be allowed to walk across the stage to receive her diploma. The request was granted.

In the following years, the number of pregnant girls at Corcoran mirrored the downward trend seen throughout the United States. The current school nurse began working there in the late 1980s. In her early years at the school, there were about 70 pregnant girls at Corcoran each year. In the 1993–1994 school year, a school district report listed 46 pregnant girls from the high school. Pregnant girls from the high school continued to use the YMED program, but the numbers of girls deciding to leave their home school declined. The number of pregnant girls in the entire Syracuse City School District was just under 300 in 1993–1994. In that same year, however, the total enrollment at the YMED program was 32, and the majority of girls were either middle school students or ninth-grade students. Attendance at YMED gradually declined until the program closed in 2000 because more and more girls chose to stay at their own schools.

In 2006, the school nurse at Corcoran reported that there were 20 pregnant girls, and all of them attended regular classes at the school. They are treated much the same as their classmates. In previous years, the school had made an exception for pregnant girls, exempting them from taking physical education. Starting in the 2006–2007 school year, however, pregnant girls were required to take physical education like all other students. The school's physical education program includes low impact sports, such as swimming and archery, which are suitable for pregnant students.

Acceptance of the pregnant students at the high school is social as well as academic. Similar to many other students at the school, the pregnant girls wear the latest fashions, and some of the girls have baby showers and invite their friends who are classmates from their high school.

Predictors, Conditions, and Risk Factors

The vast majority (82%) of adolescent girls, 15–19 years of age, who have become pregnant report that they did not intend to do so (Gutt-macher Institute, 2006). The average age of first sexual intercourse for girls is 17.4 years, and for boys it is 16.9 years (Guttmacher Institute, 2002). Detailed information on human reproduction, contraception, sexually transmitted diseases, and the HIV epidemic has led to an increase in the use of contraception by adolescents at the time of first intercourse and an overall greater use of barrier contraceptives. Still, half of the teenage girls who become pregnant do so within 6 months of the first time they have sexual intercourse (Haffner, 1995). This can be associated at least in part with inconsistent use of condoms and in a delay between the time of first sexual intercourse and use of prescription contraceptives. In 2005, among high school students who reported having had sexual intercourse, only 63% indicated that they had used a condom the last time they had intercourse (Centers for Disease Control and Prevention [CDC], 2006). Many adolescent girls who report that they use prescription contraceptives also have indicated that they waited a year or more after becoming sexually active to get a prescription (Guttmacher Institute, 1994). This is especially significant when, as mentioned earlier, half of the teenagers who become pregnant do so within 6 months of starting to have intercourse. Girls are more likely to use contraception more consistently when they experience academic success in school, when they anticipate a satisfying future, and when they are involved in a stable relationship with a sexual partner (Klein & the Committee on Adolescence, 2005). Many sexually active teenagers, however, do not have a stable relationship with a sexual partner. They often have a series of sexual partners; 12% of high school girls and 16.5% of boys report that they have had four or more sexual partners (CDC, 2006).

Which Teenage Girls Are at Risk for Becoming Pregnant?

Researchers who study teen pregnancy have identified several factors that contribute to the initiation of sexual intercourse that put adolescent girls at risk to become pregnant. These include early onset of puberty, a history of sexual abuse, poverty, lack of attentive and nurturing parents, cultural and family patterns of early sexual experience, lack of school or career goals, substance abuse, and poor school performance or dropping out of school (Klein & the Committee on Adolescence, 2005). There is a strong connection between poverty and adolescent pregnancy in the United States; 38% of adolescents live in poor or low income families, but 83% who give birth and 61% who have abortions are from poor or low income families (Klein & the Committee on Adolescence, 2005). See Table 19.4 for a summary.

Some adolescent girls become sexually active, but not by choice. Younger girls often are coerced into nonconsensual intercourse; 60% of sexually active girls under 15 years of age and 74% of girls under 14 years report that they have been coerced into having intercourse (Brooks-Gunn & Furstenberg, 1989; Centers for Disease Control and Prevention, 2006; Dailard, 2001; Haffner, 1995; Jaskiewicz & McAnarney, 1994; Kirby, 2001; Moore, Driscoll, & Lindberg, 1998).

When looking at adolescents who become pregnant, we find a strong family connection that includes mothers and older sisters. Adolescent girls who are daughters of teenage mothers are much more likely to become pregnant than the daughters of older mothers. In a 2006 report from The National Campaign to Prevent Teen Pregnancy (Hoffman, 2006), researchers found that almost 1 in 3 (33%) daughters born to teen mothers (17 or younger) became teenage mothers themselves. This compares with 1 in 9 for daughters born to mothers 20–21 years of age (Hoffman, 2006). These few years make a striking

difference. Even after taking into consideration other risk factors, such as family background and academic achievement, being the daughter of a teen mother is strongly related to the occurrence of adolescent pregnancy (Hoffman, 2006).

The adolescent pregnancy family connection also includes older sisters. Having an older sister become pregnant increases the likelihood that a younger sister also will become pregnant (Kirby, 2001). This generational and family cycle is the foundation of a number of initiatives to prevent teen pregnancy. Such programs often measure their success by the delay in age when girls become pregnant. A delay of even a few years can have a significant influence on the lives of girls participating in the program and on their younger sisters and future daughters.

After having one child during adolescence, girls are at greater risk for another pregnancy. One in 6 teenagers who already had one child gave birth to a second child during their teenage years. The rate for second births has been declining; yet, 100,000 teenagers gave birth to a second child or a higher order child in 2000.

Who Are the Fathers of Babies Born to Adolescent Mothers?

It is understandable that most of the studies and research on adolescent pregnancy are focused on girls. They are, after all, the ones who become pregnant and who have the babies. Historically, there has been much less information about the fathers of their babies. There are fewer adolescent fathers than adolescent mothers because many teenage girls are impregnated by adult men. Between 50% and 70% of adolescent girls who become pregnant do so with men 20 years of age or older (Roye & Balk, 1996). More than two thirds of the consensual partners of teenage girls are the same age as the girls or a few years older; however, some partners are more than 4 years older (Sexuality Information and Education Council of the United States, 2003).

Although the male partners of pregnant adolescent girls may be different in age than the girls, they are very similar when it comes to other important factors. Both adolescent fathers and adolescent mothers are more likely than their

Table 19.4.   Predictors of and delaying factors regarding sexual intercourse during adolescence

Predictors of sexual intercourse during early adolescence	Factors associated with delaying sexual intercourse during adolescence
Poverty	Higher family income
History of sexual abuse	Regular attendance at places of worship
Lack of attentive and nurturing parents	
Cultural and family patterns of early sexual experience	Living with both parents in a stable family environment
Lack of school or career goals	
Poor school performance or dropping out of school	
Substance abuse	

Source: Klein & the Committee on Adolescence (2005).

peers who are not parents to have poor academic performance, higher school drop-out rates, lower income, and lower income potential (Fagot, Pears, Capaldi, Crosby, & Leve, 1998; Nakashima & Camp, 1984; Xie, Cairns, & Cairns, 2001). Teenage fathers, similar to adolescent mothers, are more likely to live in poverty that has continued from generation to generation. Similarly, adult men who father children with adolescent girls also are likely to live in poverty (East & Felice, 1996). More than one third of adolescents who become fathers are born to teenage mothers themselves, which is the same statistic as for adolescent mothers. Not only are adolescent fathers and adolescent mothers similar, but adult men who father children with teenage girls tend to be more similar psychologically and sociologically to adolescent fathers than to adult men who father children with adult mothers (Nakashima & Camp, 1984).

There is an emergent interest and long overdue increase in research relating to young fathers. In many existing paradigms of support and care, the target is the mother and baby. However, researchers have found that some fathers indicate a willingness to be involved, some mothers want to have the fathers involved, and when there is partner involvement mothers display less stress (Kalil, Ziol-Guest, & Coley, 2005). In addition, positive partner support has been associated with better financial and emotional outcomes for parenting teen mothers (Bunting & McAuley, 2004). Therefore, it is essential to identify young fathers as a part of the intervention and care. For too long, young fathers have been ignored, and the results have been detrimental to their children and partners (Ferguson & Hogan, 2004).

Outcomes for Teens and Their Children

The more we learn and understand about the importance of children's early experiences and relationships, the more important it is to identify factors that affect them. Professionals dealing with young children need to understand how these factors affect teen parents and their children.

For years, researchers have studied outcomes for children of adolescent mothers. Their findings have been reported in terms of the outcomes associated or correlated with being the child of an adolescent mother. The outcomes that have been identified have been overwhelmingly negative for children. In recent years, however, researchers have asked and sought to discover whether the adolescence of the mother actually causes these adverse outcomes or whether the outcomes are likely to be the result of other factors related to the mother's life.

The following are some simplistic examples to consider:

- Would the outcomes for the child born to a 17-year-old, unmarried girl living in poverty be different from the outcomes for the child born to a 21-year-old, unmarried woman living in poverty?

- Would the outcomes for the child born to a 16-year-old, unmarried girl who never finishes high school be different from those for the child born to a 21-year-old, unmarried woman who never finished high school?

- To what extent are poverty and a mother's limited education responsible for the adverse outcomes for children, and to what extent are those outcomes caused by the adolescence of the mother?

To try to answer these questions, researchers must create and carry out complex and sophisticated studies. For example, Geronimus and Korenman (1993) examined the health disadvantages of infants with teenage mothers, comparing children born to sisters who began childbearing at different ages as a control for their study of shared neighborhood and family characteristics. Hotz, McElroy, and Sanders (1997) compared children born to adolescent mothers with children born to mothers who first conceived a child as an adolescent but miscarried. These studies and others have led to a current understanding that research does not support the idea that adolescent childbearing is automatically devastating to children; however, it also is not positive. It is a factor that is more than just marginally negative (Hoffman, 1998).

When considering the research and outcomes for children of adolescent mothers, statistics suggest that adolescent mothers are more likely to be vulnerable to the difficult and stressful life factors that place their children at risk for negative outcomes. Moreover, teen mothers may have fewer protective factors in their lives to help them cope with stress and difficult circumstances (Moore & Brooks-Gunn, 2002). Their children are affected not only by their mothers' adolescence, but also by the typical life factors that teenagers experience. If we want to understand and support the children of adolescent mothers, we must work to understand the typical development of teenagers.

There are differing opinions as to whether teen pregnancy is causal or merely correlated to adverse outcomes for children. The links between teen parenting and poor outcomes for children may or may not be causal, but they follow a kind of logic pattern. Early parenthood is an event that can contribute to adverse children's outcomes in a variety of ways (Pogarsky, Thornberry, & Lizotte, 2006).

When girls become mothers as adolescents, it is more difficult for them to develop the kind of personal capital that adults need and draw on throughout their lives for their own well-being and the well-being of their children. A prime example of such personal capital is education. Attaining an education is a major developmental task of adolescence, but women who start childbearing early are not as likely to complete high school as those who delay childbearing (Hofferth, Reid, & Mott, 2001). Being a teen parent and having low educational attainment have been linked to later financial disadvantage; that is, young mothers are poorer than women who delay childbearing (Coley & Chase-Lansdale, 1998). Both low parental educational attainment and disadvantage are associated with a variety of negative outcomes for children (Thornberry, Krohn, Lizotte, Smith, & Tobin, 2003).

Personal capital also includes the ability to form stable social and family relationships. Women who begin having children during adolescence are more likely to experience both disorder in the process of forming a family and higher levels of family dissolution (Astone, 1993). Children of young mothers, then, are more likely to experience changes in parent figures or caregivers as adults come and go in their lives. In turn, frequent changes in caregivers have been linked to a variety of problem outcomes for children (Capaldi & Patterson, 1991). For mothers, disadvantage and family disruption are associated with stress and increase the likelihood of antisocial behavior, especially drug use (Conger et al., 1992). Mothers' antisocial behavior increases the probability of similar behaviors by their children (Huesmann, Eron, Lefkowitz, & Walder, 1984). Finally, all of these characteristics are likely to be associated with styles of ineffective parenting, which is defined as low affective ties, poor monitoring, and harsh, inconsistent discipline (Dishion & McMahon, 1998).

The following are some styles of ineffective parenting that may be seen with adolescent parents.

- *Low affective ties:* Parents do not engage well with their children emotionally. They rarely show joy, tenderness, and warmth. They often do not respond to a child's emotional cues, such as crying to be comforted or needing a reassuring hug.

- *Poor monitoring:* Parents fail to attend to their children and track their actions and interactions. They poorly structure their children's activities and fail to create appropriate environments.

- *Harsh, inconsistent discipline:* Parents discipline children in ways that are abrupt and based more on the adults' frustration than on a desire to help children learn appropriate behavior. Harsh discipline is often explosive and takes the form of yelling, belittling, yanking, physical punishment, and intimidation. Because harsh discipline is so often based on the parents' feelings of frustration, it is also likely to be inconsistent. A child may get a severe spanking for a behavior one day, and the next day find that the same behavior elicits nothing more than a parental sigh (Crockenbert, 1987).

Ineffective parenting has been linked to diverse negative outcomes for children in a host of studies (Loeber & Stouthamer-Loeber, 1986). Furstenberg (2003) concluded that early child-bearing is "a disruptive event with adverse consequences for the young mothers and their families" (p. 28), but few researchers feel there is evidence that teen childbearing is, in itself, the cause of these outcomes. Finally, research consistently has shown that a mother's young age at first birth is most often associated with adverse outcomes not only for the child she bears as an adolescent, but also for the children she has when she is older (Pogarsky et al., 2003; Pogarsky et al., 2006).

Clearly, there are negative educational, financial and family stability outcomes for teens who become parents. There are medical and psychosocial risks to these young mothers. There are also several medical complications associated with teen pregnancy, including poor weight gain, anemia, and pregnancy-induced hypertension that can have a negative impact on both the mother and the baby (Carter et al., 1994). In addition, there is growing evidence that pregnant adolescents are at increased risk for domestic violence (Parker, McFarlane, & Soeken, 1994).

What Do We Know About the Children Born to Teen Mothers?

When looking at outcomes for babies, we must consider those related to health and safety, psychosocial development, and cognitive development. Babies born to adolescent mothers are at greater risk of adverse health conditions, developmental delays, and poorer developmental outcomes compared with babies born to mothers 20 years of age and older (Brooks-Gunn & Furstenberg, 1986). Many of these risks are related to the behaviors of the teenagers during pregnancy. Pregnant teens are much less likely to receive prenatal care in a timely manner. Many wait until the third trimester to begin care or have no care at all (Ventura, Martin, Curtin, Manackler, & Hamilton, 2001). They also are more likely to smoke while they are pregnant. One study in 2001 found that smoking among pregnant women more than 20 years old declined during the 1990s, but it increased among pregnant teens. Because both the importance of prenatal care and the

detrimental effects of smoking during pregnancy are well established, these factors contribute to adverse outcomes for babies of teenage mothers.

Babies born to teenagers are more likely to be born preterm (less than 37 weeks of gestation) and low birth weight. Preterm and low birth weight babies are at greater risk of serious and long-term illness, developmental delays, and death within the first year of life (Mathews, Curtin, & MacDorman, 2000; Ventura, Martin et al., 2001). A teen mother's substance abuse during pregnancy and after the birth may further affect infant development due to physiological or anatomic changes in the infant's brain or the mother's ability to nurture appropriately (Committee on Adolescence and Committee on Early Childhood and Adoption, and Dependent Care, American Academy of Pediatrics, 2001). Well-child health care and immunizations are very important to the health and well-being of infants and young children, but children of young teen mothers are less likely to see a medical provider than the children of older mothers (Hoffman, 2006).

Teen mothers, especially younger teens, may not have the maturity and skills necessary to give appropriate care to their infants (Whitman, Borkowski, Schellenbach, & Nath, 1987). Caring for infants is a challenge for many new parents, regardless of their age, marital status, education, or socioeconomic status. When parents understand how important the early years are to children's development and the implications for lifelong outcomes, they want information that will help them be good parents. A look at the parenting section in book stores, a search on the internet, a scan of parenting magazines, or a few minutes listening to a call-in radio program for parents give us a clear idea of the extent to which many parents are looking for information. Teen parents may put more time and energy into relationships with their friends and partners than into seeking information about ways to interact with their child. They often have less knowledge about child development and appropriate parenting practices, especially if they are developmentally immature. This lack of information and intuitive, positive parenting can increase the risk of child neglect or maltreatment (East & Felice, 1996).

Parents who read all the literature, visit all the web sites, and listen to knowledgeable child development experts learn that infants and young children need and thrive on warm, responsive care and appropriately stimulating experiences. The home environments of adolescent mothers and the early experiences they provide for their children, however, have been found to lack many of the characteristics that are usually associated with supportive, effective learning environments for infants and young children (Coll, Vohr, Hoffman, & Oh, 1986; Wasserman, Brunelli, Rauh, & Alvarado, 1994). Compared with older mothers of similar socioeconomic status, adolescent mothers tend not to coo, sing, and talk as much with their infants. They tend to touch and smile at their babies less. They are also more likely to be less sensitive to and accepting of their infants' behavior, and they hold less realistic developmental expectations (East & Felice, 1990). Some teen mothers use words such as *bad* or *naughty* to define their children. Furthermore, mothers with intense feelings of inadequacy and failure in the parenting role tend to withdraw emotionally and physically from their infants. This withdrawal has been linked to angry and resistant infant behaviors and troubled mother–child relationships (East & Felice, 1996).

These behaviors of teen mothers become even more important when we consider their effect on the brain development of their children. There has been an explosion of information on brain research and the importance of children's early experiences on brain development. It has been the topic of special editions of national magazines. Manufacturers of toys, equipment, and materials for young children have been quick to portray their wares as being good for young children's developing brains. It is during the early years of a child's life that the brain structures and response patterns that determine the child's learning processes, coping skills, and personality traits become established, encoded, and strengthened (Huttenlocher, 1994; Restak, 2001; Turner & Greenough, 1985). Negative environmental conditions during these critical years can have a profound influence on these nerve connections and neurotransmitter networks, potentially resulting in impaired brain develop-

ment (Perry, Pollard, Blakley, Baker, & Vigilante, 1995). Examples of such negative conditions include lack of stimulation, lack of close and affectionate interaction with the child's primary caregivers, child abuse, violence within the family, or repeated threats of physical and verbal abuse. When children grow up with inadequate stimulation from their environments, there is a "crippling effect on the development of plasticity mechanisms that is rarely outgrown" (Ebner, 1996, p. 150).

Researchers who study the development of young children often point to the importance of early relationships with children's primary caregivers, usually a child's mother. A major developmental task for infants and toddlers is to establish a close, nurturing bond with a primary caregiver. Research shows that supportive relationships have a tangible, long-term influence on children's healthy development. Such relationships contribute to optimal social, emotional, and cognitive development for infants and toddlers (Zeanah & Zeanah, 2001). Nurturing and sensitive adult–child interaction provides a context for supporting the development of curiosity, self-direction, persistence, cooperation, caring, and conflict resolution skills (Greenough, Black, & Wallace, 1987). As children grow, supportive relationships with parents and caregivers shape their self-image, provide them with resilience (a model for loving relationships), and set the foundation for learning.

Adolescent mothers' interactions with their children also have been associated with educational and social outcomes for their children. Children born to mothers who begin childbearing as teenagers have a higher risk of problematic parent–child interactions (Leadbeater, Bishop, & Raver, 1996), frequent changes in residence and in the composition of their caregiving environment (Jaffee, Caspi, Moffitt, Belsky, & Silva, 2001), lower educational achievement (Coley & Chase-Lansdale, 1998; Fergusson & Lynskey, 1997), and behavior problems (Wakschlag, Pickett, Cook, Jr., Benowitz, & Leventhal, 2002).

A study in 2004 found that the differences in the quality of caring for their children by low income, teen mothers were predictive of their children's competencies at the beginning of their school careers (Luster, Lekskul, & Oh, 2004). Michigan State University conducted a longitudinal study on motivation of children of low income, adolescent mothers because kindergarten teachers' ratings of academic motivation have been found to be predictive of educational attainment in adulthood (Luster & McAdoo, 1996). They followed 89 teen mothers and their children through kindergarten. The study found that 23%—almost 1 in 4—of the children were viewed by their first-grade teachers as relatively unmotivated (Luster et al., 2004).

In one 2000 study, children of teen mothers were more likely to score poorly on tests of academic skill and to be retained in school (Levine, Pollack, & Comfort, 2000). The findings of this study are similar to others that indicate that children of teen mothers do not do as well in school as children of older mothers. In addition, as the children of adolescent mothers grow up, they are more likely to drop out of school (Jaffee et al., 2001).

Children of teen mothers were more likely to display problem behaviors, such as truancy and fighting, compared with children of older mothers (Levine et al., 2000). A number of studies describe adverse social and behavioral outcomes for children of teen mothers, and these adolescent mothers are less likely to have appropriate expectations of their children. In turn, mothers who have inappropriate expectations for their children are likely to use harsh and rejecting discipline strategies (Fox, Baisch, Goldberg, & Hochmuth, 1987). Such strategies are linked with child anger, low self-esteem, and social withdrawal (East & Felice, 1996). Other social and behavioral child outcomes related to adolescent parenting include delinquency and violence (Pogarsky et al., 2003) and depression and anxiety (Hardy, Astone, Brooks-Gunn, Shapiro, & Miller, 1998). Overall, inappropriate expectations occur when the behaviors a parent desires or expects do not match the child's development or a specific situation. Some examples include

- Expecting an infant to stop crying on demand or to stop putting things in his or her mouth

- Expecting a toddler to try not to touch things that are within his or her reach

- Expecting a toddler not to have toileting accidents

- Expecting a preschool child to sit quietly when he or she has nothing to do

The adverse social and behavioral outcomes continue, as the children of teen mothers become older. In a study of 729 children, using data from the Rochester Youth Development Study from 1988 to 1996, boys born to mothers who began childbearing before age 19 had elevated risks of drug use, gang membership, unemployment, and early parenthood. The risks of being born to a young mother are substantial, but perhaps disproportionately so for boys (Pogarsky et al., 2006). This risk continues into adulthood and, sadly, includes an increase in the likelihood that sons of teen mothers will be incarcerated. The sons of mothers who gave birth at 17 or younger are 220% more likely to spend time in prison than the sons of mothers who delayed childbearing until their early 20s. Nearly 14% of the sons of adolescent mothers have been in prison by their late 30s, compared with 6% of the sons of mothers who were 20–21 years old when they were born. Sons of mothers who were 18–19 years of age at their birth are 40% more likely to have been in prison than the sons of mothers who delayed childbearing until their early 20s (Scher & Hoffman, in press).

What Are the Associated Costs?

Other specific adverse outcomes for children of teen mothers form the basis of a 2006 report on the public costs of teen childbearing by the National Campaign to Prevent Teen Pregnancy (Hoffman, 2006). The report estimated the public sector costs at the federal, state, and local levels that are associated with teen mothers and their partners and those costs associated with the children of teen mothers. The public costs for teen mothers are measured as the difference in the taxes that they pay because their earnings are lower and the difference in the cost of public assistance they receive (Temporary Assistance for Needy Families [TANF], food stamps, and housing assistance). Most of the costs of teen child-bearing, however, are associated with negative consequences for the children of teen mothers. These costs include public sector health care costs, foster care and other child welfare costs, in-carceration for sons of teen mothers, and lost tax revenues due to lower earnings when the children of teen mothers enter the labor force (Hoffman, 2006).

The cost of teen childbearing to taxpayers in the United States in 2004 (federal, state, and local) was at least $9.1 billion. The annual cost associated with a child born to a teen mother was $1,430. The public sector costs of young teens (age 17 and younger) having children are particularly high. These births account for $8.6 billion of costs, an average of $4,080 per mother annually (Hoffman, 2006).

To compute the true effect of teen childbearing, the researchers compared young women who are as similar as possible in all respects except for the age at which they first gave birth. They used statistical techniques that controlled for or adjusted for all the other risk factors that contributed to each specific outcome. The result was that they were able to find the average difference in economic outcomes and levels of disadvantage between young women who were identical, except for the ages at which they first gave birth (Hoffman, 2006).

Child welfare services are a major component of the public sector costs for children of adolescent mothers. These services include investigating allegations of child abuse and maltreatment and following up when abuse or maltreatment has occurred. Foster care is included in this category. Children born to adolescent mothers are one third more likely to be in foster care and 39% more likely to have a report of abuse or neglect during the first 5 years after birth than children born to mothers 20–21 years of age. After adjusting for a variety of risk factors, children of mothers who were 18–19 years old when they first gave birth are 13% more likely to be in foster care and 24% more likely to be the subject of a report of abuse or neglect than otherwise similar children born to mothers 20–21 years old. Almost 1 child in 10 of young teen mothers was the subject of a report for abuse or neglect com-

Table 19.5. Increased child welfare costs of a first birth to a teen mother compared with a first birth at age 20-21 years (costs are in billions of 2004 dollars)

Outcome measures	First birth at age 17 or younger	First birth at age 18–19 years	First birth at age 19 and younger
Foster care and/or child protective services	$1.84	$0.46	$2.30

From Hoffman, S.D. (2006, October). *By the numbers: The public costs of teen childbearing* (p. 13). Retrieved June 7, 2007, from http://www.teenpregnancy.org/costs/pdf/report/BTN_National_Report.pdf; reprinted by permission.

pared with 1 in 20 for children of mothers 20–21 years old. Table 19.5 shows the increased costs to federal, state, and local governments related to child welfare services that are incurred for children of adolescent mothers. The total of $2.3 billion dollars is shown on the right. The other two columns show the breakdown of costs based on the age of the adolescent at first birth.

These measures of the public costs of teen childbearing are both illuminating and disturbing. They remain, however, financial costs. The adolescent mothers and particularly their children are paying the life costs or the human costs of teen childbearing. We have seen that the rate of teenagers becoming pregnant and bearing children in our country is declining. We also have seen that at the current birth rate and teenage population, 4 out of 10 girls—some 900,000—in the United States will become pregnant each year. Just over half of these girls will give birth and become adolescent mothers. The concern for the well-being of their children is appropriately placed, and many programs are working to improve the outcomes for the teen mothers and their babies. These programs have been in existence for many years and have identified factors that lead to success in working with teens.

What Young Children Need and What Teens Have to Give

When we consider the needs of infants and young children and what teens have to offer based on developmental needs and tasks, there could hardly be a more obvious mismatch. We see examples of this potential disconnect in terms of physical and emotional needs and development. Infants are completely dependent on their caregivers to meet all their physical needs, which come at frequent intervals throughout the day and night. The resulting sleep deprivation is well known to almost all new parents who find it one of the most difficult aspects of early parenting. For adolescent parents, this is especially difficult because teenagers need more sleep than adults and even more sleep than they needed when they were younger—9¼ hours, according to sleep researcher Mary Carskadon (1999). Teenagers in general get an hour and a half less than that, which is not nearly enough sleep to be alert during the day (Carskadon, 1999). It is logical to expect that teenage parents who are caring for their infants will get even less sleep. Adolescent parents, then, are likely to be more sleep deprived than older parents. The effects of this sleep deprivation can have a negative impact on the adolescents' ability to respond appropriately to the needs of infants. The first sign of sleep deprivation is the inability to control emotions, especially anger. Other signs are increased levels of frustration, worry, and anxiety. In addition, when sleep-deprived people are given tasks that are physically demanding, they perceive the tasks to be more difficult than do people who are well rested. Sleep deprivation inhibits logical thinking skills and impairs decision making, self-confidence, coordination, and the ability to concentrate (The National Sleep Foundation's [NSF] Sleep and Teens Task Force, 2000). These are not only negatives for adolescents; they also influence teenagers' parenting skills as well as their children.

One of the main tasks of the adolescent stage is to develop a sense of identity. During adolescence, teens focus their attention on themselves and their identity relative to family, society, peers, and the expectations and values they have experienced thus far in their lives. Adolescence is a self-focused time for most teens. When adolescents become parents, their need to focus on themselves comes up squarely against the needs of their babies. To develop and thrive, infants need warm, responsive care from a consistent caregiver. This responsiveness requires the care-

giver first to attend to the baby and then to recognize and correctly read the baby's cues. It may be difficult for adolescents working on their identity from their own perspectives to attend to their infants, interpret their infants' cues correctly, and respond in an appropriate way. For example, a young mother may hear her baby cry, see his or her hands balled up into fists, and decide that "this baby wants to fight me," rather than understanding that the baby may want to be picked up and soothed or may be hungry or wet.

Understanding typical child development helps parents know what to expect from children of various ages and helps to explain why children do what they do. This knowledge can help parents read their children's cues and respond to them appropriately. Many adolescent mothers, however, lack specific knowledge about child development, including the ages children typically attain developmental milestones (Elster, McAnarney, & Lamb, 1983). They may, then, attribute typical behavior that they do not understand or expect with misbehavior and respond harshly to the child. For example, a child of 10 months may have just developed the pincer grasp (i.e., picking up objects with the thumb and forefinger rather than with the whole hand) and wants to use this newly developed skill to try to pick up anything from a speck of dust on the rug to the food on his or her spoon. If the child attempts to use his or her fingers to pick up applesauce, for example, a parent who is unfamiliar with this developmental milestone might think the child is deliberately trying to make a mess. A frustrated teen mother might punish her child for making a mess when he or she was actually working on mastering an important developmental task.

Programs that Help Teen Parents and Their Children

Over the years, there has been a variety of programs working to improve the outcomes for the children of adolescent mothers by providing services to them and/or their children. Some of these programs offer home visiting, some focus on early childhood education, and others have combined those services.

Children Get What Parents Bring

Early Head Start (EHS), which has been in existence since 1995, provides child development, child care, and parent support services to mostly low income families with children from pregnancy through 3 years of age. Services are provided through home visits, in center-based child care, or both (Raikes, Love, Kisker, & Chazan-Cohen, 2004). Three thousand families in 16 communities in the United States participated in a study of the effectiveness of EHS. There was a modest, consistent pattern of positive impact on participating families. Participants showed benefits in child cognitive and language development, parenting practices and beliefs, education, and employment (Love et al., 2002). Teen mothers, however, did not fare as well overall as older mothers. Adolescent mothers used fewer program services. EHS staff viewed teens as hard to serve. All parents demonstrated positive outcomes from the program in some areas, but older parents and their children showed positive results in more areas than did adolescents, especially with respect to parenting behaviors and stimulation of child language and learning. In the final report to Congress, the researchers indicated that teen mothers were less mature and less receptive than older mothers to services (Love et al., 2002),

A number of programs provide home visiting services for low income women with the goal of achieving more positive outcomes for children. Adolescent mothers and their children are well represented in such programs. Several examples of home visiting programs are The Nurse Family Partnership, Parents as Teachers, and Healthy Start/Healthy Families America. These programs begin working with women during pregnancy and continue making home visits through the child's early years. It has been difficult to measure accurately the impact of these programs on adolescent mothers and their children because some do not report directly on how teen parents compare with older mothers, some change their method of reporting program out-

comes during the course of the program, and some have multiple sites with very different methods of intervention.

Another type of program that seeks to achieve positive outcomes for children of high-risk, low income children focuses on intervention through early childhood education. Most well known of these programs is the Abecedarian project. It offered high-quality, center-based early education in North Carolina in the 1970's. Among the families in the program group, 25% were headed by mothers 17 or younger. This program provided some case management services to parents, but the primary focus was early childhood education offered at the child care center. The program provided services for more than just the early years. The continuity of services provided by Abecedarian makes it difficult to replicate. The program also has been the subject of long-term follow-up, which demonstrated noticeable gains not only in cognitive development for children of teen mothers, but also for the teen mothers themselves (Campbell, Breitmayer, & Ramey, 1986). When the target children were 15 years old, 80% of the teen mothers who had been enrolled in the early childhood program had post high school education, compared with only 28% of the mothers in the control group. More than 90% of the Abecedarian teen mothers were employed, which compared with only 66% of the teen mothers in the control group. This same effect was true for older mothers, but it was more pronounced for adolescent mothers (Ramey et al., 2000).

Jon Korfmacher (2005) of the Erickson Institute in Chicago lists four main conclusions from a review of selected intervention programs. First, teen parenting is one of many risk factors for healthy development. Second, early childhood interventions can make a positive difference in the educational outcomes of teen parents. Third, teen mothers seem to be harder to serve than those who are older, which is a recurring theme in many studies. Finally, early childhood intervention programs need to do something to work more successfully with teen parents. Research findings suggest that early childhood intervention programs must "work harder to engage teen parents in the relationships and activities that will make major positive differences in their lives and in the lives of their babies" (Korfmacher, 2005, p. 13).

A different model, one that is relationship based, may be what is needed to engage teen mothers. One example is the Ounce of Prevention Fund's network of Parents Too Soon (PTS) programs in Illinois. This program is grounded in the understanding and research that development is based on interactions. It focuses on developing positive, nurturing relationships with adolescent mothers that, in turn, will directly influence the nature of the relationships that those mothers create with their children. In particular, the staff develops relationships with mothers that are filled with mutual competence (i.e., the feelings of being secure, valued, successful, and happy), the enjoyment of learning together, and building strong connections between teenagers and themselves. The experience of being cared for in this supportive relationship and environment offers the parents a vital legacy to pass on to their children.

The program uses home visitors, doulas, and group workers to help a young mother make sense out of her changing life so she can "build her parental self" (Wechsler, 2005, p. 18). The program identifies and encourages the experiences that children and parents share that leave each feeling competent in relation to the other and eager to replicate these behaviors. It is not easy for a mother of any age to give sensitive and responsive care to a child if she has not consistently received such care. The PTS staff provide teen mothers with reliable information and nurturing experiences. The support that teen parents receive helps them to understand their own childhoods differently and to reflect on their current relationships with their parents. PTS programs translate developmental theories and intervention strategies into language and experiences.

Conclusion

The challenges of supporting and working with pregnant and parenting teens are immense, and the outcomes of interactions are significant in the future well-being of both parents and children. With the decreasing rate of teen pregnancy, it cannot be assumed the challenges are going away; and vigilance is necessary about the potential for changing issues.

Teen mothers and fathers must be considered from a developmental, behavioral, and environmental perspective. These young people are still learning about themselves and their abilities to assume more adult-like behaviors. Their brains are continuing to mature, providing teens with a growing capability to control impulses, understand their emotions and those of others, and organize and deal with the complexities of everyday life.

It is imperative to understand the multiple roles that teen parents have—the baby is not their only concern or responsibility. The vast majority of teen childbearing involves mothers who are not married. Most teen mothers have the major responsibility for childrearing; yet, a growing number of the fathers of these babies indicate a desire to be more involved, and they cannot be ignored.

When we think about implications for practice, it is essential to see the child within the context of his or her family. Teens will seek medical care for their babies, and this provides the opportunity to see teens as another focus of our care. Some babies and teen mothers will be targeted for community programs, and we must accept these parents where they are and build from that point. By identifying strengths as mothers and fathers interact with their children, we give them a foundation for learning skills.

If we are going to address the challenges of teen pregnancy and parenting, we must answer some basic questions and contextualize the issues with emerging data trends:

- What is the developmental, behavioral, and environmental status of these young parents?

- How do each of these young parents process information?

- Who is identified by these young parents as being supportive?

- What types of guidance do these young parents accept most readily?

In addressing the preceding questions, certain facts should be kept in mind:

- Overall, teen pregnancy rates are dropping in the United States; however, the United States continues to have one of the highest rates of the industrialized countries (National Adolescent Health Information Center, 2007).

- Compared with the late 1990s, fewer adolescents report being sexually experienced (National Adolescent Health Information Center, 2007).

- Almost 12% of female high school students have had four or more sex partners (Mosher, Chandra, & Jones, 2005).

- In 1991, 26.2% of sexually active adolescents used condoms; in 2005, 62.8% did (CDC, 2007).

- There has been a considerable decline in teen pregnancy rates for black, non-Hispanic teens between the ages of 15 and 19 years. In 1990, the rate was 232.7 per 1,000, but in 2002, the rate was 138.9 per 1,000 (Ventura, Abma, Mosher, & Henshaw, 2006).

- Most childbearing among females between 15 and 19 years resulted in nonmarital births. In 2004, this statistic amounted to 342,188 births outside of marriage in the United States (Martin et al., 2006).

The implications for practice are enormous in a general sense; yet, each family must be considered individually. We have to listen to young parents and build on their strengths. The true power of our work is making a difference, child by child and family by family, and recognizing that we can be agents of change.

It is important not to stereotype adolescent mothers and assume that they are all doing a poor job of parenting, based on the statistics that detail and describe the adverse outcomes of children of teen mothers. A longitudinal study at Michigan State University followed 89 adolescent mothers and their children from 1996 to 2003. All of the young mothers had very limited financial resources; yet, many of them provided high-quality care to their children in the preschool years. Project researchers and family advocates observed a range of quality in caregiving,

from neglectful to excellent (Luster, Lekskul, & Oh, 2004).

Finally, it must be remembered that "It is not easy for a mother of any age to be sensitive and responsive to a child, if she herself has not consistently received such care" (Wechsler, 2005, p. 14). In turn, relationship-based programs can help teen parents who may not have received such care. These programs do so by addressing the following (Wechsler, 2005, p. 14):

- The nurturing relationships and reliable information offered by effective teen parent programs bolster teens' development as people, while building their self-confidence as people.

- In a relationship-based program, the manner in which program staff develop positive relationships with teen parents directly influences the nature of the relationships that parents construct with their children.

- When program staff match experiences to the individual teen's thinking style, she can learn to offer mutually satisfying, developmentally appropriate experiences to her child.

REFERENCES

Astone, N.M. (1993). Are adolescent mothers just single mothers? *Journal of Research in Adolescence, 3*, 353–371.

Brooks-Gunn, J., & Furstenberg, F.F., Jr. (1986). The children of adolescent mothers: Physical, academic, and psychological outcomes. *Developmental Review, 6*, 224–251.

Brooks-Gunn, J., & Furstenberg, F.F., Jr. (1989). Adolescent sexual behavior. *American Psychologist, 44*, 249–257.

Bunting, L., & McAuley, C. (2004). Teenage pregnancy and motherhood: The contribution of support. *Child and Family Social Work, 9*(2), 207–215.

Campbell, F.A., Breitmayer, B.J., & Ramey, C.T. (1986). Disadvantaged teen age mothers and their children: Consequences of educational day care. *Family Relations, 35*, 63–68.

Capaldi, D.M., & Patterson, G.R. (1991). Relation of parental transitions to boys' adjustment problems: I. A linear hypothesis. II. Mothers at risk for transitions and unskilled parenting. *Developmental Psychology, 27*, 489–504.

Carskadon, M. (1999). When worlds collide: Adolescent need for sleep versus societal demands. *Phi Delta Kappan, 80*(5), 348–353.

Carter, D.M., Felice, M.E., Rosoff, J., Zabin, L.S., Beilenson, P.L., & Dannenberg, A.L. (1994). When children have children: The teen pregnancy predicament. *American Journal of Preventative Medicine, 10* (2), 108–113.

Centers for Disease Control and Prevention. (2006, June 9). Youth risk behavior surveillance—United States, 2005. *Morbidity and Mortality Weekly Report, 55*(SS-5). Retrieved June 15, 2007, from http://www.cdc.gov/mmwr/PDF/SS/SS5505.pdf

Centers for Disease Control and Prevention, National Center for Chronic Disease Prevention and Health Promotion. (2007). *Healthy youth! Youth online: Comprehensive results.* Retrieved April 10, 2008, http://apps.nccd.cdc.gov/yrbss

Coley, R.L., & Chase-Lansdale, P.L. (1998). Adolescent pregnancy and parenthood: Recent evidence and future directions. *American Psychologist, 53,* 152–166.

Coll, C.G., Vohr, B.R., Hoffman, J., & Oh, W. (1986). Maternal and environmental factors affecting developmental outcomes of infants of adolescent mothers. *Journal of Developmental and Behavioral Pediatrics, 7,* 230–236.

Committee on Adolescence and Committee on Early Childhood and Adoption, and Dependent Care, American Academy of Pediatrics. (2001). American Academy of Pediatrics: Care of adolescent parents and their children. *Pediatrics, 107*(2), 429–434.

Conger, R.D., Conger, K.J., Elder, G.H., Jr., Lorenz, F.O., Simons, R.L., & Whitbeck, L.B. (1992). A family process model of economic hardship and adjustment of early adolescent boys. *Child Development, 63,* 526–541.

Crockenbert, S. (1987). Predictors and correlates of anger toward and punitive control of toddlers by adolescent mothers. *Child Development, 58,* 964–975.

Dailard, C. (2001). Recent findings from the "Add Health" Survey: Teens and sexual activity. *Guttmacher Report on Public Policy, 4,* 1–3.

Dishion, T.J., & McMahon, R.J. (1998). Parental monitoring and the prevention of child and adolescent problem behavior: A conceptual and empirical formulation. *Clinical Child and Family Psychology Review, 1*(1), 61–75.

East, P.L., & Felice, M.E. (1990). Outcomes and parent–child relationships of former adolescent mothers and their 12-year old children. *Developmental and Behavioral Pediatrics, 11,* 175–183.

East, P.L., & Felice, M.E. (1996). *Adolescent pregnancy and parenting: Findings from a racially diverse sample.* Mahwah, NJ: Lawrence Erlbaum Associates.

Eaton, D.K., Kann, L., Kinchen, S., Ross, J., Hawkins, J., Harris, W.A., et al. (2006, June 9). Youth risk behavior surveillance—United States, 2005. *Morbidity and Mortality Weekly Report, 53*(SS02), 1–96. Re-

trieved June 8, 2007, from http://www.cdc.gov/mmwr/preview/mmwrhtml/ss5505a1.htm

Ebner, F. (1996). Teaching the brain to learn. *Peabody Journal of Education, 71*(4), 143–151.

Elster, A.B., McAnarney, E.R., & Lamb, M.E. (1983). Parental behavior of adolescent mothers. *Pediatrics, 71*(4), 494–503.

Fagot, B.I., Pears, K.C., Capaldi, D.M., Crosby, L., & Leve, C.S. (1998). Becoming an adolescent father: Precursors and parenting. *Developmental Psychology, 34*(6), 1209–1219.

Federal Interagency Forum on Child and Family Statistics. (2006). *America's children: Key national indicators of well-being.* Retrieved June 7, 2007, from http://www.childstats.gov/americaschildren/index.asp

Ferguson, H., & Hogan, F (2004). *Strengthening families through fathers: Developing policy and practice in relation to vulnerable fathers and their families.* Retrieved August 10, 2007, from http://www.fsa.ie/publications/strengthfathers/index.html

Fergusson, M.D., & Lynskey, T.M. (1997). Early reading difficulties and later conduct problems. *Journal of Child Psychology and Psychiatry and Allied Disciplines, 38,* 899–907.

Fox, R.A., Baisch, M.J., Goldberg, B.D., & Hochmuth, M.C. (1987). Parenting attitudes of pregnant adolescents. *Psychological Reports, 61*(2), 403–406.

Furstenberg, F.F. (2003). Teenage childbearing as a public issue and private concern. *Annual Review of Sociology, 29,* 23–29.

Geronimus, A.T., & Korenman, S. (1993). Maternal youth or family background? On the health disadvantages of infants with teenage mother. *American Journal of Epidemiology, 137,* 213–225.

Greenough, W.T., Black, J.E., & Wallace, C.S. (1987). Experience and brain development. *Child Development, 58*(3), 539–559.

Guttmacher Institute. (1994). *Sex and America's teenagers.* New York: Author.

Guttmacher Institute. (2002). *Sexual and reproductive health: Women and men* [Facts in Brief]. Retrieved June 8, 2007, from http://www.guttmacher.org/pubs/fb_10-02.pdf

Guttmacher Institute. (2006). *In brief: Facts on American teens' sexual and reproductive health.* Retrieved June 15, 2007, from http://www.guttmacher.org/pubs/fb_ATSRH.pdf

Haffner, D.W. (Ed.). (1995). *Facing facts: Sexual health for America's adolescents: The report of the National Commission on Adolescent Sexual Health.* Retrieved June 7, 2007, from http://www.siecus.com/pubs/Facing_Facts.pdf

Hardy, J.B., Astone, N.M., Brooks-Gunn, J., Shapiro, S., & Miller, T. (1998, November). Like mother, like child: Intergenerational patterns of age at first birth and associations with childhood and adolescent characteristics and adult outcomes in the second generation. *Developmental Psychology, 34,* 1220–1232.

Hofferth, S.L., Reid, L., & Mott, F.L. (2001). The effects of early childbearing on schooling over time. *Family Planning Perspectives, 33*(6), 259–267. Retrieved August 10, 2007, from http://www.guttmacher.org/pubs/journals/3325901.pdf

Hoffman, S. (1998). Teen childbearing isn't so bad after all—or is it?—A review of the new literature on the consequences of teen childbearing. *Family Planning Perspectives, 30,* 236–239.

Hoffman, S.D. (2006, October). *By the numbers: The public costs of teen childbearing.* Retrieved June 7, 2007, from http://www.teenpregnancy.org/costs/pdf/report/BTN_National_Report.pdf

Hotz, V.J., McElroy, S.W., & Sanders, S.G. (1997). The impacts of teenage childbearing on the mothers and the consequences of those impacts for government. In R. Maynard (Ed.), *Kids having kids: Economic costs and social consequences of teen pregnancy* (pp. 55–94). Washington, DC: The Urban Institute Press.

Huesmann, L.R., Eron, L.D., Lefkowitz, M.M., & Walder, L.O. (1984). Stability of aggression over time and generations. *Developmental Psychology, 20,* 1120–1134.

Huttenlocher, P.R. (1994). Synaptogenesis, synapse elimination, and neural plasticity in human cerebral cortex. In C.A. Nelson (Ed.), *Threats to optimal development: Integrating biological, psychological and social risk factors* [The Minnesota Symposia on Child Psychology Vol. 27] (pp. 35–54). Mahwah, NJ: Lawrence Erlbaum Associates.

Jaffee, S.R., Caspi, A., Moffitt, T.E., Belsky, J., & Silva, P. (2001). Why are children born to teen mothers at risk for adverse outcomes in young adulthood? Results from a 20-year longitudinal study. *Development and Psychopathology, 13,* 377–397.

Jaskiewicz, J.A., & McAnarney, E.R. (1994). Pregnancy during adolescence. *Pediatric Review, 15,* 32–38.

Kalil, A., Ziol-Guest, K.M., & Coley, R.L. (2005). Perception of father involvement patterns in teenage mother families: Predictors and links to mothers' psychological adjustment. *Family Relations, 54,* 197–211.

Kirby, D. (2001, May). *Emerging answers: Research findings on programs to reduce teen pregnancy.* Washington, DC: The National Campaign to Prevent Teen Pregnancy.

Klein, J.D., & the Committee on Adolescence. (2005). Adolescent pregnancy: Current trends and issues. *Pediatrics, 116*(1), 281–286.

Korfmacher, J. (2005). Teen parents in early childhood interventions. *Zero to Three, 25*(4), 7–13.

Leadbeater, B.J., Bishop, S.J., & Raver, C.C. (1996). Quality of mother-toddler interactions, maternal depressive symptoms, and behavior problems in preschoolers of adolescent mothers. *Developmental Psychology, 32,* 280–288.

Levine, J.A., Pollack, H., & Comfort, M.E. (2000). *Academic and behavioral outcomes among the children of young mothers* [JCPR Working Papers 193]. Chicago: Northwestern University/University of Chicago Joint Center for Poverty Research.

Loeber, R., & Stouthamer-Loeber, M. (1986). Family factors as correlates and predictors of juvenile conduct problems and delinquency. In N. Morris & M. Tonry (Eds.), *Criminal justice: An annual review of research* (pp. 29–149). Chicago: University of Chicago Press.

Love, J.M., Kisker, E.E., Ross, C.M., Schochet, P.Z., Brooks-Gunn, J., Paulsell, D., et al. (2002, June). *Making a difference in the lives of infants and toddlers and their families: The impacts of Early Head Start. Volume I: Final technical report.* Retrieved June 7, 2007, from http://www.acf.hhs.gov/programs/opre/ehs/ehs_resrch/reports/impacts_vol1/impacts_vol1.pdf

Luster, T., Lekskul, K., & Oh, S.M. (2004). Predictors of academic motivation in first grade among children born to low income adolescent mothers. *Early Childhood Research Quarterly, 19,* 337–353.

Luster, T., & McAdoo, H. (1996). Family and child influences on educational attainment: A secondary analysis of the High/Scope Perry Preschool data. *Developmental Psychology, 32*(1), 26–39.

Martin, J.A., Hamilton, B.E., Sutton, P.D., Ventura, S.J., Menacker, F., & Kirmeyer, S. (2006, September 29). Births: Final data for 2004. *National Vital Statistics Report, 55*(1). Retrieved April 7, 2008, from http://www.cdc.gov/nchs/data/nvsr/nvsr55/nvsr55_01.pdf

Mathews, T.J., Curtin, S.C., & MacDorman, M.F. (2000). Infant mortality statistics from the 1998 period linked birth/infant death data set. *National Vital Statistics Reports, 48*(12). Retrieved June 7, 2007, from http://www.cdc.gov/nchs/data/nvsr/nvsr48/nvs48_12.pdf

Moore, K.A., Driscoll, A.K., & Lindberg, L.D. (1998). *A statistical portrait of adolescent sex, contraception, and childbearing, 11.* Washington, DC: National Campaign to Prevent Teen Pregnancy.

Moore, M.R., & Brooks-Gunn, J. (2002). Adolescent parenthood. In M.H. Bornstein (Ed.), *Handbook of parenting, Vol. 3: Being and becoming a parent* (2nd ed., pp. 173–214). Mahwah NJ: Lawrence Erlbaum Associates.

Mosher, W.D., Chandra, A., & Jones, J. (2005, September 15). Sexual behavior and selected health measures: Men and women 15–44 years of age, United States, 2002. *Advance Data from Vital and Health Statistics No. 362.* Retrieved June 8, 2007, from http://www.cdc.gov/nchs/data/ad/ad362.pdf

Nakashima, I.I., & Camp, B.W. (1984). Fathers of infants born to adolescent mothers: A study of paternal characteristics. *American Journal of Diseases of Children, 138,* 452–454.

National Adolescent Health Information Center. (2007). *2007 fact sheet on reproductive health: Adolescents & young adults.* Retrieved August 13, 2007, from http://nahic.ucsf.edu//downloads/ReproHlth2007.pdf

The National Sleep Foundation's (NSF) Sleep and Teens Task Force. (2000). *Adolescent sleep needs and patterns: Research report and resource guide.* Retrieved April 7, 2008, from http://www.sleepfoundation.org/atf/cf/{F6BF2668-A1B4-4FE8-8D1A-A5D39340D9CB}/sleep_and_teens_report1.pdf

Parker, B., McFarlane, J., & Soeken, K. (1994). Abuse during pregnancy: Effects on maternal complications and birth weight in adult and teenage women. *Obstetrics & Gynecology, 84,* 323–328.

Perry, B.D., Pollard, R.A., Blakley, T.L., Baker, W.L., & Vigilante, D. (1995). Childhood trauma, the neurobiology of adaptation, and "use-dependent" development of the brain: How "states" become "traits." In M.S. Scheeringa & J.D. Osofsky (Eds.), Special Issue: Posttraumatic Stress Disorder (PTSD) in Infants and Young Children. *Infant Mental Health Journal, 16*(4), 271–291.

Piccinino, L.J., & Mosher, W.D. (1998). Trends in contraceptive use in the United States, 1982–1995. *Family Planning Perspectives, 30,* 4–10.

Pogarsky, G., Lizotte, A.J., & Thornberry, T.P. (2003). The delinquency of children born to young mothers: Results from the Rochester Youth Development Study. *Criminology, 41,* 101–138.

Pogarsky, G., Thornberry, T.P., & Lizotte, A.J. (2006). Developmental outcomes for children of young mothers. *Journal of Marriage and Family, 68,* 332–344.

Raikes, H., Love, L., Kisker, E., & Chazan-Cohen, R. (2004) What works: Improving the odds for infants and toddlers in low-income families. In J. Lombardi & M. Bogel (Eds.), *Beacon of hope* (pp. 20–43). Washington DC: ZERO TO THREE.

Ramey, C.T., Campbell, F.A., Burchinal, M., Skinner, M.L., Gardner, D.M., & Ramey S.L. (2000). Persistent effects of early childhood education on high-risk children and their mothers. *Applied Developmental Science, 4*(1), 2–14.

Restak, R. (2001). *The secret life of the brain.* Washington, DC: Joseph Henry Press.

Roye, C.F., & Balk, S.J. (1996). The relationship of partner support to outcomes for teenage mothers and their children: A review. *Adolescent Health, 19,* 86–93.

Scher, L.S., & Hoffman, S.D. (in press). Incarceration-related costs of early childbearing: Updated estimates. In R.A. Maynard & S.D. Hoffman (Eds.), *Kids having kids: Economic costs and social conse-*quences of teen pregnancy (Rev. ed.). Washington, DC: The Urban Institute Press.

Sexuality Information and Education Council of the United States. (2003, Fall). *The truth about adolescent sexuality* [SIECUS Fact Sheet]. New York & Washington, DC: Sexuality Information and Education Council of the United States.

Thornberry, T.P., Krohn, M.D., Lizotte, A.J., Smith, C.A., & Tobin, K. (2003). *Gangs and delinquency in developmental perspective.* New York: Cambridge University Press.

Turner, A.M., & Greenough, W.T. (1985). Differential rearing effects on rat visual cortex synapses. I: Synaptic and neuronal density and synapses per neuron. *Brain Research, 329*(1–2), 95–203.

United Nations, Department of Economic and Social Affairs, Statistical Office. (1998). *Demographic yearbook.* New York: Author.

Ventura, S.J., Abma, J.C., Mosher, W.D., & Henshaw, S.K. (2006). *Recent trends in teenage pregnancy in the United States, 1990–2002.* Retrieved August 13, 2007, from http://www.cdc.gov/nchs/products/pubs/pubd/hestats/teenpreg1990-2002/teenpreg1990-2002.htm

Ventura, S.J., & Bachrach, C.A. (2000, October 18). Nonmarital childbearing in the United States, 1940–99. *National Vital Statistics Reports, 48*(16). Retrieved June 7, 2007, from http://www.cdc.gov/nchs/data/nvsr/nvsr48/nvs48_16.pdf

Ventura, S.J., Martin, J.A., Curtin, S.C., Manackler, F., & Hamilton, B.E. (2001, April 17). Births: Final data for 1999. *National Vital Statistics Reports, 49*(1). Retrieved June 7, 2007, from http://www.cdc.gov/nchs/data/nvsr/nvsr49/nvsr49_01.pdf

Ventura, S.J., Mathews, T.J., & Hamilton, B.E. (2001, September 25). Births to teenagers in the United States, 1940–2000. *National Vital Statistics Reports, 49*(10). Retrieved June 7, 2007, from http://www.cdc.gov/nchs/data/nvsr/nvsr49/nvsr49_10.pdf

Wakschlag, L.S., Pickett, K.E., Cook, E., Jr., Benowitz, N.L., & Leventhal, B.L. (2002). Maternal smoking during pregnancy and severe antisocial behavior in offspring: A review. *American Journal of Public Health, 92,* 966–974.

Wasserman, G.A., Brunelli, S.A., Rauh, V.A., & Alvarado, L.E. (1994). The cultural context of adolescent child rearing in three groups of urban minority mothers. In G. Lamberty & C. Garcia-Coll (Eds.), *Puerto Rican women and children: Issues in health, growth and development* (pp. 137–160). New York: Plenum.

Wechsler, N. (2005). Passing it on: Lessons in relationships. *Zero to Three, 25*(4), 14–21.

Whitman, T., Borkowski, J., Schellenbach, C., & Nath, P. (1987). Predicting and understanding development delay in children of adolescent mothers: A multidimensional approach. *American Journal of Mental Deficiency, 92,* 40–56.

Xie, H., Cairns, B.D., & Cairns, R.B. (2001). Predicting teen motherhood and teen fatherhood: Individual characteristics and peer affiliations. *Social Development, 10*(4), 488–511.

Zeanah, C.H., & Zeanah, P.D. (2001). Towards a definition of infant mental health. In C.H. Zeanah (Ed.), *Handbook of infant mental health* (2nd ed.). New York: Guilford Press.

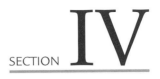

The Intersection of Best Practice in Medical Treatment and Early Education

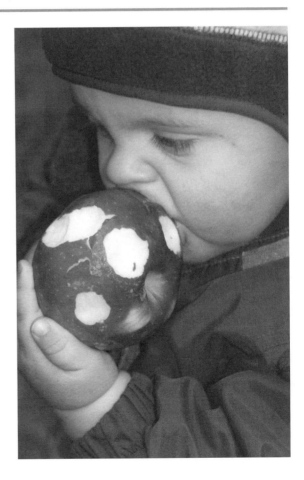

CHAPTER 20

The Neonatal Intensive Care Unit

AN ENVIRONMENT FOR BEST PRACTICE AND PARENT–PROFESSIONAL COLLABORATION

Carol Reinson and Dona Bauman

At the conclusion of this chapter, the reader will

- *Understand some of the stresses that confront families of infants admitted to neonatal intensive care units (NICU)*

- *Understand some of the perceptions that families may develop as a result of having a hospitalized newborn*

- *Understand some key concepts of family-centered care in hospital settings*

- *Understand benefits of relationship-based care for families with infants in the NICU*

- *Understand some of the developmental indicators that suggest a need for referral of newborns to early intervention directly from the NICU*

- *Be familiar with current protocols for working developmentally with infants and families in the NICU*

This chapter begins with the historical premise that there is a shared social responsibility between professional institutions in health care and education to improve the welfare of all members of society. These institutions are carefully regulated by federal and state legislation and designed to protect family rights and ensure equitable access to services (Heimer, 1999). The study of neonatal intensive care illustrates the complexity involved in linking the family, the medical community, and the educational system together to shape institutional policies and procedures collaboratively that have an impact on decision making for a newborn with medical complications.

It is widely known that the neonatal intensive care unit (NICU) experience itself creates a heightened sense of threat and considerable stress for families. The level of parental involvement in the decision-making process during transitional periods in the ongoing care of the newborn plays a key role in determining parental perceptions about the quality of care (Orfali & Gordon, 2004; Reinson, 2002). The literature reveals that parent perceptions (positive or negative) during a health care crisis may actually have an impact on an infant's long-term developmental outcome (Sydor-Greenberg & Dokken, 2000). In fact, there is definitive empirical evidence that negative parent perceptions about the health of one's child can disrupt the typical parent–child relationship, thereby contributing to the formation of the "vulnerable child syndrome," as described in medical literature (Allen, Manuel, Legault, Naughton,

& O'Shea, 2004; De Ocampo, Macias, Saylor, & Katikaneni, 2003; Gleason & Evans, 2004; McCormick, Brooks-Gunn, Workman-Daniels, & Peckham, 1993; Reinson, 2002; Thomasgard, 1998). Therefore, it is essential that all participants communicate openly and work together in partnership to form an alliance of mutual trust (McGrath, 2001). The primary goal is to promote cumulative developmental benefits through medical treatment and intervention strategies based on best practices with authentic family involvement (Gorski, 1999; Heimer, 1999; Reinson, 2002; Spoth, Kavanagh, & Dishion, 2002).

Public policymakers have long recognized that the integration of the structure of health care (e.g., physical plant, equipment, technology, personnel training) and the process of service delivery (e.g., communication patterns, caregiver perceptions and satisfaction, family inclusion in decision making) has a substantial impact on the quality of outcome (KidsGrowth Professional, 2001). This chapter will adopt a structure + process = outcome framework to explore medical and educational research on developmentally supportive, family-centered models of neonatal intensive care.

Meeting Families in the Midst of Neonatal Crisis

Health care professionals constantly strive to ensure quality, state-of-the-art medical care and a supportive environment for families during all phases of prenatal care and the delivery of a newborn. Unfortunately, perinatal complications and/or a birth crisis can occur at any time with any given family for a host of reasons. It is clearly reflected in the literature that families consider an admission to the NICU a crisis event of considerable importance, regardless of the particulars of the situation (Reinson, 2002; Spear, Leef, Epps, & Locke, 2002).

An acute medical crisis that involves a child has an urgent and dramatic emotional effect on family members. Health care workers need to remind themselves that even routine care in the NICU is not routine or normal for families

(Heimer, 1999). Nusbaum and Helton (2002) strongly recommended that professionals continually strive to be sensitive and temperate with their words, resist making any assumptions or taking situations personally, and always give their best effort when interacting with families. Indeed, the mere act of acknowledging parental stress can serve to validate a parent's emotional experience, thereby beginning the process of family adaptation to a challenging set of medical circumstances. The art of communicating sensitive news to families is enhanced when practitioners, especially physicians, engage in careful preparation, sensitive delivery, and appropriate follow-up (Olson, Edwards, & Hunter, 1987; Ramp, 1999).

Numerous studies from the 1980s to date have contributed to our collective understanding of the manifestation of parental stress during infant hospitalization (Board & Ryan-Wenger, 2003; Dudek-Shriber, 2004; Franck, Cox, Allen, & Winter, 2005; Gale, Franck, Kools, & Lynch, 2004; Miles, Funk, & Carlson, 1993; Perehudoff, 1990; Ward, 2001). It should be noted that there appears to be a predisposition or bias in the research to focus particular attention on mothers. Experts believe there may be biological and/or social role differences between mothers and fathers (Franck et al., 2005). It is thought that women embrace motherhood with their whole sense of identity and that a mother's "well-being is closely attuned to the baby's condition" (Orfali & Gordon, 2004, p. 338). For instance, it has long been demonstrated that maternal stress originates during the initial separation from the baby and that the issue of separation appears to remain a constant source of emotional turmoil throughout the course of medical treatment (Affonso et al., 1992). It is not unusual for birth mothers to display a significant degree of depression and anxiety during this time period (Spear et al., 2002).

Although there is a scarcity of research on understanding the short- and long-term impact of pediatric illness and disability on fathers, one should not assume that they play a secondary role. Fathers are increasingly involved in direct caregiving activities and serve many other vital roles, such as determining parent–child outcomes, influencing family dynamics, lessening the impact of family stress, promoting family well-being and adaptation, establishing social supports, and/or providing spousal support (Esdaile, & Greenwood, 2003; Gavidia-Payne & Stoneman, 1997; Nakamura, Stewart, & Tatarka, 2000; Reinson, 2002; Simmerman & Blacher, 2001; Young & Roopnarine, 1994). In fact, Stein (1999) portends that a perinatal crisis increases overall family vulnerability and that health care professionals should recognize that both parents have an intense desire to understand, help, and protect their children.

It is important to recognize that there has been a noticeable paradigm shift in the study of neonatal intensive care to include and highly value the family's own personal interpretation of known stressors, including actual perinatal events, infant appearance and behavior, medical procedures, staff communications and interpersonal relations, parental role alteration, environmental conditions, and social and/or family concerns during newborn hospitalization (Affonso et al., 1992; Perehudoff, 1990). The field of pediatric nursing has piloted many useful clinical instruments to evaluate family stress in an effort to address individualized family needs and improve programs to support family coping and adaptation. Although somewhat dated, the most widely known measures are Miles's *Parent Stressor Scale: Neonatal Intensive Care (PSS: NICU)* and the *Critical Care Family Needs Inventory (CCFNI)* (Leske, 1991). The CCFNI was recently adapted for use in a study, newly titled *The NICU Family Needs Inventory* (Ward, 2001). Researchers asked 52 parents to identify and rank the 10 most important need statements and the 10 least important need statements while their infants were in the NICU. Some of the items considered important were as follows (Ward, 2001):

- The parent's knowing what is being done for the infant

- The parent's being assured that the NICU staff is providing comfort for the infant (e.g., providing a pacifier, supporting the infant's body with blankets, talking softly to the infant)

- The parent's knowing what medical treatment the infant is receiving

- The staff's responding honestly to questions about the infant

- The parent's being able to visit at any time

- The parent's being assured that the infant is receiving the best care possible

- The parent's understanding the progress and expected outcome for the infant

- The parent's feeling that personnel at the hospital care about the infant

- The parent's being assured that health care providers are handling the infant gently

Clearly, the results indicated that families desired access to any and all clinical information concerning the health status of their child. They sought honest answers to their questions and assurances that medical care was being administered in a caring, humanistic manner. Families looked for every opportunity possible to remain in close proximity to their baby. However, supports that addressed the direct physical, social, and spiritual needs of the parents themselves or other immediate family members (siblings) were considered less essential. Moreover, the data also revealed that parents were not very interested in parent support groups at that point in time.

A larger study consisting of 209 mothers of premature infants used the CCFNI (Leske, 1991) to explore the relationship between maternal needs and the established priorities in a NICU environment. The findings revealed converging evidence that mothers placed the most value on accurate information about their babies and good communication practices with professionals. Mothers did not consider their own needs as important (Bialoskurski, Cox, & Wiggins, 2002). Research strongly supported professional practices that focused on and supported the diverse needs and priorities of families.

Bruns and Klein (2005) completed a retrospective evaluation survey around issues of parent satisfaction in an urban Level III NICU (i.e., critical care neonatal intensive care units, as opposed to Levels I and II hospital nurseries). The survey questions concentrated on four primary areas: the NICU environment, caregiving practices, communication opportunities, and relationships with nursing staff. The following features were rated as having a positive impact on parent satisfaction:

NICU Environment

- Open visiting hours
- Availability of a toll-free phone number
- Access to a private breast pumping room and equipment
- Privacy
- Access to child

Caregiving Practices

- NICU staff who listened to suggestions about the child's care
- Inclusion in the child's plan of care
- Opportunities for parents to learn to care for their child
- Nursing staff who supported parents to be active participants in the child's care

Communication

- Provision of information concerning medical procedures and results
- Staff who listened to parent concerns and took time with families
- Parent desires for a more regular schedule of being included in decision making
- Accessibility to talk to staff at any time

Relationships

- Recognition that parents are the primary caregivers of children
- Support for parent decisions
- Highly rated staff attributes of being helpful, caring, friendly, and comforting
- Parents being treated with respect and understanding
- Valued approachability and compassion of staff
- Staff promoting a feeling of welcome to parents

The Contemporary Touchstone of Family-Centered Care

The conceptual model of family-centered care (FCC) currently serves as a unifying framework to link together medical (primary physical morbidity) and educational factors (complex problems rooted in social, family, and environmental conditions) that are historically associated with long-term outcomes of children with special needs (Berkowitz, Halfon, & Klee, 1992). The resultant biopsychosocial model has far-reaching implications for neonatal practice. It is important that all medical and educational practitioners understand the principles of FCC in order to provide responsive and helpful services to children and their families (Lawlor & Mattingly, 1998). Within this context, FCC provides common ground for three major assumptions (Law, 1998):

1. Parents know and want the best for their children.

2. Families are diverse and unique.

3. Optimal child functioning occurs within the context of family and community.

Historically, the conceptual model of FCC slowly emerged in the 1940s and 1950s. At this time, Carl Rogers developed his landmark theories on client-centered care. He promoted a "believe in yourself" attitude and alluded to the reality that society may or may not have your best interests at heart. The belief that the experts knew what was best for any given individual or family was questioned. Over the years, there has been a clear shift away from discipline-based knowledge toward an emphasis on interdisciplinary team collaboration that includes the family's perspective. Family-centered concepts have evolved to form a centralized philosophy of care, foster humanistic attitudes and a set of practices, and provide opportunities for increased parental involvement in medical and therapeutic decision making for children with special needs (Law, 1998). Although the concept of FCC has widespread support in current thinking and many studies assert that it is critical to facilitating successful experiences for infants and their families, experts agree that health services and educational programs often are challenged to integrate family-centered principles into formal institutional policies and procedures (Bruder, 2000; Bruns & Klein, 2005; Dunst, Johanson, Trivette, & Hamby, 1991; McGrath, 2000; Woodside, Rosenbaum, King, & King, 2001).

Helen Harrison, well-known author of *The Premature Baby Book* (1993a), solicited a broad spectrum of professional and personal opinions to assist her in developing a working set of what she called The Principles for Family-Centered Neonatal Care. She included the perspectives of parent groups, attorneys, ethicists, physicians, nurses, and others with an interest in neonatal care and follow-up (Harrison, 1993b).

As previously discussed, there are numerous variables (infant and familial characteristics) to consider when designing and carrying out authentic, family-centered care in a NICU. Dunst, Boyd, Trivette, and Hamby (2002) proposed that family-centered care involves adopting a relational orientation (relationship-based care) toward families, as well as fostering participatory practice (partnership in decision making) during all phases of health care delivery. In either case, the role of communication between professionals and parents remains the primary, underlying factor that influences parent satisfaction. In addition, the NICU staff must identify and adapt common medical practices to a range of family dimensions in order to design individualized family care plans (e.g., family culture and coping mechanisms). Moreover, recommended changes in institutional policies and procedures should be based on empirical data and theoretical approaches (Atkins-Burnett & Allen-Meares, 2000).

The fields of neonatology and early intervention most recently have recognized the enormous value of enhancing the parent–child relationship and promoting infant development within the context of natural environments (McCollum, 2002). Atkins-Burnett and Allen-Meares (2000) proposed that practitioners integrate several principles of infant mental health in order to create positive change in family functioning. The following principles were identified:

- The baby's primary relationships need to support the baby's developmental needs.

- Each parent and each baby is unique in many different ways, including temperament, interaction style, and emotional make-up. Understanding this uniqueness will help in understanding the goodness-of-fit in the parent–child relationship and the areas where there may be tension or mismatch.

- The particular environmental context in which the baby and the parent reside deeply affects functioning.

- Practitioners must try to understand behavior from the inside out, to consider what it would be like to walk in that parent's shoes, what feelings, dreams, desires, and perceptions about the world led to the parent's behavior.

- Practitioners need to be aware that their own feelings and behavior affect intervention, and the interaction between parent and provider affects the parent–child relationship. Parents who feel supported in the parent–provider relationship will be more inclined to nurture and support their children. Alternatively, when the provider is directive in interactions with the parent, the parent is more likely to be directive toward the child, an interaction pattern that has negative implications for development.

The interdisciplinary principles of infant mental health have become increasingly important to practitioners who are engaged in follow-up services with children (birth to 3 years) and their families (Chandler & Yun, 2006). The related service field of occupational therapy has translated three core infant mental concepts into early intervention work with high-risk families and infants. These concepts include (Schultz-Krohn & Cara, 2000, pp. 551–552)

- Ongoing self-reflection and clinical reasoning;
- Use of non-directive suggestions; and
- Relationship-based care consisting of daily life advocacy and support.

Graham, White, Clarke, and Adams (2001) emphasized several core constructs that influence infant mental health practices, including strengthening the caregiver–child relationship by focusing on the importance of human touch and proximity to the caregiver, responsive caregiving, continuity of care, and emotional nurturance and comfort. The conceptual shift indicated here for early interventionists is to move away from child-centered treatment approaches focused solely on skill building and work toward promoting relationship-based care with the family. This area of concern is of paramount importance to early home visitors engaged in long-term, follow-up services with a newborn.

It is also important that NICU administrators carry out an appropriate program of evaluation that includes quality assurance measures that take into account the affective element of parent perspectives. The impact of policies and procedures found within a hospital environment often create a life-changing learning experience for parents. Accordingly, the health care team should examine multiple sources of quantitative and qualitative evidence on a regular basis to create both a physical and social environment that addresses the needs of the infant and his or her family. The role of caregiving and the social environment in a NICU are believed to be instrumental in providing both immediate and long-lasting benefits for the infant and family. As previously stated, it has long been recognized that health care personnel need to "be fully committed to facilitate growth of the attachment relationship between the parents and infant . . . secure attachment is essential for the infant to reach full social, emotional, and intellectual potential" (Graven et al., 1992, p. 267).

The importance of the role of social communication between an infant and caregiver arose from concern for the infant's long-term psychosocial development. Beverly Johnson (personal communication, January 2006) at the Institute for Family-Centered Care in Bethesda, Maryland, encourages health care personnel to define, design, and deliver effective human interaction in the NICU, thus developing a communication plan that promotes positive communication patterns between the mother and fetus, newborn and parents, babies and caregivers, and caregivers and NICU staff.

A Developmentally Supportive, Family-Centered Model of Neonatal Care

Since the early 1980s, several operational definitions for the term developmental care have emerged in the field. Dr. Heidelese Als of Harvard Medical Center (1998), an early pioneer in neonatology, describes developmental care as "a framework that encompasses all care procedures as well as social and physical aspects in the newborn intensive care unit. Its goal is to support each individual infant to be stable, well organized, and competent as possible" (p. 138). Historically, the field of neonatology stressed the importance of infant stimulation, which provided the premature infant with a wide range of sensory experiences. This is no longer the case. Recent studies demonstrate growing evidence that supports a developmentally supportive model of infant protection measures. As discussed in Chapter 13, Als has widely promoted the practice of reading infant cues to determine the timing and intensity of infant–caregiver interactions. In fact, she identifies the infant's primary caregiver as the primary "co-regulator," who is best suited to assist vulnerable infants with sensory processing and sensory overload issues. In addition, Als developed a synactive theory of development that is based on the premise that infant behavior is meaningful and has communicative value. She believes that sensory thresholds vary from infant to infant, day to day, and minute to minute, and that the infant functions with his or her own set of developmental expectations that are not at all age specific.

In a Cochrane Review, Symington and Pinelli (2001) described "the model of developmental care as a broad category of interventions designed to minimize the stress of the NICU environment" (p. 1). In 1997, the Developmental Care Division of Children's Medical Ventures published a concise overview for neonatal nurses regarding the developmental care of the preterm infant (Jorgensen, 1997). Jorgensen based recommendations on a thorough literature review that demonstrated enormous benefits of reducing the stress involved in a NICU environment. In particular, research continues to reveal strong evidence that the application of developmental care practices in the NICU promotes fewer days on a ventilator; earlier feeding success; shorter hospital stays; a reduction in the number of complications; increased heart rate stability; increased levels of oxygenation; improved behavioral state organization; more time in awake states; less restlessness; improved weight, length, and head circumference; lower incidence of necrotizing enterocolitis; and improved neurodevelopmental outcomes during the first 18 months of life (Als et al., 2003; Jorgensen, 1997). Moreover, the ability to read and interpret newborn neurobehavioral cues is now considered to be a reliable method for understanding the infant's moment-by-moment physiological status. Jorgensen (1997) reminds us that developmentally supportive care moves from protocol-based to process-based care in order to understand that ongoing treatment and evaluation must go hand-in-hand to meet individualized needs.

The behavior and physical appearance of a premature infant is startling and upsetting to almost every parent (Graven et al., 1992). Also, it is not uncommon for parents to experience a vast range of strong emotions, including fear, shock, and depression during the first few encounters with their premature infant. Parents attempting to hold their premature infants often experience their child arching their back and/or turning away with their eyes shielded. These behavioral responses should be not be interpreted as a sign of personal rejection, but rather the infant's attempt to screen out noxious, overwhelming stimuli. Parents need to receive educational training about reading infant cues and about available developmental interventions during the hospitalization period. The observational method of reading infant cues is congruent with the early work of Brazelton (1992), a well-known expert in the field of pediatrics. He recognized various levels of attentiveness (i.e., deep sleep, light sleep, drowsy, quiet alert, fussy, and crying) in all infants. His research concluded that the optimal

Table 20.1. Infant cues for developmental care intervention

Signs of stress and/or sensory overload	Signs of stability and receptiveness to caregiver
Color change	Stable color
Change in respiration	Regular respiration
Change in heart rate	Consistent heart rate
Extension or limpness of extremities	Flexed or tucked position
Open or gaping mouth	Hand on face
Hiccupping	Sucking
Yawning	Smiling
Looking away	Looking at caregiver
	Clear sleep states
	Relaxed tone and posture

state for learning and social interaction is the quiet alert level.

In addition to the range of emotions noted already, it is not uncommon for parents (especially mothers) to engage in vigilant watching as an attempt to monitor the NICU environment and safeguard their premature infants (Hurst, 2001). A developmental care approach offers medical personnel and parents opportunities to minimize stress and increase the infant's ability to self-regulate sensory input. Accordingly, reading nonverbal infant cues assists both parental and nursing caregivers in knowing when to interact with premature infants, thus modifying the environment to allow the child additional time to process incoming sensory information. Table 20.1 describes signs of stress and/or sensory overload versus signs of stability in newborns as a method of reading infant cues and creating developmental care interventions.

The most common developmental care interventions that provide infant protection include (Jorgensen, 1997)

- Decreasing room lighting and noise levels
- Darkening the incubator with an appropriate cover
- Assisting the infant in maintaining a flexor pattern
- Facilitating hand-to-mouth behavior and nonnutritive sucking
- Handling the child smoothly and slowly

- Not interrupting the infant's sleep whenever possible

- Grouping care and medical procedures

- Using swaddling for containment (encourages flexion)

The transition to create a developmentally supportive, family-centered model of neonatal care involves a comprehensive process in hospitals of altering the physical environment as well as elements of medical care, staff communications and relations, staff knowledge and attitude, caregiving roles during hospitalization, and education and training programs (Ballweg, 2001; Johnson, Abraham, & Parrish, 2004; Perehudoff, 1990). The Newborn Individualized Developmental Care and Assessment Program (NIDCAP) is an international organization that functions as a leader for research and training in developmental care and family-centered practice. Their formal training programs educate, implement, and monitor the ongoing performance of NIDCAP certified staff. This in-depth program requires that an entire medical team associated with a given NICU be collectively involved in the NIDCAP training. Moreover, Johnson and colleagues pointed out that

> The first step in the design planning process is to develop a collaborative team of parents, multidisciplinary health care providers, and design professionals. As a team they learn together about innovations in care and facility design through review of current literature and websites, attending conferences or seminars, and making site visits. The team should envision the ideal NICU setting, develop a vision or philosophy of care statement for the NICU, and develop goals for the design project. (2004, p. 363)

Ballweg (2001) offers additional advice on the lessons learned in making the transition to a NICU that is developmentally supportive and family centered. First and foremost, identify early an individual who is a knowledgeable change agent. Specifically, this person "needs to be able to negotiate complex systems, facilitate teams, be persistent without being a pest, and be able to deal with the psychological and emotional issues of the role" (p. 69).

Developmental Follow-Up

Parents benefit from ongoing educational information about infant behavior and developmental maturation after discharge as well as during hospitalization. It is important that parents understand that premature infants move through their own unique developmental sequences during the first 1–2 years of life that may be unlike those of typical newborns. For example, a typical infant delivered at 9 months gestation will normally exhibit physiological flexion at birth, especially in the prone position. The typical infant then will integrate flexion and develop volitional extension while prone in a cephalo–caudal fashion. However, a premature infant often is still predominantly in extension at birth. This infant must first develop the neural maturation to integrate this primitive extension pattern, achieve physiological flexion, and then begin to develop volitional extension before proceeding through the developmental sequence for gross motor skills (i.e., prone, supine, rolling, sitting, kneeling, half-kneeling, pull-to-stand, cruising, and independent walking).

The concept of adjusted age was developed to allow additional time for growth and maturation when an infant is born preterm. If an infant is born 3 months premature, then 12 weeks should be subtracted from the child's chronological age for the first 2 years. This additional time is useful when comparing a premature infant's current functional level with typical developmental schedules of maturation. Reinson (2002) found that even parents of children who were in the NICU only briefly benefited from increased educational information about child development during a series of home visits the first year. Also, there was strong evidence that developmental evaluations may have served as an intervention for children considered at risk in her study.

Often infants born early close the developmental gap between 8 to 10 months, depending on their degree of prematurity (Ensher & Clark, 1994). However, some children need to be referred during the first year for early intervention. What markers indicate to a parent or pediatrician that developmental intervention is warranted? What makes an infant high risk or low risk for developmental delay? Wallin (2003) has offered some indicators in terms of high-risk and low-risk premature infants. For example, she described high risk as including both biological factors and environmental factors. Biological high risk includes infants who have had serious medical problems while in the NICU, such as intraventricular hemorrhage, periventricular leukomalasia, seizures, bronchopulmonary dyplasia, infectious diseases, and necrotizing enterocolitis. Environmental risk refers to the intrauterine environment, the postnatal caregiving environment, or both. Wallin (2003) indicated that all other premature infants are defined as low risk, although situations always vary. Low-risk infants often have been known to develop minor to moderate disabilities that are not diagnosed until school age. In fact, Wallin (2003) stressed that sometimes low-risk, preterm babies often have poorer outcomes than full-term infants, probably as a result of a myriad of other environmental and familial influences. Wallin (2003) added further that professionals with specialized knowledge of infant development can identify many of the subtle motor, language, and cognitive delays in infants born prematurely.

It is common practice for NICUs to engage the services of a developmental specialist who has cross trained for a number of years in the fields of occupational therapy, physical therapy, early intervention, and nursing. The developmental specialist may assume a variety of roles and responsibilities depending on the current needs of the infant and/or family and NICU, including consultation and direct services to parents and staff on developmental care procedures, individualized supportive care tailored to meet the infant's immediate needs, and referral for early intervention and other community-based programs.

Soft Signs and Developmental Markers

Several developmental markers may indicate that referral to early intervention services is warranted (Blackman, 1992). These include

- Feeding issues
- "Too good" baby (never cries)

- Babies unable to calm themselves
- Babies who seem stiff when held
- Babies who appear very floppy when held
- Babies (older than 3 months) who continue to be asymmetrical in appearance
- Babies who do not vocalize during the first 6 months
- Babies who avoid eye contact with their caregivers
- Babies who do not follow a moving object after a corrected age of 3 months
- Babies who do not smile during the first 6 months
- Concerns of parents, regular caregivers, or health providers regarding child's competence or emotional well-being
- Babies who do not turn to caregiver's voice after several months.

Although clearly not happening universally at this writing, Wallin (2003) advocated for systems for tracking and monitoring the development of all premature infants and other infants at risk. Currently, there is significant variability across states in determining eligibility for early intervention services. For example, the state of Pennsylvania has five different categories of at-risk infants. Two of the five at-risk categories are babies who have been born prematurely and/or had stays in the NICU. One county in Pennsylvania registers all babies who are admitted to a NICU and invites families to fill out a parent-completed, child-monitoring developmental checklist every 4 months. Families are given the choice of either a home visit by an EI specialist and/or a short, mailed questionnaire. Parents fill out the questionnaire and then return it to the county. Service coordinators subsequently score the questionnaire and then inform the family if there is a need for further evaluation or follow-up services and referral (Reinson, Lieberman, Hurchick, Clark, & Plati, 2004).

Infants born prematurely often need to receive early intervention and/or be followed in clinical services to monitor development, in addition to regular pediatrician and well-baby visits for immunizations. One particular benefit of follow-up clinics and early intervention services is the education of parents. Moreover, follow-up clinics or early intervention can help parents of low-risk infants understand that some learning difficulties may not occur until the child enters school (Wallin, 2003).

The simple truth is that in the early stages of life, physicians and health care professionals cannot always predict with certainty which premature infants will experience positive outcomes and which children will ultimately need extensive services. Occasionally, an infant who originally demonstrates appropriate developmental signs will develop serious medical and educational issues at a later date. However, experience also has revealed that some infants who seem to have many factors working against them will show remarkable resilience. Given this knowledge, it is critical that all infants born prematurely have regular access to early intervention services. In conclusion, Glascoe and Shapiro (2007) noted five major pitfalls of developmental screening: 1) waiting until a problem is observable, 2) ignoring screening results, 3) relying on informal methods, 4) using a measure not suitable to primary care, and 5) assuming services are limited or nonexistent. These authors wrote,

> Developmental surveillance is a longitudinal process that commences with routinely eliciting and addressing parents' concerns, followed by medical history, maintaining a record of developmental progress, making accurate and informed observations about the child and parent–child interactions, identifying risk and protective factors that often predict developmental risks and resilience, and ensuring that needed interventions are promptly delivered. (Glascoe & Shapiro, 2007, pp. 2–3)

The Need for Real-Life Information: Parents as Advocates

There is growing acknowledgment in the literature to support the assumption that families represent the "most essential resource for the social, intellectual, emotional, and behavioral development of their children" (Dunlap, Newton, Fox, Benito, & Vaughn, 2001, p. 215). Numerous stud-

ies have examined the predictive value of specific family characteristics in determining the level of family involvement in educational and therapeutic programs. These variables include family functioning, marital adjustment, social supports, parenting styles, stress, and coping mechanisms (Gavidia-Payne & Stoneman, 1997). Best practices in the field of early intervention support the construct that each individual family must be respected for the level of involvement they choose for themselves. It is extremely important that health and educational professionals understand their pivotal roles in encouraging, supporting, educating, and engaging families to become involved in systemic advocacy for children with special rights (as opposed to children with special needs).

Professionals working with families during the early phases of negotiating the bureaucracy of medical care and special education need to recognize and assume responsibility for helping families to understand their vested interest in activities that empower them and their children as individuals. These activities may involve parents learning about a specific disability, networking with families of similar interest, understanding federal and state legislation, educating and training extended family, locating informal and formal support systems in the community, serving on advisory boards, presenting family perspectives to students in training, putting a face on disability rights, volunteering in educational programs, or helping parents learn just how to get through the day (O'Hanlon & Griffin, 2004; Roudebush, Kaufman, Johnson, Abraham, & Clayton, 2006).

The Parents' Perspective

In the words of one parent with three children who were admitted to a NICU:

I have had the experience of transitioning from the neonatal intensive care unit to home three times in my life. My three children were all born prematurely and spent extensive time in the neonatal intensive care unit. Their birthdays span 9 years, and during

*those 9 years technological advances in neonatal in-
tensive care occurred that allowed each one to survive
and grow up to be adults or almost adults who are or
will be productive members of society. Still even with
their excellent outcome, I remember their homecoming as a time filled with hope and fear. I also know
that if I had known what I now know about premature infants and early intervention, their homecoming
would have been a great deal easier than it was.*

For parents to feel competent enough to take
care of their premature infant at home, they must
have access to several areas of information. Information should include the medical needs of the
child, how to effectively feed the child in the way
that the parent has chosen, and how to recognize
signs of developmental delay and stress signals.
These are all areas that staff should teach or explain to assist parents in feeling comfortable with
their premature infant. Transition home from the
NICU should begin the day the child is admitted
to the NICU. It is very important that parents be
involved in this process that will gradually prepare them for caring for their baby at home. Parents need to have information about the medical
needs of their child, but they also need to know
how to feed their child and how to interact with
their child. They also need the resources that will
follow their child's development for several
years.

During the hospitalization the staff should
strive for a concept known as "mutual competence." Akers, Boyce, Mabey, and Boyce (2007)
describe a model of early intervention based on
the model of mutual competence. Bernstein, Percansky, and Wechsler (1996) define mutual competence as "any interchange through which the
parent and child feel secure, valued, successful,
happy, or enjoy learning together" (p. 118). According to Akers et al., the model of mutual competence assists a parent to nurture his or her infant by "recognizing and supporting parent and
infant capabilities and strengths" (2007, p. 45).
Supporting and assisting parents and children to
have positive parent–child interactions should
be an important goal for the NICU staff to attain.
Parents of children who are born prematurely

need to know that their infants will not respond
to them in the same manner as full-term infants.
They need to know how to interact with their infants, know the stress signals, and know that
they are not the cause of their infant turning
away during an interaction.

Parents must be ready to assume the majority of the care of the child when their child is discharged from the NICU. Sheikh, O'Brien, and
McCluskey-Fawcett (1993) reported that if parents do not feel comfortable in caring for their
child, the consequences may be problematic.
Their study, done in 1993, found a large discrep-
ancy between what nurses believed they taught
the parents and parents perceived as being taught
in order to take their child home. Browne, Langlois, Ross, and Smith-Sharp (2001) likewise indicated that many parents feel that the transition to
home is not discussed in the NICU, or, if it is, it is
not discussed until the baby is discharged. The
second chapter author recently interviewed a
parent whose premature twins were discharged
from a NICU. This parent indicated that her experience with transition included instruction in
how to change diapers, feed, take temperatures,
and CPR training. The mother reported she did
not remember being taught about any developmental needs or interactive needs of parent and
child. When asked about any follow-up that
might be provided by the NICU, the mother reported that it was too expensive for her family to
take advantage of any nursing follow-up visits.

The Education of the Handicapped Act
Amendments of 1986 (PL 99-457) is the legislation
that provides services for infants, toddlers, and
preschoolers. With the reauthorization of the legislation as the Individuals with Disabilities Education Act Amendments (IDEA) of 1997 (PL 105-17)
and subsequent reauthorization as the Individuals with Disabilities Education Improvement Act
(IDEA) of 2004 (PL 108-446), services for infants
and toddlers are now available through Part C.
State Part C programs provide therapeutic interventions and family support for families whose
children are born prematurely and are eligible
for early intervention (Akers et al., 2007).

At this writing, most states do not have adequate methods or means in place for graduates of
NICUs to make the transition from the NICU to

Part C services. The mother whose twins were discharged from the NICU remembers receiving a telephone number of the early intervention program in a packet of information, but she cannot remember where she put the phone number. Akers et al. (2007) reported that many families still do not understand the important role that Part C services can play in their children's and families' lives. Many families do not utilize the services. Some NICU staff have said that they do not want to scare parents when they are taking their children home by talking about early intervention.

Based on the concept of the protective environment, new interventions for the NICU are being explored and implemented in selected NICUs across the country. One such program described in the literature is called BEGINNINGS (Browne et al., 2001). BEGINNINGS utilizes an interim individualized family service plan (IFSP) written as early as 7–10 days after an infant is born. Browne and colleagues reported that this is a legal document used in Colorado's NICUs. The interim IFSP is developed when a family and child have needs that must be met, but an assessment has not been completed. The interim IFSP provides for transition from the NICU to the home. Initially, two service coordinators are identified: One who will work with the parents in the NICU and one who will work with the family when they make the transition into the community. The family meets with the community service coordinator and a "beginnings" connection is made that subsequently supports the family and offers continuity from one setting to another.

Another program identified in the literature is the InReach program (Akers et al., 2007). The InReach program plans for infant discharge from the moment the child is admitted to the NICU. The program has two primary goals: 1) to assist parents to learn skills in observing and interpreting their baby's behavior, and 2) to assist caregivers to become competent in these skills. Subsequently, upon discharge, a service coordinator of the Part C program is invited to participate in a discharge meeting. If the Part C service coordinator is not able to come to the hospital because of distance, then video conferencing is utilized (Akers et al., 2007).

Both of these programs are designed to support families in making connections between Part C services and the NICU, which helps them to develop a link and make the transition from the NICU to the community. In particular, both interventions are intended to assist caregivers in feeling and becoming competent as they move from the NICU to home and take on the task of parenting a high-risk, potentially challenging newborn.

Conclusion

The knowledge base that supports best practices in newborn care has become increasingly interdisciplinary in nature, with major contributions from the fields of applied science such as early intervention, early childhood special education, occupational therapy, physical therapy, speech and language pathology, nursing, medicine, and social work. The key element to all transitions is effective communication and forming a partnership with families.

Only 20%–30% of children with disabilities are identified before school entrance (Glascoe & Shapiro, 2007). Heeding the advice of Glascoe and Shapiro (2007) regarding developmental surveillance, which was quoted previously in this chapter, those figures could and should change with better outcomes for both young children and their families.

In conclusion, Ensher and Clark offered some predictions that appear to hold as true in 2008 as they did when these words were written:

> Research focused on the quality and nature of interactions between premature infants and their families has been fertile ground of inquiry over the past two decades. . . . Findings that parents may feel alienation, lack of control, poor attachment to their babies, sorrow, and tremendous stress should be no surprise. In recent years, however, researchers and developmental specialists have displayed an increasing appreciation of the individual priorities and needs of parents and a heightened sense of the important role that parents play following hospital discharge in guiding the developmental progress and physical well-being of their high risk newborns.
>
> New questions about what parents need and feel when their babies are in intensive care are a natural extension of these trends. . . . New intervention

programs directed toward involving parents while infants are in the hospital, preparing for discharge, and assisting families with the transition to home are another result. Although the specifics of planning with and for parents vary from model to model, there are common themes in research on intervention in the hospital and during the transition to home care. Five themes have emerged. First, planning with and for parents toward discharge should start in the hospital and be organized around the individual needs and priorities of a continuum of families.

Second, working with parents before and after discharge should incorporate teaching about meeting basic infant needs (such as feeding or care during oxygen therapy), as well as developmental concerns.

Third, careful follow-up is an essential component of the discharge process in order to build in continuity and support from hospital to home. In an attempt to augment traditional medical care and established approaches to monitoring infant development and teaching parenting skills, post-discharge services have been offered with a variety of follow-up services including traditional medical models, transitional units, technological assistance models, and public health and community health efforts.

Fourth, family-focused (centered) care during the transition from hospital to home ought to address changes in lifestyle commonly reported by parents of preterm and high-risk infants. Among these very real problems are excessive fatigue, loss of sleep, lack of personal time, increased personal responsibilities, and concerns over out-of-control economic burdens. Some issues may be resolved by giving families information about local and state resources, while others will require offering services to support parents in carrying out their substantial commitments in a more personally compatible and self-fulfilling way.

Fifth, linking families to anticipated educational intervention programs prior to hospital discharge is increasingly recognized as best practice ... in building on the tenet of continuity of care.

In all of these aspects of intervention, active involvement of parents in the decision-making process, before and after discharge, is a critical dimension and goal in helping a family to finally gain control after the shock and upheaval of experiencing a premature delivery. There is, in fact, a fine line between offering genuinely needed support and gradually assisting and letting go of families to make the decisions that are rightfully theirs. Ultimately, these objectives will be most readily accomplished by emphasizing the strengths and capacities of families, as opposed to reinforcing their perception of what they cannot do. While there are many ways in which the preterm infant and family experiences differ from those associated with the full-term delivery, a basic sense of parents managing their own lives in the process is essential to the well-being and integrity of all concerned. (1994, pp. 243–245)

REFERENCES

Affonso, D.D., Hurst, I., Mayberry, L.J., Haller, L., Yost, K., & Lynch, M.E. (1992). Stressors reported by mothers of hospitalized premature infants. *Neonatal Network, 11*(6), 63–70.

Akers, A.L., Boyce, G.C., Mabey, V., & Boyce, L. (2007). InReach: Connecting NICU infants and their parents with community early intervention services. *Zero to Three, 27*, 43–47.

Allen, E., Manuel, J., Legault, C., Naughton, P.C., & O'Shea, T.H. (2004). Perception of child vulnerability among mothers of former premature infants. *American Academy of Pediatrics, 113*, 267–274.

Als, H. (1998). Developmental care in the newborn intensive care unit. *Current Opinion in Pediatrics, 10*(2), 138–142.

Als, H., Gilkerson, L., Duffy, F.H., McAnulty, G.B., Buehler, D.M., Vandenberg, K., et al. (2003). A three-center, randomized, controlled trial of individualized developmental care for very low birth weight preterm infants: Medical, neurodevelopmental, parenting, and caregiving effects. *Journal of Developmental and Behavioral Pediatrics, 24*(6), 399–409.

Atkins-Burnett, S., & Allen-Meares, P. (2000). Infants and toddlers with disabilities: Relationship-based approaches. *Social Work, 45*(4), 371–379.

Ballweg, D.D. (2001). Implementing developmentally supportive family-centered care in the newborn intensive care unit as a quality improvement initiative. *Journal of Perinatal & Neonatal Nursing, 15*(3), 58–73.

Berkowitz, G., Halfon, N., & Klee, L. (1992). Improving access to healthcare: Case management for vulnerable children. *Social Work Health Care, 17*(1), 101–123.

Bernstein, V.J., Percansky, C., & Wechsler, N. (1996). Strengthening families through strengthening relationships: The ounce of prevention fund developmental training and support program. In M.C. Roberts (Ed.), *Model programs in child and family mental health* (pp. 109–134). Mahwah, NJ: Lawrence Erlbaum Associates.

Bialoskurski, M.M., Cox, C.L., & Wiggins, R.D. (2002). The relationship between maternal needs and priorities in a neonatal intensive care environment. *Journal of Advanced Nursing, 37*, 62–69.

Blackman, J. (1992). *Warning signals: Basic criteria for tracking at-risk infants and toddlers* [Brochure]. Washington, DC: ZERO TO THREE.

Board, R., & Ryan-Wenger, N. (2003). Stressors and stress symptoms of mothers with children in the PICU. *Journal of Pediatric Nursing, 18*(3), 195–202.

Brazelton, T.B. (1992). *Touchpoints: Your child's emotional and behavioral development.* New York: Perseus Publishing.

Browne, J.V., Langlois, A., Ross, E.S., & Smith-Sharp, S. (2001). BEGINNINGS: An interim individualized family service plan for use in the intensive care nursery. *Infants and Young Children, 14*(2), 19–32.

Bruder, M. (2000). Family-centered early intervention: Clarifying our values for the new millennium. *Topics in Early Childhood Special Education, 20*(2), 105–115

Bruns, D.A., & Klein, S. (2005). An evaluation of family-centered care in a level III NICU. *Infants and Young Children, 18*(3), 222–233.

Carter, J.D., Mulder, R.T., Bartram, A.F., & Darlow, B.A. (2005). Infants in a neonatal intensive care unit: Parental response. *Archives of Disease in Childhood. Fetal and Neonatal Edition, 90,* f109–f113.

Chandler, B.E., & Yun, A.R. (2006). Defining occupational therapy's role in infant mental health. *Special Interest Section Quarterly: School System, 13*(4), 1–4.

De Ocampo, A.C., Macias, M.M., Saylor, C.F., & Katikaneni, L.D. (2003). Caretaker perception of child vulnerability predicts behavior problems in NICU graduates. *Child Psychiatry and Human Development, 34*(2), 83–96.

Dudek-Shriber, L. (2004). Parent stress in the neonatal intensive care unit and the influence of parent and infant characteristics. *American Journal of Occupational Therapy, 58,* 509–520.

Dunlap, G., Newton, J.S., Fox, L., Benito, N., & Vaughn, B. (2001). Family involvement in functional assessment and positive behavior support. *Focus on Autism and Other Developmental Disabilities, 16*(4), 215–222.

Dunst, C.J., Boyd, K., Trivette, C.M., & Hamby, D. (2002). Family-oriented program models and professional helpgiving practice. *Family Relations, 51*(3), 221–230.

Dunst, C.J., Johanson, C., Trivette, C.M., & Hamby, D. (1991). Family-oriented early intervention policies and practices: Family-centered or not? *Exceptional Children, 58*(2), 115–126.

Education of the Handicapped Act Amendments of 1986, PL 99-457, 20 U.S.C. §§ 1400 *et seq.*

Ensher, G.L., & Clark, D.A. (1994). *Newborns at risk: Medical care and psychoeducational intervention* (2nd ed.). Gaithersburg, MD: Aspen Publishers.

Esdaile, S.A., & Greenwood, K.M. (2003). A comparison of mothers' and fathers' experience of parenting stress and attributions for parent-child interaction outcomes. *Occupational Therapy International, 10*(2), 115–126.

Franck, L.S., Cox, S., Allen, A., & Winter, I. (2005). Measuring neonatal intensive care unit-related parental stress. *Journal of Advanced Nursing, 49*(6), 608–615.

Gale, G., Franck, L.S., Kools, S., & Lynch, M. (2004). Parents' perceptions of their infant's pain experience in the NICU. *International Journal of Nursing Studies, 41,* 51–58.

Gavidia-Payne, S., & Stoneman, Z. (1997). Family predictors of maternal and paternal involvement in programs for young children with disabilities. *Child Development, 68*(4), 701–717.

Glascoe, F., & Shapiro, H. (2007). *Introduction to developmental and behavioral screening.* Retrieved on September 4, 2007, from http://www.dbpeds.org/articals/detail.cfm?id=5

Gleason, T.R., & Evans, M.E. (2004). Perceived vulnerability: A comparison of parents and children. *Journal of Child Health Care, 8*(4), 279–287.

Gorski, P. (1999). Is community important for health?: Examining the biopsychosocial interface. *Journal of Perinatology, 19*(6), S2–S5.

Graham, M.A., White, B.A., Clarke, C.G., & Adams, S. (2001). Infusing infant mental health practices into front-line caregiving. *Infants and Young Children, 14,* 14–23.

Graven, S.N., Bowen, F.W., Brooten, D., Eaton, A., Graven, M.N., Hack, M., et al. (1992). The high-risk, infant environment: Part 2. The role of caregiving and the social environment. *Journal of Perinatology, 12*(3), 267–275.

Harrison, H. (1993a). *The premature baby book.* New York: St. Martins Press.

Harrison, H. (1993b). The principles for family-centered neonatal care. *Pediatrics, 92,* 643–650.

Heimer, C. (1999). Competing institutions: Law, medicine, and family in neonatal intensive care. *Law & Society Review, 33,* 17–66.

Hurst, I. (2001). Vigilant watching over: Mothers' actions to safeguard their premature babies in the newborn intensive care nursery. *Journal of Perinatal and Neonatal Nursing, 15*(3), 39–57.

Individuals with Disabilities Education Act Amendments (IDEA) of 1997, PL 105-17, 20 U.S.C. §§ 1400 *et seq.*

Individuals with Disabilities Education Improvement Act (IDEA) of 2004, PL 108-446, 20 U.S.C. §§ 1400 *et seq.*

Johnson, B.H., Abraham, M.R., & Parrish, R.N. (2004). Designing the neonatal intensive care unit for optimal family involvement. *Clinics in Perinatology, 31,* 353–382.

Jorgensen, K.M. (1997). *Developmental care of the preterm infant: A concise overview* (2nd ed.). Children's Medical Ventures, Developmental Care Division.

KidsGrowth Professional. (2001). *Issue: Structure + Process = Outcomes: How quality is measured.* Retrieved on July 20, 2001, from http://www.kidsgrowthmarketplace.com

Law, M. (1998). *Family-centered assessment and intervention in pediatric rehabilitation.* Binghamton, NY: Haworth Press.

Lawlor, M.C., & Mattingly, C.F. (1998). The complexities embedded in family-centered care. *American Journal of Occupational Therapy, 52,* 259–267.

Leske, J.S. (1991). Internal psychometric properties of Critical Care Family Needs Inventory. *Heart & Lungs, 20*(3), 236–244.

McCollum, J.A. (2002). Influencing the development of young children with disabilities: Current themes in early intervention. *Children and Adolescent Mental Health, 7,* 4–9.

McCormick, M.C., Brooks-Gunn, J., Workman-Daniels, K., & Peckham, G.J. (1993). Maternal rating of child health at school age: Does the vulnerable child syndrome persist? *Pediatrics, 92*(3), 380–388.

McGrath, J.M. (2000). Developmentally supportive caregiving and technology in the NICU: Isolation or merger of intervention strategies? *Journal of Perinatal & Neonatal Nursing, 14*(3), 78–92.

McGrath, J.M. (2001). Building relationships with families in the NICU: Exploring the guarded alliance. *Journal of Perinatal & Neonatal Nursing, 15*(3), 74–83.

Miles, M.S., Funk, S.G., & Carlson, J. (1993). Parental stressor scale: Neonatal intensive care unit. *Nursing Research, 42*(3), 148–152.

Nakamura, W.M., Stewart, K.B., & Tatarka, M.E. (2000). Assessing father-infant interactions using the NCAST teaching scale: A pilot study. *American Journal of Occupational Therapy, 54,* 44–51.

Nusbaum. M.R., & Helton, M.R. (2002). A birth crises. *Family Medicine, 34*(6), 423–425.

O'Hanlon, E., & Griffin, A.T. (2004). Parent advocacy: Two approaches to change, one goal. *Zero to Three, 25,* 27–31.

Olson, J., Edwards, M., & Hunter, J.A. (1987). The physician's role in delivering sensitive information to families with handicapped infants. *Clinical Pediatrics, 26*(5), 231–234.

Orfali, K., & Gordon, E.J. (2004). Autonomy gone awry: A cross-cultural study of parents' experiences in neonatal intensive care units. *Theoretical Medicine, 25,* 329–365.

Perehudoff, B. (1990). Parents' perceptions of environmental stressors in the special care nursery. *Neonatal Network, 9*(2), 39–44.

Ramp, A. (1999). How to tell parents their child has a disability. *CEC Today, 6.*

Reinson, C. (2002, August). Parent perceptions and the assessment of developmental vulnerability. *Dissertation Abstracts International, 63/09,* 3156.

Reinson, C., Lieberman, M., Hurchick, G., Clark, K., & Plati, J. (2004, April). *Demographic characteristics of families that participate in a developmental surveillance program.* Poster session presented at the annual American Occupational Therapy Association (AOTA) Conference, Minneapolis.

Roudebush, J.R., Kaufman, J., Johnson, B.H., Abraham, M.R., & Clayton, S.P. (2006). Patient- and family-centered perinatal care: Partnerships with child-bearing women and families. *The Journal of Perinatal and Neonatal Nursing, 20*(3), 201–209.

Schultz-Krohn, W., & Cara, E. (2000). Occupational therapy in early intervention: Applying concepts from infant mental health. *American Journal of Occupational Therapy, 54*(5), 550–554.

Sheikh, L., O'Brien, M., & McCluskey-Fawcett, K. (1993). Parent preparation for the NICU-to-home transition: Staff and parent perceptions. *Child Health Care 22*(3), 701–712.

Simmerman, S., & Blacher, J. (2001). Fathers' and mothers' perception of father involvement in families with young children with a disability. *Journal of Intellectual & Developmental Disability, 26*(4), 325–338.

Spear, M., Leef, K., Epps, S., & Locke, R. (2002). Family reactions during infants' hospitalization in the neonatal intensive care unit. *American Journal of Perinatology, 19*(4), 205–213.

Spoth, R., Kavanagh, K., & Dishion, T. (2002). Family-centered preventive intervention science: Toward benefits to larger populations of children, youth, and families. *Prevention Science, 3*(3), 145–152.

Stein, M.T. (1999, July). *Professionals helping parents.* Paper presented at the meeting of The Alexis Foundation for Premature Infants and Children & Preemie-L, Directions For the 21st Century: Bridging the Gap between Parents and Professionals Conference.

Sydor-Greenberg, N., & Dokken, D. (2000). Coping and caring in different ways: Understanding and meaningful involvement. *Pediatric Nursing, 26*(2), 185–191.

Symington, A., & Pinelli, J. (2001). Developmental care for promoting development and preventing morbidity in preterm infants (*Cochrane Review*). In *The Cochrane Library, 2, 2001.* Oxford, England: Update Software.

Thomasgard, M. (1998). Parental perceptions of child vulnerability, overprotection, and parental psychological characteristics. *Child Psychiatry and Human Development, 28*(4), 223–240.

Wallin, C.M. (2003). Is there any such thing as a low-risk preemie? *Zero to Three, 24*(3), 26–30.

Ward, K. (2001). Perceived needs of parents of critically ill infants in a neonatal intensive care unit (NICU). *Pediatric Nursing, 27*(3), 281–286.

Woodside, J., Rosenbaum, P., King, S., & King, G.

(2001). Family-centered service: Developing and validating a self-assessment tool for pediatric service providers. *Children's Health Care, 30*(3), 237–252.

Young, D., & Roopnarine, J. (1994). Father's childcare involvement with children with and without disabilities. *Topics in Early Childhood Special Education, 14*(4), 488.

CHAPTER 21

Home and School Programs for Infants and Young Children with Special Needs

Deborah A. Bryden and Gail L. Ensher

At the conclusion of this chapter, the reader will

- *Understand the essentials of an individualized family service plan (IFSP) and an individualized education program (IEP) in offering services for young children and their families*

- *Understand the mandate for multidisciplinary teamwork on behalf of young children and their families*

- *Understand some of the essentials of best practices in developing educational programs for young children in early intervention, preschool, kindergarten, and the early primary grades*

- *Understand some of the unresolved issues and essentials of best practice in helping young children make the transition from early intervention to pre-K to kindergarten and into the early primary grades*

The Individuals with Disabilities Education Improvement Act (IDEA) of 2004 (PL 108-446) is the culmination of years of legislation to ensure services for all children, including a free appropriate public education (FAPE). Overall, IDEA is organized into four parts. Part A focuses on general provisions. Part B addresses assistance for the education of all children with disabilities (school age and preschool programs; ages 3–21 years). Part C deals specifically with infants and toddlers with disabilities (ages birth–2 years). Part D describes national activities for improving the education of children with disabilities (i.e., support programs).

Since 1975, when Congress approved mandatory special education legislation known as the Education for All Handicapped Children Act (PL 94-142), several major amendments have been passed that specify, clarify, and add new dimensions to the legislation. In particular and more relevant to the education of young children, in 1986 Congress passed a major set of amendments to the Education for All Handicapped Children Act, extending all rights and protections of the law to preschoolers with disabilities. The provisions of this set of amendments, which became the Education of the Handicapped Act Amendments of 1986 (PL 99-457), required states to provide a free, appropriate public education to children with disabilities ages 3 through 5 years by the school year 1990–1991. In addition, these amendments provided grants to states so they could offer interdisciplinary educational services both to infants and toddlers with disabilities and to their families from birth through the age of 2 years (Salvia, Ysseldyke, & Bolt, 2007).

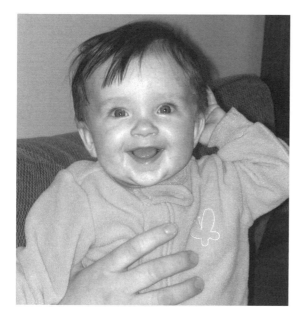

Mandates of Statewide and Federal Legislation

The 2004 reauthorization of IDEA makes specific reference to the following with respect to provisions for young children and their families:

- "Appropriately identify infants and toddlers with disabilities that are in need of services" (IDEA Infant & Toddler Coordination Association, 2004, p. 3).

- "[Ensure] appropriate early intervention services based on scientifically based research, to the extent practicable, are available to all infants and toddlers with disabilities and their families . . ." (IDEA Infant & Toddler Coordination Association, 2004, p. 3).

- [Enact] a public awareness program focusing on early identification of infants and toddlers with disabilities, including the preparation and dissemination by the lead agency . . . to all primary referral sources, especially hospitals and physicians . . . to be given to parents, especially to inform parents with premature infants, or infants with other physical risk factors associated with learning or developmental complications, on the availability of early intervention services . . ." (IDEA Infant & Toddler Coordination Association, 2004, p. 3).

- Provide a new state birth to 6 option, including the possibility of serving age 3 until elementary school admission. The IFSP should include "a description of the appropriate transition services for the infant and toddler" (p. 6).

- Finally, the legislation made several changes to the content of the IFSP including "a statement of the measurable results or outcomes expected to be achieved for the infant or toddler and the family including pre-literacy and language skills, as developmentally appropriate for the child, and the criteria, procedures, and timelines used to determine the degree to which progress toward achieving the results or outcomes is being made and whether modifications or revisions of the results or outcomes or services are necessary" (IDEA Infant & Toddler Coordination Association, 2004, p. 6).

Early Intervention in the State of New York

Each state varies in terms of compliance and funding sources for early intervention. In New York State, the legislature created the Early Intervention Program in Article 25 of the Public Health Law in 1992. Some of the responsibilities of the Department of Health, as a lead agency (New York State Department of Health [NYSDOH], 2005a, p. 1), include

- Administering and monitoring the statewide early intervention program
- Providing training and technical assistance to everyone involved in the early intervention program
- Keeping an updated statewide central directory of early intervention services, resources, and experts
- Implementing a system of payments for early intervention services
- Safeguarding parent rights under the early intervention program

Establishing Eligibility

The following sections are a review of the steps that occur in the early intervention (EI) program in New York State (Westchester Institute for Human Development, 2005).

Referral   Parents who have concerns about their child's development make contact with their county department of health. An EI service coordinator is immediately assigned to the family. Their role initially is to visit the family and obtain a social history. This includes medical and developmental background information as well as parent concerns.

Evaluation   Evaluation is the next step in the process, and this includes a core assessment of five developmental areas. These include

1. Cognitive development, which is defined as attention to the environment that is essential for learning, learning rate and style, memory, early learning milestones, and play skills

2. Communication, which encompasses skills that prepare for later speech, including feeding skills, cooing, babbling, and jargoning (nonsense syllables that have the intonation of adult speech); important language milestones, such as first words, putting words together, and coordinating gesture and words to communicate; skills in terms of how a child forms and combines words

3. Social-emotional development that is defined as the ways in which the child relates to others; attention and concentration; self-soothing and self-regulation skills; how the child experiences and expresses thoughts and feelings; how well the child can tolerate frustration and ask for help so as to get along with others

4. Self-help and/or adaptive skills that encompass early self-care skills that one might ex-

pect at different ages, including the child's ability to signal hunger in early infancy to dressing oneself in the preschool years

5. Physical and/or motor skills that include health and vitality, and fine and gross motor skills (movements of the small and large muscles, respectively)

Eligibility for EI services requires that a child have one of the following:

*   A 12-month delay in one developmental area

*   A 33% delay in one area

*   A 25% delay in two of the five areas

Evaluation team members generally consist of a psychologist, a special education teacher, a speech language therapist, and an occupational or physical therapist (if there are motor concerns). All results are discussed with parents by the team and Early Intervention service coordinator. The evaluation report includes pertinent background information, medical and developmental history information, family concerns, observations, assessment results, and clinical recommendations.

Developing an Individualized Family Service Plan

One of the cornerstone dimensions of both federal and state legislation that focuses on infants and toddlers is the full partnership and involvement of families in all aspects of the planning and implementation processes. Thus, if a child is found to be eligible for services, an IFSP is developed. It is important to note that regulations require that the IFSP meeting be held within 45 days of the initial referral (with the exception of

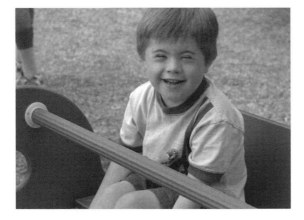

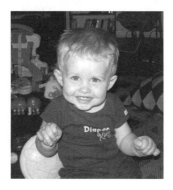

extenuating circumstances). Participants in this initial meeting should include the parent(s), the evaluator(s), the early intervention official (EIO), the service coordinator, and any other members the parent(s) would like present. An interpreter is required for families whose dominant language is not English. Parents participate directly in the written plan for their child.

The specified plan subsequently is reviewed at least every 6 months (or earlier by parent request). Monitoring of all service providers, evaluators, and service coordinators is required by the county health department. County agencies are state monitored. Periodic site visits take place to assess IFSP certifications and overall compliance with regulations. An essential requirement is that parents must be fully informed of all procedures at all times (in the dominant language). There are procedural safeguards in the regulations that are specific to notice, confidentiality, due process, mediation, and impartial hearings.

Families Learning About Disability and Their Common Questions

When families first learn that their infant or child has a disability, it is inevitably a difficult event.

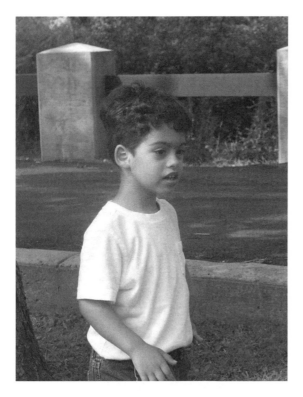

Dependent on the nature and severity of the problem, people deal with information and situations very differently. There are, however, some questions that are common across families, and these might include some of the following (South Carolina Department of Disabilities and Special Needs [SCDDSN], 2006, p. 5):

- What caused my child's disability?
- Did I do anything to cause my child's disability?
- What did I do to deserve this?
- How could God allow this to happen?
- What will my child be able to do?
- Will my child need support forever?
- Who will take care of my child when I am gone?
- How will my child's disability affect my marriage?
- How will my spouse, my other children, my extended family, my friends, accept this child? Will they love my child?
- Will I be able to provide for my child's needs?
- Will I be a good parent?
- Can I love this child?
- Will my child outgrow those special needs?

These questions are ones that parents may voice directly to the provider. Not infrequently, these questions extend beyond the scope of teacher and/or therapist roles into areas of expertise that require counseling and support staff. Also, individual reactions may be very different from one home to the next. Thus, the provider's role requires a great deal of flexibility, open-mindedness, excellent listening, and communication skills.

Knowledge of various emotions that can occur initially (and may be ongoing) is critical. The following are some of the typical reactions that may be a result (SCDDSN, 2006, p. 6):

- Denial: "This cannot be happening to me, to my child, to our family."
- Anger: Aggression toward the child, personnel, or family members.
- Fear: Suspicion of the unknown and future.
- Guilt: Concern about what caused the problem
- Confusion: Not fully understanding new terminology or what is happening. Confusion results in an inability to make decisions and mental overload.
- Powerlessness: Inability to change what is happening.
- Disappointment: Imperfection poses a threat to their ego and values.
- Rejection: Rejection directed at the child, person or family.

As these feelings are shared openly with providers, it is critical that providers not falsely soften or minimize the situation. It is important to be both sensitive and realistic. Providing information about local support groups, respite agencies, and perhaps the names and numbers of other families may be helpful.

At times, issues regarding a young child may not be apparent to the caregiver. It then becomes a challenge to the child care provider to address situations in a professional, productive manner. Parents may be appreciative and open-minded, but at the same time hesitant, distant, and distressed.

Here are some things to consider, when discussing difficult issues with families (Child Care Information Services—Northeast, 2006, p. 1):

- Address issues when they first develop. Putting off a conversation usually makes it harder to bring up later. Do not wait until parent conferences to discuss serious problems.
- Set up a time to talk in a private place, where you will not be overheard or interrupted.
- Think about the things that you want to say and how you want to present information.
- Be specific about what the issues are; give concrete examples of things you have observed or have documented.
- Listen to the parent's observations and explanations. Ask questions so that you can understand the situation and the parent's point of view.
- End the conversation on a positive, solution-finding note. Make a plan for the next steps to be taken.
- Confidentiality is imperative; issues discussed with parents must be held in confidence.

Pediatricians also play a role in the early intervention process, both with referral and ongoing support. Therefore, it is crucial that pediatricians are familiar with the rules and laws of early intervention in order to help parents (American Academy of Pediatrics [AAP], 2006). If a parent suspects concerns, based on the skills of previous children, it is important to pursue assessment, even if the pediatrician disagrees.

Working Together

Service provision for young children may occur in home, at the child care site, or perhaps a combination of both. Ideally, providers need oppor-

tunities to work with anyone who has direct contact with the children. Regardless of the setting, individuals need respect and positive support for the work they are doing. Understanding the family dynamics is critical to the child's success. Because many families now involve single parents who need to work or two parents who both need to work, scheduling may require some evening or weekend hours (Clifford & National Training Institute for Child Care Health Consultants Staff, 2006).

Per the National Center for Family-Centered Care (1990), individual family strengths and needs drive service delivery, and the following dimensions should be incorporated into the process of building relationships:

- Recognize that family is constant in a person's life, while service systems fluctuate.
- Facilitate family/professional collaboration at all levels of services.
- Honor racial, ethnic, cultural, and socioeconomic diversity of families.
- Recognize individual family strengths and respect diverse methods of coping.
- Share complete and unbiased information with families on a continuing basis and in a supportive manner.
- Encourage family-to-family support and networking.
- Recognize and meet developmental needs of infants, children, adolescents and adults, and their families, into service systems.
- Create policies and programs that offer families emotional and financial support.
- Offer accessible, flexible, culturally competent, and responsive services.

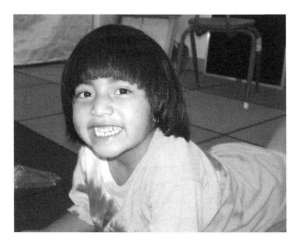

Despite the multiple positive considerations of working in homes, there is, of course, potential for conflict. Personality conflicts frequently fall into three basic categories: perception, emotions, and communication (SCDDSN, 2006). In-home providers require special qualities, such as flexibility, good communication skills, and perhaps an ability to change one's style entirely, depending on the situation. There also are some drawbacks and limitations to home service, based on a survey from the Texas Interagency Council for Early Childhood Intervention (Campbell, 1999, pp. 2–4); these include travel time, cancellations, safety issues, and, at times, a lack of appropriate equipment and materials.

The SCDDSN emphasized several points for developing partnerships (2006, pp. 14–15), including this pertinent point to bear in mind: "While families of people with disabilities may at times be families in crisis, they are not disabled families. They have capacities for creative problem-solving and coping that professionals must respect, promote, and encourage."

In addition, remember the following:

- For there to be an effective partnership between individuals, families, and professionals, there must be mutual respect, joint decision-making, sharing of feelings, flexibility, and honesty in dealing with each other.

- Meet the needs of the individual and/or family at their level and at their pace. Respect the family's dignity and privacy. (We are visitors in their homes.)

- Be knowledgeable about resources available to the individual and the family.

- Be willing to admit that you do not have all the answers and be willing to seek information and assistance from others.

- Connect individuals and families to others with similar experiences.

- Do not keep individuals or families waiting.

- If you do not agree with an individual or family: 1) focus on the individual's best interest, 2) emphasize what's right rather than who's right, and 3) begin with areas of agreement and work from there.

- If you are faced with a situation or complaint you cannot handle, speak with other team members.

Moreover, remember

All of us have dreams, visions and anticipations for the future. Like everyone else, people with disabilities and their families have great expectations. Like everyone else, they too need help to be able to have their expectations come true. Professionals and other people without disabilities also need to have great expectations for people with disabilities. Great expectations include feeling control over one's life, finding meaning in one's life, feeling appreciated for one's own value. (Beach Center on Families and Disability, 1990)

Arstein-Kerslake and colleagues (1999, p. 38) also provided pertinent thoughts that often reflect attitudes of parents toward the professionals in the parent–professional partnership.

Transitions to New Settings and New Programs

An important service component is helping young children make transitions. The following sections discuss this process at various stages.

Moving from Early Intervention to Preschool

Parents, the early intervention service coordinator, and the child's providers all play a significant role in the transition process from EI to the preschool process. According to the New York State Department of Health (NYSDOH), the following factors need to be considered during this process (2005b, p. 9):

- Review the progress made by the child and family, and consider whether any services may be needed when the child exits the Early Intervention program.
- Determine whether a referral is appropriate for Preschool Special Education programs and services.
- Determine whether the child and family may need services from other programs under the auspices of the NYSDOH, or services administered by other state or local agencies. . . . .

- Ensure that a transition plan is in place within required timelines to maintain continuity of services, as appropriate, for the child and family.
- Identify community resources needed by and available to assist the child and family.

Together, caregivers and providers make a decision as to whether to refer a child for services at the preschool level. In the process, it is important to keep in mind that the New York State Education Department is the oversight agency, that the respective school district must maintain a register of children in early intervention who are potentially eligible for the Committee on Preschool Special Education (CPSE), that the CPSE reviews referrals made by the EI team to determine child eligibility, and, finally, that the CPSE develops an IEP if a child is determined to be eligible for further services (Songer & Menapace, 2007b).

Parent–Provider Partnerships

Parents hold important visions for their children as they move from the toddler stage to preschooler. Both families and professionals may want to work together and write their expectations down for later review. The following from the Beach Center on Families and Disability (1990) is one example:

Parent Vision for Their Children

- We want our children to be happy.
- We want our children to progress developmentally.
- We want our children to be safe and free from ridicule.
- We want our children to have appropriate social skills.
- We want our children to have friends who love them for who they are.
- We want our children to be invited to birthday parties.
- We want our children to feel loved and accepted by our community.
- We want our children to reach their greatest potential.
- We want our children to be involved in fun after-school activities with neighborhood friends.
- We want our children to have the same opportunities that their same-age peers and siblings have.

Using the New York State system as an example, there are several options available for preschoolers that include Head Start centers, regular preschool programs, child care centers, and special class integrated setting (SCIS) options for children with a continued need for intensive teacher and services provisions. It is critical that parents visit various program options as early as possible (even before the multidisciplinary transition evaluation). Service coordinators and parents also should contact the chairperson on preschool special education in the district where they reside to learn about the process and available options. Once the transition evaluation is completed, a CPSE is held to review the results and determine the most appropriate programming. Parents who have toured various programs can voice their interest(s) at this point.

Per new New York state and federal guidelines, a transition conference needs to be held to determine whether a child should be referred to preschool special education programs and services and to review program options that are available, if a child is found to be eligible (Songer & Menapace, 2007b). The transition conference must be held at least 90 days before a child is first eligible for preschool services. Subsequently, in order to proceed, parents must provide consent to the committee on special education for evaluation of the child, including review of existing information and assessments and new evaluations, as deemed necessary. Ideally, as part of the pro-

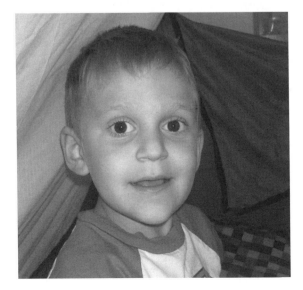

cess, the service provider(s) should tour various preschool options with parents to assist in the decision-making process.

Transitions to new settings and new programs are difficult for all involved. Often, parents feel a very close bond with those providing services at the time of transition. After all, the initial providers helped them through the first stages of dealing with the diagnosis, if there is one, and its implications for future years. According to Arstein-Kerslake and colleagues (1999), a celebration eases the transition process. A get-together to acknowledge everyone's work, accomplishments, and close friendships helps to close one door and open the next.

Eligibility for Committee on Preschool Special Education

Although there are some similarities between early intervention and preschool services, there also are some significant differences. The transition from a few to several hours of programming per week to a half day, center-based program of 12–15 hours per week, for some, brings rewarding and welcoming change. The special education teacher is thus able to address cognitive, self-help, social and adaptive development, and attend to carry over of speech, physical, or occupational therapy goals. The parents are not isolated; rather they have a more consistent team approach to meeting their children's needs.

Criteria for eligibility in moving from EI to pre-K are based on the following:

- A 12-month delay in one or more functional areas

- A 33% delay in one functional area

- A 25% delay in at least two functional areas

- At least 2.0 standard deviations below the mean in one functional area, or at least 1.5 standard deviations below the mean in each of two functional areas (defined as adaptive behavior, cognitive development, motor abilities, speech and language development, and social emotional behavior)

Moreover, a child can be deemed eligible by meeting the criteria for a developmental diagno-

sis of autism, deafness, deaf-blindness, hearing impairment, orthopedic impairment, other health impairment, traumatic brain injury, and visual impairment, including blindness (Songer & Menapace, 2007a). Subsequently, eligibility is determined and an IEP is developed. Formal assessment for qualification for preschool services in New York State includes all areas of development (i.e., motor, cognitive, speech and/or language, adaptive, social and/or emotional, and physical). Typically, such evaluations involve a physical examination, an individual psychological assessment, social history, observation in a natural setting (e.g., home, child care site), and other appropriate measures in areas that affect learning and behavior.

Service Options for Preschoolers with a Disability

Preschool children with a disability and their families have several options for receiving services, including home, nursery schools, child care centers, pre-K sites, and special education preschool settings. Services may be provided as

- Related services by one or more of the following professionals, including occupational, physical, or speech therapists and special education itinerant teachers for a specified number of times per week, as determined by the CPSE (Songer & Menapace, 2007b)

- With a special education itinerant teacher (SEIT) who works with the child, the child's family, and/or a regular education teacher to adapt programs to the child's needs (Songer & Menapace, 2007)

- A special class in an integrated setting (SCIS) where a child with special needs is placed in an inclusive program with typically developing children and children with special needs

- A special class of no more than 12 children, all of whom have been identified with special needs (Songer & Menapace, 2007b)

As with services in the early intervention program, parents or families are a central part of the decision-making process and hold rights to raise questions and/or disagree with any aspect of that process. Finally, like the EI plan, services are reviewed on a regular basis to ensure that plans and programs are appropriate to the needs of children and their families.

Moving to Kindergarten and Beyond

As described by a number of scholars who have written about families and individuals with special needs, transitions are one of the most challenging periods or stages during the life cycle that parents face (Entwisle & Alexander, 1998; Fowler, Schwartz, & Atwater, 1991; Kagan, Carroll, Comer, & Scott-Little, 2006; Kraft-Sayre & Pianta, 2000; La Paro, Pianta, & Cox, 2000; Mangione & Speth, 1998; Pianta & Cox, 1999; Pianta & Kraft-Sayre, 2003; Turnbull, Turnbull, Erwin, & Soodak, 2006). Families of children with and without special needs often feel an array of emotions as they send their sons and daughters to kindergarten for the first time, ranging from excitement and enthusiasm to fear and concern about the future. For children with a disability, as they transition from age level to age level, there can be significant issues of continuity between home and school and between school- and service-based programs. Valuable relationships formed in the earliest years, which for many families have become a foundation of security, will change. Regulations and requirements for eligibility from infancy and the toddler years necessarily differ as children advance into kindergarten and the early primary years of school. Whether appropriate or not, families may find that the supports they were offered at the pre-K stages of programming will lessen, often dramatically as their children grow older, and despite the best intent of transition and annual conferences, services may become less connected, minimally aligned, and less collaborative. However, there are positives to balance the sense of uncertainty and the unknown. For example, the comfort zone of known relationships will expand for parents and children, and new friendships will emerge. The challenges of reality hopefully will open wider doors to the development of maturity, problem solving, and new experiences.

Along with the many expected and often unexpected changes and challenges, some tenets remain common to promising, best practices. Most importantly, these relate to the bedrock of strong linkages and communication among home and school, families, and educational staff. Indeed, those who have written extensively about this stage of development for families and children have strongly suggested that the transition to school "sets the tone and direction of a child's school career" (Pianta & Kraft-Sayre, 1999, p. 47). Moreover, Pianta and Cox, concerning what they described as the "changing nature of the transition to school" (1999, p. 363), wrote,

Clearly, a key transition point for children is the transition to formal schooling. Entwisle and Alexander's . . . landmark study stands as a stark reminder of the importance of this transition. In this study, the trajectories of children's school adjustment (among both children at risk and not at risk) were nearly fixed by third grade. The influence of schools in modifying individual differences in children's competencies had declined considerably by third grade. This early school transition period can be thought of as a sensitive period (Bornstein, 1989) for developing the skills, knowledge, and attitudes critical to later school success. As a sensitive period, these years take on unique importance in establishing the developmental "infrastructure" on which later experience will build. Minor adjustments in the trajectory of child adjustment in this period may have disproportionate effects on the direction of the child's school career.

Because a sensitive period is one in which considerable fluidity occurs, both positive and negative consequences can be strongly influenced. Retention, peer problems, difficult relationships with teachers, and problems learning to read are just some of the early "downward" deflections that can easily be translated into increasingly intransigent patterns of failure (e.g., Pianta, Steinberg, & Rollins, 1995; Shepard & Smith, 1989). However, evidence strongly suggests that "upward" deflections of school outcome pathways can also be initiated during the early childhood period and have long-lasting effects (e.g., Lazar, Darlington, Murray, Royce, & Snipper, 1982; Ramey & Campbell, 1991; Schweinhart et al., 1986).

Viewing formal schooling as a context for development and melding developmental with educational research and theory is a conceptual leap that may enhance previous efforts to understand this important period. Such an approach puts the child, family, and school at center stage; leads to the recognition that individual indicators of the child have limited usefulness; and focuses attention on the processes and mechanism accounting for child outcomes that are considered to be desirable. How do early developmental functions emerge in the transition to formal schooling? What are the roles of family, school, and community in the transition process? How is the transition process influenced by the quality of adaptation in earlier transition periods? These are the major questions that such a framework suggests and that a new generation of research must address. (p. 367)

Programs of Promise

Meeting the needs of young children of all abilities, within the context of increasingly diverse homes and complex American schools, will continue to be a challenging goal of the highest priority. How that priority translates into programs of promise will vary from state to state, community to community, school to school, program to program, family to family, and even child to child. This truism we know all too well from the long and rich legacy of early childhood programs that have been developed since the early days of Head Start in the 1960s. The formidable questions that emerge from the history that precedes us are these: What have we learned that will enable us to replicate and enhance programs of promise for all children across the range of abilities? When the early years of the educational process grow into the later primary grades and adolescence, have we left students and their families in a better place that will enable them to realize their fullest potentials and enable them to adapt to an ever-changing world with high stakes and high demands?

Where Have We Been?

The litany of programs in early childhood education is extensive and diverse. The overarching efforts of these programs from infancy to the early primary grades have resided in the common goal of supporting, facilitating, and enhancing the development of young children. To cite just a few, this research has included programs focused on the following:

- Changing the negative trajectories of poverty (Brooks-Gunn, 2003; Bryant & Maxwell, 1997;

Farran, 2005; Halpern, 2000; Loeb, Fuller, Kagan, & Carrol, 2004; Votruba-Drzal, Coley, & Chase-Lansdale, 2004)

- The effects of child care on children with and without disabilities (Belsky et al., 2007; Johnson et al., 2003; Love et al. 2003; National Institute of Child Health and Human Development Early Child Care Research Network, 2003; Paulsell, Nogales, & Cohen, 2003)

- Early intervention with special populations, such as children who were exposed prenatally to drugs and alcohol (Olson & Burgess, 1997; O'Malley & Streissguth, 2003); children who have been neglected and abused (Barnett, 1997); children who were infected with HIV (Cohen, Grosz, Ayoob, & Schoen, 1997); children who were born at early gestational ages (Als, 1997; Blair & Ramey, 1997); children who were born into families with teen parents (Reichman & McLanahan, 2001); and children who have parents with developmental disabilities (Feldman, 1997)

- The effects of early intervention for children with specific disabilities, such as autism, Down syndrome, cerebral palsy, hearing and visual impairments, among others (Calderon & Greenberg, 1997; Dawson & Osterling, 1997; Fewell & Deutscher, 2002; Mahoney & Perales, 2003; Spiker, Hebbeler, & Mallik, 2005; Spiker & Hopmann, 1997)

- Developmental systems, curricula, and strategies for teaching (Als et al., 2003; Dodici, Draper, & Peterson, 2003; Justice & Pullen, 2003; National Association for the Education of Young Children [NAEYC], & the National Council of Teachers of Mathematics [NCTM], 2003; Raver, 2002; Rosenkoetter & Barton, 2002)

- Perceived and evidence-based benefits of the education of mixed groups of children at differing ages, of varying abilities, and in different settings and environments (Cross, Traub, Hutter-Pishgahi, & Shelton, 2004; Garfinkle & Schwartz, 2002; Grubbs & Neimeyer, 1999; Hanson et al., 2001; Lieber et al., 2000; Rafferty, Boettcher, & Griffin, 2001)

- Changes in children and families, given varying intensities and protocols of service and resources (Brorson, 2005; Melnyk et al., 2001)

- Changes in children and families, given the benefit of primary prevention and long-term follow-up (Bailey et al., 2005; Kaplan-Samoff, 2001; McCormick et al., 2006; Palfrey et al., 2005; Ramey et al., 2000)

- Studies of factors that appear to offer young children protection and resilience in the face of adversity (Osofsky & Thompson, 2000; Shonkoff & Phillips, 2000)

Themes of Effective Programs

There are different agendas, different goals, and very different approaches to the rich and myriad efforts in early childhood special education. At the same time, there are at least a few cornerstone qualities or themes that appear to be foundational to effective programs for young children and their families across the life span from birth through the age of 8 years and probably beyond. It is beneficial to summarize the commonalities or threads that, from our perspective, augur well for effective outcomes for both families and their young children.

Effective Programs Recognize that Behavior Is Communication   Whether early intervention is focused on infants in the neonatal intensive care unit (NICU), children who have been abused and neglected, children with autism or sensory processing disorders, multirisk families with substance abuse, or teenage parents, effective programs are mindful that "behavior is communication" (Songer, 2005) and use this tenet as a fundamental principle. Developmentally, we need to meet both children and adults where they are by observing the behaviors that they display, building on their reservoirs of strength, and, likewise, taking into consideration areas of need. In essence, teachers, physicians, therapists, and researchers must listen to and understand the audiences with whom they are working in order to facilitate positive steps toward change. The principle sounds simple; however, it often is challenging to implement in light of diversity, the call to set aside our own perspectives and the

requirement to value the priorities of others. For example, in working with families for whom English is not the primary language or with children who are not using words to express themselves or with preterm infants in intensive care, professionals are compelled to rely on behavioral cues and other ways of reading and interpreting, rather than verbal context.

Effective Programs Are Consistent   We know that early childhood programs can effect positive change for families and children over time. How long and in what ways those gains are maintained are issues that are dependent upon a number of variables, including the extent to which programs and professionals are able to build in consistencies of support, resources, strategies, as well as meeting other needs of children within the context of their families in their ever-changing life cycles. In so doing, families and communities need to be at the forefront of ongoing intervention programs. Early childhood professionals may skillfully employ specific interventions, but these are most powerful and most likely to be sustained when they interface with the daily lives of children and families at home. Accordingly, professionals must build corridors and bridges between programs and existing realities that provide for adaptability in the face of unexpected events, crises, and individual uniqueness. Otherwise, the short-term gains of a given day may be washed out within weeks, months, and most certainly years. This is the plague that has daunted early childhood education since the inception of Head Start.

Effective Programs Are Monitored and Interpreted Along Multiple Dimensions   Evaluation is a given in our work with children and families. Yet, capturing those changes and developments that make a difference in the lives of children and families is an exceedingly demanding task that requires new and innovative perspectives. Much has been written about the assessment of young children and measurement of systematic gains. Historically, these have focused heavily on program content, which is determined on the basis of norm-referenced tests, in large part because these are the variables that

are more easily contained and analyzed. Much harder to address are issues concerning process, the temperament of children, ease in family caregiving, interactions with playmates and siblings, abilities of children to adapt to change and transition, abilities of infants and children to calm themselves, capacities of families to facilitate positive self-esteem in their children, the enjoyment of children in communicating with families and schoolmates, the feelings of young children with positive school achievement, and the salience and impact of informal community supports for families. In the long-term, these are the qualities that often differentiate the skills and abilities of young children and their families to maintain their positive gains as they encounter new situations and new pieces of learning.

In addition to the complexities of capturing the dynamics of differentiating qualities of children, Warfield and Hauser-Cram (2005, pp. 354–355) pointed out the evolving needs of viewing early intervention within an ecological, multiple interacting systems context. Warfield and Hauser-Cram further described the need for a multiple tiered approach as follows:

> First, it uses a broad and inclusive definition of evaluation . . . (Jacobs & Kapuscik, 2000, p. 3). Thus, the purpose of evaluation from the perspective of the multi-tiered approach is to address questions about program processes as well as the program's impact on outcomes.
>
> Second, the multi-tiered approach is a developmental model designed so that the demands for technical expertise increase from tier to tier. This allows those new to program evaluation to develop their skills over time and build evaluation capacity into a program's daily operations. Third, the model emphasizes that no one standard evaluation strategy is appropriate for all programs, services, or interventions.
>
> Individualized evaluation plans need to be developed for each situation in order to maximize the fit between the program's capacity for evaluation and the goals of the evaluation. Thus, a wide range of methodologies should be utilized including qualitative approaches (e.g., focus groups, case studies, observation studies) (Patton, 1987) and mixed method approaches that integrate quantitative and qualitative methods (Caracelli & Greene, 1997; Hauser-Cram, Warfield, Upshur, & Weisner, 2000).
>
> Finally, the multi-tiered approach generates studies that can establish accountability. Evaluations

can document accountability by presenting data on the extent to which the program is identifying and serving those who are entitled to services, providing the range of services it is mandated to provide, and establishing some reasonable match between participant need and service receipt. (2005, pp. 356–357)

Thus, as recent legislation focused on infants and young children has demanded that our parameters be expanded to seeing the child within the context of family, likewise, contemporary programs must widen their boundaries to evaluate their impact and effectiveness in partnership with medical, social, and therapeutic services, as well as the community at large. Such data collected over time and in a broader circle of neighborhoods may help us to answer the important questions of why some children and families seem to be resilient in the face of adversity and others are not.

Effective Programs Build on Fundamental, Developmental Strength   The field of special education traditionally has been steeped in a philosophy of a deficit orientation that tenaciously poses the question of "What is wrong with the child?" Such an approach toward children and their families of looking for trouble rarely leads to effective programming.

Alternatively, an examination of the experiences, people, and programs that have engendered and sustained positive change shows that those are the opportunities that have capitalized and built upon fundamental, developmental strengths within children and families. One case in point is the Jowonio School, an inclusive setting in Syracuse, New York, which has served hundreds of families and young children with a range of abilities since 1970. Nationally and internationally, the school is known, in particular, for its work with toddlers and preschool children with severe autism disorders. Aside from the expert clinical and educational services offered, the program has been recognized repeatedly by families, staff, and teachers-in-training as a uniquely welcoming and nurturing facility that has facilitated and witnessed remarkable growth in the children served. This is in large part because of the conviction that positive change is a potential to be realized in every individual, regardless of apparent limitations.

Effective Programs Facilitate Decision Making in Partnership

Buttressed by the new legislation and amendments of 2004 in early childhood special education, professionals have increasingly acknowledged the centrality and wisdom of making decisions in partnership with families. Realistically, the power and relevance of early intervention resides directly with primary caregivers and the degree to which service providers utilize that strength in carrying out programs. Agendas and priorities of families may vary from the desires, goals, and objectives of professionals. However, services are best implemented when closely aligned with the wishes and understanding of the families of children for whom they are intended.

There are circumstances in the medical arena when the intentions of families (e.g., with a religious base) cannot be honored because of the survival and well-being of the child. In such instances, medical staff must skillfully work with families, with the hope of broadening opposing perspectives into compliance without the addition of legal resources. The balance between family dynamics and professional expertise and helping is always an evolving, delicate balance that must be refined and enhanced.

It is true that families bring very different skills, points of view, resources, and coping styles to relationships. However, within this context, "effective intervention should become part of the family's social support system that empowers and strengthens the family in its caregiving role, instead of merely the provision of a specific educational or therapeutic treatment" (Kelly, Booth-LaForce, & Spieker, 2005, p. 244). Inevitably, this theme or guiding principle for early intervention is closely connected to the following tenet: that professionals and effective programs recognize and validate the reality that families are "the constant" in the lives of their children (Songer, 2008). Simply stated, the voices of caregivers must be heard and acknowledged throughout various scenarios of program implementation. As much as professionals desire to support and offer assistance, they will not be

there in subsequent years. As service providers, all of our efforts must be undergirded with the basic recognition that we need to leave families with stronger, more resilient capacities to carry on their caregiving responsibilities with their children in our absence. Otherwise, we have created a need for dependence that unforgivably leaves them vulnerable and helpless.

Effective Programs Survey and Use Accessible, Community Resources

McWilliam (2005) wrote, "As soon as families are enrolled in early intervention, someone needs to figure out what resources families need in order to accomplish their priorities" (p. 215). Families do not reside or raise children in isolation. They live within the context of communities with resources that may or may not be offered. Families do best when they are connected to others and are able to access friends, services, information, and support, according to their needs. Over time, these needs and resources will change. Those programs that are most effective recognize the fact that they cannot provide everything for a given child and family.

Professional staff in early childhood special education have the responsibility for the delivery of specific services; however, they need to be knowledgeable about resources that are readily accessible for families, such as medical and counseling specialists, quality respite and child care facilities, specialized programs (e.g., WIC), and centers where parents and caregivers can obtain information about particular areas of need (e.g., Medicaid waivers, public health nurses, centers for developmental evaluation, the processes of early intervention). In addition, connecting families with other families in similar circumstances with whom they can interact and share are invaluable resources for parents so that they do not feel alone. Often these informal connections are just as important, and in some instances more vital, than are the program-specific services because they exist where families live and stay long after children have grown out of particular settings. Accordingly, one of the most helpful tools for professionals is a list of 10–12 web sites that they can access for current information on local, state, and federal levels that can be shared with colleagues and families of children for whom they are providing services. (See the list of web sites in the resources appendix at the end of this book.)

Effective Programs Are Adaptable to Settings, Communities, and Individuals   The nature of much of our work is change, and finding that right match for families is crucial if we are to be effective in what we do. This guiding principle for programs interfaces closely with others discussed here in the tapestry of service delivery. That is, we are remiss if we proceed as if one way of doing things fits all. Professionals are called upon daily to adapt to changing cultures, regulations and legislation, family dynamics, patterns of learning among children, resources available within communities, new treatments and interventions within their respective fields of expertise, and a myriad of other variables that are constantly evolving.

Effective Programs Are Centered on Relationships   Whether working with families on primary prevention or children with established special needs, the most effective programs always are centered on relationships. With some families, these connections are short term; with others, they last for 1–2 years or more. In the absence of strong relationships, however, little can be accomplished. In addition, we must be mindful of the lessons communicated in the following poem:

Meet Me Where I Am

Meet me where I am
And have meaningful expectations
Identify and explore what I am passionate about
And use my passions to build
Know what stresses me
and minimize or remove the stressors
Read my behavioral cues
And interpret them as communication
Understand that I have bad days
And acknowledge that it's not just my disability
    talking
Recognize my "all systems go" signals
And support my flight
Know that I am a unique individual
And see this as my greatest asset
Meet me where I am
And support MY dreams!
—Nancy S. Songer (1999)

Conclusion

In the case of most families, we are meeting them at one of the most fragile times in their lives. Families live through the hopes and dreams for their children, and when a part of that is taken away or tarnished, their lives are never the same. Through relationships with caring and helpful individuals, they are able to move on to refurbished hopes and dreams with renewed strength and energy.

This does not mean that the pathways will be easy. This does not mean that the burdens and responsibilities are lifted from their own, rightfully placed shoulders. This does mean, though, that professionals will be honest and straightforward and offer the best advice known at the time. They will support and hold back, as necessary, so that when they must leave, families are able to sustain their own lives and provide the love and caregiving so necessary to realize the potentials of their children.

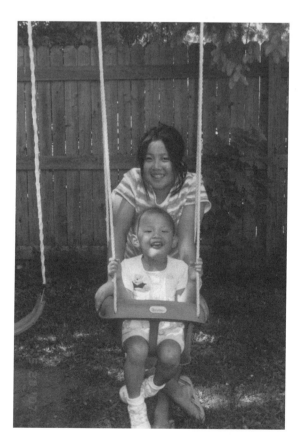

REFERENCES

Als, H. (1997). Earliest intervention for preterm infants in the newborn intensive care unit. In M.J. Guralnick (Ed.), *The effectiveness of early intervention* (pp. 47–76). Baltimore: Paul H. Brookes Publishing Co.

Als, H., Gilkerson, L., Duffy, F.H., McAnulty, G.B., Buehler, D.M., Vandenberg, K., et al. (2003). A three-center, randomized, controlled trial of individualized developmental care for very low birth weight preterm infants: Medical, neurodevelopmental, parenting, and caregiving effects. *Journal of Developmental & Behavioral Pediatrics, 24*(6), 399–409.

American Academy of Pediatrics. (2006). The ABC's of early intervention for pediatricians. Retrieved on October 11, 2007, from http://www.ny2aap.org/nyabcei.html

Arstein-Kerslake, C., Arstein-Kerslake, G., Androvich, T., Androvich, B., McGuire, A., & McGuire, P. (1999). *Handbook on family involvement in early childhood special education programs* (pp. 1–54). Sacramento: California Department of Education.

Bailey, D.B., Jr., Hebbeler, K., Spiker, D., Scarborough, A., Mallik, S., & Nelson, L. (2005). Thirty-six-month outcomes for families of children who have disabilities and participated in early intervention. *Pediatrics, 116*(6), 1346–1353.

Barnett, D. (1997). The effects of early intervention on maltreating parents and their children. In M.J. Guralnick (Ed.), *The effectiveness of early intervention* (pp. 147–170). Baltimore: Paul H. Brookes Publishing Co.

Beach Center on Families and Disability. (1990, Spring). *Families and Disability Newsletter, 2*(1).

Belsky, J., Burchinal, M., McCartney, K., Vandell, D.L., Clarke-Stewart, K.A., & Owen, M.T. (2007). Are there long-term effects of early child care? *Child Development, 78*(2), 661–701.

Blair, C., & Ramey, C.T. (1997). Early intervention for low-birth-weight infants and the path to second-generation research. In M.J. Guralnick (Ed.), *The effectiveness of early intervention* (pp. 77–97). Baltimore: Paul H. Brookes Publishing Co.

Brooks-Gunn, J. (2003). Do you believe in magic?: What we can expect from early childhood intervention programs. *Social Policy Report (a publication of the Society for Research in Child Development), XVII*(1), 3–15.

Brorson, K. (2005). The culture of a home visit in early intervention. *Journal of Early Childhood Research, 3*(1), 51–76.

Bryant, D., & Maxwell, K. (1997). The effectiveness of early intervention for disadvantaged children. In M.J. Guralnick (Ed.), *The effectiveness of early intervention* (pp. 23–46). Baltimore: Paul H. Brookes Publishing Co.

Calderon, R., & Greenberg, M. (1997). The effectiveness of early intervention for deaf children and children with hearing loss. In M.J. Guralnick (Ed.), *The effectiveness of early intervention* (pp. 455–482). Baltimore: Paul H. Brookes Publishing Co.

Campbell, D. (1999, June). Early intervention at home. *ADVANCE,* 1–5.

Child Care Information Services—Northeast. (2006). *Discussing difficult issues.* Retrieved October 25, 2007, from http://www.ccisnephila.com/forproviders/discussingdifficultissues.html

Clifford D., & National Training Institute for Child Care Health Consultants Staff. (2006). Overview of the field of child care version 3. Chapel Hill: National Training Institute for Child Care Health consultant, Department of Maternal and Child Health, University of North Carolina.

Cohen, H.J., Grosz, J., Ayoob, K.T., & Schoen, S. (1997). Early intervention for children with HIV infection. In M.J. Guralnick (Ed.), *The effectiveness of early intervention* (pp. 193–206). Baltimore: Paul H. Brookes Publishing Co.

Cross, A.F., Traub, E.K., Hutter-Pishgahi, L., & Shelton, G. (2004). Elements of successful inclusion for children with significant disabilities. *Topics in Early Childhood Special Education, 24*(3), 169–183.

Dawson, G., & Osterling, J. (1997). Early intervention in autism. In M.J. Guralnick (Ed.), *The effectiveness of early intervention* (pp. 307–326). Baltimore: Paul H. Brookes Publishing Co.

Dodici, B.J., Draper, D.C., & Peterson, C.A. (2003). Early parent–child interactions and early literacy development. *Topics in Early Childhood Special Education, 23*(3), 124–136.

Education for All Handicapped Children Act of 1975, PL 94-142, 20 U.S.C. §§ 1400 *et seq.*

Education of the Handicapped Act Amendments of 1986, PL 99-457, 20 U.S.C. §§ 1400 *et seq.*

Entwisle, D.R., & Alexander, K.L. (1998). Facilitating the transition to first grade: The nature of transition and research on factors affecting it. *The Elementary School Journal, 98*(4), 351–364.

Farran, D.C. (2005). Developing and implementing preventive intervention programs for children at risk: Poverty as a case in point. In M.J. Guralnick (Ed.), *The developmental systems approach to early intervention* (pp. 267–304). Baltimore: Paul H. Brookes Publishing Co.

Feldman, M.A. (1997). The effectiveness of early intervention for children of parents with mental retardation. In M.J. Guralnick (Ed.), *The effectiveness of early intervention* (pp. 171–191). Baltimore: Paul H. Brookes Publishing Co.

Fewell, R.R., & Deutscher, B. (2002). Attention deficit hyperactivity disorder in very young children: Early signs and interventions. *Infants and Young Children, 14*(3), 24–32.

Fowler, S.A., Schwartz, I., & Atwater, J. (1991). Perspectives on the transition from preschool to kindergarten for children with disabilities and their families. *Exceptional Children, 58*(2), 136–145.

Garfinkle, A.N., & Schwartz, I.S. (2002). Peer imitation: Increasing social interactions in children with autism and other developmental disabilities in inclusive preschool classrooms. *Topics in Early Childhood Special Education, 22*(1), 26–29.

Gartner, A., Lipsky, D.K., & Turnbull, A.P. (1991). *Supporting families with a child with a disability: An international outlook.* Baltimore: Paul H. Brookes Publishing Co.

Grubbs, P.R., & Neimeyer, J.A. (1999). Promoting reciprocal social interactions in inclusive classrooms for young children. *Infants and Young Children, 11*(3), 9–18.

Halpern, R. (2000). Early childhood intervention for low-income children and families. In J.P. Shonkoff & S.J. Meisels (Eds.), *Handbook of early childhood intervention* (2nd ed., pp. 361–386). Cambridge, England: Cambridge University Press.

Hanson, M.J., Horn, E., Sandall, S., Beckman, P., Morgan, M., Marquart, J., et al. (2001). After preschool inclusion: Children's educational pathways over the early school years. *Exceptional Children, 68*(1), 65–83.

IDEA Infant & Toddler Coordination Association. (2004, December 1). *Washington update: Summary of changes made to Part C by IDEA reauthorization of 2004.* Retrieved June 5, 2008, from http://www.ideainfanttoddler.org/Wash_Update_Reauth.pdf.

Individuals with Disabilities Education Improvement Act (IDEA) of 2004, PL 108-446, 20 U.S.C. §§ 1400 *et seq.*

Johnson, D.J., Jaeger, E., Randolph, S.M., Cauce, A.M., Ward, J., & National Institute of Child Health and Human Development Early Child Care Research Network. (2003). Studying the effects of early child care experiences on the development of children of color in the United States: Toward a more inclusive research agenda. *Child Development, 74*(5), 1227–1245.

Justice, L.M., & Pullen, P.C. (2003). Promising interventions for promoting emergent literacy skills: Three evidence-based approaches. *Topics in Early Childhood Special Education, 23*(3), 99–113.

Kagan, S.L., Carroll, J., Comer, J.P., & Scott-Little, C. (2006, September). Alignment: A missing link in early childhood transitions? *Young Children,* 26–32.

Kaplan-Samoff, M. (2001). Healthy steps: Delivering developmental services for young children through pediatric care. *Infants and Young Children, 13*(3), 69–76.

Kelly, J.F., Booth-LaForce, C., & Spieker, S.J. (2005). Assessing family characteristics relevant to early intervention. In M.J. Guralnick (Ed.), *The developmental systems approach to early intervention* (pp. 235–265). Baltimore: Paul H. Brookes Publishing Co.

Kraft-Sayre, M.E., & Pianta, R.C. (2000). *Enhancing the transition to kindergarten: Linking children, families, &*

schools. National Center for Early Development & Learning, Kindergarten Transition Studies, University of Virginia.

La Paro, K.M., Pianta, R.C., & Cox, M.J. (2000). Teachers' reported transition practices for children transitioning into kindergarten and first grade. *Exceptional Children, 67*(1), 7–20.

Lieber, J., Hanson, M.J., Beckman, P.J., Odom, S.L., Sandall, S.R., Schwartz, I.S., et al. (2000). Key influences on the initiation and implementation of inclusive preschool programs. *Exceptional Children, 67*(1), 83–98.

Loeb, S., Fuller, B., Kagan, S.L., & Carrol, B. (2004). Child care in poor communities: Early learning effects of type, quality, and stability. *Child Development, 75*(1), 47–65.

Love, J.M., Harrison, L., Sagi-Schwartz, A., van Ijzendoorn, M.H., Ross, C., Ungerer, J.A., et al. (2003). Child care quality matters: How conclusions may vary with context. *Child Development, 74*(4), 1021–1034.

Mahoney, G., & Perales, F. (2003). Using relationship-focused intervention to enhance the social-emotional functioning of young children with autism spectrum disorders. *Topics in Early Childhood Education, 23*(2), 77–89.

Mangione, P.L., & Speth, T. (1998). The transition to elementary school: A framework for creating early childhood continuity through home, school, and community partnerships. *The Elementary School Journal, 98*(4), 381–397.

McCormick, M.C., Brooks-Gunn, J., Buka, S.L., Goldman, J., Yu, J., Salganik, M., et al. (2006). Early intervention in low birth weight premature infants: Results at 18 years of age for the Infant Health and Development Program. *Pediatrics, 117*(3), 771–781.

McWilliam, R.A. (2005). Assessing the resource needs of families in the context of early intervention. In M.J. Guralnick (Ed.), *The developmental systems approach to early intervention* (pp. 215–233). Baltimore: Paul H. Brookes Publishing Co.

Melnyk, B.M., Alpert-Gillis, L., Feinstein, N.F., Fairbanks, E., Schultz-Czarniak, J., Hust, D., et al. (2001). Improving cognitive development of low-birth-weight premature infants with the COPE Program: A pilot study of the benefit of early NICU intervention with mothers. *Research in Nursing & Health, 24,* 373–389.

National Association for the Education of Young Children (NAEYC) & the National Council of Teachers of Mathematics (NCTM). (2003). *Early childhood mathematics: Promoting good beginnings.* Retrieved April 16, 2008, from http://www.naeyc.org/about/positions/psmath.asp

National Center for Family-Centered Care. (1990). *What is family-centered care?* Alexandria: VA: Association for the Care of Children's Health.

National Institute of Child Health and Human Development Early Child Care Research Network.

(2003). Does amount of time spent in child care predict socioemotional adjustment during the transition to kindergarten? *Child Development, 74*(4), 976–1005.

New York State Department of Health. (1997). Title II-A of Article 25 of the Public Health Law, November, 1–54.

New York State Department of Health. (2005a). *Early intervention program–Shaping futures* (pp. 1–2). Albany, NY: Author.

New York State Department of Health. (2005b, February). *The transition of children from the New York State Department of Health Early Intervention Program to the State Education Department Preschool Special Education Program or other early childhood services* (February; pp. 1–98). Albany, NY: Author.

Olson, H.C., & Burgess, D.M. (1997). Early intervention for children prenatally exposed to alcohol and other drugs. In M.J. Guralnick (Ed.), *The effectiveness of early intervention* (pp. 109–145). Baltimore: Paul H. Brookes Publishing Co.

O'Malley, K., & Streissguth, A. (2003). Clinical intervention and support for children aged zero to five years with fetal alcohol spectrum disorder and their parents/caregivers. Retrieved June 15, 2004, from http://www.excellence-earlychildhood.ca/documents/OMalley-StreissguthANGxp_rev.pdf

Osofsky, J.D., & Thompson, M.D. (2000). Adaptive and maladaptive parenting: Perspectives on risk and protective factors. In J.P. Shonkoff & S.J. Meisels (Eds.), *Handbook of early childhood intervention* (2nd ed., pp. 54–75). Cambridge, England: Cambridge University Press.

Palfrey, J.S., Hauser-Cram, P., Bronson, M.B., Warfield, M.E., Sirin, S., & Chan, E. (2005). The Brookline Early Education Project: A 25-year follow-up study of a family-centered early health and development intervention. *Pediatrics, 116*(1), 144–152.

Paulsell, D., Nogales, R., & Cohen, J. (2003). *Quality childcare for infants and toddlers: Case studies of three community strategies. Final Report.* Cambridge, MA: Mathematical Policy Research, Inc. and ZERO TO THREE Policy Center.

Pianta, R.C., & Cox, M.J. (1999). The changing nature of the transition to school: Trends for the next decade. In R.C. Pianta & M.J. Cox (Eds.), *The transition to kindergarten* (pp. 363–379). Baltimore: Paul H. Brookes Publishing Co.

Pianta, R.C., & Kraft-Sayre, M. (1999, May). Parents' observations about their children's transitions to kindergarten. *Young Children,* 47–52.

Pianta, R.C., & Kraft-Sayre, M. (2003). *Successful kindergarten transition: Your guide to connecting children, families, & schools.* Baltimore: Paul H. Brookes Publishing Co.

Rafferty, Y., Boettcher, C., & Griffin, K. (2001). Benefits and risks of reverse inclusion for preschoolers with and without disabilities: Parents' perspectives. *Journal of Early Intervention, 24*(4), 266–286.

Ramey, C.T., Campbell, F.A., Burchinal, M., Skinner, M.L., Gardner, D.M., & Ramey, S.L. (2000). Persistent effects of early childhood education on high-risk children and their mothers. *Applied Developmental Science, 4*(1), 2–14.

Raver, C.C. (2002). Emotions matter: Making the case for the role of young children's emotional development for early school readiness. *Social Policy Report (a publication of the Society for Research in Child Development), XVI*(3), 3–18.

Reichman, N.E., & McLanahan, S.S. (2001). Self-sufficiency programs and parenting interventions: Lessons from New Chance and the Teenage Parent Demonstration. *Social Policy Report (a publication of the Society for Research in Child Development), XV*(2), 3–13.

Rosenkoetter, S., & Barton, L.R. (2002, February/March). Bridges to literacy: Early routines that promote later school success. *Zero to Three,* 33–38.

Salvia, J., Ysseldyke, J.E., & Bolt, S. (2007). *Assessment in special and inclusive education* (10th ed., pp. 49–65). Boston: Houghton Mifflin.

Shonkoff, J.P., & Phillips, D.A. (Eds.). (2000). *From neurons to neighborhoods: The science of early childhood development.* Washington, DC: National Academies Press.

Songer, N.S. (2005). PowerPoint presentation for course *Guiding Challenging Behavior,* School of Education, Syracuse University, Syracuse, NY.

Songer, N.S. (2008). PowerPoint presentation for course *Families of Children with Special Needs,* School of Education, Syracuse University, Syracuse, NY.

Songer, N.S., & Menapace, T. (2007a). *Transition from CPSE to CSE.* Syracuse, NY: The Mid-State Central Early Childhood Direction Center, Syracuse University.

Songer, N.S., & Menapace, T. (2007b). *Transition from EI to CPSE.* Syracuse, NY: The Mid-State Central Early Childhood Direction Center, Syracuse University.

South Carolina Department of Disabilities and Special Needs. (2006). *Working with families who have special needs.* Columbia, SC: Author.

Spiker, D., Hebbeler, K., & Mallik, S. (2005). Developing and implementing early intervention programs for children with established disabilities. In M.J. Guralnick (Ed.), *The developmental systems approach to early intervention* (pp. 305–349). Baltimore: Paul H. Brookes Publishing Co.

Spiker, D., & Hopmann, M.R. (1997). The effectiveness of early intervention for children with Down syndrome. In M.J. Guralnick (Ed.), *The effectiveness of early intervention* (pp. 271–305). Baltimore: Paul H. Brookes Publishing Co.

Turnbull, A., Turnbull, R., Erwin, E., & Soodak, L. (2006). *Families, professionals, and exceptionality: Positive outcomes through partnerships and trust* (5th ed.). Upper Saddle River, NJ: Prentice Hall.

Votruba-Drzal, E., Coley, R.L., & Chase-Lansdale, L. (2004). Child care and low-income children's development: Direct and moderated effects. *Child Development, 75*(1), 296–312.

Warfield, M.E., & Hauser-Cram, P. (2005). *Monitoring and evaluation in early intervention.* Retrieved October 11, 2007, from http://www.wihd.org/learlyi/ earlyi/assess.html

Westchester Institute for Human Development. (2005). *Early childhood services.* Retrieved on October 11, 2007, from http://www.wihd.org/learlyi/ earlyi/assess.html

CHAPTER 22

Putting It All Together

Gail L. Ensher, David A. Clark, and Nancy S. Songer

At the conclusion of this chapter, the reader will

- *Be knowledgeable about some basic tenets relating to best practices in working with professionals across diverse disciplines*

- *Be knowledgeable about some basic tenets relating to best practices in working with diverse populations of families who come to us with different backgrounds, from different cultures, and from different ethnic ancestries*

- *Be knowledgeable about some basic tenets relating to best practices in working with diverse populations of young children (from birth through 8 years of age) who come to us with different challenges, with varying abilities, and from different cultures and ethnic backgrounds*

In writing this last chapter, we do not assume to have the final word on best practices in early childhood special education. It is our intent, however, to share with our readers a few closing thoughts that hopefully will translate into meaningful relationships and work with infants and young children, families, and other professional colleagues. Accordingly, we see the following as some of the key, although unresolved issues that continue to plague research, policies, and program implementation in our respective fields:

- Training programs rightfully focus on the intervention and education of young children; however, they need to address with equal effort adult–adult interactions with families and other professionals.

- Problems faced by families and young children could be greatly reduced, or at least minimized, if our educational and mental health programs had a more primary focus on prevention and education. For example, we must ask why in this country of such technological advances the rate of prematu-

rity continues to exceed that of many developing nations. Prevention is the best form of intervention (Songer, 2008).

- In early childhood (birth through 8 years), our respective fields need to be interactive and intersecting. Yet, often this is not the way in which we proceed to treat, educate, and/or work with young children and their families. Despite our rhetoric about collaboration, too frequently we continue to offer services in isolation that lack coherence and context.

- With so many mothers and fathers in the work force, we are greatly in need of quality, accessible, and affordable child care for young children in this country. We now have the data, as reflected in numerous research studies, that documents the critical importance of the experiences that infants and preschoolers (with and without special needs) have in child care settings. If the interactions are positive and nurturing, children do well; if they are not, children suffer the adverse consequences.

- There still remains a wide disparity in performance, social and/or mental health concerns, and learning opportunities afforded to children and families across different ethnic groups and diverse cultures in the United States. In particular, individuals from underrepresented groups continue to be overrepresented in populations struggling with substance abuse, violence, child abuse and neglect, lack of prenatal care, infectious diseases, and adolescent pregnancies. Welfare has not adequately addressed these ongoing issues. In addition, we know that the single most important marker in this country relative to how well young children do in school remains maternal education.

- The United States reflects a widening economic gap, which continues to have serious implications for families and their young children in accessing and affording routine health care. Clearly, this issue is closely connected to issues of prevention; disparities in opportunities across diverse ethnic groups and cultures; and the medical, social, and/or developmental consequences for young populations.

- Finally, since the new millennium, the world has witnessed some of the worst natural and man-made disasters ever experienced, and they have entered our homes via television and the Internet. On September 11, 2001, people worldwide stood paralyzed by the catastrophic destruction and loss of life as two planes hijacked by terrorists crashed into the World Trade Center buildings in New York City, a third plane was flown into the Pentagon building in Arlington, Virginia, and a fourth plane crashed under attack in the fields of Shanksville, Pennsylvania. Thousands of people lost their lives in the December 26, 2004, Indian Ocean tsunami, which was witnessed worldwide through the media. In the summer of 2005, natural disasters struck again with the ravages of Hurricanes Katrina and Rita that left thousands of people homeless. Finally, the stream of information about the devastation from the war in Iraq has been a daily occurrence in our living rooms since the official declaration of war in Iraq by

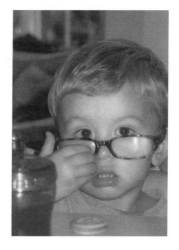

the United States in 2003. In response, parents and professionals everywhere across this country have been left wanting in terms of how to explain such devastation and violence to young children.

What Have We Learned About Pathways to Best Practices?

The following highlights some central guidelines and issues that we hope readers will take with them into their teaching, work with families and young children, writing, and research.

Teaming Among Professionals

In everything that we do as professionals in education, clinical disciplines, and medical fields, it is essential that we work in teams with colleagues and family members. Conflicts and differences of opinion are inevitable; however, how we make decisions, integrate families into teams, resolve conflicts, and resolve differences in priorities that differ from those of families are all concerns that must be addressed.

Thus, translating into best practice, team members at minimum need to

- Be knowledgeable about resources locally, statewide, and on a national level that serve to support work with other professionals, families, and young children

- Know about child development and the ranges of performance appropriate at various ages throughout the early childhood period from birth through 8 years

- Be knowledgeable about their own respective disciplines and be able to offer this information, jargon free, to colleagues and families

- Be familiar with the language of related disciplines of team members who likewise provide services to families and children

- Know their own values and priorities, but be able to set these aside in order to listen to and acknowledge other points of view of professional colleagues and families

- Be knowledgeable about legislation appropriate to early childhood education (e.g., regulations relating to criteria for qualification for services; processes for developing individualized family service plans and individualized education programs; family qualification for specialized programs, such as Medicaid; guidelines for reporting to child protective services)

- Know how to help families realize their own strengths in caring for and raising their own children

- Know how to help families see the strengths in their children

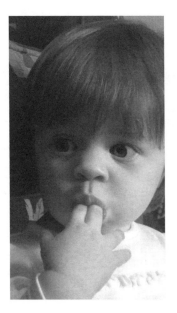

- Understand how family perceptions (about disability, child rearing, receiving help from outsiders) vary across cultures

- Know how to offer services to families and young children in a variety of settings, including hospitals, child care centers, schools, and homes

- Know current research and evidence-based studies in one's respective field of training

Partnering with Families

We enter fields of endeavor, such as pediatrics, teaching, or a clinical discipline, because we want to work with children. What we initially do not realize is that much of our efforts inevitably will be focused on interacting and interfacing with families. In recent years, partnerships with caregivers and parents have been increasingly recognized as being central to working with young children; however, the identification and implementation of those skills and abilities required for best practices with families are the more difficult tasks to accomplish. As physicians, educators, social workers, nurses, clinicians, and therapists, we believe that the following represent a beginning toward best practices with families:

- We need to understand family systems and the development of families in different places—that is, premature births, special needs, death, chronic illness, abuse by parents, caregivers with disabilities, teenage mothers and fathers, siblings with a disability, various cultures or religions that differ from our own, families of affluence, and families struggling to make ends meet. The possibilities and dynamics are almost limitless, and professionals must be flexible and adaptable to individual needs and situations in order to meet families where they are and to respond genuinely to their needs at that given time in their lives.

- Early environments matter and, as professionals, we need to assume a proactive position that moves ahead preventively with services and/or resources, rather than waiting until remediation becomes necessary. Often, such a position and perspective will require that we go against prevailing views that we should delay until problems can be documented. Abundant research now indicates that waiting probably is contraindicated. Young children will do better if their families know what to do, are healthy, and are supporting their development in the earliest months and years of their lives. Moreover, we know that "the astonishing developmental achievements of the earliest years occur naturally when parents and other caregivers talk, read, and play with young children and respond sensitively to their cues. Efforts to protect early brain development are best embedded in an overall strategy of general health promotion and disease prevention" (Shonkoff & Phillips, 2000, pp. 412–413).

- We need to know how to talk to each other—one professional to another—so that communication and information offered to families is consistent. Repeatedly, families have reported to us that they do not know who to believe and what to do because the advice and direction that they receive, sometimes within the same organizations or agencies, are so disparate. Agendas and priorities can always be changed, but we make life much more difficult for families when we send different messages for intervention and programming.

- We need to know how to facilitate families assuming a genuine role in carrying out medical and educational interventions for their children. Primary caregivers and parents need to know that they have some control over what is happening or taking place in services offered to their children. In the neonatal intensive care unit, for example, parents can participate in kangaroo care for their children, which likely will result in closer attachment, earlier feeding, and hopefully an earlier discharge to home. In home-based programs, families are the lifelong teachers who will maintain the gains over the months to come. In school-based programs, parents will bring home the lessons learned in school. In short, interventions are fully re-

alized through the constant caregivers in the lives of children.

- We need to know how to help parents and caregivers problem solve in determining their own family needs and available resources without intruding. This means that we take seriously their expressed concerns and priorities, always inform them as to whether and when we are gathering data concerning their family, always maintain confidentiality with respect to their family needs, discuss what seems to be working and not, and discuss what is happening at home from their perspective, not only ours (Songer, 2008). In the end, their points of view will drive the success of any attempted intervention efforts, and they will let us know whether our endeavors have been successful.

- Many of the children referred for early intervention services display challenging behaviors. Thus, for many families, one of their primary needs is helping them to guide the behavior of their children in maximally positive, nurturing ways that will enhance development within the context of a healthy home environment. As noted in Chapter 21, "Behavior is communication" (Songer, 2008).

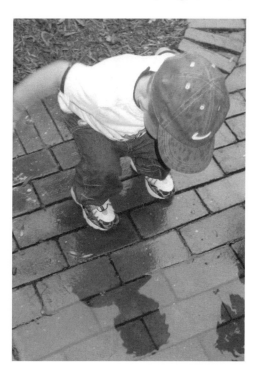

Offering the Best of What We Know to Infants and Young Children with Special Needs

Although there is much that still remains to be studied in early childhood special education, this field and related areas of research have yielded valuable insights relating to working with infants, young children, and their families. In closing, these are a few of the findings to date that seem to represent the best of what we know.

- Shonkoff and Phillips (2000, pp. 360–361) stated so well the need for the individualization of service delivery. They wrote,

  For young children whose development may be compromised by an impoverished, disorganized, or abusive environment, as well as for those with a documented disability (who themselves represent a remarkably heterogeneous population), interventions that are tailored to specific needs have been shown to be more effective in producing desired child and family outcomes than services that provide generic advice and support (Brooks-Gunn et al., 2000; Farran, 1990, 2000; Guralnick, 1998). Furthermore, programs that directly target the everyday experiences of children appear to be more effective in improving their acquisition of skills than those that seek to promote child development indirectly by enhancing the general quality of the caregiving environment (Farron, 2000). Similarly, services that are focused explicitly on parenting behaviors have greater impact on parent–child interactions than do generic parent education efforts (Brooks-Gunn et al., 2000).

- As we need to be consistent with families in our communication and relationships, similarly we need to be consistent with infants and young children in our strategies, interventions, and across settings. Translated into practice, this guideline means developing connections between hospital staff and caregivers when children are hospitalized, developing connections between service providers representing different disciplines in early intervention, and using coherent approaches in school settings and classrooms. Perhaps one of the most significant barriers to maintaining gains from year to year in early educational programs is the fragmentation of services for families and for children and the lack of preparation for both as they transition throughout their educational experiences. New personnel who will be responsible for programming need to know what has gone before so that they can build on strengths and meet continuing challenges.

- Appropriate assessment is a large part of planning and implementing programs for young children and their families. Children need to be observed over time, in different settings, with their peers, and with familiar and unfamiliar adults in order to gain the full picture of their performance and behavior. Strategies for observation and evaluation must be much broader in scope than those traditionally used in the past, and they must incorporate a heavier focus on temperament, social-emotional behavior and mental health, attending abilities, the nature of interaction with known and unknown individuals, play with and without peers and adults, compliance and abilities to follow directions, and the scaffolding of support needed to accomplish various tasks. Such considerations are equally as important as the developmental and content variables that continue to encompass a large measure of evaluation processes for young children.

- Guiding behavior is one of the major challenges and, at the same time, opportunities that teachers have in working with young children. Teachers and clinicians always need to be mindful that changing behavior means to teach. When something is not working, positive alternatives need to be taught. Limiting behavior is seldom a long-term, successful solution (Songer, 2008).

- Development is not a linear acquisition of skills and concepts. In developing effective programs for young children (with and without disabilities), we always need to consider concentrating on foundational and functional abilities, rather than attempting to teach splinter skills out of context.

- When we teach young children, we always should expect the improbable—the highest

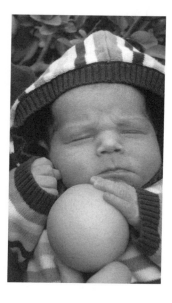

level of learning and behavior. This does not mean that we do not make accommodations and adaptations within the parameters of reality; however, when there is a good fit between curriculum and/or program and child, the child will learn. Multiple variables will intercede to facilitate (and sometimes deter) this process, and inevitably there will be steps backward because development never has a straight trajectory. Yet, if the teaching and learning environment overall is nurturing, appropriate, positive, and expectant, the possibilities are limitless in realizing a child's fullest potential!

Conclusion

Conditions in 2008 show that we live in an ever-changing world. A decade ago, we would not have thought it possible to save babies at 23 weeks of gestation. A decade ago, we would not have thought it possible to have reduced the vertical transmission rate of HIV from mother to newborn to approximately 1%. A decade ago, we were markedly less diverse in our schools and communities than we are today. A decade ago, more than 50% of the mothers in our communi-

ties were not working, with the vast majority of children younger than 5 years in caregiving situations outside of the home. A decade ago, many mothers were not waiting until their 30s to start their families, with multiple births now a common occurrence in our neonatal intensive care nurseries. A decade ago, we would not have thought that more than 50,000 U.S. women wishing to conceive would be requiring in vitro fertilization. A decade ago, families were less fragmented than they are today. A decade ago, the world was a less violent, less fearful place to live.

Thus, as we look to the decade ahead, our biggest challenge will be keeping abreast of this ever-changing, uncertain world for both young children and their families. Very likely in the decade ahead, the technologies for saving newborns will become even more sophisticated and refined. Very likely in the decade ahead, the social issues in the United States across diverse cultures and ethnic groups with different languages will continue to grow. Very likely in the decade ahead, teen pregnancies (although now reflecting a slight decline) will remain on our radar screen to be resolved, especially among adolescents younger than 16 years of age. Very likely in the decade ahead, this country will continue to struggle with mental health concerns for young children and their families.

So, when we look down the pathways that have gone before us, the key question will be, "What have we learned from best practices of the past that will guide us in looking ahead so that we leave both families and children in a better place tomorrow?"

REFERENCES

Shonkoff, J.P., & Phillips, D.A. (Eds.). (2000). *From neurons to neighborhoods: The science of early childhood development*. Washington, DC: National Academies Press.

Songer, N.S. (2008). PowerPoint presentation for course *Guiding Challenging Classroom Behavior*, School of Education, Syracuse University, Syracuse, NY.

Resources for More Information

ORGANIZATIONS PROVIDING OBSTETRIC, PEDIATRIC, AND HEALTH CARE INFORMATION

Academic Pediatric Association
http://www.ambpeds.org

American Academy of Pediatrics
http://www.aap.org

American College of Obstetricians and Gynecologists
http://www.acog.org

Association for Infant Mental Health
http://www.aimh.org.uk

Autism Society of America
http://www.autism-society.org

Centers for Disease Control and Prevention
http://www.cdc.gov

Centers for Medicare and Medicaid Services
http://www.cms.hhs.gov

Children's Defense Fund
http://www.childrensdefense.org

Children's Futures
http://www.childrensfutures.org

David and Lucille Packard Foundation
http://www.packard.org

Families USA
http://www.familiesusa.org

Family Voices, Inc.
http://www.familyvoices.org

Guttmacher Institute
http://www.guttmacher.org

Immunization Action Coalition
http://www.immunize.org

Institute for Child Health Policy
http://www.ichp.ufl.edu

Kaiser Family Foundation
http://www.kaisernetwork.org

National Association of Children's Hospitals and Related Institutions
http://www.nachri.org

National Initiative for Children's Healthcare Quality
http://www.nichq.org

National Institute of Child Health and Human Development
http://www.nichd.nih.gov

National Institutes of Health
http://www.nih.gov

The Robert Wood Johnson Foundation
http://www.rwjf.org

Wisconsin Council on Children and Families: *The Facts About Baby's Brain*
http://www.wccf.org/brain_baby_facts.php

ZERO TO THREE: National Center for Infants, Toddlers and Families
http://www.zerotothree.org

Pediatric Research Societies

American Pediatric Society, Society for Pediatric Research
http://www.aps-spr.org

Safe Kids Worldwide
http://www.safekids.org

State Issues

National Conference of State Legislators
http://www.ncsl.org

National Governors Association
http://www.nga.org

Statehealthfacts.org
http://www.statehealthfacts.org

INFORMATION ON INTERVENTION AND EARLY CHILDHOOD SPECIAL EDUCATION

American Speech-Language-Hearing Association
http://www.asha.org

Center for Parent Education and Family Support: *Topic 3: Parent and Child Temperament*
http://www.cpe.unt.edu/roper/module1/block1_topic3.html

The Central New York Early Childhood Direction Center: *Developmental Checklists: Birth to Five*
http://ecdc.syr.edu/Developmental_Checklists.html

The Central New York Early Childhood Direction Center: *Developmental Checklists: Birth to Five, Spanish Translation*
http://ecdc.syr.edu/Developmental_Checklists.html

Maine's Network of Child Care Resource Development Centers: *Growing Ideas: Social and Emotional Development in Young Children*
http://www.ccids.umaine.edu/ec/growingideas/socemolg.pdf

National Association for the Education of Young Children
http://www.naeyc.org

National Dissemination Center for Children with Disabilities
http://www.nichcy.org

National Early Childhood Technical Assistance Center
http://www.nectac.org

National Early Childhood Technical Assistance Center: *Promoting Social, Emotional and Behavioral Outcomes of Young Children (served under IDEA)*
http://www.nectac.org/~calls/2007/challengingbehavior/challenge.asp

National Institute for Early Education Research: *Promoting Children's Social and Emotional Development Through Preschool Education*
http://nieer.org/resources/policyreports/report7.pdf

Sensory Integration International
http://www.sensoryint.com

Society for Research in Child Development
http://www.srcd.org

The Whole Child: *Social and Emotional Development*
http://www.pbs.org/wholechild/abc/social.html

Index

Page numbers followed by *f* indicate figures; those followed by *t* indicate tables.